PHARMACOLOGY FOR MIDWIVES

Pharmacology for Midwives

The Evidence Base for Safe Practice

2nd Edition

Sue Jordan

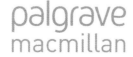

palgrave
macmillan

First edition 2002
Reprinted nine times
Second edition 2010

Published by
PALGRAVE MACMILLAN

Palgrave Macmillan in the UK is an imprint of Macmillan Publishers Limited,
registered in England, company number 785998, of Houndmills, Basingstoke,
Hampshire RG21 6XS.

Palgrave Macmillan in the US is a division of St Martin's Press LLC,
175 Fifth Avenue, New York, NY 10010.

Palgrave Macmillan is the global academic imprint of the above companies
and has companies and representatives throughout the world.

Palgrave® and Macmillan® are registered trademarks in the United States,
the United Kingdom, Europe and other countries.

ISBN-13: 978–0–230–21558–0

This book is printed on paper suitable for recycling and made from fully
managed and sustained forest sources. Logging, pulping and manufacturing
processes are expected to conform to the environmental regulations of the
country of origin.

A catalogue record for this book is available from the British Library.

A catalog record for this book is available from the Library of Congress.

10 9 8 7 6 5 4 3 2 1
19 18 17 16 15 14 13 12 11 10

Printed in China

This book is dedicated to my family

Contents

List of Implications for Practice

List of Figures

List of Tables

List of Boxes

List of Contributors

Nick Clerk, Glan Clwyd Hospital, North Wales NHS Trust, Rhyl, Wales

Richard Griffith, School of Human and Health Sciences, Swansea University, Swansea, Wales

Billy Hardy, Department of Professional Education, University of Glamorgan, Wales

Bronwyn Hegarty, Educational Development Centre, Otago Polytechnic, New Zealand

Sue Jordan, School of Human and Health Sciences, Swansea University, Swansea, Wales

Jennifer Sassarini, Department of Developmental Medicine, University of Glasgow, Scotland

Mike Tait, School of Human and Health Sciences, Swansea University, Swansea, Wales

Foreword

As a researcher with a specific interest in the appropriate use of technology in childbirth that includes the use of any drugs or medication ingested by a pregnant woman and her unborn child, I welcome the invitation to write this Foreword.

This second edition of *Pharmacology for Midwives* is indeed timely and extremely valuable in our chemical society in which there is an increase in prescribed medication, self-medication, over the counter medicines, internet purchasing and street medication. I would like to congratulate Sue Jordan and her distinguished contributors on producing a book that I believe has a long shelf life, clinical relevance and is a superior production to the first edition published in 2002.

This edition has improved content and depth, with substantive new sections on immunology and mental health medication as well as up-to-date legal and professional data. The section on the use of antidepressant medication is particularly welcome, with the increasing number of mental health problems requiring medication in pregnancy and in the postnatal period making it valuable to other members of the multiprofessional team and indeed to those who wish to increase their knowledge in this area.

Midwives in hospitals, stand-alone midwifery units and community midwifery units need to be able to put their hands on a ready reference book about pharmacology and pregnancy that meets the needs of busy clinicians. Therefore, it is essential for books to be user-friendly, relevant and written for the audience who are going to use them.

I believe this is a book that every midwife will open at some stage in their career and this makes it a precious purchase. However, it should be made available on every midwifery unit and in every library for easy access. In addition, it should be included in the book lists for all student midwives and those studying Midwife Prescribing because it is uniquely relevant to midwifery practice and is a key text holding a privileged place in the current market.

I have no doubt about the longevity of this book and its relevance to current practice and sincerely recommend it to all midwives and health professionals who care for and about the health and wellbeing of pregnant women.

DR MARLENE SINCLAIR
Professor of Midwifery Research
Institute of Nursing Research
University of Ulster

Preface

Management of medicines during pregnancy, labour, and the postnatal period is an increasingly important aspect of the midwife's role. Responsibilities include: drug administration; prescribing specified drugs under locally agreed protocols or as independent prescribers; and monitoring the woman, fetus and neonate for adverse drug reactions. Midwives are often the professionals providing women with information and advice on medicines, for example for pain relief in labour and management of the third stage of labour. Although information on medicines is widely available, women rely heavily on professionals for interpretation of this information and advice tailored to their own unique circumstances (Watkins and Weeks, 2009). It is essential, therefore, that midwives, and other registrants, understand the uses, doses, adverse effects, interactions, precautions, and contraindications of the drugs they administer (NMC, 2007).

Traditionally, midwifery practice has been primarily concerned with caring for healthy, 'low-risk' women during normal childbirth. However, increasing numbers of women with pre-existing medical conditions and serious complications of pregnancy are achieving successful pregnancy outcomes under medical and midwifery care, and midwives are involved in administration of an increasing number of drugs to a client group whose conditions necessitate close monitoring. Practice is constantly evolving in response to internal and external pressures. Changing socioeconomic conditions, government policy, and developments in technology all impact on maternity service provision. Many midwives working in consultant units may assume many of the functions previously undertaken by junior doctors. In contrast, government policy and consumer pressure have encouraged team working and caseload practice in the community, with the midwife rather than the doctor undertaking the role of lead professional in the provision of maternity care. Across this continuum runs an acknowledgement of the increased responsibility and autonomy of midwifery practice that is pertinent to the administration, monitoring, and management of medication.

The tragedy of thalidomide in the 1960s highlighted the potential for iatrogenic morbidity. The response of the pharmaceutical industry has been to recommend caution when administering drugs to pregnant or breastfeeding women. For both ethical and practical reasons, involving women who are pregnant or breastfeeding in research, particularly randomized controlled trials, is difficult. Difficulties are accentuated when evidence of harm is sought (Jordan, 2007). Therefore, much drug administration is based on custom and practice rather than research evidence. These uncertainties surrounding pharmacological research and knowledge, together with increased public awareness and burgeoning professional concern, make drug administration, and the associated information sharing, difficult aspects of the midwife's role.

It is estimated that some 10% (3.8–16.6%) of inpatient admissions are associated with a harmful incident: 15.1% of these are linked to medication (de Vries et al., 2008) and over half are preventable (Sari et al., 2007). In the UK, 14,156 of 72,482 (19.5%) medication incidents voluntarily reported in 2007 were described as resulting in harm, and 37 deaths were attributed to medication error (NPSA, 2009). Medication errors may be defined as:

> any preventable events that may cause or lead to inappropriate medication use or patient harm while the medication is in the control of the health care professional, patient, or consumer.

Such events may be related to professional practice, health care products, procedures, and systems, including prescribing; order communication; product labelling, packaging, and nomenclature; compounding; dispensing; distribution; administration; education; monitoring; and use. (NCC MERP, 2005: 4)

Although several professionals may be involved in medication incidents, nurses and midwives are the professionals closest to the patient and the final link in the medication chain (Jordan, 2009). We have categorized three underlying causes of medication errors: education, medication systems, and pressures in the workplace (Griffith et al., 2003). While this book, in the main, relates to education, we hope that it will stimulate consideration, and further research, of systems for medication management: most particularly, work is needed to link medication administration with medication monitoring, and electronic record keeping may be one vehicle for this (Jordan et al., 2009a).

This book aims to help by reviewing the available literature on drugs commonly prescribed during pregnancy, labour, and the puerperium, and highlighting problems frequently experienced as well as indicating others that may be encountered only occasionally. We hope this will assist midwives in discharging their responsibilities effectively (and safely) in respect of drug administration and monitoring.

SUE JORDAN
PROFESSOR DAME JUNE CLARK

Acknowledgements

Sue Jordan wishes to thank: Chris Ruby, midwifery lecturer, for help with the early stages of the first edition, Simon Emery, consultation obstetrician and gynaecologist, Rena McOwat, midwifery lecturer (retired), Vicky Whittaker, midwifery lecturer (retired), Kate Isherwood, midwife, Alison Schooler, midwifery lecturer, Cheryl Davies, pharmacist, Scot Pegler, pharmacist, Sue Philpin, senior lecturer, Fiona Murphy, senior lecturer, Maria Andrade, lecturer, Yamni Nigam, lecturer, for help with the first edition; Stephen Storey, librarian, Lynda Thompson, Senior Commissioning Editor, Dr John Gammon, Deputy Director, Professor Melanie Jasper, Head of School of Human and Health Sciences, Professor Gareth Morgan, Head of Medical School, for support with the project.

The authors and the publishers are also grateful to the following for their kind permission to use the following copyright material:

Oxford University Press for Figure 1.1, adapted from Grahame-Smith and Aronson (1985) *The Oxford Textbook of Clinical Pharmacology and Drug Therapy*, and Figure 4.2, from Harries et al. (2008) Anaesthesia for Caesarean section, in Clyburn et al. (eds) *Obstetric Anaesthesia*; Elsevier for Figure 1.2, adapted from McKenry and Salerno (1995) *Pharmacology in Nursing*, 19th edn, St Louis, Mosby; McGraw-Hill for Figure 1.7, adapted from Benet (1996) General principles, in Hardman et al. (eds) *Goodman & Gilman's: The Pharmacological Basis of Therapeutics*, 9th edn; Springer Science+Business Media for Figure 2.2, from Hughes (1992) Analgesia methods during labour and delivery, *Canadian Journal of Anesthetics*, 39: 5 and Professor S.C. Hughes at the Department of Anesthesia, San Francisco General Hospital, who gave his permission for the use of this figure in the first edition; Massachusetts Medical Society for Figure 2.3 from Eltzschig et al. (2003) Regional anesthesia and analgesia for labor and delivery, *The New England Journal of Medicine*, 348(4): 319–32; *Nursing Standard* and RCN Publishing Company for Figure 14.1 from Story and Jordan (2008) An overview of the immune system, *Nursing Standard*, 23: 15–17, 47–56 (Figure 2).

Every effort has been made to trace all the copyright holders, but if any have been inadvertently overlooked the publishers will be pleased to make the necessary arrangements at the first opportunity.

Using this Book

This book aims to offer an understanding of the principles of drug actions and their relevance to practice. Following an introduction to pharmacology, the book details the drugs commonly administered in labour, where the midwife often takes much of the responsibility. To assist readers in evaluating the evidence, some findings are quoted in detail. The later parts of the book present an overview of situations where care will usually be shared or managed by obstetricians.

In several chapters, in order to explain drug actions and side effects, we have been encouraged to offer readers an explanation of the underlying physiology and pathophysiology. We hope that readers will find these sections informative as few books for midwives discuss common disorders such as asthma, diabetes, epilepsy and mental illness, which all occur in at least 1% of the UK population. Where our explanations are incomplete, referencing in the text signposts further reading.

For a variety of reasons, including practical considerations, this book has been limited to drugs commonly prescribed during pregnancy. We have therefore been unable to include drugs prescribed by specialists in unusual circumstances such as the management of cancer or arthritis in women who are pregnant. We have not included drugs sold as 'herbal remedies' as, in the main, the evidence base is not well documented.

In the UK, practitioners rely heavily on the *British National Formulary* (BNF) and this is reflected in the text. Some drugs are known by more than one name, and have been dual named in the text. A glossary of terms is appended.

Features of this book
Implications for practice

The tables summarize and highlight the links between pharmacology and clinical practice for the most commonly used drugs. As far as possible they have been adapted from published guidelines, which are referenced in the text. They aim to provide the busy practitioner with an easily accessed practice checklist or guideline and meet the NMC requirement to inform women of common adverse effects and procedures to follow (NMC, 2007b: 30).

Practice points

Over three hundred practice points are provided throughout the text. These sections are designed to provide an immediate link to practice so that the relevance of the text is not lost to the reader.

Case reports

The core sections of the book contain illustrative case reports, instances where pharmacology could have been applied to practice to influence the outcome for an individual woman.

Quick reference for major drugs

Appendix I provides a summary of uses, side effects, cautions and interactions for the most commonly used drugs. This is intended not only to highlight common problems but also to provide a reference point for those seeking information on rarer conditions and drug interactions.

List of Abbreviations

ACEI	angiotensin converting enzyme inhibitor
ACTH	adrenocorticotrophic hormone
ADH	antidiuretic hormone
ADR	advance drug reactions
AED	antiepileptic drug
AIDS	acquired immune deficiency syndrome
ANS	autonomic nervous system
ARDS	acute/adult respiratory distress syndrome
BMI	body mass index
BP	blood pressure
	British Pharmacopoeia
CEMACH	Confidential Enquiry into Maternal and Child Health
CESDI	Confidential Enquiry into Stillbirths and Deaths in Infancy
CI	confidence interval
CNS	central nervous system
CSE	combined spinal epidural
CTZ	chemoreceptor trigger zone
CVS	cardiovascular system
DIVC	disseminated intravascular coagulopathy
DH	Department of Health
DNA	deoxyribonucleic acid
DVT	deep vein thrombosis
ECG	electrocardiograph
ECT	electroconvulsive therapy
EEG	electroencephalograph
FBC	full blood count
FEV_1	forced expiratory volume in 1 second
FVC	forced vital capacity
GABA	gamma amino butyric acid
GFR	glomerular filtration rate
GI	gastrointestinal
HDN	haemorrhagic disease of the newborn
HELLP	haemolysis, elevated liver enzymes, low platelets
HR	heart rate
IUGR	intrauterine growth retardation
LFT	liver function test
LMW	low molecular weight
MAOI	monoamine-oxidase inhibitor
MCHRC	Maternal and Child Health Research Consortium (CESDI authors)
MHRA	Medicines and Healthcare products Regulatory Agency
MI	myocardial infarction
MIC	minimum inhibitory concentration
mOsm/kg	milliosmoles per kilogram

NCC	National Collaborating Centre for Women's and Children's Health
NICE	National Institute for Health and Clinical Excellence
NSAID	nonsteroidal anti-inflammatory drug
OR	odds ratio
OTC	over the counter (drugs sold by a pharmacist)
PCA	patient-controlled analgesia
PE	pulmonary embolus
PEFR	peak expiratory flow rate
pO_2	partial pressure (concentration) of oxygen
pCO_2	partial pressure (concentration) of carbon dioxide
PPH	postpartum haemorrhage
RCT	randomized controlled trial
RNA	ribonucleic acid
RR	relative risk
SIADH	syndrome inappropriate ADH (excessive secretion of ADH)
SSRI	selective serotonin uptake inhibitor
TB	tuberculosis
TCA	tricyclic antidepressant
TFT	thyroid function test
TSH	thyroid-stimulating hormone
UTI	urinary tract infection
VC	vomiting centre
im	intramuscular
iv	intravenous
sc	subcutaneous

Notes on dosage abbreviations

1,000 nanograms (ng)	= 1 microgram (μg)
1,000 micrograms	= 1 milligram (mg)
1,000 milligrams	= 1 gram (g)

Micrograms and nanograms should not be abbreviated as confusion is likely to arise (BNF, 2009).

Quantities less than 1 gram should be written as milligrams.
Quantities less than 1 milligram should be written as micrograms.

> For example, 500 mg is better than 0.5 g
> 500 micrograms is better than 0.5 mg
> This minimizes the use of the decimal point, which is easily misread.

Part I
Introduction to Pharmacology

Introduction

The administration of medicines is always undertaken with due regard for the relevant bioscience principles, evidence base and legal considerations. This first part of the book outlines these issues in relation to current midwifery practice.

Emboldened terms can be found in the Glossary.

CHAPTER 1

Principles of Pharmacology

Sue Jordan

This chapter briefly describes the state of the evidence base in midwifery pharmacology; it continues with an account of pharmacological principles, terms and definitions as they relate to midwifery practice.

Chapter contents

- The evidence base for pharmacological interventions
- Drug therapy
- Getting the drug into the body
- Pharmacokinetics: how the body handles the drug
- Pharmacodynamics: actions of the drug on the body
- Therapeutics: effects of the drug on the person

Pharmacology is the science dealing with the interactions between a living system and chemicals introduced from outside the system. A drug may be defined as any small molecule that, when introduced into the body, alters body function by interactions at the molecular level.

The evidence base for pharmacological interventions

When assessing the contribution made by drugs to healthcare, the available evidence could be considered under the headings **placebo** and **nocebo** effects, empirical evidence and rational/scientific evidence.

Placebo and nocebo effects

The 'power of the placebo' should not be underestimated (Beecher and Boston, 1955; Turner et al., 1994). The nonspecific effects of treatment (placebo/nocebo) interact, probably at a biological level, with disease, therapeutic interventions and psychosocial factors. It is important to separate the results of the placebo effect from other treatment effects and the natural course of the condition or disease.

Empirical

Many remedies or treatments are given on an empirical or 'trial-and-error' basis, as they have been for thousands of years. For example, salicylates, as willow bark or aspirin, have long been used to relieve the symptoms of headache. Many of the questions about why drugs work or do not work are still unanswered.

Monitoring for **adverse effects** of drugs is based on empirical evidence. For example, on administering a drug known to lower blood pressure, such as nifedipine or bupivacaine, it would seem sensible to monitor blood pressure at regular intervals. Case data suggest that this approach can contribute to care (Jordan and Torrance, 1995; Jordan, 1998; Jordan et al., 2002). Despite the absence of randomized controlled trials on the outcomes of monitoring patients for adverse effects, failure to monitor may be considered a medication error (NCC MERP, 2005).

Rational or scientific

The 'gold standard' in scientific research is the randomized controlled trial (RCT). However, it is important that pragmatic randomized controlled trials: have adequate numbers of participants to account for clustering; are conducted in a representative population; and are free from crossover (Jordan and Segrott, 2008). Sample sizes for clinical trials are calculated on the basis of the projected positive outcomes, and therefore may be insufficient to detect adverse effects. Practice based on the results of randomized controlled trials can only claim to be evidence based in relation to the primary outcomes of the trials. Medicine's stated goal is for practice to be based on rational, scientific evidence, largely derived from meta-analyses of the findings of randomized controlled trials (EBM Working Group, 1992). In some areas, this has been achieved and research is ongoing, but identification and attribution of adverse effects may not be possible until large databases have been assembled and post-marketing surveillance has been undertaken (Jordan, 2007).

Example
Meta-analysis of 15 trials involving 5,888 women suggests that antibiotic treatment of asymptomatic bacterial vaginosis does not reduce the incidence of preterm birth, premature rupture of membranes or low birth weight. However, some benefits were seen if antibiotics were administered before 20 weeks' gestation. Therefore, future trials will recruit women at entry to antenatal services (McDonald et al., 2007).

Several initiatives are underway to assist the transfer of research findings to clinical practice and guide the adoption and purchase of therapies, for example the Cochrane Collaboration and the National Institute for Health and Clinical Excellence (NICE). The success of the clinical effectiveness initiative depends on keeping practitioners informed of research findings and their relevance to practice.

Example
Although we have been aware of the potential benefits of magnesium sulphate infusions in eclampsia for many years, clinicians were deterred from its use by the difficulties of measuring **serum** magnesium levels and the dangers of respiratory arrest. The significant development that led to the widespread adoption of magnesium sulphate in eclampsia was the randomized controlled trial involving 1,687 women with eclampsia (Eclampsia Trial Collaborative Group, 1995). Significantly fewer convulsions occurred in women treated with magnesium sulphate than either diazepam or phenytoin; the use of phenytoin was associated with significantly more adverse outcomes in women and infants.

The evidence base in practice

Library searches for this book have revealed the dearth of research evidence on which medication management and monitoring are based. For example, in midwifery, for the past four decades, we have faced an epidemic of bottle feeding. In a small study (n = 127), the onset of lactation was delayed by at least 13 hours if medication was administered during labour (Hildebrandt, 1999). However, the impact on breastfeeding of many commonly prescribed medications, such as prochlorperazine and oxytocin, is almost unknown. To address such issues, and be in a position to target appropriate breastfeeding advice, we shall require research funding and funding bodies sympathetic to the interests of women and children.

Absence of trials of medication monitoring means that the guidelines suggested are often based on bioscience principles, empirical evidence and case data. Nevertheless, it is hoped that this information will assist busy practitioners in their discussion with clients, thus empowering women in making what can be difficult decisions, both in normal childbirth and in situations where women's needs are rather more specialized.

Drug therapy

The interactions between the drug and the person receiving it can be divided into four stages:

- Getting the drug into the body
- Getting the drug around, about and out of the body – **pharmacokinetics**
- Actions of the drug on the body – **pharmacodynamics**
- Effects of the drug on the person – therapeutics.

Getting the drug into the body

Two issues are considered here:

- compliance/adherence/concordance
- drug formulation (pharmaceutical considerations).

Compliance

Compliance, adherence or concordance with medication is the extent to which clients adhere to prescribed regimens and associated professional advice. Although studies on compliance give conflicting results, it is estimated that up to 50% of patients make major errors and 16–17% are noncompliant (Buxton, 2006). Direct questioning is not always successful at detecting noncompliance (Sackett et al., 1991), but can be useful (Jordan, 2002).

Associations with non-adherence include:

- women who consider themselves to be healthy
- fear of harming the unborn child
- living alone
- taking more than three drugs
- more than two drug administrations per day
- reduced oesophageal motility, for example dehydration.

Drug formulation

The formulation of a medicine refers to its physical and chemical composition. This includes both the specified active ingredients and other chemicals present, the excipients or 'packing chemicals'. The formulation determines the drug's **bioavailability**, or the proportion of the dose that reaches its destination (Wilkinson, 2001: 5). Excipients stabilize the active ingredient or modify its release. Excipients are listed in the product information, but exact quantities may not be divulged.

Excipients may be responsible for **adverse drug reactions**. For example:

■ The sodium content of many antacid indigestion remedies and some proprietary analgesics may be enough to precipitate fluid retention and breathlessness/pulmonary oedema in pregnancy or in people with incipient heart failure.
■ Potassium ions in some multivitamin preparations or some medicines, such as co-amoxiclav, may be harmful to patients with renal failure or those taking long-term nonsteroidal anti-inflammatory drugs (NSAIDs) or angiotensin converting enzyme inhibitors (ACEIs).
■ Aspartame, an artificial sweetener contained in some medicines, for example co-amoxiclav (some brands), some calcium supplements and some proprietary medicines, could be harmful to people with phenylketonuria (a genetic condition).
■ Oral medicines containing sugar promote dental caries (Mentes, 2001). Medicines available in 'sugar-free' forms contain sorbitol, which can cause diarrhoea. The calorie content of sugar-free medicines can be important for any patient following a closely monitored diet, for example some antibiotics and some preparations of paracetamol (Lebel et al., 2001).
■ **Hypersensitivity** responses or allergies may be caused by excipients.

Excipients may differ between brands; therefore the rate of release of active ingredient may be different, and brands may not be **bioequivalent**. Important examples include: antiepileptic drugs, lithium preparations, antipsychotic medications, ciclosporin, and thyroid hormone preparations. Where a condition, such as epilepsy, is controlled with a certain branded product, changing to another brand or (cheaper) generic drug may result in loss of disease control (Chappell, 1993).

Liquids and solids

The physical formulation of a drug affects its rate of absorption. Before being absorbed, **tablets** must disintegrate and active ingredients must dissolve. The rate at which this occurs depends on formulation, including the size of the particles in the preparation. For example, drugs will be absorbed more rapidly and completely from liquids than tablets. This can be useful: for example paracetamol liquid relieves pain more rapidly than tablets (Rang et al., 2007); liquid risperidone (2 mg) has been suggested as an alternative to parenteral antipsychotic administration in some acute situations (Currier and Simpson, 2001).

Also, it is possible that a greater proportion of the drug will be absorbed when several tablets are taken than when the same dose is taken as a single tablet. For example, bioequivalence between single and multiple fentanyl buccal tablets is not established (Darwish et al., 2006).

Delayed-release preparations

Many drugs come in tablets or capsules that delay the release of active ingredients. Modified-release preparations are sometimes prescribed to allow less frequent dosing, usually once or twice a day, rather than 3 or 4 times. However, their bioavailability is sometimes less than normal release medicines, and close observation is needed when substitutions are made, particularly with antiepileptic medication. **Enteric-coated** preparations are designed so that the drug is not released in the stomach. This protects the stomach and ensures that the drug reaches the lower gastrointestinal tract. Examples include NSAIDs, and preparations to treat Crohn's disease.

Practice point

■ Any damage to the surface of delayed-release preparations may affect release of the medication and drug delivery. If such tablets or capsules are chipped or broken, they should not be administered without advice from a pharmacist. Pharmacists should also be consulted before these preparations are crushed or broken.

The storage requirements of each preparation depend on the formulation, and the data sheet for each product and brand should be consulted for instructions on storage.

Pharmacokinetics: how the body handles the drug

This section addresses the questions:

■ Is the drug getting to the desired site of action (absorption and distribution)?
■ Is the drug getting out of the body (elimination)?
■ Is there a risk of accumulation and toxicity?

The actions and adverse effects of any drug depend on the concentration of the drug in the tissues.

Therapeutic range

Every drug has a 'therapeutic range' or a desirable range for the concentration of drug in plasma and tissues. Above the therapeutic range, toxic effects are more likely to appear. Below the therapeutic range, the drug is less likely to have the desired effect (Figure 1.1). For some drugs, this range is narrow, and the therapeutic concentration is close to the concentration at which adverse effects appear, for example lithium, digoxin, antiepileptic drugs, warfarin, insulin, opioids, ciclosporin, and tacrolimus. Therefore, people receiving these drugs must be monitored closely. For some drugs, such as carbamazepine, lamotrigine, lithium, phenytoin, and gentamicin, the plasma concentrations are measured regularly, to increase the likelihood of benefits and reduce adverse effects. However, for most drugs, the therapeutic effects are assessed more indirectly by observation, for example insulin regimens are monitored by measurement of blood glucose concentrations. For other drugs, the therapeutic range is wide in most individuals, and there is a larger 'safety margin' between therapeutic dose and toxic dose. For example, in people not suffering from epilepsy, penicillins and folic acid are relatively safe, even in overdose.

Timing of drug administration

For a medicine with a narrow therapeutic range, dose intervals are calculated to prevent more than twofold fluctuations in plasma concentrations. If strict adherence to dosage intervals fails, both toxicity and therapeutic failure are likely. For example, where these drugs require administration twice each day, they should be given 12 hours apart.

Where medicines must be given 4 times a day, that is, every 6 hours, this will usually involve disturbing sleep. Flucloxacillin, co-fluampicil or erythromycin may be prescribed for administration every 6 hours. If administration is irregular, the plasma concentration of the drugs may at times fall so low as to be ineffective, allowing regrowth of microorganisms; at other times, as dosing intervals are compressed, plasma concentrations may become so high that toxicity ensues (for example gastrointestinal disturbance). Administration every 6 hours presents practical problems. For example, oral erythromycin, 4 times per day, is sometimes prescribed for urinary tract infections antenatally. It is also advisable to administer oral erythromycin 1 hour before or after meals. Therefore, it is not easy to calculate the timing of erythromycin administration to provide maximum clinical effect (Figure 1.1).

In this example, the drug is scheduled to be administered 4 times per day or every 6 hours. If this is done strictly, for example at 6.00 am, 12 noon, 6.00 pm and midnight, although the concentrations fluctuate, they remain within the therapeutic range. This is illustrated:

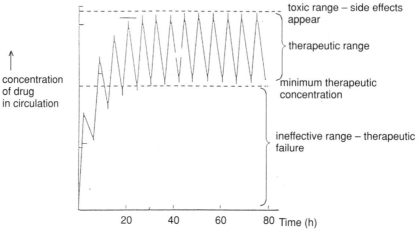

However, if the ward is busy, the dosing may be rescheduled to accommodate other tasks, with the result that the drug is administered at 10.00 am, 2.00 pm, 6.00 pm and 10.00 pm. Therefore, the concentrations fluctuate wildly. At times the drug is below the minimum therapeutic concentration and ineffective, but at other times it causes toxicity, as illustrated:

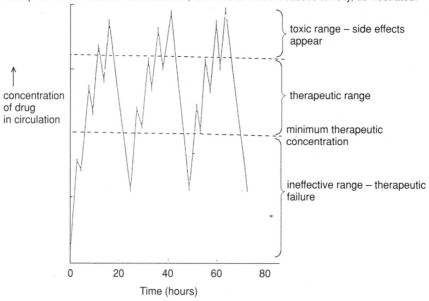

Figure 1.1 'Peaks and troughs' of bolus dose administration
Source: Adapted from Grahame-Smith and Aronson (1985) © 1985 By permission of Oxford University Press

For other drugs, where the therapeutic range is wide in most individuals, dose intervals may be calculated to permit fluctuations in plasma concentrations of up to sixfold. Deviations from the prescribed schedule are likely to cause therapeutic failure, but not toxicity (Wilkinson, 2001).

The concentration of any drug in the plasma and tissues depends on the way the drug is treated by the body.

The body handles all drugs in three stages (Figure 1.2): absorption, distribution, and elimination. These processes are affected by pregnancy. The clinical significance of these changes is greatest for women taking regular antiepileptic therapy (Chapter 18).

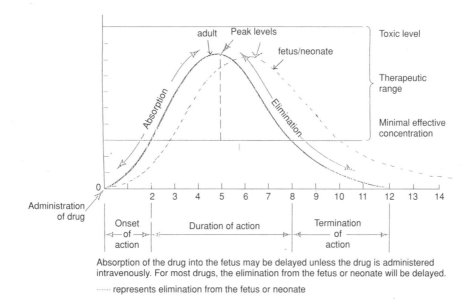

Absorption of the drug into the fetus may be delayed unless the drug is administered intravenously. For most drugs, the elimination from the fetus or neonate will be delayed.

----- represents elimination from the fetus or neonate

Figure 1.2 Changes in plasma concentration of a drug following a single dose
Source: Adapted from McKenry and Salerno (1995). Reproduced with permission from Elsevier

Absorption

Absorption is the process by which a drug is made available to the body fluids for distribution. Together with drug formulation (above), absorption affects the extent to which a drug reaches its destination or its bioavailability (Wilkinson, 2001: 5). The absorption of a drug depends on the route of administration (Figure 1.3), and the way the drug molecules move across cell membranes throughout the body. Regardless of the route of administration, drugs enter the circulation; the rate and extent is reduced by topical administration. Important barriers to drug absorption and distribution include: the gut wall, capillary walls, cell membranes, the **blood/brain barrier**, the placenta, and the blood/milk barrier.

Most drugs are given orally because this is convenient. A few drugs, including aspirin and alcohol, are partially absorbed straight from the stomach; most others are passed into the small intestine before being absorbed. Pain, particularly migraine (Box 4.5) and labour pain, reduces gastric motility, delaying the absorption of oral medications.

Practice point

■ Migraine sufferers are advised to take analgesia, usually paracetamol, at the first warning of an attack. During a migraine attack, analgesics such as paracetamol and antiemetics such as metoclopramide cannot be absorbed efficiently because they are not passed into the small intestine. Under these circumstances, liquid paracetamol or buccal preparations can be useful.

Route

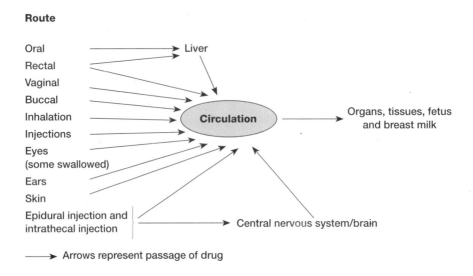

Figure 1.3 Routes of administration

The presence of food in the stomach influences the absorption of many drugs, such as iron (Chapter 10), antimicrobial agents (Chapter 13) and nifedipine (Chapter 7). Food can affect drug absorption and bioavailability by: binding the drug, increasing gastric acidity, impairing transport across the intestine, and altering elimination. Meals with high fat content cause release of bile salts and a hormone (cholecystokinin), which slows the gastrointestinal tract, possibly increasing drug absorption (Genser, 2008).

Food, antacids or guar gum may bind to drugs, keeping them within the intestines, and decreasing absorption, to a varying degree (Baxter, 2006). Examples include: erythromycin stearate, tetracyclines/doxycycline, iron preparations, indinavir, ampicillin, and ciprofloxacin. For other drugs, for example nifedipine, lithium, and lovastatin, the drug/food interaction is beneficial, in that it prevents the sudden onset of drug actions.

Co-administration with food may ameliorate nausea, but sometimes at the cost of reduced or delayed absorption, for example carbamazepine, iron (Chapter 10), or aspirin. For most drugs, it is important to *maintain a constant relationship between medication and meals*, so that plasma concentrations of the drug do not vary from day to day.

The decline in gastrointestinal motility associated with pregnancy (due to increased progesterone and decreased motilin) delays the absorption of certain drugs from the gastrointestinal tract. This may reduce the efficacy of antiepileptics (Chapter 18) and single dose 'rescue' medication, such as analgesia or antiemetics, where a fast response is important.

Drugs administered orally pass to the liver, where they are metabolized, whereas drugs administered by other routes pass directly into the circulation. The proportion of drug passing straight into the circulation cannot be predicted with rectal, epidural or spinal administration (Figure 1.3; Chapter 2).

Distribution

Distribution is the movement of the drug around the body (Figure 1.4). It is affected by:

- plasma protein binding
- the lipid solubility of the drug, that is, whether it dissolves in fatty tissues
- the binding properties of the drug

- blood flow to the organs and the state of the circulation
- the life cycle: pregnancy, lactation, infancy
- disease, for example pre-eclampsia or heart failure.

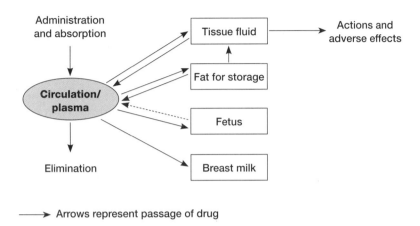

Arrows represent passage of drug

Note: return of metabolites from fetus to mother varies between drugs.

Figure 1.4 Drug distribution and body compartments

The increase in plasma volume (by up to 50%) in pregnancy may dilute the concentration of medicines. The cardiovascular system returns to its pre-pregnancy state some 3 months after birth.

Plasma proteins

Drugs are bound to the plasma proteins to a varying extent. Some drugs (for example warfarin, nifedipine, antiepileptics, and antidepressants), some hormones, calcium ions, and bilirubin circulate largely bound to plasma proteins, particularly albumins. Normally, the free and bound forms are in equilibrium or a state of balance. Only the free drug is biologically active. The bound drug acts as a storage reservoir. The availability of albumin for binding is reduced in pregnancy, neonates, malnutrition and burns. This increases the effects, and adverse effects, of some drugs such as antiepileptics. Drugs that are highly protein bound pass into breast milk less completely; therefore, some drugs such as warfarin and valproate, which are problematic during pregnancy, may not preclude breastfeeding, with specialist advice (Anderson, 2006). Protein binding is a source of drug interactions. Some drugs, for example aspirin, displace bilirubin from its binding sites on plasma albumins.

Lipid solubility

Lipid solubility is the extent to which the drug dissolves in the body's fatty tissues (Figure 1.4). It is possible to visualize the body as chemically composed of fluid compartments plus fatty tissues. Most drugs are spread throughout the body's fluid compartments and pass into the fatty tissues to a greater or lesser extent. Because of its high myelin content, the brain can be regarded as a fatty tissue. The extent to which the drug spreads throughout the body is referred to as the 'volume of distribution'.

Examples

The benzodiazepines (for example diazepam, temazepam) have a high volume of distribution and pass into all fatty tissue. When these drugs are discontinued, the effects of withdrawal may be prolonged. This is attributed to the drugs dissolving extensively in the fat and passing out into the circulation gradually over time.

When anaesthetic gases, such as nitrous oxide, are administered, they dissolve in fatty tissues. In women with generous deposits of adipose tissues, more of the gas enters the body fat, leaving less in the circulation. Therefore, such women require larger doses to achieve effective analgesia. Also, when the inhalation is discontinued, they take longer to recover since the drug, which has passed into the body fat, takes time to clear (Chapter 4).

Drugs that are highly lipid soluble pass into the brain and cross the placenta easily. For example, the higher lipid solubility of fentanyl and diamorphine allow them to pass into the brain and the fetus more readily than morphine.

Binding characteristics

A few drugs have unusual binding characteristics. For example, tetracyclines bind to growing bones and teeth and cannot be given to anyone who is growing, pregnant or breastfeeding. The antimalarial chloroquine can bind to the retina of an adult or fetus. A high dose can cause retinal damage. Pregnant women should seek specialist advice regarding travel to countries where malaria is endemic.

Blood flow to the tissues

Some tissues receive a better blood supply than others; for example, the blood flow to the brain is much higher than that to bone. The local and general state of the circulation determines the distribution of drugs. In **shock**, the distribution of the circulation, and any drugs administered, is impaired. Drugs administered orally, subcutaneously or intramuscularly may not be absorbed adequately. The circulation is preferentially redistributed to the heart, brain and lungs. Therefore any drug administered will be circulated into these organs, bypassing others. Because the volume of the circulation is restricted, the drugs will be at a high concentration in the tissues they do reach. This can be critical when administering drugs with a narrow safety margin such as magnesium sulphate (Chapter 9).

Practice points

- If a patient with a compromised circulation, for example due to pre-eclampsia or blood loss, receives an intramuscular injection, the drug may not be absorbed. If the circulation is restored, by administration of fluids, the injection may be suddenly absorbed, resulting in a concentration above the therapeutic range. Because both beneficial and adverse effects may be unpredictably delayed, intramuscular injections are not given to patients with cardiovascular compromise.
- A compromised circulation may reduce the blood supply to the intestines, reducing absorption of oral medication. Therefore, such patients usually receive intravenous medication.

The life cycle
The placenta

The placenta is not an effective barrier to the passage of drugs, and the blood/brain barrier is underdeveloped in the fetus. Permeability may be further increased by cytokines released during stress associated with hypoxia and labour (Rosenberg, 2002). Lipid soluble drugs such as anaesthetic gases and some opioids (including fentanyl) cross the placenta rapidly. However, the passage of other drugs is regulated by the placenta. Drugs of high molecular weight, such as heparins, are too large to enter the fetus, and some drugs are metabolized and inactivated by the placenta, for example prednisolone. The placenta contains several transporter proteins that: maintain homeostasis; protect the fetus from potentially toxic substances (Freyer, 2008); and supply the fetus with amino acids for growth. Nicotine and cocaine block these transporters, restricting fetal growth (Magee and Koren, 2007). The transporter proteins show genetic variation, making some fetuses genetically vulnerable to increased drug exposure and adverse effects: examples include olanzapine and phenytoin (Newport et al., 2007; Wells, 2007).

For some drugs, such as cocaine, clearance from amniotic fluid may be limited, allowing the drug to be absorbed through the fetal skin for the first 24 weeks and swallowed; this may explain why regular use may be damaging (Chapter 20).

Highly charged (ionized) molecules cross the placenta with difficulty. If a drug enters the fetus and is then metabolized into a charged molecule, it may become 'trapped' because of the difference in **pH** (acidity) between fetus and mother. The relative acidity of the fetus may be accentuated if hypoxia occurs during birth. In this way, opioids administered to the woman can be trapped and accumulate in the fetus, causing adverse effects (Chapter 4).

As the placenta thins towards the end of pregnancy, the amount of drug reaching the fetus increases. The infant may be born experiencing the adverse effects of the mother's medication or withdrawal syndromes, some of which are potentially dangerous.

Practice point

■ Where the midwife has been able to obtain a history of drug misuse, delivery under specialist supervision should be advised and neonatologists alerted (Chapter 20).

Neonates

The blood/brain barrier is not fully developed in the fetus or the neonate. Therefore drugs absorbed during delivery or taken in with breast milk may enter the infant's brain with relative ease while remaining undetectable in the blood.

The body of the neonate contains a relatively high proportion of water and a low proportion of fat. Any fat-soluble drugs are therefore distributed into a small volume. For example, vitamin K is administered to neonates in its fat-soluble form. The relatively low body fat content of neonates limits its distribution. Any water-soluble drugs will be diluted over a relatively larger body volume. This means that neonates, particularly premature infants, receive different drug doses from adults, even when body weight is taken into consideration.

Example

Naloxone (Narcan®) may be administered to neonates in a dose of 10 micrograms/kg (subcutaneous, intramuscular or intravenous injection) repeated every 2–3 minutes as necessary, whereas the corresponding adult dose is 1.5–3 micrograms/kg. The alternative single-dose regimen involves a higher dose (BNF, 2009).

Lactation

Most drugs pass into breast milk, but the concentrations are often too small to be harmful (Table 1.2). The amount of drug passing into breast milk varies between women, during feeds, with the age of the infant and use of a breast pump. The relative dose, as a proportion of body weight, received by the infant depends on the drug administered: for example, the dose of lithium is 80% of maternal dose. The relative maturity of the infant's liver and kidneys is also considered (Lawrence and Schaefer, 2007). The content and composition of breast milk can also be affected by the mother's diet and any exposure to environmental toxins such as weedkillers.

Disease and drug distribution

Drug distribution is compromised in conditions affecting the cardiovascular system (above), thyroid or gastrointestinal disease.

Drug elimination or clearance

Drug elimination includes:

- metabolism
- excretion
- elimination half-life (a measure of rate).

The route of elimination varies between drugs. Most drugs are metabolized in the liver and excreted *via* the kidneys, although bile is also an important route of excretion, for example for oestrogens and corticosteroids (Figure 1.5). A few drugs (for example magnesium and lithium) are eliminated unchanged, whereas others are extensively metabolized. Some metabolites are active, for example those of carbamazepine and opioids, while others may cause adverse effects, for example pethidine/meperidine (Chapter 4). Alcohol is unusual in that 5–10% is eliminated unchanged *via* the lungs, sweat and urine.

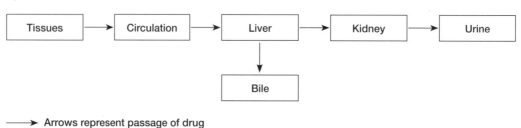

⟶ Arrows represent passage of drug

Hepatic or renal failure will impair the body's ability to eliminate most drugs (as in eclampsia or severe pre-eclampsia). Drugs will also accumulate if the woman or neonate is dehydrated. If the drug accumulates, adverse effects will intensify.

Figure 1.5 Usual routes of drug elimination

The efficiency of drug elimination is measured by 'clearance', which is the volume of body fluid from which a drug is removed each minute (Buxton, 2006).

Drug metabolism

Elimination of many drugs depends on metabolic processes and the associated enzymes. Most metabolism takes place in the liver, but the gastrointestinal tract and the central nervous system contain enzymes responsible for the metabolism of some drugs. These metabolic processes allow the body to deal with and detoxify foreign substances. All drugs given orally must pass through the liver to reach the circulation. (This is known as 'first pass metabolism'.) Drugs administered by other routes reach the liver after passing round the general circulation. There are no tests to assess the liver's ability/capacity to metabolize and eliminate medication.

Metabolism in the liver occurs in two stages:

1 The products of digestion are transformed by metabolism or detoxification.
2 The metabolites are then rendered soluble in water (by **conjugation**), so that they can be excreted *via* the kidneys.

Both these processes depend on enzymes. Activity of liver enzymes is affected by:

- Genetic makeup, for example the therapeutic response and ability to eliminate selective serotonin reuptake inhibitor (SSRI) antidepressants varies according to the presence or absence of specific genes, and is impaired in some 10% of Caucasians, who may develop adverse effects, such as agitation or euphoria, at low or normal doses (Serretti and Artioli, 2004; Bray et al., 2008). The response to warfarin depends on the genetic variants of the enzymes metabolizing and responding to warfarin (Schwarz et al., 2008).
- Liver impairment, for example in women or infants with malnutrition, cirrhosis of the liver, hepatitis or HELLP syndrome. Drugs eliminated by the liver, such as erythromycin and metronidazole, will be administered in lower doses (Quintiliani and Quintiliani, 2008).
- The liver's environment, that is, what reaches the liver from the gut and the circulation.
- The life cycle.

Rate of metabolism
During pregnancy, the rate of metabolism increases in some enzymes and decreases in others. Only some women will be affected by changes in metabolism associated with pregnancy, depending on the genetically determined forms of enzymes they have inherited and their ability to metabolize the drug when not pregnant.

Depending on what has been ingested, the liver enzymes can be accelerated (induced) or slowed down (inhibited). If enzymes are accelerated, drugs will be removed too rapidly, and signs and symptoms of the illness will return. However, if enzymes are inhibited or blocked, drugs could accumulate. Some drugs, foods and herbs can interfere with the rate of these metabolic processes, thereby increasing or decreasing the effects of certain drugs (Wilkinson, 2005). Retiming administration of medicines will not prevent these drug/food interactions.

1 Enzyme induction/acceleration and drug loss
Liver enzymes adapt to their environment, that is, they become accustomed to whatever is ingested: diet or drugs. Regular ingestion of some drugs (including rifampicin, carbamazepine and alcohol), foods (for example barbecued meats and caffeine), or herbs (for example St John's wort), or exposure to tobacco accelerates the action of enzymes in the gut lining and the liver. This process of enzyme induction takes days or weeks. It means that any drugs or hormones eliminated by the enzymes affected are metabolized away more rapidly and become less effective. Examples of drugs affected include diazepam, clozapine, steroids, and warfarin. To accommodate the patient's regular use of enzyme-inducing substances, the prescriber may increase the medication dose.

Example
Some drugs, including some antiepileptics, rifampicin, rifabutin, some antiretrovirals, and St John's wort, render standard dose oral contraceptive pills (combined and progestogen only) ineffective, and alternative methods of contraception are advised. For effective contraception, women taking some antiepileptics need

a higher daily dose of oestrogen than is available in most combined oral contraceptives (at least 50 micrograms rather than 30 micrograms); also emergency hormonal contraception in standard dose is unlikely to be effective (BNF, 2009). About 25% of unplanned pregnancies in women taking antiepileptic medication can be attributed to 'pill failure' (Fairgrieve et al., 2000).

Pregnancy increases or induces the metabolism of some drugs, such as lamotrigine, carbamazepine, some antiretrovirals, codeine, chlorpheniramine, erythromycin, benzodiazepines, morphine, nicotine, and methadone, reducing their effectiveness. Some women may find that they need to smoke more cigarettes towards the end of pregnancy or that they need higher doses of nicotine replacement therapy (Anderson, 2006).

Practice point

■ Women using these medicines long term should be observed for signs of therapeutic failure; those using single-dose 'rescue' therapy should be informed that they may find their usual dose is less effective.

Enzyme induction occurs to a limited extent in the fetus (Wells, 2007).

2 Enzyme inhibition/slowing and drug accumulation
Activity of certain enzymes in the gut lining and liver is stopped suddenly or inhibited not only by certain drugs, such as keotconazole, ritonvair (for HIV/**AIDs**), fluoxetine, alcohol (in high doses), erythromycin, cimetidine, and St John's wort, but also by grapefruit or grapefruit juice and possibly other fruit juices containing furanocoumarin (or furocoumarin) derivatives. This reduces the metabolism and elimination of several drugs: 200–250 ml grapefruit juice can double the **bioavailability** of most calcium channel blockers (except diltiazem, but including nifedipine), suddenly increasing the concentration in the tissues and the actions and adverse effects. The effect lasts some 24 hours (Dresser et al., 2000, 2002). Further work in this area will probably expand the list of foods and drugs affected, but currently includes carbamazepine, warfarin, amphetamines, some statins, nifedipine, sildenafil, zopiclone, diazepam, midazolam, pimozide, ergotamine (including LSD), ciclosporin, sertraline, and erythromycin (Jordan et al., 2003; Genser, 2008).

Practice points

■ Product information sheets should always be checked for drug/food interactions.
■ It may be advisable to remove grapefruit and grapefruit juice from hospital menus. Alternatively, menus should be checked against medication charts.

Examples of enzyme inhibition include:

■ Concurrent administration of cimetidine with pethidine (meperidine) impairs the metabolism and elimination of the opioid, which may then accumulate and cause severe adverse effects such as respiratory depression. This drug interaction is not shared by ranitidine.
■ Amphetamines, including dexamphetamine and methylphenidate, may inhibit the metabolism of SSRIs, leading to euphoria, hypomania or mania.
■ Drug/food interactions are a particular problem with warfarin (Lake and Jordan, 2005).

During pregnancy, some drugs are metabolized more slowly, and the risk of adverse effects increases, for example olanzapine, clozapine, haloperidol, citalopram, and caffeine (Anderson, 2006).

Practice point

■ Women taking these drugs should be reviewed for adverse effects, using a recognized adverse effect profile (Jordan, 2008), and the need for dose reduction should be discussed with prescribers.

The fetus and neonate (particularly premature infants) metabolize and eliminate drugs more slowly than adults. The fetus may be unable to detoxify some compounds and reactive products of metabolism that may bind DNA, RNA or proteins; this may explain why the fetus is vulnerable to radiation damage, including radioiodine therapy (Wells, 2007). By about 2 months of age, the neonate is able to eliminate drugs as well older children (Ginsberg, 2002).

Examples
Following administration during labour, it can take a neonate 2–3 days to clear the metabolites of meperidine (pethidine), during which time the neonate may be irritable (Chapter 4).

Breastfed infants in the first few months of neonatal life are less able to metabolize the caffeine their mothers ingest. For example, if a mother takes several cups of filtered, boiled or strong coffee, she may feel no ill effects, but the caffeine can accumulate in the infant, making him or her unduly irritable and unable to concentrate on feeding. Women should be aware that some over the counter analgesics contain appreciable amounts of caffeine.

Drug excretion
Most drugs are dependent on the kidneys for excretion. The functioning of the kidneys can be considered as two processes: glomerular filtration (measured as glomerular filtration rate (GFR)) and tubular secretion and reabsorption.

Drug excretion may rely on either or both of these processes, depending on the drug involved. GFR is usually considered the best overall measure of the kidneys' ability to eliminate drugs in health and disease (Levey et al., 1999). GFR is the volume of fluid filtered into the nephrons every minute, that is, the sum of the volume of filtrate formed each minute in all the functioning nephrons in the kidneys. It represents about 20% of the plasma flowing through the kidneys. The normal GFR for a standard male (of body surface area $1.73m^2$) is 100 ml/min; the value for a female is 90% of this. A GFR below 60 ml/minute/$1.73m^2$ surface area indicates renal disorder, and is associated with increased risk of cardiovascular disease (Stevens and Levey, 2005) (Box 1.1).

Pregnancy and GFR
In normal pregnancy, the circulating volume expands by about 50%, therefore renal plasma flow and GFR rise by 30–100% in the second trimester, but decline towards term. This increases the elimination of certain drugs (Tomson and Battino, 2007). Therefore, doses and dose frequency of ongoing therapeutic regimens will need to be increased, particularly antiepileptic drugs and low molecular weight heparins (Chapter 8). By the fourth week of pregnancy, GFR has risen 20%; therefore, increased drug elimination and decreased drug effects may occur before the woman realizes she is pregnant (Perrone et al., 1992).

Examples
The elimination of ampicillin and other penicillins is increased, and therefore higher doses (at least 500 mg of ampcillin every 8 hours) are administered regularly if infections are to be treated effectively (Chapter 13).

The increase in elimination, combined with the increased circulating volume, reduces the plasma concentration of antiepileptic medication, particularly lamotrigine, levetiracetam, and oxcarbazepine. This may make pregnant women more vulnerable to seizures, particularly should any dose be missed or delayed.

Practice point

■ For women with epilepsy, seizure frequency may worsen during pregnancy and after birth. Therefore, careful monitoring of antiepileptic therapy and compliance is required. This should include venous blood samples to assess the plasma concentrations of antiepileptic drugs.

The circulating volume contracts during the 48 hours following birth, but renal function does not return to the pre-pregnant state for some 6 weeks (Freyer, 2008). Drug concentrations vary over the first 6–8 weeks (Walker et al., 2009), but may be at pre-pregnant values by 1–2 weeks postpartum: women have reported symptoms associated with lamotrigine toxicity (sedation and incoordination) at this time (Tomson and Battino, 2007). Breastfeeding may delay the return to pre-pregnancy drug elimination rates (Morrell, 2003).

Practice point

■ Close monitoring for the effects and adverse effects of medicine with a structured list should be maintained during this time (Jordan, 2008).

Box 1.1 Measurement of renal function

For several drugs, prescribers will wish to know the GFR before initiation of therapy. If the GFR is too low, some drugs, such as magnesium, lithium, and metformin, will not be given. For other drugs, a reduced dose will be prescribed at prolonged intervals, for example gentamicin. GFR should also be checked during therapy to assess any changes.

GFR is usually assessed from measurement of serum creatinine concentration. Because creatinine is freely filtered by the kidneys, it offers useful approximations of the 'clearing ability' of the kidneys. Creatinine concentration is conveniently measured from venous blood samples. It rises above normal when 50% of nephrons have been damaged. If patients are reviewed regularly, serial measurements of **serum** creatinine highlight any changes in kidney function, provided patients maintain relatively constant body mass and dietary intake (Rodrigo et al., 2002).

Practice points

■ During pregnancy, as GFR rises, concentration of serum creatinine falls: *any value above 70 micromoles/litre (µmol/l) indicates renal compromise and should be reported without delay*. This is particularly important in the interpretation of results of laboratory investigations for women with pre-eclampsia or urinary tract infections (Chapter 9). (Normal non-pregnant range is 62–124 micromoles/litre, varying slightly between laboratories.)

■ The prescriber should be informed if the serum creatinine concentration increases, as drug doses will normally need to be reduced, and the prescriber may wish to order further investigations of kidney function.

Laboratory reports may estimate the eGFR. This is the GFR standardized for body surface area, taking into account age and gender (JSC, 2006), but is not used in pregnancy (NCC, 2008a). Calculating the GFR from a full creatinine clearance test involves 24-hour urine collection; this is time-consuming and vulnerable to human error. However, relying solely on the measure of creatinine concentration from the venous blood sample may not give sufficient accuracy. An estimation of GFR (and the patient's ability to clear drugs) can be obtained from the Cockcroft and Gault formula (BNF, 2009). This takes into account three factors known to influence GFR: age, weight and gender:

$$GFR = \frac{(140 - age) \times (wt \text{ in kg}) \times 1.04 \text{ (for females)} \text{ (males} \times 1.23)}{Serum \text{ (creatinine) in micromoles/litre}}$$

The value should be compared to pregnancy norms.

If GFR falls, the elimination of most drugs is impaired, causing accumulation and even toxicity. Therefore, those administering medications, particularly magnesium sulphate, should be aware of the circumstances likely to be associated with a low GFR and impaired renal elimination.

GFR (and therefore urine output and drug elimination) are affected by:

- changes in blood flow to the kidneys, for example dehydration (including the use of diuretics), shock, heart failure, administration of NSAIDs or ACEIs
- renal disorders and loss of nephrons, for example repeated urinary tract infections, pre-eclampsia and hypertension.

Practice point

- If people are acutely ill, blood flow and renal function can change rapidly, affecting drug concentrations. If the volume of urine is too low, the kidneys are at risk of damage. Urine output <0.5 ml/kg/hour indicates that the circulation is seriously compromised and renal blood supply and oxygen delivery are inadequate (Jevon and Ewens, 2002). Urine output below 30 ml/hr should be reported to the doctor managing the patient, because renal damage may be occurring, and drugs may rapidly accumulate and reach toxic concentrations (Berman et al., 2008).

The neonate and GFR

The kidneys of the fetus eliminate drugs slowly into the amniotic fluid, which is then ingested through the mouth, further reducing clearance. Renal reserve is low in neonates and declines steadily from early adulthood. The GFR of the neonate is only 30–40% of adult values (Surf et al., 1998). Therefore, there is a danger that certain drugs, such as magnesium, may accumulate following maternal administration. These neonates should be observed for signs of muscle weakness, including respiratory depression, for 48 hours after birth. Other drugs, such as lithium, may accumulate during breastfeeding.

Elimination half-life

The elimination **half-life** for each drug is the time taken for the concentration of the drug in plasma and the amount of drug in the body to fall to half its maximum value (Buxton, 2006: 16) (see Figure 1.6).

Half-life is used to calculate the:

- dose interval
- time to eliminate a drug
- time taken from initiation or change of therapy before the concentration of the drug reaches a 'steady state' (below) (Buxton, 2006; Endrenyi, 2007).

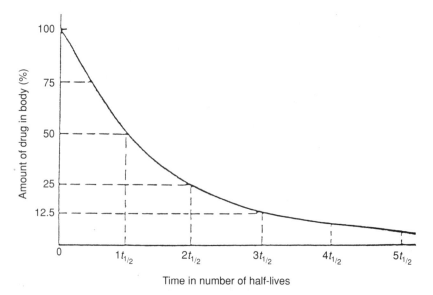

Most drugs follow this pattern of elimination:
• during the first half-life, 50% of the drug is eliminated from the body
• after 3 half-lives, 87.5% or $\frac{7}{8}$ of the drug has been removed
• after 4–5 half-lives, this dose of the drug has effectively disappeared.

Figure 1.6 Graph to illustrate elimination half-life following a single intravenous dose

A drug's half-life depends on its biological properties. Duration of action of a drug increases in direct proportion to its half-life. For most drugs, dose has less impact on the duration of action than half-life. If the dose is doubled, the peak plasma concentration will double, and the duration of action will increase by one half-life. Therefore, attempts to extend the duration of action by increasing the dose are unlikely to be successful, because the increase in peak plasma concentration is likely to cause intolerable adverse effects. For example:

- if a drug should be administered every 4 or 6 hours, administering a double dose at bedtime will prolong duration of action, but not necessarily double it
- administering 100 mg pethidine rather than 50 mg prolongs the duration of action, but does not double it.

Dose interval
For some drugs, to maintain the drug concentration within the therapeutic range (Figure 1.1), doses are administered approximately every half-life. If drug administration intervals are much longer than this, the fluctuations in the concentration of the drug in the plasma may lead to therapeutic failure (Buxton, 2006).

Elimination time
Fifty per cent of a dose will be eliminated 1 half-life after discontinuation. For example, tetrahydrocannabinol (the active ingredient of cannabis) has a half-life of 50 hours, and so will be detectable in blood and urine samples for several days after ingestion. In contrast, diamorphine/heroin has a half-life of 1.25 ± 0.25 hours, and will be cleared from the body in a much shorter time. Therefore, samples can detect non-prescription use of cannabis, but not heroin.

Steady state

With repeated dosing, drugs accumulate in the body (Figure 1.7). The time taken for this to happen depends on the drug's elimination half-life. For most drugs in normal doses, repeated administration at regular intervals will result in a relatively constant plasma concentration or a 'steady state'. At this concentration, the rate of drug elimination is equal to the rate of administration: what goes in, goes out. The time taken to achieve 'steady state' is between 3 to 5 times the elimination half-life. After 4.3 half-lives, 95% of the steady state concentration value will be reached (Endrenyi, 2007). The full effects of the drug and dose-related adverse effects often do not appear until the steady state is reached. If the half-life of the drug is known, it will be possible to predict when dose-related adverse effects are most likely to appear for the first time.

Practice point

■ Patients should be monitored for adverse effects 3–5 half-lives after starting a new drug.

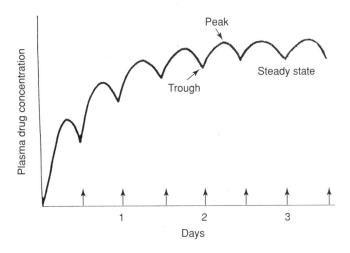

The figure shows repeated twice-daily oral dosing of a drug with a half-life of 12 hours. The drug accumulates for 3–5 half-lives, then reaches a steady state, where the amount of drug eliminated equals that administered.

Figure 1.7 Diagram to illustrate the accumulation of a drug with repeated dosing
Source: Adapted from Benet (1996) © 1996 By kind permission of McGraw Hill Education

In emergency situations, it is not possible to wait for 3–5 half-lives for a drug to reach the steady state concentration. Therefore a high dose will be administered, to achieve a therapeutic concentration rapidly. This is known as a 'loading dose'. Examples include management of eclampsia or pre-eclampsia with magnesium sulphate, and management of **cardiac dysrhythmias.**

For a few drugs, including phenytoin, alcohol, some SSRIs, and salicylates (including aspirin), elimination or disappearance from plasma does not depend on a single half-life, as described above. This is because the enzymes and carrier molecules responsible for drug elimination become 'saturated' and eliminate the drug at a constant rate. Such drugs are more likely to have a prolonged duration of action. For example, adults, on average, eliminate alcohol at a rate of 8–10 g (150–220 mmol)/hour (this is approximately equivalent to half a pint of beer, a glass of wine or a measure of shorts). Consequently, if 10 pints (or equivalent) are consumed, high concentrations of alcohol may persist in the body the following day (Masters, 2001). This pattern of drug elimination is also observed following overdose of several drugs, particularly aspirin.

Where drugs alter absorption or elimination of other drugs, as outlined above, these are termed 'pharmacokinetic interactions'. While the mechanisms are predictable, the impact on the individual varies depending on the drug involved.

Pharmacodynamics: actions of the drug on the body

Most drugs work as a result of specific physiochemical interactions between drug molecules and the recipient's molecules. These chemical reactions may alter the way the cells are functioning, which in turn may lead to changes in the behaviour of tissues, organs and systems. Drugs modify the existing functions of the body; they cannot introduce new functions.

Most drug molecules work *via*:

- **receptors** in cell membranes or within cells
- **ion** channels in cell membranes, for example local anaesthetics or calcium antagonists
- enzymes in cells, for example NSAIDs, or extracellular fluid, for example ACEIs, or plasma, for example heparin.

Locks and keys

Many drugs work by acting on specific receptor proteins, ion channels or enzymes. These are components of cell membranes or cytoplasm, which normally respond to the body's hormones (systemic and local), neurotransmitters or other chemical mediators – the endogenous **ligands**. The three-dimensional shape of receptors (ion channels or enzymes) matches the specific shape of hormones or neurotransmitters. For example, insulin only fits into and binds with insulin receptors, and thyroxine with thyroxine receptors. Therefore, thyroxine receptors are activated only by thyroxine and not by insulin, and *vice versa*. This idea of specificity, based on the three-dimensional shape or structure of hormone or neurotransmitter and receptor, is referred to as the 'lock and key hypothesis' (Clark, 1933). It describes how hormones and neurotransmitters (keys) fit and interact with their corresponding receptors (locks) (Figure 1.8).

Some drugs are direct replacements, for example insulin or thyroxine. Others imitate the actions of the body's own hormones or neurotransmitters and provide an artificial boost to certain receptors, for example opioids, oxytocin, or **beta agonist** bronchodilators, such as salbutamol. These drugs have the same, or similar, three-dimensional structures as hormones or neurotransmitters and can bind to their receptors in their place, and modify the actions of the cells and body systems controlled by the receptor. Drugs that 'fit into' binding sites on receptors may either activate them (agonists) or block and inactivate them (antagonists).

An **agonist** will bind to a receptor and alter its functioning (Figure 1.8a). For example salbutamol, prescribed for asthma or tocolysis, is a beta$_2$ agonist, while pethidine (meperidine) is an opioid agonist. Agonists usually augment the normal function of the receptors to which they bind. For example, pethidine stimulates the opioid receptors, increasing analgesia, sedation and constipation. Likewise, beta agonists mimic some of the actions of the sympathetic nervous system, increasing heart rate, dilating bronchioles and relaxing the uterus (Chapters 7 and 15).

An **antagonist** will bind to a receptor, blocking it and preventing the agonist reaching its site of action (Figure 1.8b). For example, naloxone (Narcan®) blocks the opioid receptors and reverses the actions of pethidine, reducing respiratory depression, analgesia, and sedation; however, *when naloxone is administered, pain may return*. Similarly, beta blockers (propranolol, atenolol, or labetolol) block the actions of the sympathetic nervous system, slow and stabilize the heart rate, and induce bronchoconstriction.

Practice point

■ Beta blockers are contraindicated for people who suffer from asthma, due to the risk of a life-threatening narrowing of the airways (BNF, 2009: 86).

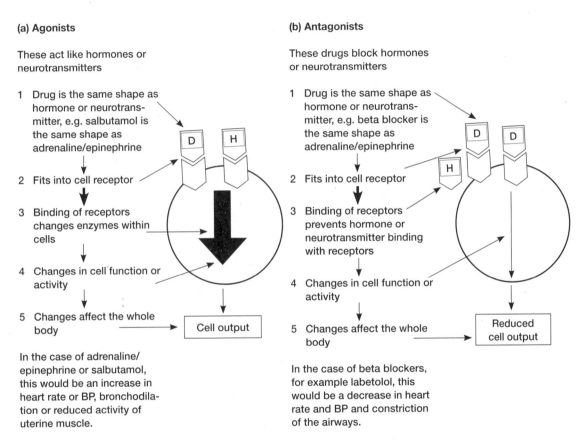

(a) Agonists

These act like hormones or neurotransmitters

1 Drug is the same shape as hormone or neurotransmitter, e.g. salbutamol is the same shape as adrenaline/epinephrine

2 Fits into cell receptor

3 Binding of receptors changes enzymes within cells

4 Changes in cell function or activity

5 Changes affect the whole body → Cell output

In the case of adrenaline/epinephrine or salbutamol, this would be an increase in heart rate or BP, bronchodilation or reduced activity of uterine muscle.

(b) Antagonists

These drugs block hormones or neurotransmitters

1 Drug is the same shape as hormone or neurotransmitter, e.g. beta blocker is the same shape as adrenaline/epinephrine

2 Fits into cell receptor

3 Binding of receptors prevents hormone or neurotransmitter binding with receptors

4 Changes in cell function or activity

5 Changes affect the whole body → Reduced cell output

In the case of beta blockers, for example labetolol, this would be a decrease in heart rate and BP and constriction of the airways.

Key: D represents drug; H represents hormone or neurotransmitter.

Figure 1.8 Diagram to illustrate the mode of action of drugs acting on receptors (simplified, not to scale)

Some drugs have intermediate actions, and are 'partial agonists' (see Galbraith et al., 2007), for example the opioid buprenorphine, prescribed as an analgesic and used in substance misuse teams.

Some drugs are specific for one receptor type (for example ranitidine), whereas others block more than one type of receptor, for example prochlorperazine (Stemetil®). Drugs that act on several types of receptors have diverse adverse effect profiles, affecting many systems of the body. This is well illustrated by prochlorperazine (Chapter 5) and antipsychotics (Chapter 19).

Drugs bind to their target receptors, ion channels or enzymes, and may continue to exert their effects when they have disappeared from the plasma. Therefore, doses can often be administered at intervals longer than the half-life (Holford, 2001).

Hormones, neurotransmitters and their analogous (lookalike) drugs are described as 'the first messengers' in a complex signalling cascade. Once a hormone or drug has bound to its receptor, this affects the cell's enzymes and activities *via* 'second messengers'. These include a variety of substances such as intracellular calcium ions. A few drugs, lithium and magnesium, are small enough to move inside cells and act on the enzymes and metabolic pathways inside the cells, bypassing the receptors. These drugs have adverse effects that affect many different cells and systems.

A drug's actions on the developing fetus may be different to that in the adult, and there are many examples of drugs harming the fetus while not affecting the mother. For example, warfarin acts on an enzyme only found in developing fetal epiphyses (growing part of bones), and antiepileptic drugs cause the accumulation of a chemical that disrupts DNA synthesis (Morrell, 2003).

Dose–response relationships

There is often considerable individual variation in the changes in body function brought about by drugs, and drug doses have to be adjusted to individual needs. However, there is usually a relationship between drug dose and patient response, that is, the higher the dose, the greater the effect on the body. This is explained by the link between drug concentration, occupancy of receptors and physiological changes (Rang et al., 2007). Drug molecules may be viewed as competing with the body's own endogenous hormones or neurotransmitters for the limited number of sites on receptors. Therefore, they are more likely to be effective at high doses, when they literally outnumber the body's own molecules.

There is often a minimum effective dose, below which no effects are observed. For some drugs, there are maximum doses, above which no further beneficial effects are observed. Examples include inhaled corticosteroids and many drugs prescribed in mental health. In theory, this is linked to the idea that when all receptors are occupied by the drug, no further changes are possible and higher doses are unlikely to confer additional benefit.

Practice point

■ If women with serious mental illness are prescribed drugs above the dosages stated in the BNF, there is little additional benefit, but the risk of adverse effects is increased. Therefore, much additional patient monitoring, including regular ECGs, is required (BNF, 2009).

In other instances, the patient will lack the necessary enzymes to respond to a drug, and increased dosing will have no beneficial effects. For example, about 10% of Caucasians lack the enzyme needed to convert codeine to morphine; if morphine is not formed, there is no analgesia; another 10% are unduly sensitive to warfarin, and will require very low doses to achieve target coagulation levels.

Practice point

■ These genetic variations are unpredictable. It may be helpful to seek a personal or family history of previous experience of unusual reactions to prescribed drugs.

Most reactions between drugs and receptors, ion channels or enzymes are reversible, and eventually wear off when the drug is discontinued. One exception to this is aspirin. One of the actions of aspirin is to bind with and inhibit the platelet enzymes responsible for synthesizing the chemicals that promote clotting. This binding is irreversible. The effect of aspirin on the coagulation process takes several days to wear off, and clotting only returns to normal when new platelets have been synthesized in the bone marrow, which takes up to a week. Therefore, if aspirin is administered within a week of birth, the risk of postpartum haemorrhage is increased.

Changes in response

The cells' receptors are continually being renewed by their protein-synthesizing machinery. When a drug is administered over a period of time, the cells or their receptors may adapt: the number of receptors available on the cell surface may change in response to the presence of drugs.

Tolerance or desensitization

The continued presence of an agonist drug may reduce the number of relevant receptors available. This desensitization or down regulation of receptors is believed to be responsible for the loss of response seen with continued use of opiates, oxytocin or beta$_2$ agonists (bronchodilators).

Practice points

- Prolonged administration of oxytocin, for example for augmentation of labour, may render the uterine muscle unresponsive and atonic. As a result, the uterus may not contract following birth, increasing the risk of postpartum haemorrhage. In these circumstances, the uterus will not respond to oxytocin and other agents (for example prostaglandins and ergometrine) will be needed to combat the haemorrhage (Plested and Bernal, 2001; Robinson, 2003; McEwan, 2007).
- Patients who rely on beta$_2$ agonists (such as salbutamol) to control their asthma run the risk that, when their asthma worsens, these drugs will no longer work, and their symptoms will only be controlled by high doses of corticosteroids.

Supersensitivity

Conversely, the continued presence of an antagonist or blocking drug may increase the number of receptors. Therefore, if an antagonist is abruptly discontinued, the tissues may be unduly sensitive. For example, abrupt withdrawal of beta blockers makes the myocardium unduly responsive to stress, which increases the risk of a heart attack.

Withdrawal

If a drug has been used long term, abrupt withdrawal may cause a predictable pattern of adverse effects. Therefore, gradual discontinuation is usually recommended, particularly for corticosteroids, antiepileptic drugs, beta blockers, antidepressants, benzdiazepines, and other drugs prescribed for mental illness.

Infants born to mothers taking antidepressants, antipsychotics, antiepileptics, long-term opioids, or drugs of abuse may show symptoms of withdrawal on delivery.

Pharmacodynamic drug interactions

Where drugs act on the same or similar receptors, ion channels or enzymes or have similar actions or adverse effects, their actions are intensified if they are co-administered. For example, administration of more than one sedative can depress the central nervous system, affecting the performance of skilled tasks or causing sedation and respiratory depression.

Practice point

- Co-administration of alcohol with antihistamines (for hay fever or colds), some antidepressants, some antiemetics, cannabis, antipsychotics, antiepileptic drugs, opioids (including codeine), or benzodiazepines intensifies sedation. Ability to drive will be affected, but blood alcohol levels may not be. At higher doses, alcohol is not eliminated for 12 hours or more, and therefore this interaction may occur the day after the intake of a high dose of alcohol (Baxter, 2006).

Similarly, certain foods or herbs may intensify a drug's adverse reactions. For example: the irritant effects of chilli pepper may combine with those of ACEIs to produce a troublesome cough; similarly, liquorice intensifies the fluid retention of oestrogens or corticosteroids, sometimes causing clinically significant hypertension and potassium loss.

Therapeutics: the effects of the drug on the person

Not all treatments are effective, and patients need to be monitored to detect non-response. Sometimes the underlying physiological problems may worsen, rendering a previously effective regimen useless, as is occasionally seen in women with pre-eclampsia. More predictably, therapeutic failure may be induced by a drug interaction, for example if a patient with hypertension self-medicates with ibuprofen or another NSAID.

Even if a drug is working on the body's cells, there may be no noticeable response. Clinical response shows considerable individual variation. This is not always predictable, and idiosyncratic reactions can occur. For example, some women are unduly sensitive to oxytocin, and therefore infusions are commenced using a very low dose (BNF, 2009). Clinical effects also depend upon age, gender, pregnancy, disease state, drug interactions, weight, height, and genetic makeup. Women are at greater risk of adverse drug reactions than men. This may be due to differences in body composition (women have less muscle mass and reduced kidney function) or hormone balance, and, generally, women require lower doses of drugs than men, even when body weight is taken into consideration (Routledge, 2004).

Adverse effects

An adverse drug reaction is defined as any untoward and unintended response in a patient or investigational subject to a medicinal product, which is related to any dose administered (ICH, 1996). A more precise definition is:

> An appreciably harmful or unpleasant reaction, resulting from an intervention related to the use of a medicinal product, which predicts hazard from future administration and warrants prevention or specific treatment, or alteration of the dosage regimen, or withdrawal of the product. (Edwards and Aronson, 2000: 1255)

Serious **adverse events** or reactions are defined as untoward medical occurrences that at any dose:

- result in death
- are life-threatening
- require or prolong hospitalization
- result in persistent or significant disability or incapacity
- result in congenital anomalies (ICH, 1996).

Types of adverse drug reactions

Adverse drug reactions can be broadly divided into those which are dose related and predictable, and those which are neither. Some authorities (Edwards and Aronson, 2000) include withdrawal reactions and therapeutic failure as adverse drug reactions. It may be appropriate to consider the effects of drugs administered in pregnancy and labour in a separate category, as transgenerational adverse effects.

Dose-dependent adverse effects

Dose-dependent adverse effects are often the drug's main adverse effects. Severity is usually related to dose administered. Since such effects are often highly significant and entirely predictable, appropriate monitoring systems must be in place. For example, without adequate monitoring, anticoagulants can cause bleeding, and insulin can cause hypoglycaemia. With other drugs, the link between drug actions and adverse effects is less obvious and requires rather more understanding of physiology. For example, metoclopramide and prochlorperazine (Stemetil®) are dopamine antagonists. They are useful antiemetics because they block the excitatory action of dopamine on the vomiting centre. However, they also block the actions of dopamine in the areas of the brain that control posture and movement (the basal ganglia). For metoclopramide, this limits the dose that can be administered (Chapter 5).

Adverse effects related to subsidiary actions

Many drugs act on more than one type of cell receptor, potentially causing diverse adverse effects. The outcomes are predictable, and appropriate monitoring should be in place. For example, oxytocin acts on the oxytocic receptors of the uterus, but it also acts on the antidiuretic (ADH) receptors in the nephrons. This gives it the potential to trigger water retention and fluid overload. Therefore, fluid balance records should be maintained (Chapter 6). Similarly, prochlorperazine acts on muscarinic receptors in addition to dopamine receptors. By blocking the action of muscarinic receptors, prochlorperazine is responsible for drying the body's secretions such as saliva.

In pregnancy, the subsidiary actions of drugs on the uterus assume great importance. Any drugs that stimulate uterine contractility should be avoided, including misoprostol and all drugs chemically related to ergotamine (Chapter 6). This last group includes some drugs prescribed for migraine, such as sumatriptan, which authorities advise to avoid in pregnancy (BNF, 2009).

Practice point

■ Medicines for migraine are often prescribed on an 'as needed' basis, to be stored and administered only during an attack of migraine; the woman must be careful not to continue use of such medicines during pregnancy (Box 4.5).

Less predictable adverse effects: hypersensitivity/hypersusceptibility responses

Some of the rarest and most serious adverse events are unpredictable, idiosyncratic allergic or **hypersensitivity** responses, which may occur with any drug at any dose in any situation. They are not related to the known physiological actions of the drug, but are initiated when drugs trigger the immune system of susceptible people, hence the term 'hypersusceptibility' adverse drug reactions.

There are four types of hypersensitivity reactions (Table 14.1):

■ Type I: Immediate hypersensitivity response, **anaphylaxis** (Box 1.2)
■ Type II: Antigen/antibody reactions (Chapter 14) damaging red cells, white cells or platelets
■ Type III: Antigen/antibody reactions in other organs, which sustain damage
■ Type IV: Cell-mediated allergic reactions and delayed hypersensitivity.

Individuals with a history of **atopic** disorders, such as asthma or eczema, are particularly vulnerable to type I reactions.

Mild drug reactions usually take the form of an erythematous rash or an urticarial ('nettle') rash. Serious hypersensitivity responses, such as anaphylaxis, bone marrow depression and **haemolysis**, are rare but can be fatal (Rang et al., 2007). In all cases, it is important that the offending drug is discontinued. However, a rash caused by infection should not be mistaken for a hypersensitivity response (CEMACH, 2007). Once someone has experienced even a mild allergic skin reaction to a drug, including itching and urticaria, they are likely to be sensitized and more likely to have an anaphylactic reaction at the next exposure (Box 1.2). A rash without either itching or wheals may be a type II, III or IV reaction, and not associated with anaphylaxis. In the case of penicillin, doctors may determine this by skin testing; the tests predict 60% of clinical hypersensitivity responses (Midtvedt, 2008).

Practice point

■ All allergic reactions are recorded in detail and displayed prominently on patients' notes. Documentation of a drug rash should include any itching, urticaria (hives or nettle rash) or wheals, as these are features of a type I reaction, which could progress to anaphylaxis.

Almost any medication, allergens in food, latex or insect stings can induce a hypersensitivity response; common offenders include antimicrobials (particularly intravenous), NSAIDs, hormone preparations, dextrans, heparin, vaccines, blood products, iron injections, and local anaesthetics. Where drugs have similar chemical structures, *some cross-allergies exist:* for example, 5–15% of people allergic to penicillins will also be allergic to cephalosporins.

Occasionally, excipients (packing chemicals) used in tablets or injections may be responsible for hypersensitivity responses. For example, zinc or other components of insulin injections may be responsible for rashes at injection sites. Benzyl alcohol (contained, for example, in some diclofenac and interferon alfa injections) has caused severe reactions in premature infants (BNF, 2009).

Box 1.2 Anaphylaxis and angioedema

The most immediate type of hypersensitivity response is anaphylaxis. Cases where infant death followed maternal anaphylaxis after administration of a general anaesthetic for Caesarean section are reported (MCHRC, 2000). Anaphylaxis is characterized by the sudden onset of urticarial rash (hives), flushing, tissue swelling (particularly around the mouth), obstruction of the respiratory tract, bronchoconstriction (narrowing of the airways), and/or hypotension or diarrhoea. Bronchospasm, causing sudden and worsening difficulty in breathing, may be the first indication of a problem. Dilatation of blood vessels may cause hypotension, which may be followed by circulatory collapse and incontinence. The patient may visibly swell and lose consciousness as blood pressure plummets. Other presentations are possible. Death is most likely to occur from oedema obstructing the airways (angioedema) (Sampson et al., 2006).

Practice point

■ Anaphylaxis may occur within seconds or up to 1 hour after injection. Therefore, observation for at least 15 minutes when the first dose of a new intravenous drug is given is vital.

The management of anaphylaxis is described in the current edition of the BNF. This involves stopping the drug, calling help, maintaining the airway, positioning the patient, administering drugs as directed in national guidelines (oxygen, adrenaline and rapid-acting antihistamines), monitoring vital signs, preparing fluid for resuscitation, and organizing immediate transfer to hospital. Adrenaline is usually given intramuscularly into the lateral thigh using the 1 in 1000 solution, repeated, if necessary, 5 minutes later. Lower doses are prescribed for self-administration, for example as EpiPen®, to those who develop anaphylaxis to insect stings or foods.

In extreme emergencies, if the circulation is inadequate, adrenaline may be given by slow intravenous injection using the 1 in 10,000 solution injected over 5 minutes (Sampson et al., 2006; Lack, 2008a, 2008b).

Practice point

■ Two different strengths of adrenaline/epinephrine solution are available. Should the stronger (1 in 1,000) solution be administered intravenously, fatalities could occur.

In anaphylactic shock, cardiac output is so low that adrenaline can only enhance the blood supply to the placenta, therefore concerns regarding vasoconstriction by adrenaline are misplaced (MCHRC, 2000). Paediatricians may occasionally administer adrenaline to neonates during resuscitation: the intravenous route is recommended, but tracheal administration may be possible if intravenous access cannot be established (ILCOR, 2006).

Adrenaline can have adverse effects. It is only administered to seriously ill patients, with extreme caution and close monitoring of vital signs and ECG. Practitioners monitor for:

• cardiac arrhythmia
• sudden rise in BP, which could cause cerebral haemorrhage
• vomiting (and subsequent choking)
• pulmonary oedema
• hyperglycaemia.

Adrenaline may not be effective in patients taking beta blockers/antagonists (such as atenolol or labetolol) and intravenous salbutamol or glucagon may be needed (Sampson et al., 2006). Beta blockers prevent adrenaline reaching the beta receptors; therefore, there may be no response from the beta receptors, and no relief of obstructed airways. Beta blockade allows adrenaline to act on only the alpha receptors, causing a sudden, severe rise in blood pressure and bradycardia. Extra care may also be needed for patients prescribed drugs that block alpha receptors (such as clonidine for pain or hypertension) (Baxter, 2006). In theory, other drugs that block alpha receptors, such as antipsychotics or tricyclic antidepressants, could cause similar problems.

Intravenous antihistamine (chlorphenamine/chlorpheniramine) is also administered and continued for 24–48 hours to prevent relapse, together with close observation (BNF, 2009). It is estimated that 10% of patients with anaphylaxis will not respond to treatment (Sampson et al., 2005).

Practice point

■ Although patients often respond rapidly, recovery takes some 24–48 hours, and close observation to ascertain the need for repeat doses is essential during this time.

A few drugs, vancomycin and opioids, can cause histamine release. This is associated with severe flushing and hypotension. This reaction may be confused with anaphylaxis, but requires different management (Aronson, 2006).

Transgenerational adverse effects

Pregnancy, childbirth, breastfeeding and developing infants may be affected by medicines or environmental exposure. The impact of medication on the fetus may include congenital anomalies, cell damage, prematurity, low birth weight and developmental delay. Since the ova of female infants are formed before birth, there is potential for prenatal exposures to affect subsequent generations.

Manufacturers of many drugs and herbal remedies advise against use in pregnancy and lactation on the grounds that there are insufficient human data to demonstrate safety. No drugs have been subjected to randomized controlled clinical trials for **teratogenicity** in human pregnancy. Therefore, no drug has been demonstrated as 'safe'. The evidence for transgenerational adverse drug reactions is largely derived from observation studies, case reports of incidental exposure, national databases (mainly from Scandinavian countries), and animal studies.

Drugs in pregnancy

It is estimated that 4.9% of births and 4.2% of live births in Wales from 1998 to 2007 were associated with congenital anomalies (CARIS, 2008). The causes of most, about two-thirds, congenital anomalies remain unknown, and less than 1% are attributable to prescribed drugs (Ruggiero, 2006). Exposure of either parent to a medicinal product *at any time during conception or pregnancy* should be reported in association with congenital anomalies (ICH, 1996). All reported congenital anomalies in Europe are collated to monitor perinatal health across Europe, and detect abnormal clusters of problems (Macfarlane et al., 2003). However, attributing causation relies on data on prescribed medicines being accurately reported to those maintaining the databases.

Relatively few drugs are known to cause congenital anomalies, but only drugs that have been used for many years in thousands of women with no evidence of harm can be designated 'generally regarded as safe'. No teratogenic drugs are harmful to the developing fetus in all cases. Estimates vary as to the incidence of congenital anomalies: up to 30% with warfarin, up to 16% with sodium valproate (Aronson, 2006).

Some drugs can damage cells, causing organ failure, cancers or DNA changes. For example, infants whose mothers received the antiretroviral drugs zidovudine and lamivudine in pregnancy have shown DNA changes, but to date these have not been associated with human cancers (Poirier et al., 2004). *Some authorities suggest that infants exposed to antiretroviral drugs* in utero *are monitored to detect any problems at the earliest opportunity.* Table 1.1 at the end of the chapter outlines some of the drugs known to be potentially harmful to the fetus.

The vulnerability of the fetus is usually considered in stages:

- *Pre-implantation*, days 0–14, when any damage to the fertilized embryo is believed to be 'all or nothing': either the embryo dies or it successfully implants.
- *Cell division*, the first 14–17 days of gestation, when drugs that impair cell division (such as cytotoxic drugs) should be avoided: they are most likely to cause abortion at this time.
- *Organ differentiation*, days 18–55, when most organs form and major structural congenital anomalies can arise if crucial enzymes are affected, making the first trimester a period of vulnerability for several drugs, for example lithium, vitamin A, and warfarin. However, the central nervous system, inner ear and palate continue developing after this.
- *During the later stages of pregnancy*, the central nervous system, eyes, teeth, and external genitalia continue to develop and the blood supply and functioning of the placenta become more vulnerable. The blood vessels in the placenta may be constricted by nicotine, cocaine, amphetamines or beta blockers, restricting fetal growth. The functioning, rather than the structure, of organs may be damaged throughout pregnancy by several drugs, including alcohol, cocaine, insulin, furosemide (frusemide), and antithyroid agents. Problems may only become apparent in long-term studies, for example: children of mothers taking sodium valproate are more likely to require special needs education (Freyer, 2008); and retinoids (isotretinoin for acne) in late pregnancy can cause neurobehavioural deficits. However, not all children exposed to medicines *in utero* are monitored during childhood and adolescence.

Drug administration during pregnancy and breastfeeding is based on assessment of risks and benefits. Prescribing is likely to be restricted if drug exposure is known to result in a consistent pattern of similar anomalies, or the incidence of congenital anomalies is above the rate in the population, 4%. The risks of fetal damage depend on several factors as well as the chemical composition of the drug (Lipkin, 1993):

- stage of pregnancy
- amount or dose of drug ingested
- number of doses: a single dose may be less damaging than repeated exposure
- other agents to which mother and fetus are exposed
- mother's nutritional status
- genetic makeup of mother, fetus and placenta.

Some of these factors predict the risk of congenital anomalies associated with phenytoin (Wells, 2007). The picture is complicated by epidemiological work that links congential anomalies, particularly cleft lip, cleft palate, and congenital heart malformations, with adverse life events associated with severe maternal stress during the first trimester (Hansen, 2000), and stillbirth with high levels of psychological stress (66 stillbirths in 19,282 respondents) (Wisborg et al., 2008).

Some two-thirds of congenital anomalies, including most cardiac anomalies and neural tube defects, can be detected *in utero* by expert ultrasound screening. This procedure is likely to help women who need to take medicines for long-term conditions, such as epilepsy or bipolar disorder, or who have inadvertently been exposed to potentially harmful drugs (Tomson and Hiilesmaa, 2007).

Drugs in childbirth

Drugs given during childbirth may have long-term effects on the woman and infant. Antibiotics given during childbirth may alter the microorganisms in the neonate's colon, which, in turn, might affect the regulation of the immune system, possibly increasing the risks of **atopy** (Russell and Murch, 2006; Jordan et al., 2008). Also, opioid analgesics given in labour may pass into the infant, reducing ability to coordinate and suckle correctly, painlessly and effectively; high doses reduce the chances of successful breastfeeding (Jordan et al., 2005; Jordan, 2006) (Chapter 4). Women may be helped by extra support and informed explanations as to why they may be experiencing difficulties.

Breastfed infants

Drugs that can be administered to neonates are usually suitable for nursing mothers, for example paracetamol. For a few drugs, such as lithium or clozapine, there are reports of serious adverse reactions in infants. For some medicines, there is relatively little information, and very little research has been undertaken. Due to the absence of data, many manufacturers advise against breastfeeding. However, the short- and long-term benefits of breastfeeding to infant and mother should be considered, including:

- lower incidence of infection
- reduced risk of diabetes
- the impact on brain growth and sensory acuity
- reduced risk of breast cancer (Lawrence and Schaefer, 2007).

Women who wish to breastfeed may need help to consult pharmacy information services.

Table 1.2 lists some drugs known to be harmful during breastfeeding.

Conclusion

For many older drugs, the impact in pregnancy has been ascertained through observation and laboratory investigations. In contrast, there are relatively few observation studies and reports of the effects of maternal medications on breastfed infants. The movement of drugs administered in labour between mother and neonate has not been fully investigated, despite the known sedative effects of many analgesics and recognition of the importance of early initiation of breastfeeding.

There are also relatively few data describing how the physiological changes associated with labour and the puerperium, in normal and difficult labours, may be responsible for either therapeutic failure or adverse drug reactions, including easily overlooked or unattributed events, such as suboptimal neonatal behaviour. It is hoped that the framework for the bioscience principles outlined here will offer a useful guide to the practitioner. More detailed accounts are available in medical textbooks.

Further reading

- Galbraith, A., Bullock, S., Manias, E. et al. (2007) *Fundamentals of Pharmacology*, 2nd edn. Addison Wesley, Harlow.
- Jordan S. (2008) *The Prescription Drug Guide for Nurses*. Open University Press/McGraw-Hill, Maidenhead.
- Rang, H., Dale, M., Ritter, J. and Flower, R. (2007) *Pharmacology*, 6th edn. Churchill Livingstone, Edinburgh.
- Schaefer, C., Peters, P.W. and Miller, R.K. (eds) (2007) *Drugs during Pregnancy and Lactation: Treatment Options and Risk Assessment*, 2nd edn. Elsevier, Oxford.

Table 1.1 Some drugs known to be potentially harmful to the fetus

For a more complete list, the midwife should refer to the current BNF, and consult the manufacturers if uncertainty persists. Some drugs entail additional monitoring. Further examples are given in the relevant chapters. Drugs not included in this list are not proven to be safe.

Drug	Potential problem
ACEIs, e.g. enalapril, captopril, lisinopril	Renal damage, skull defects, olighydramnios
Alcohol (including some cough remedies)	Poor growth and learning disabilities. Fetal alcohol syndrome with very heavy use. Withdrawal syndrome in neonates
Amiodarone	Growth restriction, cardiac arrhythmia, congenital hypothyroidism
Amitriptyline, tricyclic antidepressants	Neonatal irritability when used near term
Amphetamines (includes 'ecstasy')	Neonatal irritability and poor feeding when used near term. Tachycardia. Growth restriction and anomalies
Anabolic steroids	Masculinization of female fetus. Adrenal suppression
Antiepileptics	Increased risk of anomalies and growth restriction with all drugs studied
Antihistamines	Manufacturers advise avoid on the basis of animal studies
Antimalarials *Specialist advice mandatory*	Any risks of congenital anomalies are outweighed by harmful effect of malaria. Extra folate supplements may be recommended with prophylactic regimens. Doxycycline is not recommended
*Antithyroid agents	Neonatal goitre and hypothyroidism
*Antipsychotics	Neonatal withdrawal problems and posture and movement disorders if used near term
	Atypical antipsychotics associated with gestational diabetes and low birth weight. Neonatal withdrawal problems/irritability and (rarely) seizures if used near term
	Older drugs: only isolated reports of congenital anomalies
Aspirin	Near term, bleeding complications, delayed or prolonged labour
	High doses in last trimester, possible premature closure of ductus arteriosus, pulmonary hypertension, kernicterus.
	Low dose for prevention of pre-eclampsia, no associations with congenital anomalies
Azathioprine	Risk of spontaneous abortion, possible risk of low birth weight, premature birth or abnormal white cell counts in neonate
Barbiturates	Congenital anomalies reported. Vitamin deficiencies and bleeding
	Dangerous withdrawal syndrome and respiratory depression in neonates
Benzodiazepines	Possibility of facial clefts, GI anomalies, vision defects, microcephaly. Respiratory depression, poor muscle tone or withdrawal syndrome in neonate
Beta blockers	Intrauterine growth retardation. Neonatal hypoglycaemia, respiratory problems

Drug	Potential problem
Buspirone (for anxiety)	Teratogenic in animals. Manufacturer advises avoid
*Cancer chemotherapy and radiotherapy	Risk of miscarriage, growth delay. Risk depends on individual drug
Carbamazepine	Possibility of neural tube defects (1%), microcephaly, hypospadias, facial or digit anomalies, vitamin deficiencies
Carbenoxolone, in mouthwashes and gels (Bioplex mouthwash®, Bioral gel®) and liquorice	Maternal fluid retention and oedema. Avoid
Chloral hydrate	This acts like alcohol, best avoided
Chlorpromazine	Possible hypotension during labour
Clomiphene	Possible association with neural tube defects (Elizur et al., 2008)
Cocaine	Placental abruption, premature rupture of membranes, developmental delay, intrauterine growth retardation, necrotizing enterocolitis and seizures in newborns, congenital anomalies
Cyclophosphamide	Growth restriction. Skull and CNS deformities. Conception not advised within 3 months of use in women and men
Danazol	Masculinization of the neonate
Diuretics (all)	Impaired blood supply to placenta, growth restriction
	Inner ear damage possible with furosemide (frusemide)
	Prolonged labour, thrombocytopenia, electrolyte disturbances, hypoglycaemia in neonate, with thiazides
Ephedrine, in OTC 'cold cures'	Fetal tachycardia. Possible link to anomalies such as ventricular septal defect, gastroschisis, if used in early pregnancy
Fluoride in high concentrations	Mottling of teeth with extreme exposure
Gabapentin	Toxicity in animal studies
General anaesthetics	Considered safe for patients. During childbirth, risk of respiratory depression in neonates. Possibly a small increase in miscarriage and developmental delay with repeated occupational exposure to anaesthetic gases
*Gold salts, for rheumatoid arthritis	Teratogenic in animal studies. Manufacturer advises contraception during and for 6 months after treatment discontinuation
Ibuprofen	Manufacturers advise avoid, including topical use. Regular use may be associated with in utero constriction of ductus arteriosus, lung or kidney damage and oligohydramnios. Delayed labour
*Indometacin	Manufacturers advise avoid. Possible in utero constriction of ductus arteriosus, lung or kidney damage and oligohydramnios. Delayed labour
Iodine, topical povidone iodine	Neonatal goitre and hypothyroidism. Povidone iodine is best avoided (Velasco et al., 2009). Radioactive iodine contraindicated in women of child-bearing age
*Isotretinoin, retinoids, for acne, including topical preparations, acitretin for psorisasis	**Teratogen**. Microcephaly, hydrocephalus, facial, cardiac, eye and ear defects reported in 35% of infants following oral use. Also spontaneous abortion, premature birth, developmental delay. Avoid. Requires effective contraception for 1 month before treatment and 5 weeks after discontinuation of isotretinoin, or 3 years for other retinoids

Drug	Potential problem
Ketamine	Not recommended. Risk of hypertension and panic attacks. Animal studies suggest fetotoxicity
*Lamotrigine	Possibility of cleft palate, hypospadias, GI anomalies
*Levetiracetam	Possibility of low birth weight. Toxicity in animal studies
*Lithium	Possibility of polyhydramnios, cardiac anomalies or arrhythmia, goitre, neonatal jaundice, stillbirth. Detailed ultrasound investigations recommended. Risks of toxicity in neonates if dose not reduced at delivery
**Live vaccines MMR, BCG, varicella	Fetal infections
Smallpox	Fetal death
Lysergic acid diethylamide (LSD)	Possibility of limb, eye or CNS anomalies
Metformin	No evidence of teratogenicity to date, when used in conjunction with polycyctic ovary syndrome for first 6–8 weeks of pregnancy
Methotrexate	Growth restriction, CNS and skull anomalies. Conception not advised within 3 months of use in women and men
Mercury	Methyl mercury is associated with cerebral palsy, mental retardation. Mercury and mercury amalgams (in filled teeth) have not been shown to be harmful, but dental assistants should observe hygiene practices
Mineral oils (as laxatives)	Vitamin deficiencies possible, particularly vitamin K
Mifepristone	Used for termination of pregnancy. Should this fail, manufacturer advises discontinuation of pregnancy. Risk of congenital anomalies
Misoprostol	Used for termination of pregnancy. Uterine contractions. Risk of miscarriage, avoid. Congenital anomalies, e.g. facial paralysis, defects of extremities in association with use in first trimester
NSAIDs	Regular use may impair fertility. Regular use in pregnancy may be associated with heart, lung and kidney problems. Possible risk of congenital anomalies. At term, prolonged labour and risk of bleeding
Nicotine	Intrauterine growth retardation, premature labour, *placenta praevia*, placental abruption. Possible associations with cleft palate and childhood cancers
Opioids	With regular use: behaviour problems, neurodevelopmental delay, low birth weight, premature labour, withdrawal syndrome in neonates. Maternal withdrawal may lead to premature rupture of membranes
Oral contraceptives/emergency contraception	Possible small risk of Down's syndrome or cardiovascular anomales, with accidental first trimester exposure, not supported by all epidemiological studies
Oral hypoglycaemics	Insulin offers better glycaemic control. Congenital anomalies with sulfonylureas in older studies
Paracetamol	Possible association with asthma with heavy use. Considered safe at usual doses
*Phenytoin	Possibility of facial, finger and cardiac anomalies, microcephaly. Vitamin deficiencies

Drug		Potential problem
Quinine (in tonic water, for cramps)		Very high doses may damage eyes and ears. Risks of untreated malaria are much greater
†Sibutramine		Some reports of spontaneous abortion (Sequeira, 2008)
SSRI antidepressants		Some studies have found increased incidence of congenital anomalies, particularly cardiac defects with paroxetine
		Neonatal withdrawal (irritability, tremor, shivering, respiratory distress) or bleeding when used towards term
		Manufacturers advise to avoid unless benefits outweigh risk
Statins to lower cholesterol		Congenital anomalies of CNS and limbs reported. Avoid
Sulfasalazine (for inflammatory bowel disease)		Additional folate supplements needed. Small risk of haemolysis in infant. An alternative drug is usually sought
Theophylline, in some 'cold cures' such as Franol®		Irritability, vomiting or cyanosis in neonate. Avoid in third trimester. Possible link to pre-eclmpsia and cardiac abnormalities
*Topiramate		Toxicity in animal studies
Triptans, sumatriptan, related drugs for migraine		Teratogenicity in animal studies. Manufacturers advise avoid (see ergometrine). No evidence of congenital anomalies following use of sumatriptan
*Valproate		Neural tube defects (up to 3%), learning difficulties, bone, facial, eye, CNS anomalies. Risks probably greater than with other antiepileptic therapy
*Vigabatrin		Possibility of cleft palate, neural tube or cardiac defects
Vitamins, large doses	A	Older studies suggest congenital anomalies. Medical supervision recommended
	D	Therapeutic doses unlikely to be harmful. High doses cause hypercalcaemia in mother and fetus. Topical calcitrol not recommended
Warfarin		High risk of fetal damage (Chapter 8), haemorrhage

Key: * Specialists will always be involved in the prescription of these drugs; ** vaccination in pregnancy, with any preparation, is only indicated where protection is needed without delay (DH, 2006). Administration should follow discussion of the risk and benefits with specialists (contacts are given in the BNF, Ch. 14); † the marketing authorization for sibutramine was suspended in January 2010.

Table 1.2 Breastfeeding: some drugs known to be potentially harmful

For a more complete list, the midwife should refer to the current BNF, and consult the manufacturers if uncertainty persists. Some drugs entail additional monitoring. Further examples are given in the relevant chapters. Drugs not included in this list are not proven to be safe.

Drug	Potential problem
ACEIs	Impaired kidney function, observe for oedema
Alcohol (including some cough remedies)	Sedation, poor suckling, feeding problems. A single drink over 30 minutes not shown to be harmful. Avoid feeding within 2 hours of drinking
Amiodarone	Hypothyroidism. Avoid
Anabolic steroids/androgens	Masculinizes infant. Impairs lactation. Avoid
Antifungals	Many manufacturers advise avoid
Antihistamines, particularly clemastine	Sedation. Manufacturers advise avoid
Antimicrobials	May affect gut flora, causing diarrhoea. Hypersensitivity responses possible (Chapter 13)
Antipsychotics	Possible sedation. CNS damage reported in animal studies. Most manufacturers advise avoid (Chapter 19)
Aspirin	Risks of bleeding and Reye's syndrome
Beta blockers	Monitor infant for bradycardia, hypothermia, hypoglycaemia
Bromocriptine	Suppresses lactation
Bronchodilators, e.g. salbutamol	Restlessness, tachycardia
Buprenorphine	May inhibit lactation. Manufacturer advises avoid with long-term use. Risk of sedation
Caffeine (large doses), theophylline (e.g. OTC medication, Franol®)	Large doses (>300 mg caffeine/3 cups of coffee/6 cups of tea) cause jitteriness, inattentive/poor feeding and poor sleeping, particularly in first 3 months
Cannabis	Delayed motor development
Cimetidine, ranitidine	Cimetidine may affect male infants, manufacturer advises avoid (Chapter 12). Ranitidine not known to be harmful, but enters breast milk
Clarithromycin	Manufacturers advise avoid.
Cocaine	Irritability and trembling. Avoid
Codeine	Isolated cases of accumulation and sedation
Combined oral contraceptives	Diminish milk supply, particularly in malnourished mothers. Progesterone only pill considered safe
Corticosteroids	If mother's dose is more than 40 mg prednisolone daily, the infant's adrenals may be suppressed
Cytotoxic drugs	Damage to bone marrow, white blood cells and infection. Avoid
Diuretics	May impair milk production
Ergometrine, ergotamine (LSD)	May impair milk production (Chapter 6). Ergotamine may affect the infant's circulation, avoid
Fluoxetine (Prozac®)	Irritability, GI upsets. Risk of hypersensitivity responses and bleeding. Manufacturer advises avoid
Gold salts	Pass into milk. Manufacturers advise avoid

Drug	Potential problem
Ibuprofen	Some manufacturers advise to avoid, including topical use. Not known to be harmful
Immunosuppressants	Manufacturers advise avoid. Small amounts of drug in milk, but some infants may be slow in eliminating drugs. Very few cases reported
Iodine, including topical preparations	Hypothyroidism in neonate. Avoid
Isotretinoin, retinoids for acne	Risk of damage to sight, hearing, bones or liver. Increased skin fragility. Risk of convulsions. Avoid, including topical preparations
Lithium	GI upset. Risk of damage to CNS and kidneys. Manufacturers advise avoid
Loperamide	High concentration in breast milk
Metformin	Manufacturer advises avoid. Present in milk. No problems reported in the few cases available
Methadone	Sedation (Chapter 20)
Metoclopramide	Manufacturer advises avoid. Used to stimulate milk production. No problems reported in the few cases available
Metronidazole, tinidazole	Pass into breast milk. Avoid high dose metronidazole, and tinidazole
Monoclonal antibodies	Manufacturers advise avoid breastfeeding during and after therapy. Very few cases reported
Nicotine, including patches	Milk let down inhibited. Irritability, poor feeding, GI upset
NSAIDs	Naproxen reported to affect coagulation. One case of seizures with indoemticin. Single doses not known to be harmful
Quinolones/fluoroquinolones	High concentrations in breast milk. Manufacturers advise avoid
Sedatives: benzodiazepines, antipsychotics, prochlorperazine, some tricyclic antidepressants (doxepin), alcohol, opioids	Difficulty establishing feeding. Neonate becomes too drowsy, and muscle tone is too weak. May fail to gain weight and length appropriately
SSRIs	No long-term data. Amounts in milk small. Weight, restlessness, irritability and lethargy should be monitored. Manufacturers of citalopram and escitalopram advise avoid. Manufacturer of paroxetine states breastfeeding can be considered. Manufacturer of sertraline states discontinuation of breastfeeding should be considered
Stimulant laxatives, e.g. senna	Diarrhoea in infant possible
Stimulants: ephedrine (cold cures), amphetamines	Neonate becomes irritable and sleeps poorly. Avoid
Sumatriptan and related preparations for migraine	Withhold breastfeeding for 12 or 24 hours after administration. Risk of vasoconstriction.
Sulfasalazine	Small risk of haemolysis in infant
Sulphonylureas, e.g. glipizide	Small risk of hypoglycaemia in infant
Tetracyclines	Teeth discolouration. Avoid
Vitamins A and D, high doses	Possible risk of damage to liver and bones

Note: The current BNF, the manufacturers' literature (www.medicines.org.uk), the Drugs and Lactation database (www.toxnet.nlm.nih.gov/cgi-bin/sis/htmlgen?LACT) and Schaefer et al. (2007) contain more complete information. Further examples are given in the relevant chapters on antimicrobials and anticonvulsants.

CHAPTER 2

Administration of Medicines

Sue Jordan

This chapter outlines the routes of medication administration commonly encountered in midwifery, as shown in Figure 1.3.

Chapter contents

- Oral administration
- Buccal/sublingual administration
- Rectal administration
- Vaginal administration
- Injections
- Intravenous administration
- Epidural and **intrathecal administration**

For eye and ear drops, see Further reading

Oral administration

Most drugs are given orally, for convenience. All **tablets** and **capsules** should be swallowed with a full glass of water, with the patient sitting upright and remaining upright for 30 minutes (McKenry and Salerno, 2003). This prevents prolonged contact between the drug and the linings of the mouth and oesophagus, which are vulnerable to corrosive substances, such as bisphosphonates, aspirin, doxcycline, iron, and potassium salts. **Enteric-coated** NSAID tablets or slow-release potassium tablets can cause localized ulcers further down the gastrointestinal tract.

Crushing or dispersing tablets alters their **bioavailability**, usually by hastening absorption; this sudden rise in drug concentration may cause serious **adverse drug reactions** (Schier et al., 2003). If a tablet is crushed or a capsule is opened, fine particles may be released into the air. This can cause:

- adverse reactions to the skin or absorption through the respiratory tract of the administrator, for example cytotoxics, hormones, steroids, and prostaglandins
- growth of resistant microorganisms in non-disposable equipment or in the lungs or skin of the administrator (antibiotics only) (Wright, 2002).

■ Crushing a modified-release preparation will liberate a larger dose than expected, increasing the risk of adverse drug reactions.
■ Crushed or dispersed tablets may have a most unpalatable taste.
■ If a non-dispersible tablet is left in water before administration, it could become inactive.
■ Crushed or dispersed tablets should not be mixed together, because their ingredients may interact.
■ Cutting tablets is likely to give an inaccurate dose, which may affect clinical response.
■ If a preparation is not licensed to be crushed or dispersed, this could be construed as 'tampering' with the product and render its use unlicensed (Griffith, 2005).

Administration in relation to food is an important consideration (see Chapter 1, Absorption; Jordan et al., 2003).

Buccal/sublingual administration

Buccal or sublingual administration allows rapid drug absorption. This can be useful in emergencies, including recurrent seizures, angina, or hypoglycaemia. The oral cavity contains several large veins, which, indirectly, drain into the superior vena cava and pass into the systemic (general) circulation without passing through the liver. Therefore, drugs absorbed from the oral cavity are not broken down (metabolized) by the liver and quickly reach the circulation in relatively high concentrations (Figure 1.3). For example, peak plasma concentrations of sublingual misoprostol are approximately double those of oral misoprostol, which may account for the increased uterine contractility associated with this route (Souza et al., 2008).

Case report

A teenage girl was administered sublingual nifedipine for hypertension. Her heart rate rose and palpitations occurred almost immediately.

Practice points

■ Hypertension can be controlled more reliably with intravenous than sublingual nifedipine (Maggioni et al., 2008).
■ Women should be advised against biting into capsules, because this releases the drug into the oral cavity, where it could be rapidly absorbed, resulting in high concentrations and adverse effects. For example, patients should not bite nifedepine capsules, without medical supervision, because the large amount of nifedepine released into the circulation could dangerously lower blood pressure, jeopardizing the blood supply to the uterus.

If no clinical changes have occurred 5 minutes after sublingual administration, it is likely that the drug has been ineffective and the prescriber should be notified. Eating, drinking or smoking will interfere with sublingual absorption. Buccal or sublingual tablets can cause mucosal irritation.

Rectal administration

Despite cultural considerations and practical difficulties, the rectal route may be useful for short-term drug administration, if other routes are not available. Laxatives, antiemetics, analgesics, and treatments for ulcerative colitis are sometimes administered this way.

The mucosal lining of the rectum is delicate, and does not provide an effective barrier to transmission of infection. The excipients necessary for absorption may be irritant (Tucker, 2007), therefore suppositories may irritate the delicate rectal lining, particularly with repeated use, for example carbamazepine and NSAIDs. The rectal capillaries are fragile and rectal administration is associated with increased risk of bleeding, particularly if the patient is already vulnerable to bleeding, for example if anticoagulants are administered (Wilkinson, 2001).

Practice point

■ Suppositaries are not given to patients who are at high risk of infection or bleeding (Hayes et al., 2003).

The position of the veins in the rectum determines drug absorption. The upper part of the rectum is drained by the superior rectal vein, which passes to the liver. The lower rectum is drained by the middle and lower rectal veins (the haemorrhoidal veins), which enter the systemic circulation directly, bypassing the liver. Therefore, drugs administered into the lower rectum bypass the liver, and act more rapidly than oral preparations. However, the exact position of the suppository may vary, and an unpredictable quantity of drug may enter the upper rectum and pass to the liver, delaying or reducing the activity of the drug (Figure 1.3). The rectum is normally empty, but the presence of any faeces can interfere with drug absorption, making it less predictable (Tucker, 2007). For example, absorption of metronidazole is about 50% less when administered rectally rather than orally.

Practice point

■ The amount of medication absorbed by this route may be irregular, incomplete and unpredictable (Wilkinson, 2001) or slow (Holmér Pettersson et al., 2006), and the patient should be observed for signs and symptoms of both over- and underdosing.

To assist drug distribution, the patient should remain lying for 15 minutes, and be reassessed afterwards.

The walls of the rectum contain numerous sensory nerve endings of the vagus nerve. If this is stimulated it may:

■ increase peristalsis
■ induce an urge to defaecate
■ slow the heart rate.

Practice points

■ Suppositories are not administered to patients with undiagnosed abdominal pain, as any obstruction could be worsened or an inflamed appendix could rupture.
■ Suppositories must be inserted above the anal sphincter to be retained. The anal sphincter can be identified by asking the client to 'bear down'. The suppository should be inserted some 1.5 inches above this (Smith et al., 2008).
■ Patients with **cardiac dysrhythmias** (irregularities) or a recent heart attack should not receive drugs per rectum (rectally) (Hayes et al., 2003).

Vaginal administration

Drugs (tablets, capsules, pessaries, solutions, sprays, ointments, foams, and creams) administered *per vaginam* are absorbed *via* the dense venous plexus in the vaginal walls into the internal iliac veins and pass into the circulation without being metabolized in the liver, and may pass into the fetus. Local irritation may occur, particularly if excipients include polyethylene glycols (Tucker, 2007). Rate and extent of absorption varies with drug formulation, **pH**, leakage, recipient's age, and state of the menstrual cycle (Hassain and Ahsan, 2005). Systemic absorption of misoprostol is slower and more sustained with vaginal than oral or sublingual administration (Souza et al., 2008).

Injections

The most effective and rapid strategy for drug administration is directly into a vein. Other injections, into muscle, subcutaneous fat or the dermis, are used when a drug cannot be given orally or topically, or if urgent treatment is needed, and it is not possible to establish intravenous access. Safety devices reduce the risk of needlestick injury (Pratt et al., 2007). Sites for intramuscular and subcutaneous injections should be clean; whether further skin preparation is necessary is uncertain, and local policy should be followed (Lister, 2004).

Intramuscular injections

Intramuscular injections are used in emergency care, during labour, and for the administration of antipsychotic medication where adherence to long-term oral regimens is problematic. They can be painful, and absorption may be erratic.

Muscles are well supplied with blood vessels. To avoid inadvertent administration into a vein, the syringe plunger should be drawn back for 5–10 seconds to check that no blood enters the syringe before the drug is injected (Smith et al., 2008). Intramuscular injections are avoided in patients at high risk of bleeding, for example those taking anticoagulants. Injections should not be given into immobile limbs, for example after bupivacaine administration, because their circulation is compromised. Observing the site 2–4 hours later will help to detect any problems.

Intramuscular injections are notoriously painful and are avoided, unless essential. Pain increases with:

■ needle diameter (not length)
■ skin stretch
■ volume injected
■ chemical nature of the drug
■ muscle tension
■ administration into subcutaneous fat (Palmon et al., 1998; McKenry et al., 2006).

In order to reduce pain:

■ restrict the volume injected
■ inject slowly, at a maximun rate of 1 ml/10 seconds to minimize tissue stretch
■ administer injection with muscles relaxed
■ offer a warm compress to reduce pain, particularly after penicillin injections.

Intramuscular injections are given using the Z-track technique. This seals the drug in the muscle. However, this seal will be disrupted by massaging or tight clothing.

Absorption may be reduced in people with diabetes, for whom intramuscular doses of penicillins should be increased.

Injection sites

Intramuscular injections can be administered into the lateral thigh, the deltoid, the ventrogluteal region, or the dorsogluteal region.

Deltoid

The deltoid muscle offers a convenient site for the administration of subcutaneous injections. However, only small volumes should be administered into this muscle: up to 1 ml (Rodger and King, 2000). The radial nerve and brachial artery pass close to the lower deltoid. *Therefore, all injections in this region must be administered above the level of the axilla. If the radial nerve is damaged, this will cause permanent wrist drop.*

The blood supply to the deltoid muscle is greater than the other injection sites. Therefore, injections administered here are absorbed and eliminated more rapidly than other intramuscular sites, which renders the deltoid muscle unsuitable for depot injections.

Gluteal region

Some intramuscular injections are administered into the gluteal region, for example antipsychotic depots, diclofenac, and magnesium. The large muscle mass in this region offers two injection sites: dorsogluteal and ventrogluteal. The sciatic nerve lies close to the dorsogluteal site, and is vulnerable to injury. In most people, the sciatic nerve is beneath the muscle piriformis (part of gluteus medius). However, in some people, part of this nerve emerges above (0.5%) or within (12.2%) the muscle piriformis. In this unusual position, the nerve is vulnerable to damage from injections placed in the 'upper, outer quadrant' of the buttock.

Practice point

■ When injecting into the dorsogluteal site, it is important to identify the bony landmarks (the greater trochanter and the posterior spine of the iliac crest) and place the injection above an imaginary line joining the two, above the buttock area.

The dorsogluteal (or buttock) area contains much adipose tissue, which can extend below the gluteal muscles. This can cause confusion when dividing the area into quadrants to locate the dorsogluteal injection site, and allows an injection to be placed too low, that is, close to the sciatic nerve.

Both the ventrogluteal site and the useable area of the dorsogluteal site contain the gluteus medius muscle. Up to 2.5 ml can be injected here. Authorities consider the ventrogluteal site preferable to the dorsogluteal site, because there are fewer nerves and muscles in close proximity (Rodger and King, 2000; Smith et al., 2008).

The thigh

The thigh contains the bulkiest muscles of the body. The vastus lateralis in the lateral aspect of the anterior thigh is relatively distant from major nerves and blood vessels, but has been associated with femoral nerve injury. It is able to accommodate up to 5 ml of injection in an adult (1.0 ml in children under 3 and 2.5 ml in those under 15) (Hayes et al., 2003). However, patients report more pain from injections administered into the thigh than the buttock (McKenry and Salerno, 2003), and any scars and nodules are immediately visible to the recipient. In the front of the thigh, the medial aspect of the vastus medialis is close to the femoral artery, femoral vein and saphenous nerve, and this is not usually recommended for intramuscular injections.

Depth of adipose tissue

Absorption from intramuscular or subcutaneous injections may be unusual in both obese and emaciated recipients (Wilkinson, 2001). The depth of the subcutaneous fat depends on the individual, their age, fat stores, and gender. In the dorsogluteal site, this ranges from 0.5 to 6 inches (1.2–14.4 cm). For many women, even those around 8–9 stone (50–60 kg), the subcutaneous fat in the gluteal region is greater than 2 inches (4.8 cm) (n = 213; Cockshott et al., 1982). In the ventrogluteal site, the depth of subcutaneous fat varies less between individuals, and is about 3.75 cm (1.6 inches) (Workman, 1999). The thick layer of adipose tissue in the dorsogluteal region in some individuals means that in many people, standard needles of 35 mm deposit the medication in fat, not muscle (Cockshott et al., 1982). At the dorsogluteal site, some 35/61 (57%) women and 8/39 (21%) men were affected, while fewer patients (10/61, 16% women; 2/39, 5% men) had problems at the ventrogluteal site (Nisbet, 2006).

Subcutaneous injections

Subcutaneous injections are given to administer a range of drugs, including vaccines, insulin, and heparin. The usual sites are the abdomen, lateral thigh or upper arm, but other sites are available. Needles are inserted at 45 or 90 degrees. When shorter, fine gauge needles are used, for example for insulin pen injections, the needle can be inserted at 90 degrees. Many prepackaged preparations have short needles, and instructions for administration at 90 degrees. However, if the needle is more than 1 inch (2.4 cm) long, or the subcutaneous layer is thin, a shallow angle of 45 degrees is recommended (for example with syringe drivers), to ensure that the injection does not penetrate the muscle.

The depth of subcutaneous tissue varies between individuals. A survey of 65 adolescents (38 girls) found that the depth of subcutaneous fat varied between 7 and 26 mm on the outer arm, 7 and 31 mm on the abdomen, and 9 and 30 mm on the anterior thigh. Where the subcutaneous layer is thin, insulin injections administered at 90 degrees with a standard 12.5 mm needle could be placed in muscle, affecting absorption and causing tissue atrophy (Shin and Kim, 2006).

Practice point

■ The depth of the subcutaneous layer should be assessed for each patient. Skin folding and/or 6 mm needles may be necessary for thin patients. If less than 1 inch (2.4 cm) of tissue can be grasped, the subcutaneous injection should be administered at 45 degrees (Berman et al., 2008).

The subcutaneous fat contains numerous blood vessels. To avoid inadvertent administration into a vein, the syringe plunger should be drawn back to check that no blood enters the syringe before the drug is injected (Smith et al., 2008). However, this is not advised when administering insulin or heparin (Hayes et al., 2003). Massaging the site may increase trauma to the small vessels. Bruising after a subcutaneous injection can be reduced by the application of ice. During pregnancy the peripheral circulation is dilated, which may enhance the absorption of drugs given by subcutaneous or intramuscular injections.

Practice points

■ Women with diabetes should be alerted to the added risks of hypoglycaemia in early pregnancy (Carlson and Byington, 1998) (Chapter 19).
■ To avoid complications at the injection site, if repeated subcutaneous injections are administered, sites 1 inch (2.4 cm) apart should be defined in each area, and injections rotated.

Intravenous administration

The intravenous route, using either central or peripheral lines, is used for the infusion of fluids and electrolytes, drug administration, and parenteral nutrition. Intravenous infusion is the fastest and most certain route of drug administration.

Practice point

■ Because of the rapid absorption of intravenous drugs, it is important that they are administered strictly on time. Delays and subsequent 'bunching' of administration cause exaggerated 'peaks and troughs' in drug concentrations (Figure 1.1).

Intravenous administration may be by continuous infusion, intermittent infusion or as bolus doses. These are not interchangeable: a patient died when a 60-minute intravenous infusion of vancomycin was mistakenly administered as a bolus dose (Cousins, 1995).

Continuous intravenous infusions

Continuous infusion aims to establish and maintain a steady concentration of drug in the circulation. The drug is administered as a dilute solution, to reduce irritation of the vein. However, it is important to ensure that the drug is compatible with the infusate. For example, furosemide (frusemide) is incompatible with glucose/dextrose solutions, and amiodarone is incompatible with sodium chloride.

Intermittent infusion

Intermittent infusion may cause the concentration of the drug in plasma to 'peak and trough', and fall above and/or below the therapeutic range. This can cause both toxicity and therapeutic failure. This could occur, for example, in patients treated with intravenous antibiotics or heparin. Penicillins and cephalosporins are not sufficiently chemically stable for continuous infusion, and are given by intermittent infusion.

Bolus doses

Injection are usually given *via* existing intravenous access. A single bolus injection will produce a very high concentration of the drug in the plasma. The drug rapidly reaches the therapeutic range, which is useful in emergencies. If the drug is administered too rapidly, the concentration is likely to overshoot the therapeutic range and enter the toxic range. If the drug is administered slowly, the concentration rises less rapidly. With care, the rate of infusion can be adjusted to optimize the therapeutic effects and minimize **adverse effects**.

Bolus doses must be given slowly enough to allow the flow of infusate to continue and dilute the drug. The rate of administration will depend on the drug. Generally, unless the patient has suffered a cardiac arrest, or a severe haemorrhage, no dose should be administered in less than 1 minute (BNF, 2009). Most drugs can be administered over 1–5 minutes. **Anaphylaxis** is more likely if drugs are administered too rapidly.

The rapid administration of drugs is likely to cause:

■ trauma to the veins
■ serious adverse drug reactions
■ fluid overload, if large volumes of fluid are administered.

Drugs are rarely added to infusions. If this is necessary, the drug must be *mixed thoroughly*. This involves detaching the container from the giving set. Without thorough mixing, delivery will be uneven. If potassium or magnesium are allowed to settle or 'layer' at the bottom of an infusion bag, a high concentration will be delivered. This will reach the heart quickly and may cause a cardiac event. The use of ready-prepared solutions is safer (BNF, 2009).

Case report

Magnesium sulphate was administered for tocolysis in a healthy 20-year-old woman. The solution was prepared by injecting magnesium sulphate into the intravenous infusion bag. The woman complained of feeling slightly hot. The infusion was stopped when the respiratory rate was five/minute and BP was 135/45 mmHg. Venous blood sampling revealed a high concentration of magnesium (6.95 mmol/l). Oxygen and calcium gluconate were administered, and the situation was 'rescued', with no long-term consequences. Investigations revealed that the magnesium had not been thoroughly mixed prior to administration (Cao et al., 1999).

This case illustrates the importance of thorough mixing if magnesium sulphate is added to an infusion bag.

Incompatibilities

Many drugs interact with the infusate or other drugs, resulting in loss of effect, toxicity or other actions. Therefore, whenever possible, *only 1 drug should be added to any infusion container and never to blood products, mannitol, or sodium bicarbonate. Only specially formulated preparations can be added to amino acids or fat emulsions* (BNF, 2009). More detailed information is available in hospital pharmacies.

When infusates are incompatible, chemical reactions occur; this may cause solid particles to form in the giving set. For example, furosemide (frusemide) and dextrose/glucose interact and may form a visible precipitate, causing solid white particles to appear in the infusion line. Unfortunately, this may not become apparent immediately. The longer drugs or chemicals remain in contact with each other, the greater the chance of incompatibilities arising. Precipitates can cause thrombophlebitis or, if the infusion leaks, skin sloughing.

Many drugs are incompatible with components of total parenteral nutrition, and should not be administered in the same giving set (BNF, 2009). Double-lumen intravenous catheters allow the separation of drugs and feed (Chadwick and Forbes, 1996). A Y-site connection may not be suitable for administration of unstable drugs, such as acyclovir and ondansetron (Thomson et al., 2000). Specialist advice should be sought.

Practice points

- Infusions should be checked regularly for signs of incompatibility: cloudiness, colour change, or crystallization. However, *the absence of visual changes does not exclude the possibility of incompatibility*. For example, the combination of heparin and gentamicin is incompatible, but there may be no visible changes to the infusion. This mistake may only be realized when the infection fails to respond to the antimicrobial, or a thromboembolic event occurs.
- To reduce the risk of chemical reactions causing drug incompatibilities, the giving set should be changed every 24 hours if it is used to administer a drug (BNF, 2009).
- It is often necessary to contact the pharmacy for information on incompatibilities.

See Appendix 6 of the BNF and the product literature for information on compatibilities and infusion rates.

Cannulation

For ease of venous access, it is important that the site to be cannulated should be vasodilated. It is therefore important to ensure that the area is warm.

Pain

Venepuncture and venous cannulation may be painful. For many patients, this may be reduced by the application of local **anaesthetic** cream. Repeated venous access may result in fibrosis around the veins, for example in women who regularly undergo blood tests or inject recreational drugs.

EMLA® (eutectic mixture of local anaesthetics) is a mixture of lidocaine/lignocaine and prilocaine, which may be applied to the skin surface to provide analgesia for venepuncture, cannulation, or intraspinal needle insertion (Sharma et al., 1996; Koscielniak-Nielsen et al., 1998; Harris et al., 2001). A thick layer under an occlusive dressing will provide analgesia if applied 45–60 minutes before the procedure. Tetracaine (amethocaine) gel is an alternative; analgesia is expected within 30 minutes. Tetracaine causes vasodilation, whereas lidocaine (lignocaine) can cause vasoconstriction, which is important when obtaining venous access (Russell and Doyle, 1997). There is a small risk of adverse drug reactions, mainly local irritation, but also from systemic absorption (Chapter 4). Application to mucous membranes, wounds or areas of atopic dermatitis must be avoided (BNF, 2009). If it is not possible to wait 30–45 minutes before securing intravenous access, topical vapo-coolant sprays may reduce pain by lowering the skin temperature and interrupting the transmission of the pain sensation (Hijazi et al., 2009).

Maintaining venous access

The intravenous infusion site must be checked for patency at every use.

Maintaining patency of a vein

An injection port must be 'flushed' with 2 ml of fluid before and immediately after every use to ensure complete delivery, and at least every 24 hours to prevent clot formation (Ben-Arush and Berant, 1996). If venous access is failing, resistance to the injection will be felt at this time. Sodium chloride 0.9% or dilute heparin solution (for example Hepsal®) are used to maintain venous patency. If heparin (10–200 units every 4 hours) is used, the patient may experience the adverse effects of heparin (Chapter 8). Saline flushes have been shown to be as effective as heparin in maintaining venous patency for catheters left in place for up to 48 hours (Sweetman et al., 2007). Due to the potential for dosage errors and adverse effects, heparin flushes are not recommended for venous access in adults (Toft, 2009).

Extravasation

Leakage (or extravasation) of **isotonic** fluid in small amounts is not damaging, but fluid containing drugs may be extremely irritant. Severe tissue necrosis and skin breakdown, requiring skin grafting, may follow the extravasation of noradrenaline/norepinephrine, adrenaline/epinephrine, or cytotoxic drugs. Fluids containing potassium or glucose are also highly irritant.

The extent of any extravasation can be limited by frequent checks and transparent dressings. An extravasated drug is an emergency. Product literature should be consulted.

Phlebitis

Phlebitis is inflammation of a vein, usually due to damage to the wall, which causes the release of inflammatory mediators and clot formation. Redness, pain and oedema usually occur 2–3 days after insertion of the needle. If the venous catheter is not removed, infection will result. Phenytoin, erythromycin, and diazepam are particularly irritant, as are high concentrations of potassium, multivitamins, dextrose, and amino acids. Phlebitis is more likely when the infusion is acid or alkaline, is very concentrated or contains penicillins and vancomycin.

Precautions taken to reduce extravasation and phlebitis include:

- ensuring the intravenous line is patent
- avoiding compromised circulations, for example veins that have been traumatized by venepuncture
- avoiding wrists and digits, because these are hard to immobilize
- selecting a site that allows proximal access
- checking for leaks before giving the drug
- observing the infusion site for swelling or redness
- asking the woman to report any burning, itching or pain
- using a dressing that allows inspection
- flushing the drug through with a few millilitres of saline.

Practice point

- The site of infusion is an important source of potential discomfort, which can disturb much-needed sleep in the puerperium. This can be minimized by regular observations of the site and resiting as needed.

Infections

Intravenous lines are notorious sources of infection. Strict asepsis is always necessary when handling intravenous giving sets (BNF, 2009). The use of ready-prepared infusions is less likely to introduce infection than ad hoc/extemporaneous additions to infusions on the ward. Similarly, ready-prepared infusions for administration over 30–60 minutes are preferable to manual intravenous injections.

The incidence of infection can be reduced by:

- replacing intravenous cannulae every 48 hours
- hand disinfection with soap and water before handling intravenous cannulae
- use of gloves
- disinfection of the patient's skin
- leaving only sterile tape in contact with the entry site
- firmly anchoring the intravenous catheter
- transparent dressings to allow site inspection
- change of dressing if moisture visibly collects under the dressing
- assessing the site at least daily for signs of redness
- asking the patient to examine the site for signs of redness
- assessing the patient for signs and symptoms of fever (Wilson, 1994; Berman et al., 2008).

Infection is more dangerous with a central line (see Pratt et al., 2007).

How the body handles intravenous drugs

Intravenous administration means that all the drug administered is absorbed. There is no need to take account of any uncertainties in dose or timing due to individual differences involving the gut or the liver enzymes. Doses can be calculated and adjusted to the patient's needs more precisely than with other routes of administration.

Although the intravenous route minimizes potential problems with drug absorption, consideration must be given to potential problems with drug distribution and elimination (Chapter 1). When giving any drug, distribution will be reduced and the chances of toxicity increased in renal failure, heart failure, and **shock**; patients with severe pre-eclampsia or eclampsia are particularly at risk.

Circulatory overload

If the amount of fluid in the blood vessels is increased beyond the heart's capacity to pump it, the circulation becomes overloaded and blood backlogs into the pulmonary veins. This causes pulmonary oedema and breathlessness, which may progress to acute/adult respiratory distress syndrome (ARDS or 'shock lung'), followed by systemic oedema and heart failure. Women with pre-eclampsia/eclampsia or diminished renal or cardiac reserve are at particular risk of circulatory overload. This is a particular danger with the administration of oxytocin or isotonic solutions (for example 0.9% sodium chloride, Ringer's lactate @ 275 **mOsm/kg**) or **hypertonic** solutions (for example dextrose 5% in 0.45% saline @ 406 mOsm/kg). None of these fluids contain clotting factors or oxygen-carrying pigments; therefore, overuse can impair coagulation and the availability of oxygen in the tissues.

Practice points

- Flow rate is checked at regular intervals, when the woman changes position and if the height of the infusion stand is altered. If an infusion is falling behind schedule, only minor adjustments to the rate may be made, that is, within 30%, without consulting a doctor (Loeb et al., 1993). Too rapid an infusion may cause circulatory overload.
- Large volumes of cold fluids or blood products may adversely affect the myocardium or impair the clotting mechanisms (CEMACH, 2007).
- Rapid resuscitation is particularly dangerous in seriously ill women (CEMACH, 2007).
- A record of all fluids administered must be kept. Even small imbalances can cause overload in vulnerable patients such as neonates or those with severe pre-eclampsia. Many problems could be avoided by checking vital signs and state of hydration before and during administration of infusions (Clayton and Stock, 1993: 111). The frequency with which acute/adult respiratory distress syndrome appears as a cause of maternal death forced Department of Health assessors to issue a terse warning regarding the risks of circulatory overload in pre-eclamptic women (DH, 1998: 45); however, further cases have been reported (CEMACH, 2005: 84).
- If large volumes of fluids are infused, the need to replace clotting factors and red cells should be discussed with the multidisciplinary team (CEMACH, 2005).

Case reports

Circulatory overload can cause acute/adult respiratory distress syndrome (ARDS), particularly in eclamptic/pre-eclamptic women.

1 At 27 weeks gestation, a woman developed HELLP syndrome. During transfer between hospitals, the fetus died *in utero*. While labour was being induced, excessive amounts of fluid were transfused. This caused pulmonary oedema, and positive pressure ventilation was needed to maintain oxygenation prior to Caesarean section. The lung damage was so severe that acute/adult respiratory distress syndrome followed (DH, 1998: 42).

This case illustrates the dangers of fluid retention associated with oxytocin (Chapter 6). In pre-eclampsia, the vessels are so damaged, and the vascular space is so reduced, that excess fluid readily passes into the tissue spaces, causing pulmonary oedema and further damage leading to acute/adult respiratory distress syndrome.

Circulatory overload can cause heart failure.

2 A woman who was wheezing, with raised pulse and respiratory rates was given intravenous fluids and salbutamol. The signs and symptoms of heart failure and circulatory overload were not recognized and she suffered a cardiac arrest.

In this case, administration of intravenous fluids exacerbated pre-existing peripartum cardiomyopathy (CEMACH, 2007: 126).

Excessive water intake from infusions or oral intake may dilute the sodium concentration in circulating fluids. This is potentially dangerous and may prolong labour by inhibiting oxytocin secretion (Chapter 6) (Moen et al., 2009).

Practice point

■ Oral fluid intake should be recorded alongside intravenous fluids.

Raised intracranial pressure

If hypotonic solutions are administered, in effect excess pure water is infused, which will pass into cells, causing them to swell. This can damage the cells of the brain or the cardiac conduction system. **Hypotonic** solutions (for example 0.45% saline @ 154 mOsm/1) are not given to patients at risk of raised intracranial pressure: for example those with eclampsia, severe pre-eclampsia, head injury or cerebrovascular accident.

Transfer to fetus

Electrolytes and glucose from intravenous infusions are transferred to the fetus. Intravenous glucose may cause fetal hyperglycaemia, followed by rebound hypoglycaemia (Philipson et al., 1987).

Protein deficiency

The osmotic activity of plasma proteins is important in maintaining the distribution of body water. When reduced concentrations of plasma proteins are present, for example due to liver disease, malnutrition or burns, they are unable to hold water in the blood vessels. The water is then likely to enter body cavities, tissue spaces and cells. Therefore, such patients should not receive hypotonic infusions.

Lactate infusions

Lactate (as in Ringer's lactate) is metabolized into bicarbonate by the liver. Therefore administration of lactate is avoided in:

■ alkalosis, for example hyperventilating women
■ liver disease, for example HELLP syndrome.

Actions of the drugs

In general, drug actions are not affected by the route of administration. However, the onset of adverse drug reactions may be much more rapid when drugs are administered intravenously, and extra precautions are needed. Ampicillin, diazepam, and potassium are taken as illustrative examples.

Ampicillin

Intravenous administration poses several potential problems not normally encountered with oral administration:

- in an infusion, ampicillin is incompatible with many other drugs, for example gentamicin
- ampicillin is inactivated by contact with tetracyclines or erythromycin
- heparin may be potentiated by contact with ampicillin
- fits can occur if injections are too rapid, especially in neonates and patients with renal impairment
- hypersensitivity responses can be severe.

Diazepam

Intravenous diazepam is very important in seizure control. However, it can cause several problems not usually seen with oral administration:

- Respiratory depression can occur in susceptible individuals and other sedatives (for example pethidine) are potentiated. Therefore, respiratory support should be available for emergency use.
- Diazepam cannot be diluted or mixed with other drugs or infusions.
- Diazepam tends to precipitate onto plastic tubing, and is therefore given directly into a vein if possible.
- Diazepam is an irritant; consequently, small veins are avoided, and leakage is hazardous. There is a high risk of thrombophlebitis.
- After a large dose, withdrawal symptoms, such as anxiety, insomnia, photophobia, tinnitus, or nausea, can last for several weeks.

Case report

This case illustrates the importance of careful supervision of all intravenous infusions.

A 39-year-old woman had given birth and had developed a fever, for which an antibiotic was prescribed, to be administered diluted in 0.9% saline or water for injection. Unfortunately, strong potassium chloride solution was mistakenly substituted and administered intravenously. An immediate cardiac arrest occurred. Despite instant attempts at resuscitation, the woman sustained massive brain damage. The health authority settled the claim.

It is recommended that potassium chloride is kept securely away from the general drug stock, and extensive checks are carried out before it is ever infused (Cousins, 1994).

Hypersensitivity responses

Most hypersensitivity responses are harmless skin eruptions, presenting as an itchy 'nettle' rash and swelling around the infusion site. However, bronchospasm and anaphylaxis can occur. Not only the drug but the preservative of the infusion can trigger a hypersensitivity response, for example sulphites can precipitate an asthma attack (Box 1.2).

Epidural and intrathecal administration

The term 'intraspinal or neuraxial injection' is used to refer to administration within the spinal column, that is, to encompass epidural, spinal and combined spinal epidural administration (Wildsmith, 1996). In childbirth, this is closely aligned with 'regional analgesia', which is defined as blocking the passage of pain impulses through a nerve by depositing an analgesic drug close to the nerve trunk, cutting off sensory innervation to the region it supplies (Eltzschig et al., 2003). A needle is inserted into the lumbar spine in the L3–L4 or L4–L5 intervertebral spaces (lumbar vertebrae are numbered L1–L5). These are usually selected because the spine of L4 can be readily identified as lying between the highest points of the iliac crests. Drugs may be administered into the epidural space or the intrathecal (subarchnoid) space (Figure 2.1).

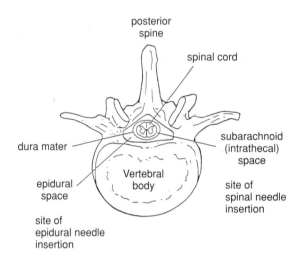

Figure 2.1 Transverse section of the spine

The problems encountered are those attributed to the route of administration, plus the **side effects** of the drugs themselves. Epidural or combined spinal epidural analgesia is usually achieved and maintained with bupivacaine and fentanyl, with diamorphine reserved for urgent situations (NCC, 2004).

Epidural anaesthesia

Epidural anaesthesia entails injection into the fat in the narrow space between the dura and the bony canal. (Figures 2.1 and 2.2). The drug circulates in the epidural space, diffuses through the dura, where it acts on the nerve roots (local anaesthetics) or **receptors** in the spinal cord (opioids) and circulates in the subarachnoid space (Figure 2.3).

Obese women have reduced epidural and subarachnoid space, due to the pressure of adipose tissue; therefore,they may require less analgesia, and doses should be increased very gradually (Soens et al., 2008).

Sufficient opioid or local anaesthetic is injected to be absorbed into the circulation, *via* the epidural veins, the azygous vein and hemiazygous veins, in proportion to the total dose used (Figure 2.3). The drug then passes into the fetus. Epidural veins are engorged during pregnancy and enlarge further during contractions. Therefore, drug absorption is increased at delivery or when the mother is spontaneously pushing, and 'top-up' injections are usually avoided at this time.

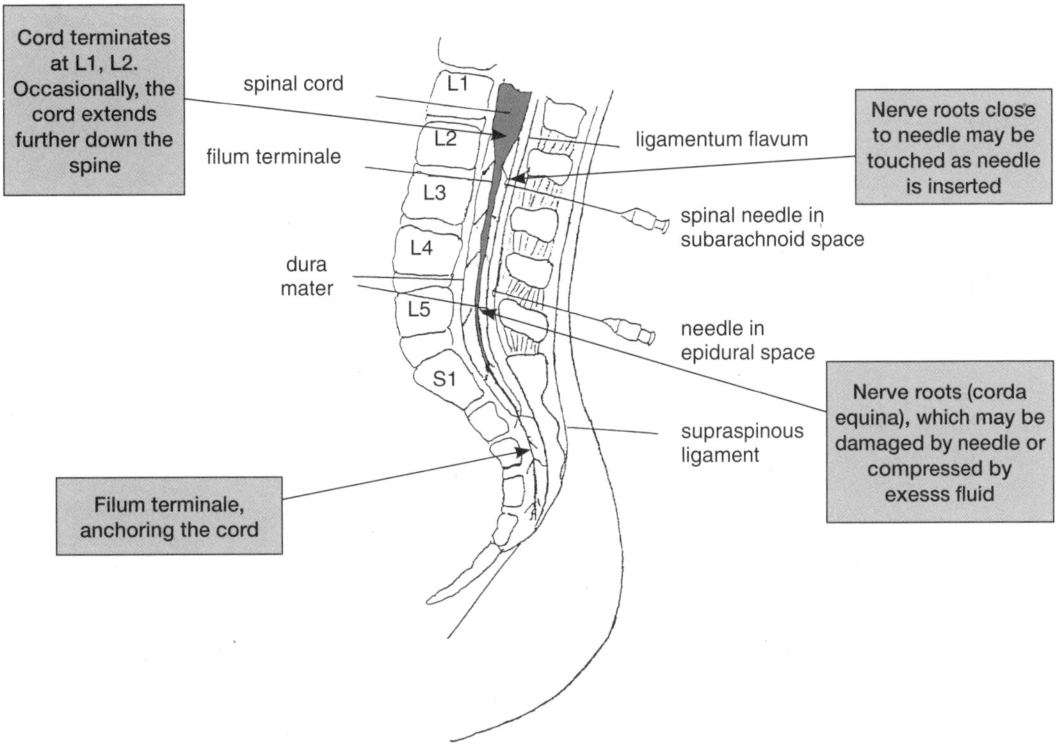

Figure 2.2 Diagram of the lumbosacral spine, showing needle placement for subarachnoid and lumbar epidural analgesia
Source: Adapted from Hughes (1992) ©1992 With kind permission from Springer Science+Business Media

The drug also passes from the epidural veins to the brainstem and occipital cortex *via* the:

- basivertebral venous plexuses in the bodies of the vertebrae
- anterior internal vertebral venous plexus
- veins on the anterior surfaces of the vertebrae, which communicate with the venous sinuses draining the brain.

The presence of the drug in the brainstem causes respiratory or cardiovascular depression, nausea and itching associated with intraspinal/regional opioids (Eltzschig et al., 2003). Individual variation in venous drainage and posture may influence the amount of drug reaching the brain (Schreiber et al., 2003; Doepp et al., 2004).

Following a test dose and initial administration, ongoing epidural analgesia may be by:

- bolus injection on request
- patient controlled administration (PCA), with lockout
- a constant infusion device
- scheduled bolus injections (*Drugs and Therapy Perspectives*, 1996).

Intermittent boluses, administered by professionals or patients, are preferred to continuous infusions (NCC, 2007: 126).

The anaesthetist may administer the initial bolus injection, with subsequent bolus doses given by midwives. Although scheduled bolus injections provide more effective analgesia, they call for more careful monitoring of the level of sensory blockade (Box 4.2), and risk the administration of higher doses (Howell, 1995a).

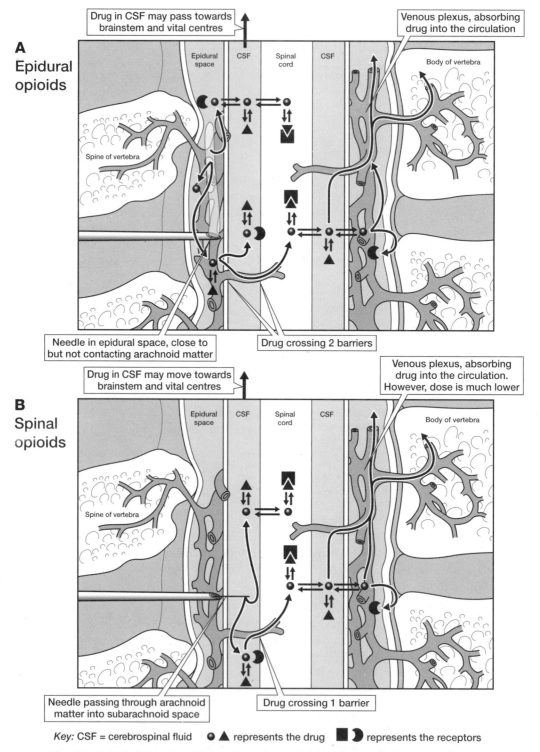

A Epidural opioids

Drug in CSF may pass towards brainstem and vital centres

Venous plexus, absorbing drug into the circulation

Epidural space | CSF | Spinal cord | CSF

Body of vertebra

Spine of vertebra

Needle in epidural space, close to but not contacting arachnoid matter

Drug crossing 2 barriers

B Spinal opioids

Drug in CSF may move towards brainstem and vital centres

Venous plexus, absorbing drug into the circulation. However, dose is much lower

Epidural space | CSF | Spinal cord | CSF

Body of vertebra

Spine of vertebra

Needle passing through arachnoid matter into subarachnoid space

Drug crossing 1 barrier

Key: CSF = cerebrospinal fluid   ● ▲ represents the drug   ■ ◗ represents the receptors

Figure 2.3 Epidural and intrathecal administration and drug circulation
Source: Eltzschig, H., Lieberman, E., Camann, P., Camann, W (2003) Regional anesthesia and analgesia for labor and delivery, *The New England Journal of Medicine*, **348**(4): 319–32
© 2003 Massachusetts Medical Society. All rights reserved

Addition of adrenaline (epinephrine)

When added to epidural analgesia, adrenaline vasoconstricts the epidural venous plexus, thereby reducing the systemic absorption of local anaesthetic and increasing duration and intensity of analgesia (Norris et al., 1994; Collis et al., 2008). It acts directly on the pain pathways to enhance analgesia and on the motor neurones to further inhibit their functions. Bupivacaine is usually administered without adrenaline (plain), but adrenaline is added to lidocaine/lignocaine if perineal analgesia is required quickly (Brownridge, 1991). The addition of adrenaline to bupivacaine may increase the placental transfer of bupivacaine, due to changes in protein binding. Therefore the addition of adrenaline reduces maternal, but not fetal, exposure to local anaesthetic (Reynolds, 1993a).

The side effects and interactions of adrenaline militate against its use:

- Adrenaline is a vasoconstrictor and reduces placental blood flow. In women where placental blood flow is already compromised, for example by chronic hypertension or pregnancy-induced hypertension, adrenaline may further jeopardize the fetal blood supply and cause fetal heart decelerations (Hollmen, 1993). However, this is a secondary consideration in the emergency management of anaphylaxis (Box 1.2).
- Adrenaline can precipitate cardiac dysrhythmias or alterations in maternal blood pressure, which can decrease placental perfusion.
- Adrenaline may prolong the first stage of labour (Dounas et al., 1996).
- Adrenaline interacts dangerously with:
  - volatile general anaesthetic gases, causing dysrhythmias
  - oxytocin, causing hypertension
  - beta blockers, causing hypertension (BNF, 2009; Box 1.2; Chapter 9).

Case report

A young primipara in normal labour received epidural analgesia containing adrenaline. When labour failed to progress, an oxytocin infusion was commenced. Over the next 2 hours, the woman became hypertensive, drowsy and comatose, and developed a hemiparesis. Following an emergency Caesarean section, the woman made a full but gradual recovery in intensive care. This involved transfer to a tertiary centre for several weeks.

If administering bupivacaine with adrenaline, professionals need to consider the interactions of both components.

Spinal/intrathecal anaesthesia

This entails injection into the subarachnoid space (Figures 2.1, 2.2). Analgesics act on the lower part of the spinal cord and the nerve roots (Shennan et al., 1995). Typically, a very thin needle is advanced through the lumen of the epidural needle to allow the drug to be placed in the cerebrospinal fluid (CSF) (Figure 2.3). In labour, this is associated with more technical difficulties and catheter failures (Arkoosh et al., 2008).

Practice points

- The drug may circulate in the CSF and reach the vital centres in the brain stem up to 11 hours later, causing delayed respiratory depression. Thus observations should be maintained for 24 hours (Chapter 4, Implications for practice, Opioids).
- The reduced CSF volume in obese patients makes this more likely, and extra vigilance is needed (Soens et al., 2008).

From the subarachnoid space, the drug diffuses into the epidural space, where it is:

■ absorbed into the circulation
■ passed to the brain rapidly *via* the epidural veins or more slowly *via* the CSF (Eltzschig et al., 2003).

Headache, pruritus, fetal bradycardia and, in older studies, respiratory depression may occur more commonly with intrathecal than epidural analgesia (Sweetman et al., 2007; Collis et al., 2008).

Combined spinal epidural (CSE) analgesia

Low spinal anaesthesia, combined with epidural anaesthesia, is currently preferred to general anaesthesia for most Caesarean sections (DH, 1996; NCC, 2004). The combined spinal epidural technique allows lower doses and concentrations of both drugs to be administered, and reduces requests for additional pain relief, but may not confer benefit overall (Simmons et al., 2007). When an opioid, usually fentanyl, is combined with bupivacaine or ropivacaine, the dose of local anaesthetic is lower. This may permit ambulation during labour and reduce the incidence of:

■ unpleasant motor blockade
■ paresis or paralysis of the lower body
■ instrumental deliveries caused by higher doses of epidural local anaesthetics (NCC, 2007).

CSE analgesia does not circumvent all the problems associated with traditional epidural analgesia:

■ incidence of hypotension and headaches is not improved by the addition of opioids (Simmons et al., 2007)
■ Caesarean section rates are not improved (Traynor et al., 2000; NCC, 2007)
■ the common adverse effects of opioids, such as nausea, vomiting and itching, may still be troublesome
■ the potential for local problems, such as meningism, is increased.

Careful monitoring is still required to avoid hypotensive episodes, which are potentially damaging to the fetus (Shennan et al., 1995), and neonatal resuscitation may be required more frequently (Comet Group, 2001). Meta-analysis indicates that CSE increases acidity in the umbilical artery when compared to low-dose epidurals, but differences are not considered clinically important (Simmons et al., 2007).

Administration of intraspinal/regional analgesia

The technical complexities of administration and the need for specialist skills and support counterbalance the advantages of regional analgesia (Reynolds, 1993b). 'Test doses' are mandatory. Epidurals are more likely to fail if:

■ the first dose fails
■ presentation is posterior
■ pain occurs during placement
■ the epidural is given for less than 1 hour or more than 6 hours (Le Coq et al., 1998)
■ the woman is obese (Soens et al., 2008).

Problems associated with the insertion of regional analgesia include:

■ failure to flex the spine
■ twisting the spine, for example due to sitting on a sloping bed
■ need for reinsertion (4.7%) (Paech et al., 1998)
■ estimating distance from skin to epidural space, which ranges between 2.5 and 10 cm (usually 4–6 cm). This increases with obesity in the lower back and decreases in the sitting position

■ locating the midline in obese women. This is easier in a sitting position. Ask the woman to point to the midline.

Practice point

■ Women may need help to remain still during insertion, for example by ensuring that feet do not slip, and beds are flat (Collis et al., 2008).

Problems after insertion include:

■ kinking of lines
■ blockage of catheters
■ accidental removal of lines
■ infection
■ systemic absorption
■ movement of catheters with change of position (Soens et al., 2008).

Complications of intraspinal or regional drug administration

Intravascular injection

The prominent venous plexus in the epidural space makes inadvertent intravascular injection a potential hazard of epidural analgesia, occurring in 0.02–0.04% of women (NCC, 2004). An accident of this type may cause cardiac toxicity and profound hypotension (Chapter 4).

Headache

Headache may occur on insertion, due to air entry into the CSF. Later onset headache may be due to dural puncture, not recognized at insertion.

Unintentional dural puncture

Unintentional dural puncture occurs in some 0.19–3.6% of women in UK units (Baraz and Collis, 2005), rising to 11% if complex regimens or larger needles are used (NCC, 2004). Normally the brain is cushioned on a bed of CSF. As the dura is punctured by the epidural needle or catheter, CSF may leak, reducing intracranial pressure. If CSF is lost:

■ the brain will pull on pain-sensitive trabeculae, causing headache, particularly in the upright position
■ blood vessels overfill to compensate for the loss of volume of CSF. Vasodilation stimulates pain receptors, causing headache
■ regeneration of CSF normally takes 5–10 days
■ serious (extremely rare) complications include herniation of the brain through the foramen magnum.

Seventy per cent of women experience severe headache, which worsens on standing (Eltzschig et al., 2003); this may be accompanied by tinnitus, photophobia, nausea, or neck stiffness (Sweetman et al., 2007).

Practice points

■ Epidural needles and catheters are not inserted or advanced if women are moving or during contractions, because dural puncture at this time would cause ejection of CSF at high pressure

(Clyburn et al., 2008b). Pressure in the CSF rises during pregnancy, and may reach very high levels during contractions.

■ If dural puncture has occurred, CSF may appear in the needle. CSF is a clear fluid, which may be distinguished from saline by the presence of glucose (identified by a glucose reagent strip) (Collis et al., 2008).

Following dural puncture:

■ women are usually encouraged to increase fluid intake, including caffeinated beverages, to restore CSF volume. Caffeine is a vasoconstrictor. The dose required is equivalent to 3–5 cups of strong coffee, enough to induce cardiac dysrhythmias or seizures in susceptible people (Chapter 19, Implications for practice: epilepsy in pregnancy)
■ headache should be monitored (it may become chronic)
■ regular paracetamol should be offered; if this fails, more powerful analgesia may be offered
■ to manage pain, doctors may request sumatriptan, strong opioids, or ACTH
■ on discharge, women should be advised to: contact the services if headache or backache return, or weakness, numbness or fever develop; avoid straining, heavy lifting or straining at stool; intake plenty of liquids
■ women may be advised to take laxatives to avoid straining at stool
■ most units advise early mobilization (Baraz and Collis, 2005).

Dural puncture may be managed by insertion of an intrathecal catheter to allow immediate analgesia for labour, reduce the incidence and severity of headache, and avoid a second dural puncture (Baraz and Collis, 2005).

Severe post-dural puncture headache for 24 hours, which is hindering mobilization, may require an epidural 'blood patch' (Wildsmith, 1996; Pang and O'Sullivan, 2008). This is the epidural injection of 15–20 ml of the patient's own blood. It alleviates pain in some 70% of women. If a blood patch is performed to treat a headache, the epidural needle must be reintroduced; this prospect may deter some women from accepting the treatment. A blood patch may be complicated by a second dural puncture and backache. Prophylactic blood patch is the administration of 15 ml blood after birth but before removal of the epidural needle. This has been shown to reduce, but not eliminate, the need for a second procedure (Howell, 1995b).

Dural puncture headache is unlikely to be responsible for neurological problems or speech difficulty, and such clinical signs and symptoms are indications to summon immediate medical assistance (CEMACH, 2005).

Backache

Tenderness at the puncture site is anticipated for 5–7 days (Pang and O'Sullivan, 2008). The puncture site may take a few weeks to heal. Prolapsed intervertebral disc, subdural abscess, epidural abscess, and epidural haematoma have been reported in association with epidural analgesia; the first symptom of these serious conditions is backache (Forster et al., 1996; Evans and Misra, 2003; Collis and Harries, 2005; Ruppen et al., 2006). Recognizing these serious conditions is difficult and requires urgent specialist input.

Practice point

■ Indications of serious problems include deep-seated back pain, bladder or bowel dysfunction, or fever (Harries et al., 2008).

The relationship between new long-term backache and epidural analgesia during labour remains controversial, but effects beyond 7 days are not substantiated by current studies (Anim-Somuah et al.,

2005; NCC, 2007). Whereas retrospective studies have indicated that this association exists (MacArthur et al, 1990; Russell et al, 1993), a randomized controlled trial (RCT) involving 306 women (Howell et al., 2001), with follow-up (Howell et al., 2002), and an RCT with a high crossover rate (n = 1292) (Orlikowski et al., 2006) found no association between new onset, long-term backache and either the use of epidural analgesia or the dose of bupivacaine administered. Previous backache was significantly associated with new onset, long-term backache (Russell et al., 1993; Butler and Fuller, 1998).

Practice point

■ Attention to posture before, during and after labour may reduce long-term backache (Reynolds, 1993b).

Epidural haematoma

An epidural haematoma may form if insertion of the intraspinal needle causes bleeding and bruising. This can compress vital structures, for example in the spinal cord. The incidence is estimated to be around 5/million insertions (Ruppen et al., 2006).

Practice point

■ To reduce the risk of epidural haematoma, the woman should be examined for signs of bleeding (Chapter 8), and coagulation and platelet count should be checked before the procedure if:
  ■ HELLP syndrome is even a remote possibility (Yerby, 2000)
  ■ anticoagulants have been administered (Chapter 8)
  ■ low molecular weight heparin has been administered within the last 24 hours
  ■ other haematological disorders are present.

Spinal analgesia is hazardous if the woman has disseminated intravascular coagulation (Richardson, 2000).

The presence of blood in the CSF or epidural space, whether due to haematoma, bleeding or a blood patch, could cause an inflammatory reaction, and in very rare instances involve the meninges, leading to back pain and neurological problems (Rice et al., 2004).

Abscess formation

Abscess formation in association with regional analgesia or blood patches is very rare (20–37 per million epidurals). A typical presentation may be back or leg pain, with or without fever, arising 4–16 days after birth. Cases have occurred where needle insertion was difficult, oral corticosteroids were prescribed, and/or the epidermal barrier was disrupted by flaking skin, itching and scratching (Collis and Harries, 2005; Cummings and Dolak, 2006). It is suggested that, in view of the risk of contaminated bed linen, transmission of skin microorganisms may be reduced by 'double spraying', that is, spraying the skin with antiseptic, wiping, respraying, and allowing to dry (Cummings and Dolak, 2006). Although difficult, prompt recognition of abscess formation allows antibiotic therapy to be administered and prevent permanent impairment of mobility, bowel and bladder function (Evans and Misra, 2003).

Accidental total spinal anaesthesia

Accidental total spinal anaesthesia can occur if the dura is accidentally punctured and an epidural dose is administered intrathecally. Since the epidural dose is at least 10 times greater than the spinal (intrathecal) dose, the local anaesthetic may inhibit the vital centres, causing loss of consciousness, respirations and blood pressure (Pang and O'Sullivan, 2008). Therefore, initial doses of local anaesthetics are regarded as test doses (NCC, 2007).

Neurological deficit

It is estimated that serious persistent neurological complications arise in around 4/million women receiving epidural analgesia in childbirth (Ruppen et al., 2006). Neurological deficit may arise from either accidental damage to nerve roots or spinal cord during injection or chronic inflammatory reactions to impurities injected (Rice et al., 2004). There have been rare cases of incomplete recovery from the blockade of sensory, motor and sympathetic neurones. If the woman reports a 'shooting pain' down the nerve, into the leg, it is likely that the needle has contacted a nerve root. Contact between needle and spinal cord causes intense pain and sometimes paralysis (Figure 2.2) (Collis et al., 2008). Septic and aseptic meningitis, and reversible bilateral hearing loss have been reported (Sweetman et al., 2007). *Herpes* infection of the skin may be associated with viral meningitis (Harries et al., 2008).

Case report

This case illustrates the rare complication of septic meningitis.

A healthy 22-year-old primigravida received epidural analgesia with fentanyl. Following uncomplicated delivery, she was discharged 24 hours postpartum with a healthy infant. She returned 48 hours later, vomiting and febrile but alert and complaining of headache. She rapidly deteriorated and developed neck rigidity. Despite treatment, she died 4 weeks later.

Puncture of the skin and dura may allow entry of microorganisms into the cerebrospinal fluid, and, in very rare cases, can bring about infection (Choy, 2000).

Practice points

- Vomiting, headache and fever alert practitioners to possible serious complications.
- New long-term headache requires urgent attention (Reynolds, 1993b).
- To minimize the potential for error, all intraspinal drugs must be:
  - double-checked
  - freshly prepared
  - administered slowly
  - sterile.
- Sprays used on the skin should not contaminate instruments. Chlorhexidine or alcohol could cause chemical meningitis (Collis et al., 2008).

Some intraspinal drug regimens are complex, and involve more detailed calculations than are normally performed in hospital practice. The possibility of error should be reduced if all intraspinal infusions are:

- prepared in the pharmacy under sterile conditions
- standardized
- prescribed on charts reserved for spinal infusions
- accompanied by charts detailing the clinical monitoring required (Cousins, 1996).

Problems may be minimized by regular monitoring, including:

- maintaining maternal non-supine position

- BP, heart rate every 5 minutes for first 30 minutes, every 15 minutes until at least 2 hours postpartum and hourly for 16 hours if opioids are administered
- maternal respirations
- the height of sensory block
- the height of motor block until complete recovery
- continuous fetal heart monitoring
- pulse oximetry.

Protocols vary between institutions (Arkoosh, 1991; Brownridge, 1991; Norris et al., 1994; Stienstra et al., 1995; *Drugs and Therapy Perspectives*, 1996; DH, 1996; Hall, 1996) (Chapter 4).

Box 2.1 Intraspinal/regional analgesia: cautions and contraindications

- History of hypersensitivity responses to drugs administered
- Bacteraemia or septicaemia (causes hypotension)
- Infection or inflammation at insertion site, for example meningitis, lumbar TB, spinal metastases
- Raised intracranial pressure
- Coagulation disorders, including:
  - current use of anticoagulants (see Epidural haematoma; Chapter 8)
  - pre-eclampsia with bleeding abnormalities
- Haemorrhage or anticipated haemorrhage, for example bleeding disorders, low platelet count, severe renal disease
- Hypovolaemia (low circulating volume)
- Neurological disorders
- Previous spinal surgery
- Some serious heart conditions (hypotension may be a problem)
- No intravenous access (Collis et al., 2008)

   Administration of regional analgesia requires skilled and experienced personnel. When life-threatening incidents have occurred, they have usually been associated with lapses in standards of administration and management (Brownridge, 1991; DH, 1996, 1998).

Conclusion

While usually uneventful, administration of medicines remains a high-risk activity and a focus for clinical supervision, with potential for clinically important errors. To minimize the risk of harm, collaborations between higher education institutions and clinical areas have become mandatory (NMC, 2009).

Further reading

- Berman, A., Snyder, S., Kozier, B. and Erb, G. (2008) *Kozier and Erb's Fundamentals of Nursing*, 8th edn. Pearson, Upper Saddle River, NJ.
- Hayes, D., Hendler, CB., Tscheschlog, B. et al. (eds) (2003) *Medication Administration Made Incredibly Easy*. Lippincott, Williams & Wilkins, Springhouse, PA.
- Smith, S., Duell D. and Martin, B. (2008) *Clinical Nursing Skills: Basic to Advanced Skills*, 7th edn. Pearson/Prentice Hall, Englewood Cliffs, NJ; selected chapters.

CHAPTER 3

Law, Medicines and the Midwife

Richard Griffith

This chapter describes the statutory framework for the control of medicines and discusses the implications for midwives.

Chapter contents

Introduction

Medicines are used for their therapeutic benefits but they also have great potential to harm those who take them. Drugs such as thalidomide (*J* v. *Distillers Co (Biochemicals)* (1969) 8 CL 99) and Opren (*Nash* v. *Eli Lilly & Co* [1993] 1 WLR 782) demonstrate the tragic consequences that may follow medication administration. Therefore the law regulates the arrangements for the supply of medicines to patients. The Medicines Act 1968, s. 58A requires that medicines that represent a danger to the patient be classified as prescription only and their administration be supervised by an appropriate practitioner. Midwives who meet such conditions as specified in law can become appropriate practitioners (Medicines Act 1968, s. 58(1)). However, unlike doctors who can prescribe from one national formulary, non-medical prescribers can have up to seven different roles when prescribing or administering medicines to patients, each with its own requirements and limitations. In order to practise safely and avoid legal and professional liability, midwives must ensure that each time they prescribe or administer medicines to a patient, they have the proper authority to do so. For example, a practice nurse was cautioned by the Nursing and

Midwifery Council's conduct and competence committee when she prescribed drugs to patients when she did not have the authority to do so. The committee stressed that while the role of non-medical prescribers was expanding, public protection demanded they could only prescribe and administer medicines where they had the legal authority to do so (NMC, 2003).

Accountability

As registered practitioners, midwives are accountable or answerable for their actions to four main legal sources. A range of sanctions may be applied for failing to adequately meet the required standard in each case.

The profession

A midwife who is found guilty of professional misconduct is liable to removal from the professional register. The Nursing and Midwifery Council (NMC) has the authority to hold midwives to account through the Nursing and Midwifery Order 2001. The professional standard required of a midwife by the governing body is given in the NMC's (2008a) *Code, Standards of Conduct, Performance and Ethics for Nurses and Midwives* and is further elaborated by the *Midwives Rules and Standards* (NMC, 2004). Some 214 nurses and midwives were issued with striking off orders for professional misconduct in 2007/8. Of the allegations investigated by the NMC, some 14% concerned direct contact with patients and 9.87% with maladministration of medication (NMC, 2008b).

The employer

Midwives have legal binding contracts of employment with their employers, which require, among other duties, that they obey the reasonable requests of the employer and work with due care and skill. The contract further requires that midwives are duty bound to account for their actions and to disclose any misdeeds. An employer may therefore hold an employee to account through reasonable disciplinary policies and procedures that ultimately may lead to dismissal.

As a result of the control employers exercise over their employees, the law holds them vicariously liable for any **tort** committed by an employee during the course of their employment, which has the effect of indemnifying the employee against damages for harm caused to another in the course of their employment. Independent midwives are self-employed and do not have this protection.

The client

A mother or child who feels they have been harmed by the carelessness of a midwife can seek redress though the civil court system. This remains a lengthy and costly process and is still a relatively rare occurrence, although the NHS annual compensation bill runs at some £500m. The great majority of clients will usually complain to the midwife's employer or the NMC rather than go to law. However, when a case is successfully brought, the award of damages can run into millions of pounds. In *T (A Minor)* v. *Luton & Dunstable Hospital NHS Trust* (Unreported, 23 November 1998), T suffered cerebral palsy as a result of a prolonged delivery, during which placental abruption and type II (late) heart decelerations went unnoticed. The NHS trust accepted that it was vicariously liable and agreed damages amounting to some £1,736,347.

Society

We are all accountable to society through the criminal law. A midwife who breaks the law is as liable to prosecution as any other person. The statutes concerned with the regulation of medicines, such as the Medicines Act 1968 and the Misuse of Drugs Act 1971, carry criminal penalties if breached. It is therefore vital that midwives are within the law when working with medicines.

Summary

The four spheres of accountability regulating the practice of the midwife are not mutually exclusive. It is entirely possible that a midwife might be removed from the professional register, dismissed from her post, sued by a patient and receive a fine, community penalty or imprisonment. It is essential therefore that the midwife understands that the notion of accountability is always considered as a whole through all four spheres. This will ensure safe and effective practice that will benefit the patient and avoid being called to justify one's actions.

The legal regulation of medicines

Medicines Act 1968

The principle statute regulating the use of medicines is the Medicines Act 1968. This provides an administrative and licensing system to control the sale and supply of medicines to the public. Before a drug can be marketed for sale to the public, it must have a 'marketing authorization' issued by the secretary of state for health. A marketing authorization cannot be issued unless the Commission on Human Medicines (CHM), under the auspices of the Medicines and Healthcare products Regulatory Agency (MHRA), has been consulted (s. 2, Medicines Act 1968). The MHRA is charged by the 1968 Act with looking at matters such as the quality of the drug and its usefulness for the purpose for which it is marketed. It is further charged with the promotion of the collection of data on adverse reactions to drugs (s. 4, Medicines Act 1968).

Drugs that have a marketing authorization are categorized into three types for the purpose of supply to the general public.

General sales list drugs

General sales list drugs may be sold through a variety of outlets without the need for a registered pharmacist; they are commonly known as over the counter (OTC) drugs. Examples include paracetamol and aspirin.

Pharmacy only

Pharmacy only medicine can only be purchased under the supervision of a registered pharmacist in a retail pharmacy. Examples include ranitidine, cimetidine and piriton.

Prescription only

Prescription only medicines can only be obtained from a registered pharmacist by prescription from a registered doctor, dentist or eligible non-medical prescriber. They cannot normally be supplied unless a prescription has been issued from an appropriate practitioner. The criteria for determining which products should be available on prescription only are regulated by European Directive 92/26/EEC. These medicines are listed in article 3 of the Prescription Only Medicines (Human Use) Order 1997. Under the Medicines (Products Other Than Veterinary Drugs) (Prescription Only) Order 1983, in exceptional circumstances, pharmacists may supply 5 days' emergency treatment of a prescription only medicine.

Appropriate practitioners

The Medicines Act 1968, s. 58(1) bestows prescribing authority to registered medical practitioners, dentists and vets who are able to issue prescriptions from their relevant formularies. The Medicinal Products: Prescribing by Nurses etc. Act 1992 and the Health and Social Care Act 2001, s. 63 extended the range of appropriate practitioners. The Medicines for Human Use (Prescribing) (Miscellaneous Amendments) Order 2006 introduced three categories of non-medical prescriber:

- independent prescriber
- independent/supplementary prescriber
- community practitioner prescriber.

Under the 2006 regulations, registered midwives, whose names in each case are held on the NMC professional register, with an annotation signifying that they have successfully completed an approved programme of preparation and training, can become an independent and/or supplementary prescriber.

Definitions

Administration

Administration is not generally defined but accepted as involving the drug being given by a practitioner or a practitioner supervising the patient taking the dose. The Prescription Only Medicines (Human Use) Order 1997 defines parenteral administration as administration by breach of the skin or mucous membrane.

Supply

Section 131 of the Medicine Act 1968 defines supply as supplying a drug in circumstances corresponding to retail sale. However, if a midwife were providing any prescription only medicine for patients to take away and administer themselves, that would amount to supply. For example, a midwife supplying a medicine under a patient group direction must issue the medicine in a prepacked form suitable for the patient to take away. The midwife cannot issue a note for a pharmacist to supply the medicine.

Prescription

Prescription means a prescription issued by an appropriate practitioner under or by virtue of the NHS Act 1977, that is, written on the proscribed form and signed and dated by the practitioner, for example FP10.

The form of a prescription

Article 15 of the Prescription Only Medicines (Human Use) Order 1997 requires that a prescription must be completed and signed in ink, or be otherwise indelible, on the statutory form and must contain the following information:

- the name and address of the patient
- the drug described clearly
- the signature of the prescriber
- the date of signing.
- the address of the appropriate practitioner
- the status of the appropriate practitioner, for example midwife independent prescriber.

Administration of prescription only medicine

A drug categorized as a prescription only medicine can normally only be administered by or under the direction of an appropriate practitioner. Section 58(2)(b) of the Medicines Act 1968 states that:

> No person shall administer otherwise than to himself any such medicinal product unless he is an appropriate practitioner or a person acting in accordance with the directions of an appropriate practitioner.

However, article 9 of the Prescription Only Medicines (Human Use) Order 1997 limits the restriction on the administration of prescription only medicines to those that are for parenteral administration:

> The restriction imposed by s 58(2) (b) shall not apply to the administration to human beings of a prescription only medicine which is not for parenteral administration.

Midwife as appropriate practitioner

The National Health Service (Miscellaneous Amendments Relating to Independent Prescribing) Regulations 2006 introduced independent prescribing and extended the range of medicines that can be prescribed. It allows midwives with this status to prescribe any licensed medicine, including issuing private prescriptions, for any medical condition that an independent prescriber is competent to treat and this includes some controlled drugs. As appropriate practitioners for the purposes of the Medicines Act 1968, s. 58(2), midwives who are independent prescribers can also give directions for the administration of any product they are legally allowed to prescribe as long as they are satisfied that the person to whom they give the instructions is competent to administer the medicine.

All registered midwives can train to be independent prescribers. However, the NMC (2006) *Standards of Proficiency for Nurse and Midwife Prescribers* state that practitioners must have at least 3 years' post-registration experience before undertaking the course. Midwives who successfully complete the programme must register their prescribing qualification with the NMC before they can start prescribing.

Controlled drugs

Non-medical independent prescribers can only prescribe a limited range of controlled drugs for specified medical conditions that generally fall outside the scope of midwifery practice:

- diamorphine, morphine, diazepam, lorazepam, midazolam, or oxycodone for use in palliative care
- buprenorphine or fentanyl for transdermal use in palliative care
- diazepam, lorazepam, midazolam for the treatment of tonic-clonic seizures
- diamorphine or morphine for pain relief in respect of suspected myocardial infarction, or for relief of acute or severe pain after trauma, including in either case postoperative pain relief
- chlordiazepoxide hydrochloride or diazepam for treatment of initial or acute withdrawal symptoms, caused by the withdrawal of alcohol from persons habituated to it
- codeine phosphate, dihydrocodeine tartrate or co-phenotrope.

Prescribing borderline substances, off-label medicines or unlicensed medicines

Borderline substances are mainly foodstuffs, such as enteral feeds and foods that are specially formulated for people with medical conditions. They also include some toiletries, such as sun blocks. Independent prescribers are able to prescribe these products but should limit their prescriptions to the substances on the approved list of the Advisory Committee on Borderline Substances, which is published as Part XV of the *Drug Tariff* and can also be found in the BNF.

The terms 'off-label' or 'off-licence' medicines describe the use of licensed medicines in a dose, age group, or by a route not in the product specification. Midwives who are independent prescribers can prescribe off label but in doing so take full responsibility for their prescribing. They will be accountable for harm caused to the patient by off-licence prescribing or administration. For example, the Department of Health (2003) reported an incident of off-license administration where a nurse crushed an antibiotic tablet and inserted it into an intravenous infusion because the patient had swallowing difficulties. The patient collapsed and required 4 days' therapy in intensive care.

Regardless of the midwife's prescribing authority, an off-licence prescription or administration will not give the practitioner the protection from liability for unsafe products normally given by the Consumer Protection Act 1987, which holds the producer liable for a defective product. Where a patient is harmed by a medicine prescribed or administered off licence, liability in negligence could arise for the practitioner.

Unlicensed medicines are those that do not have a product licence because, for example, there may not be enough commercial interest in marketing the medicine in the UK. This can happen if there are only a small number of patients who would use the medicine. Such medicines are often available from specialist manufacturers or made up by pharmacists as patient-specific formulations, often known as 'specials'. Independent prescribers cannot prescribe unlicensed medicines.

Supplementary prescribers

Supplementary prescribing was introduced in April 2003 and is a voluntary prescribing partnership between the independent prescriber, who must be a doctor or dentist, and the supplementary prescriber, who can be a midwife, to implement an agreed patient-specific clinical management plan.

The Prescription Only Medicines (Human Use) Order 1997 requires that to be lawful, supplementary prescribing by a registered midwife must only occur where:

- the independent prescriber is a doctor (or dentist)
- the supplementary prescriber must be a registered midwife, whose name is recorded in the relevant register, with an annotation signifying that they are qualified to order drugs, medicines and appliances as a supplementary prescriber
- there must be a written clinical management plan relating to a named patient and to that patient's specific conditions
- agreement to the plan must be recorded by both the independent prescriber and the supplementary prescriber before it begins
- the independent prescriber and the supplementary prescriber must share access to, consult and use the same common patient record.

Following diagnosis by the doctor and agreement of the clinical management plan, the supplementary prescriber may prescribe any medicine for the patient that is referred to in the plan until the next review by the independent prescriber. There is no formulary for supplementary prescribing and no restrictions on the medical conditions that can be managed under these arrangements. The scope of supplementary prescribing is very broad and any prescription only medicine, pharmacy medicine, general sales list medicine or controlled drug, whether licensed or unlicensed, can be issued as long as it is part of the agreed clinical management plan.

The NMC (2006) argues that because of the bureaucracy of developing individual plans for each patient, supplementary prescribing has been used as a blanket authority to prescribe medication. However, the MHRA (2003), who is responsible for ensuring that the law concerning medicines is complied with, states that using the same clinical management plan for all patients with the same condition is unlawful and does not meet the legislative requirements of supplementary prescribing.

To be lawful, a clinical management plan must contain:

- the name of the patient to whom the plan relates
- the illnesses or conditions that may be treated by the supplementary prescriber
- the date on which the plan is to take effect and when it is to be reviewed by the doctor or dentist who is a party to the plan
- reference to the class or description of medicinal product that may be prescribed or administered under the plan
- any restrictions or limitations as to the strength or dose of any product that may be prescribed or administered under the plan, and any period of administration or use of any medicinal product that may be prescribed or administered under the plan

■ relevant warnings about the known sensitivities of the patient to, or known difficulties of the patient with, particular medicinal products

■ the arrangements for notification of:

    ■ suspected or known adverse reactions to any medicinal product that may be prescribed or administered under the plan

    ■ suspected or known adverse reactions to any other medicinal product taken at the same time as any medicinal product prescribed or administered under the plan

■ the circumstances in which the supplementary prescriber should refer to, or seek the advice of, the doctor or dentist who is a party to the plan (Prescription Only Medicines (Human Use) Order 1997).

A supplementary prescriber who issues a prescription in contravention of the regulations could face prosecution under the regulations and a misconduct charge from the NMC, as well as disciplinary proceedings from their employer.

The training for supplementary prescribing is incorporated into non-medical independent prescribing courses (NMC, 2006).

Alternatives to prescriptions for the supply and administration of medicines

As well as granting prescribing authority, the Medicines Act 1968 and its regulations allow for the supply and administration of prescription only medicines by midwives without a prescription through the use of patient group directions, patient-specific directions and specific exemptions under the Prescription Only Medicines (Human Use) Order 1997.

Patient group directions

A patient group direction is a written instruction for the supply or administration of a licensed medicine in an identified clinical situation where the patient may not be individually identified before presenting for treatment. Since 2003, independent hospital agencies and clinics registered under the Care Standards Act 2000, prison healthcare services, police services and defence medical services have also been able to use patient group directions.

A patient group direction is drawn up locally by doctors, pharmacists and other health professionals and must meet the legal criteria set out in Box 3.1.

Box 3.1 Legal requirements for a valid patient group direction

The legal requirements for a valid patient group direction include:

- The name of the body to which the direction applies
- The date the direction comes into force and the date it expires
- A description of the medicine(s) to which the direction applies
- The clinical conditions covered by the direction
- A description of those patients excluded from treatment under the direction
- A description of the circumstances under which further advice should be sought from a doctor (or dentist, as appropriate) and arrangements for referral made
- Appropriate dosage and maximum total dosage, quantity, pharmaceutical form and strength, route and frequency of administration, and minimum or maximum period over which the medicine should be administered
- Relevant warnings, including potential adverse reactions
- Details of any follow-up action and the circumstances
- A statement of the records to be kept for audit purposes
- Names and signatures of registered practitioners entitled to supply and/or administer medicines under the patient group direction

Source: Prescription Only Medicines (Human Use) Amendment Order 2000

Each patient group direction must be signed by a doctor and a pharmacist, and approved by the organization in which it is to be used, typically a primary care or NHS trust.

Patient group directions can only be used by registered healthcare professionals, including midwives, acting as named individuals, and a list of individuals named as competent to supply and administer medicines under the direction must be included.

A patient group direction can include a flexible dose range for the midwife to select the appropriate dose for the patient. Medicines can also be used off licence, provided such use is supported by best clinical practice and the patient group direction contains a statement detailing why this is necessary.

The Misuse of Drugs Regulations 2001 were amended in 2003 to allow some controlled drugs to be supplied and/or administered under a patient group direction. These include:

■ diamorphine, but only for the treatment of cardiac pain by nurses working in coronary care units and A&E departments of hospitals
■ all drugs listed in Schedule 4 of the 2001 Regulations (mostly benzodiazepines), except anabolic steroids
■ all drugs listed in Schedule 5 of the 2001 Regulations, that is, low strength opiates such as codeine.

The National Prescribing Centre (NPC, 2004) suggests that the supply and administration of medicines under patient group directions should be reserved for the limited number of situations where this offers an advantage for patient care without compromising patient safety. It further suggests that particular caution should be used when deciding whether to use a patient group direction for an antibiotic, as antimicrobial resistance is a public health issue of great concern and care should be taken to ensure that any strategy to control increasing resistance will not be jeopardized. For example, a patient group direction should not allow the supply or administration of a medicine for minor viral diseases that are unaffected by antibiotics, such as treating sore throats in the absence of good evidence of bacterial infection.

In summary, a patient group direction:

■ is a direction approved by senior doctor and pharmacist
■ must be developed according to strict legal criteria
■ can only allow medicines to be supplied and administered by registered professionals who sign up to the direction
■ does not need patients to be specifically named
■ requires suitability for treatment to be assessed by a registered health professional who then supplies and administers the medicine
■ should be limited to mainstream practice
■ has limited scope for dose variation.

The registered professional acting in accordance with a patient group direction is accountable for the supply and administration of the medicine. They must hand over the medicines to the patient and cannot issue a note for collection from a pharmacy or some other person.

Patient-specific directions

A patient-specific direction is a written instruction for medicines to be supplied for administering to a named patient. Examples are an instruction on a ward drug chart, or an instruction by a GP in medical notes for a midwife to administer a medicine.

A patient-specific direction is individually tailored to the needs of a single patient and it should be used in preference to a patient group direction wherever appropriate.

Authority for patient-specific directions

The Prescription Only Medicines (Human Use) Order 1997 authorizes the use of patient-specific directions and article 12 allows any appropriate practitioner (including midwives with independent prescribing authority) to write a written instruction for the supply and administration of a prescription only medicine in a hospital.

Article 12A of the 1997 Order gives an exemption for the supply and administration of prescription only medicines by a national health service body where the medicine is supplied for the purpose of being administered to a particular person in accordance with the written directions of a doctor, even though the direction does not satisfy the conditions for a valid prescription.

A patient-specific direction differs from a prescription. To be lawful, a prescription must meet the requirements of article 15 of the 1997 Order. A patient-specific direction is lawful even if it does not meet these requirements and a midwife is entitled to administer medicines in accordance with a patient-specific direction.

In summary, a patient-specific direction:

- is a written instruction by a doctor (or other appropriate practitioner in a hospital)
- does not have to comply with prescription requirements
- must be patient specific
- can be administered by any capable person who may not be a registered health professional
- indicates that the doctor is responsible for assessing the patient
- must be accompanied by a list of named patients.

Liability for harm rests with the doctor who will be judged on the appropriateness of the patient-specific direction and the appropriateness of delegation.

Specific exemption for the supply or administration of medicines under the Medicines Act 1968

The Medicines Act, s. 58(2)(b) requires that the administration of a prescription only medicine be done by or under the direction of an appropriate practitioner. This normally requires a prescription. However, midwives have an exemption from the Medicines Act s. 58(2)(b) to supply or administer medicines when attending a woman in labour.

Relevant Aspects of the Prescription Only Medicines (Human Use) Order 1997 – SCHEDULE 5
Article 11(1)(a)

EXEMPTION FOR CERTAIN PERSONS FROM SECTION 58(2) OF THE ACT

PART I EXEMPTION FROM RESTRICTIONS ON SALE OR SUPPLY

Persons exempted	Prescription only medicines to which the exemption applies	Conditions
Registered midwives	Prescription only medicines containing any of the following substances: Chloral hydrate Ergometrine maleate Pentazocine hydrochloride [Phytomenadione] Triclofos sodium	The sale or supply shall be only in the course of their professional practice and in the case of ergometrine maleate only when contained in a medicinal product which is not for parenteral administration

Note: these are not usually the first choice medicines, and some, such as oral ergometrine, are no longer in the BNF (2008). The medicine in square brackets was added by the Prescription Only Medicines (Human Use) Amendment (No 3) Order 1998.

Article 11(2)

PART III EXEMPTIONS FROM RESTRICTION ON ADMINISTRATION

Persons exempted	Prescription only medicines to which the exemption applies	Conditions
Registered midwives	Prescription only medicines for parenteral administration containing any of the following substances but no other substance specified in column 1 of Schedule 1 to this Order: [Diamorphine] Ergometrine maleate Lignocaine Lignocaine hydrochloride [Morphine] Naloxone hydrochloride Oxytocins, natural and synthetic Pentazocine lactate Pethidine hydrochloride Phytomenadione Promazine hydrochloride	The administration shall be only in the course of their professional practice and in the case of promazine hydrochloride, lignocaine and lignocaine hydrochloride shall be only while attending on a woman in childbirth

Note: the medicines in square brackets were added by the Prescription Only Medicines (Human Use) Amendment Order 2004.

Exemption for the administration of a prescription only medicine in an emergency

In addition to the specific exemptions for midwives in schedule 5 of the 1997 Order, a general exemption on restriction from parenteral administration is allowed for the following medicinal products for the purpose of saving life in an emergency, and there is no specific restriction on who is entitled to administer these medicines:

- Adrenaline injection 1 in 1000 (1 mg in 1 ml)
- [Atropine sulphate and obidoxime chloride injection]
- [Atropine sulphate and pralidoxime chloride injection]
- Atropine sulphate injection
- [Atropine sulphate, pralidoxime mesilate and avizafone injection]
- [Chlorphenamine injection]
- [Dicobalt Edetate injection]
- Glucagon injection
- [Glucose injection 50%]
- Hydrocortisone injection
- [Naloxone hydrochloride]
- [Pralidoxime chloride injection]
- [Pralidoxime mesilate injection]
- Promethazine hydrochloride injection
- Snake venom antiserum
- Sodium nitrite injection
- Sodium thiosulphate injection
- Sterile pralidoxime.

Note: the medicines in square brackets were added later by the Prescription Only Medicines (Human Use) Amendment (No 3) Order 2004. It should be noted that pralidoxime mesilate and avizafone injection are not in the BNF.

Similar arrangements exist for the supply of prescription only medicines in an emergency.

Misuse of Drugs Act 1971

Controlled drugs are prescription only medicines that are further regulated by the Misuse of Drugs Act 1971. In health contexts, the Misuse of Drugs Regulations 2001 categorize controlled drugs into five numbered schedules:

1 No health purpose (for example lysergic acid)
2 Opiates (for example pethidine and diamorphine) and major stimulants (cocaine and amphetamines)
3 Barbiturates and minor stimulants; for example temazepam, which is one of the most widely abused prescription drugs in the UK, is categorized for criminal purposes under the Misuse of Drugs Regulation 2001 as a class C drug (class A if prepared for injection), and it is an offence to possess or supply it without a prescription. Unlike the other benzodiazpines, it is therefore a schedule 3 drug for health purposes and subject to controlled drug prescribing and recording requirements
4 Benzodiazapine tranquillizers and anabolic steroids
5 Preparations with minimal risk of abuse.

Drugs from schedules 2 and 3 can only be dispensed on prescription. A valid prescription must be written indelibly, be dated and signed by the prescriber. The dose and name and address of patient must be stated. For schedules 1–3, the dose of the drug must be in words and figures.

Special record keeping requirements apply for controlled drugs. Drugs in schedules 1 and 2 of the 1985 regulations must have a record, kept in a bound register, of each time the drug is obtained or supplied. Midwives may possess and use specified controlled drugs under a midwives' supply order signed by a doctor or supervisor of midwives. The order must state the name and occupation of the midwife, why the drug is required and the total quantity to be obtained. Currently, the Prescription Only Medicines (Human Use) Order 1997 allows a midwife to possess and administer diamorphine, morphine, pentazocine and pethidine hydrochloride under these arrangements. For schedule 2 controlled drugs, the midwife must record supplies received and administered in a book solely used for that purpose. A midwife is not entitled to destroy surplus supplies of controlled drugs but is able to surrender them to a medical officer identified in an agreed local policy.

Professional requirements

Although the general legal requirements for the supply and administration of prescription only medicines have exemptions for registered midwives, a midwife must have regard to her professional accountability and obligations when supplying or administering medicines.

Midwives rules and code of practice

The Nursing and Midwifery Council (2004), through the *Midwives Rules and Standards*, regulates a midwife's professional practice with regard to the supply and administration of medicines. While the rules acknowledge that midwives may be supplied with certain medicines listed in schedule 5 of the Prescription Only Medicines (Human Use) Order 1997, the regulatory body stresses that the actual drugs used by the midwife in practice are agreed in a local policy in collaboration with a senior midwife, medical and pharmacy staff.

Midwives are also required to limit the administration of medicines and dosages to those they have been trained to use and administer. Furthermore, a midwife shall administer medication by means of apparatus only if it meets the requirements for use by a midwife (NMC, 2004).

Requirements relating to controlled drugs

When administering a controlled drug in the NHS, a midwife is required to comply with locally agreed health authority policies and procedures. The NMC (2004) acknowledges that this might include a standing order signed by a consultant and senior midwife authorizing the administration of controlled drugs and medicines for the midwife's use in her practice in an institution.

A prescription for controlled drugs that has been issued directly to the expectant mother is regarded in law as her property. As such, the midwife cannot lawfully possess such drugs and cannot return unused drugs to the pharmacist. It is the responsibility of the mother to destroy unused controlled drugs, and the midwife should encourage the mother to do this in her presence. A record must be kept of any advice the midwife gives, any action taken and the quantities of controlled drugs (NMC, 2004).

Civil liability

Negligence

It can be seen that considerable flexibility is afforded midwives in the supply and administration of medicines during the course of their practice. The standard required of the midwife is that of the 'ordinary [person] professing to have and exercise that particular skill or art' (J McNair in *Bolam* v *Friern HMC* [1957] 1 WLR 582). In *Whitehouse* v. *Jordan* [1981] 1 All ER 267 (HL), the House of Lords confirmed that this standard applied to errors in the course of treatment, including childbirth and surgery. In **common law**, there are several cases where a health professional has been found liable in negligence for falling below the required standard.

Parenteral administration of medicines usually involves the use of an injection. The breaking of a needle during an injection is a matter that would require an explanation but has not, to date, given rise to liability in negligence, but failure to deal with the aftermath of a broken needle has done so. In *Gerber* v. *Pines* (1939) 79 Sol Jo 13, a GP was held to be negligent for failing to inform a woman that a piece of needle remained in her after it broke during an injection. In *Henderson* v. *Henderson* (1955) 1 BMJ 672, a surgeon was found negligent after causing scarring when he persisted in trying to remove a needle that broke during suturing. Negligence can also occur where a practitioner injects into the wrong site. In *Daly* v. *Wolverhampton Health Authority* (1986) CLY 1050, liability was conceded where an injection caused a permanent neuroma. Similarly, a midwife was found liable when she injected pethidine into the inside of the woman's leg, damaging a superficial nerve (*Walker* v. *South Surrey District Health Authority* (1982) CAT, 17 June 1982). A further cause of action in negligent injection giving might arise from giving the injection at a time when a skilful practitioner would wait.

Failure in communication in relation to drug administration has also been shown to be negligent. In *Collins* v. *Hertfordshire County Council* [1947] 1 KB 598, the mishearing of a prescription resulted in a lethal dose being administered. Allowing the administration of 4 extra injections of streptomycin above the 30 prescribed, resulting in permanent loss of balance, rendered a ward sister liable in negligence (*Smith* v. *Brighton & Lewes Hospital Management Committee* (1958) The Times, 2 May).

In *Dwyer* v. *Roderick* (1983) The Times, 12 November, a doctor was found liable in negligence when an incorrectly written prescription resulted in an overdose of the drug. Similarly, in *Prendergast* v. *Sam & Dee Ltd* (1989) The Times 14 March, both the doctor and pharmacist were found liable in negligence when an illegibly written prescription resulted in the wrong drug being supplied to the patient.

A further failure in communication that can render a midwife liable in negligence is a failure to inform a patient of the **side effects** of a drug. In *Goorkani* v. *Tayside Health Board* (1991) 3 Med LR 33, a man who had already lost the sight of one eye was given drug therapy to prevent deterioration in the other eye. His doctor did not warn him that the drug carried the risk of infertility as a side effect of long-term prescription and he became infertile. The court held that the doctor had failed in his duty of care to warn his patient of the risk of infertility arising from extended treatment. It is hoped that this book will assist the midwife here by outlining the common adverse reactions and risks associated with medicines commonly used by midwives. It is essential therefore that a midwife adheres to the standards of prescribing required by law and the profession in order to avoid liability in negligence or a charge of professional misconduct.

Congenital Disability (Civil Liability) Act 1976

As well as the common law duty of care owed towards the mother, a midwife also owes a duty to the unborn child. The 1976 Act allows a child born alive to sue a person for negligence for damage caused to it in the womb. This would include a midwife who, through carelessness, harmed the child before or during birth. On the grounds of public policy, s. 1(1) of the Congenital Disabilities (Civil Liability) Act 1976 excludes the child's mother from liability under the Act even if the child was born disabled as a result of her misuse of drugs, alcohol or tobacco. The one exception to this rule is where the mother is responsible for a traffic accident that causes harm to her unborn child while driving a motor vehicle. This exception is introduced as, although technically suing the mother, the damages to the child are paid by the vehicle's insurers. For health professionals, no such exemption exists. If there is a breach in the standard of care to the mother that causes harm to the unborn child, they are liable if the child is born alive. In *Richards* v. *Swansea NHS Trust* [2007] EWHC 487, a child suffered cerebral palsy as a result of a delayed emergency Caesarean section. The court held that the trust had failed to meet the standard set by the profession in failing to adhere to the Royal College of Obstetricians' guidance on emergency Caesareans and were liable to pay damages to the child. At the time of writing, the exact sum is undisclosed, but is likely to exceed £1m.

Conclusion

The legal regulation of medicines and the professional and contractual regulation of midwifery practice seek to protect the public from harm. Nevertheless, midwives are afforded considerable discretion and flexibility within these frameworks to exercise professional judgement when supplying and administering medicines. When informing their decision making, midwives would do well to heed the requirements of the statutory framework on medicines, professional guidance on the use of medicines, and court decisions on negligent care. In this way, midwives will ensure that their practice meets the standards required by the accountability bestowed upon them by the law, their profession, their employers and their moral obligation to the women in their care.

Further reading

■ Griffith, R.A. and Tengnah, C.A. (2008) *Law and Professional Issues in Nursing.* Learning Matters, London.
■ Mason, J.K. and Laurie, G. (2005) *Mason and McCall Smith's Law and Medical Ethics*, 7th edn. Oxford University Press, Oxford.

Orders referred to in this chapter

Medicines for Human Use (Prescribing) (Miscellaneous Amendments) Order 2006 (SI 2006/915)
Misuse of Drugs Regulations 2001 (SI 2001/3998)
Nursing & Midwifery Order 2001 (SI 2002/253)
Prescription Only Medicines (Human Use) Amendment (No 3) Order 1998 (SI 1998/2081)
Prescription Only Medicines (Human Use) Amendment (No 3) Order 2004 (SI 2004/2693)
Prescription Only Medicines (Human Use) Amendment Order 2004 (SI 2004/2)
Prescription Only Medicines (Human Use) Order 1997 (SI 1997/1830)

Part II

Drugs in Labour

Introduction

For myriad reasons, few deliveries take place without some form of pharmacological intervention. Ideally, all labours would require no more than inhalational analgesia, but, in practice, such labours are the minority, and even Entonox® is not without its hazards. Administration of analgesia would appear to be linked with use of antiemetics and possibly uterotonics/oxytocics. This core section of the book describes the drugs regularly administered to healthy women in labour. Knowledge of the potential adverse effects of the drug administered will empower the midwife to monitor for adverse reactions and to take timely remedial action.

Emboldened terms can be found in the Glossary.

CHAPTER 4

Pain Relief

Sue Jordan

This chapter describes the analgesics commonly administered to labouring women, starting with the least invasive and progressing to the most technically complicated. Opioids are considered together, as their actions are similar, regardless of route of administration. Nonsteroidal anti-inflammatory drug (NSAIDs) are frequently prescribed to provide pain relief postpartum. Clonidine, ketamine, and neostigmine are being investigated for use in childbirth.

Chapter contents

- Pathophysiology of pain
- Inhalational analgesia
- Opioids (for example pethidine/meperidine, morphine, fentanyl)
- Local anaesthetics (for example bupivacaine, lidocaine/lignocaine)
- Summary: pain relief in labour
- Pain relief in pregnancy and the puerperium: NSAIDs (for example ibuprofen and aspirin) and paracetamol

---

Many women request pain relief during labour and a wide range of pharmacological and non-pharmacological options exist. These should be carefully discussed with the woman during antenatal visits so that she is able to choose a method of pain relief appropriate to her individual needs. This decision should then be documented in the case notes. Nevertheless, it is recognized that women's requirements for pain relief are not always predictable and may change during labour, and therefore the midwife should be able to discuss with the woman the specific advantages and disadvantages of all the pharmacological options available (Dickersin, 1989; Simpkin, 1989).

Pathophysiology of pain

Authorities define pain as: 'an unpleasant sensory and emotional experience associated with actual or potential tissue damage, or described in terms of such damage' (IASP, 1986: S217). The experience of pain is individual and contextualized; there is not always a clear relationship between tissue damage and pain experience. Pain scores offer a useful communication tool to assist in assessing the need for analgesia (Fairlie et al., 1999; Collis et al., 2008).

Practice point

■ Analgesia should be monitored using a 'pain scale', such as a visual analogue scale or a verbal rating scale.

The individual's learned experience is an important determinant of pain perception and the development of pain syndromes (Loeser and Melzack, 1999). Therefore, experience in previous deliveries will influence each woman's analgesic requirements.

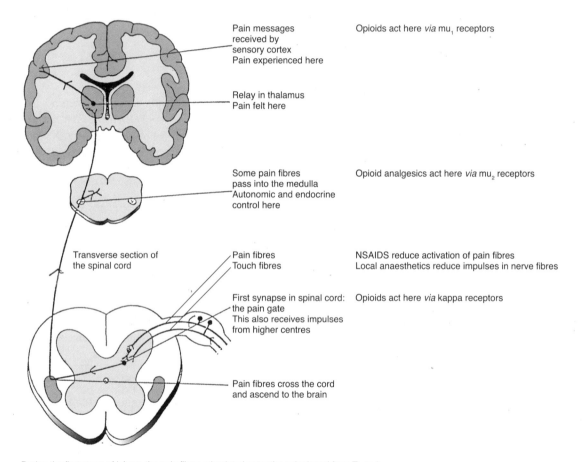

Pain messages received by sensory cortex
Pain experienced here

Opioids act here *via* mu₁ receptors

Relay in thalamus
Pain felt here

Some pain fibres pass into the medulla
Autonomic and endocrine control here

Opioid analgesics act here *via* mu₂ receptors

Transverse section of the spinal cord

Pain fibres
Touch fibres

NSAIDS reduce activation of pain fibres
Local anaesthetics reduce impulses in nerve fibres

First synapse in spinal cord: the pain gate
This also receives impulses from higher centres

Opioids act here *via* kappa receptors

Pain fibres cross the cord and ascend to the brain

During the first stage of labour, the pain fibres stimulated enter the spinal cord from T_{10} to L_1.
During the second stage of labour, the pain fibres from the perineum are stimulated and enter the spinal cord from S_2 to S_4.

Figure 4.1 Diagram to illustrate the pain pathways
Source: Adapted from Jordan (1992)

The anatomy of the pain (or nociceptive) pathways is outlined in Figure 4.1. Aspects most relevant to pharmacology include:

■ Specific pain nerve fibres in the tissues are stimulated by inflammatory mediators, including kinins, histamine and prostaglandins released from cell membranes when tissues are damaged. The production of prostaglandins is inhibited by NSAIDs.

- The passage of pain impulses depends on action potentials in the neurones of the pain pathways. These are blocked by local **anaesthetics**.
- The integration of pain fibres, touch fibres and descending analgesic tracts occurs in the dorsal horn of the spinal cord, the 'pain gate' (Melzack and Wall, 1996). This is one site of opioid action.
- The pain pathways synapse in the reticular formation in the brainstem. Here they activate the sympathetic nervous system and increase:
  - level of arousal and consciousness
  - respiration
  - heart rate
  - blood pressure
  - emesis
  - sweating/perspiration.
- Anaesthetic gases (for example nitrous oxide) and opioids act in the brainstem.
- The pain pathways can overwhelm the cerebral cortex, to the exclusion of other considerations. The cerebral cortex is one site of opioid action.

Consequences of pain

Severe, unrelieved pain may not only provide the woman with a negative experience of childbirth, but can also have adverse physiological consequences:

- *Increased rate and depth of respirations* (see nitrous oxide): Hyperventilation rapidly reduces the carbon dioxide (CO_2) in the body, leading to vasoconstriction of the maternal and placental circulations, jeopardizing the fetus. Between contractions, the lack of carbon dioxide reduces the respiratory drive and decreases respirations. This can lead to hypoxia of mother and fetus.
- *Tachycardia:* The increase in heart rate increases both the work and the oxygen needs of the heart, while simultaneously reducing coronary blood flow. Ischaemic changes in the ECG are not uncommon in labour. Tachycardia can reduce **cardiac output**. In labour, cardiac output must increase to meet the work requirements of the muscles. If cardiac output declines, insufficient oxygen will be delivered to the muscles for aerobic respiration to take place; therefore lactic acid will accumulate, making the woman acidotic.
- *Hypertension:* Any sudden rise in blood pressure (BP) can threaten the cerebral circulation. The physiological changes of pregnancy render cerebral blood vessels especially vulnerable to hypertensive episodes.
- *Gastric stasis and emesis:* Pain causes gastric stasis and disturbances of the autonomic nervous system. Intense pain may lead to nausea and vomiting.

Practice point

- Even if a woman has received no analgesia, close observations of vital signs must be maintained.

Pain relief in labour

Midwives often take responsibility for administration of analgesia, either as initial or subsequent 'top-up' doses. The woman, the condition of the fetus and the parameters of the labour are assessed to ascertain whether it is clinically appropriate to administer any drug before doing so.

Inhalation analgesia

Inhalation analgesia is achieved by the use of anaesthetic gases in sub-anaesthetic concentrations. The widespread use of inhalation analgesia in childbirth for over 100 years has established its relative safety. Nevertheless, administration of inhalation agents requires close supervision (Clyburn and Rosen, 1993). In the UK, only nitrous oxide is in regular use for inhalation analgesia in childbirth, although other anaesthetic agents (for example isoflurane and enflurane) may be employed for Caesarean section and surgical procedures. Therefore, the principles of inhalation anaesthesia, relevant to all gaseous agents, will be outlined, with a more detailed review of nitrous oxide. Nitrous oxide is administered as Entonox®, using premixed cylinders of 50% nitrous oxide in 50% oxygen as a homogenous gas (BOC, 2004).

Uses of inhalation agents

Nitrous oxide, as Entonox®, is normally available in all settings and provides intermittent analgesia during uterine contractions (NCC, 2007). Women find it to be a more effective analgesic than pethidine (meperidine) or TENS machines, but less effective than epidural analgesia (Reynolds, 1993b).

Actions of inhalation agents

The precise mechanism of action of anaesthetics remains uncertain. Although the chemistry of anaesthetic gases is diverse, they share the properties of lipid solubility and the ability to bind to cell membranes at certain sites. This interaction with cell membranes affects ion channels, the functioning of neurotransmitters at **synapses** and the transmission of nerve impulses in the central nervous system. Anaesthetics potentiate the actions of inhibitory neurotransmitters, particularly in the brainstem, thalamus and hippocampus (memory centre) (Evers et al., 2006). The brainstem contains a network of neurones, which transmits sensory input to the cerebral cortex, in a nonspecific manner, to control states of arousal and consciousness. Gradual suppression of brain activity here results in the four stages, or depths, of anaesthesia: analgesia, delirium, surgical anaesthesia and finally depression of the vital centres of the medulla. Depth of anaesthesia is assessed by response to verbal commands and reflex responses (Carmichael et al., 2007).

Practice point

■ An incorrect dose of an inhalation agent may produce a stage of anaesthesia that is not clinically desirable. The depth of anaesthesia should therefore be monitored in women receiving **general anaesthetics** (NCC, 2004).

How the body handles inhalation agents

The effect of an inhalation agent depends not only on how much is absorbed but also on the concentration of gas reaching the brain. This is determined by:

■ concentration of the inspired gaseous mixture
■ pulmonary ventilation delivering the gas to the lungs
■ transfer across the respiratory (alveolar) membrane into the bloodstream
■ solubility of the gas in blood
■ loss of the gas into other body tissues
■ cardiac output and the blood supply to the brain.

Concentration of inspired gas

Nitrous oxide is not sufficiently powerful to produce surgical anaesthesia when used alone. Concentrations of 50% nitrous oxide are needed for effective analgesia. If this is administered with air, rather than oxygen, hypoxia will ensue. Should high concentrations be administered (for example following improper storage, below), hypoxia is an urgent consideration. When nitrous oxide was inhaled with air from the pre-1965 standard obstetric analgesic machine, oxygen concentrations as low as 1.8% were inhaled and the women were so hypoxic they became cyanosed (Cole, 1975).

Practice point

■ Improper storage of cylinders could allow administration of concentrations of nitrous oxide greater than 50%, reducing the percentage of oxygen available. If this is suspected, oxygen saturation should be assessed.

Pulmonary ventilation

Increases in **ventilation** will increase the delivery of gas to the blood and hasten the effects of inhalation analgesia. Women given nitrous oxide tend to overventilate in order to maximize pain relief. The inherent danger is that they will exhale too much carbon dioxide, lowering the carbon dioxide concentration in the blood, which causes:

■ vasoconstriction of the placental bed and hypoxia in the fetus
■ maternal hypoventilation between contractions, leading to fetal hypoxia
■ cerebral vasoconstriction, making the woman dizzy
■ **alkalosis**, which may induce tetany.

Practice points

■ It is important that the respirations of all women are supervised during the administration of inhalation agents, and instructions are given to breathe slowly and fairly deeply (Clyburn and Rosen, 1993: 180; Bryant and Yerby, 2004).
■ Tetany usually begins as painful involuntary spasms of the muscles of the hands and feet. If the early signs go unnoticed, it may develop into spasm of the larynx and obstruction of the airway.
■ Any reports of dizziness, tingling or twitching in the woman's hands or feet should be an indication to monitor breathing patterns closely for signs of overbreathing.
■ The prolonged use of nitrous oxide from early labour should be avoided (Reynolds, 1993b).
■ Women with diseases of the nerves or muscles (such as disseminated sclerosis) may be unable to benefit fully from nitrous oxide inhalation.
■ Obesity reduces vital capacity and adversely affects other aspects of respiratory and cardiovascular function. Difficulties are compounded by pregnancy. Administration of general anaesthetics to obese women is complicated, and some anaesthetists opt to insert epidural catheters early in labour (Soens et al., 2008).

Solubility of the gas in blood

The solubility of the gas in blood determines the rate at which the gas is absorbed and eliminated from the body. Gases such as nitrous oxide, which dissolve in blood to a minimal extent, act on the brain very quickly, giving rapid analgesia (within 20–60 seconds) and are excreted rapidly. Due to its relatively low solubility in lipids (fats), nitrous oxide is rapidly eliminated from the blood and tissues with high blood flow, including the brain.

Transfer

The amount of gas transferred into different tissues depends on the flow of blood, the concentration of the gas and the nature of the tissue, since gases dissolve more readily in some tissues than in others. Anaesthetics have a tendency to accumulate in fat (Chapter 2).

The **blood/brain barrier** is freely permeable to anaesthetics and the brain is well perfused, therefore the concentration of gas in the brain is approximately equal to that in the blood. The analgesic effects of nitrous oxide are experienced some 25–35 seconds after administration and persist for about 60 seconds after inhalation ceases.

Being lipid soluble, inhalation agents cross the placenta. The concentration of nitrous oxide in the fetus reaches 80% of maternal values within 3 minutes of administration.

Cardiac output

Cardiac output is important in determining blood flow to lungs and all tissues; the distribution of inhalation agents may be impaired in women with pre-eclampsia or a compromised cardiovascular system (Nagelhout, 1992).

Elimination of inhalation agents

Nitrous oxide is rapidly eliminated through the woman's and neonate's lungs after birth. This is an advantage over other analgesics, which depend on the immature liver and kidneys for removal. In both mother and neonate, it is estimated that the effects of Entonox® wear off after 2–3 minutes, although removal from tissues with low blood flow, such as fat, takes longer (Kennedy and Longnecker, 1996).

Nitrous oxide

Nitrous oxide is colourless, odourless, heavier than air and non-explosive. It strongly supports combustion, and should not be allowed to contact lighted cigarettes, oils, greases, tars or many plastics. Should a fire occur, normal fire extinguishers are effective (BOC, 2004).

Adverse effects of nitrous oxide

The **adverse effects** of nitrous oxide are considered in relation to:

1 Immediate exposure of woman and fetus/neonate
2 Long-term exposure of staff.

1. Immediate exposure

Nitrous oxide is not a muscle relaxant and, unlike other anaesthetic gases, it has no effect on smooth muscle, including the uterus (Evers et al., 2006). All anaesthetic gases depress the nervous system. This involves both the higher functions and the vital centres of the medulla and brainstem.

Central nervous system (CNS) depression (obtunding)

Nitrous oxide produces some maternal sedation. Self-administration provides some safeguard against overdosage: as the woman becomes drowsy, the mask or mouthpiece falls away. The manufacturers suggest that administration will cease before the laryngeal (gag) reflex is lost (BOC, 2004). However, overuse of inhalation agents can result in depression of the central nervous system, including the laryngeal reflex. If the laryngeal reflex is suppressed, and unable to protect the airway, there is a danger of aspiration of stomach contents, should any vomiting occur (Zelcer et al., 1989; Clyburn and Rosen, 1993).

Practice points

- Close observation of the woman for any signs of sedation is extremely important.
- Women in established labour should not be left alone (NCC, 2007).

CNS depression, dizziness, light headedness and confusion are usually mild, although it is recommended that no one should drive or use machinery for at least 12 hours following the use of Entonox® analgesia (BOC, 2004). Only in very high concentrations does medullary paralysis (stage four of anaesthesia) occur, depressing respiratory and cardiovascular systems (Rang et al., 2007).

Neonatal CNS depression is a potential hazard with all inhalational and induction agents, including prolonged administration of nitrous oxide (Capogna and Celleno, 1993). In normal doses, nitrous oxide is eliminated so rapidly that neonates do not suffer adverse effects (Brownridge, 1991).

Hallucinations

Vivid dreams and hallucinations represent the delirium stage (stage two) of anaesthesia and women should be warned that these may occur transiently, since the feelings of dissociation produced may be very unpleasant (Bushnell and Justins, 1993). Some of the analgesic properties of nitrous oxide are attributed to its effect on the affective and cognitive dimensions of pain (Carstoniu et al., 1994). Some people may find inhalation pleasurable and overuse Entonox® in early labour.

Nausea

Nausea is a common adverse reaction to nitrous oxide and vomiting may occur (NCC, 2007).

Hypoxia

When high concentrations of nitrous oxide have been administered for some time, 'diffusion hypoxia' may occur on abrupt discontinuation and resumption of breathing air. This is due to large volumes of nitrous oxide entering the alveoli and diluting the available oxygen. Therefore, for a brief period, the woman and neonate are inhaling a concentration of oxygen below 20%.

Practice point

- The resulting hypoxia can be prevented by administration of supplementary oxygen when nitrous oxide is discontinued to both the neonate at birth and the woman in the early recovery period (Clyburn and Rosen, 1993; Evers et al., 2006).

Hypoxia is a particular danger if nitrous oxide is used without adequate supervision or if the woman has a pre-existing respiratory disease (Rang et al., 2007). All anaesthetics tend to depress the vital centres, but the effects of nitrous oxide are subtle and may be easily overlooked (Evers et al., 2006). The use of nitrous oxide may worsen any existing fetal hypoxia and exacerbate any placental insufficiency. Zelcher et al. (1989) suggest that if the fetal heart rate is abnormal, the use of nitrous oxide is ill-advised. In one study (n = 40), inhalation of Entonox® throughout the first and second stages of labour resulted in a higher incidence of maternal hypoxia than epidural analgesia (Arfeen et al., 1994). Pulse oximeters were used to detect hypoxia in this study.

Patients with pre-existing coronary artery disease may experience increased myocardial ischaemia (Aronson, 2006).

Practice points

■ A pulse oximeter assists in assessing the situation, since it provides continuous or intermittent measurement of maternal haemoglobin saturation without causing discomfort. However, it *cannot detect changes in carbon dioxide concentrations.*

■ Use of a pulse oximeter is advised if administration of nitrous oxide has been prolonged, the woman has dark skin, opioids are co-administered or any uncertainty exists (DH, 1996; Evers et al., 2006).

2. Adverse effects related to prolonged exposure (mainly staff)

Vitamin B$_{12}$

After 6 hours' exposure, nitrous oxide inactivates vitamin B$_{12}$ (Rang et al., 2007). The effect persists for several days. After brief exposure, this is rarely clinically significant. However, nitrous oxide should be avoided if pre-existing vitamin B$_{12}$ deficiency exists, for example in pernicious anaemia (Rang et al., 2007). Aronson (2006) reports two cases of peripheral nerve damage following 80 and 180 minutes of nitrous oxide exposure in patients who were subsequently found to have pernicious anaemia. Excessive use over several months led to reversible spinal cord degeneration in a further case (Doran et al., 2004). Administration of Entonox® more frequently than every 4 days (which is unlikely to occur in midwifery) should be accompanied by routine examination of the red and white blood cells for evidence of B$_{12}$ deficiency (BOC, 2004).

Fertility

There is a possibility that prolonged occupational exposure to nitrous oxide may impair male or female fertility and increase the incidence of spontaneous abortions and preterm birth (Burm, 2003; BOC, 2004; Olfert, 2006). Nitrous oxide in low analgesic doses is **teratogenic** in rodents (Rice, 1993); the doses causing congenital anomalies or pregnancy loss would be equivalent to a thousand parts per million, which would only be found in theatres without scavenging equipment (Burm, 2003). Use of, or exposure to, nitrous oxide during the first trimester may be harmful to the fetus, but is not absolutely **contraindicated**, for example following trauma (BOC, 2004).

Practice point

■ Because of the possible effects on staff, the concentration of nitrous oxide in the atmosphere should be maintained below a specified level and monitored regularly. Gas should not be allowed to escape into the atmosphere at any time, for example by ill-fitting masks or uncuffed endotracheal tubes (Burm, 2003).

BOC (2004) recommends that the concentration of nitrous oxide should not exceed one hundred parts per million (ppm). However, more stringent criteria of 50 or 25 ppm are set in some

North American guidelines. These levels are unlikely to be exceeded with effective ventilation and air conditioning plus the scavenging of waste gases (Burm, 2003).

Practice point

■ Healthcare workers should protect themselves by ensuring that all gas cylinders are functioning correctly (not leaking) and avoiding the area within one foot of the client's face while the client is exhaling or administering nitrous oxide (McKenry and Salerno, 2003).

Storage of Entonox®

Entonox® in cylinders may separate into nitrous oxide and oxygen if the temperature falls below −6°C (for example if it is stored outside). It is unsafe to administer in this condition: initially oxygen would be administered, and the base of the cylinder would contain 100% nitrous oxide. To ensure homogenization, cylinders should be stored horizontally above 10°C for 24 hours before use; if this is not possible, the manufacturers' guidelines should be consulted (BOC, 2004). Incorrectly stored cylinders may administer insufficient oxygen. Entonox® delivered by pipeline has a lower critical temperature, −30°C, which is unlikely to be reached in the UK.

Interactions: nitrous oxide

The respiratory and cardiovascular depressant actions of opioids may be compounded by nitrous oxide, causing transient maternal hypoxia (Evers et al., 2006). Most gaseous anaesthetics sensitize the heart to the action of adrenaline/epinephrine, risking **cardiac dysrhythmias**, but nitrous oxide is free from this effect.

Cautions: nitrous oxide

- Nitrous oxide has the capacity to enter any pockets of gas trapped within the body and expand them. It is therefore contraindicated in any situation where abnormal quantities of gas are trapped within the body, due to the risk of gas retention, for example in women with sinus infections or middle ear occlusion, where rupture of the tympanic membrane may occur (BOC, 2004; Aronson, 2006). A case is reported where nitrous oxide ruptured internal iliac artery occlusion balloons during a Caesarean hysterectomy (Welters and Leuwer, 2008). Nitrous oxide may also diffuse into air bubbles formed by regional analgesia, hindering the spread of local anaesthetic (Sweetman et al., 2007), or causing pressure effects (Aronson, 2006).
- Nitrous oxide may impair levels of consciousness. It should not be administered to women whose level of consciousness is already impaired.
- To reduce the risk of cross-infection, including hepatitis C, appropriate microbiological filters should be placed between the patient and the breathing system; supplying clean masks and mouthpieces may not be sufficient (AAGBI, 1996; Bajekal et al., 2000; Chilvers and Weisz, 2000; Pediani, 2003).
- Pulmonary hypertension may be worsened, and nitrous oxide is not recommended (Evers et al., 2006).
- Nitrous oxide is not advised for women with vitamin B_{12} deficiency (Rang et al., 2007), or women with sickle cell disease, which is associated with low vitamin B_{12} concentrations (Aronson, 2006).

Summary

Although it is not always effective, nitrous oxide combined with oxygen has relatively few adverse effects and these can be minimized if administration is supervised and monitored by the midwife. Rapid elimination from maternal and neonatal circulations (Olofsson and Irestedt, 1998) and observation data indicate that it does not interfere with breastfeeding (Jordan et al., 2009b). Women should be advised that nitrous oxide is more likely to make pain tolerable than offer complete analgesia, but is unlikely to lengthen or complicate labour. It remains a flexible and useful method of pain relief during parturition, but should not be overused in early labour.

Implications for practice: Entonox®

Although the use of nitrous oxide is generally safe, careful supervision of the woman and her breathing pattern is important.

Potential problem	Management and care suggestions
Sedation	Supervise closely. Self-administration
	Be alert for vomiting
Maternal and fetal hypoxia	Use premixed oxygen with nitrous oxide
	Ensure the cylinder is correctly stored and fully mixed
	Supervise – ensure slow, even inspirations
	Use a pulse oximeter, for example if opioids are co-administered
	Avoid prolonged use
	Advise discontinuation when the peak of the contraction has passed
	Monitor fetal HR intermittently
	Be prepared to administer oxygen to the neonate
Dizziness, tetany	Prevent hyperventilation
	Discontinue should tingling in hands and feet occur. Specifically question the woman about this
Nausea	Supervise closely. Position to avoid aspiration
Hallucinations, dissociation	Warn recipients. Avoid overuse
Vitamin B_{12} deficiency	To avoid this arising in women without B_{12} deficiency, limit maternal administration to 24 hours
Affects on reproduction	Monitor the concentration in the environment. Avoid excessively close staff contact with gas
Risk of fire	Avoid contact with cigarettes, greases and oils

Opioids

Opioid drugs, such as pethidine (meperidine), are used extensively in labour. The term **opioid** is used to describe any preparation acting on the body's opioid **receptors**, which normally respond to endorphins, enkephalins and other endogenous opioids. Thus morphine, diamorphine, pethidine, meptazinol, codeine, buprenorphine (Temgesic®), pentazocine (Fortral®), fentanyl and its derivatives, and the 'morphine **antagonists**' such as naloxone (Narcan®) are all opioids. In the absence of evidence favouring any particular opioid (Fairlie et al., 1999), the opioid offered may be based on institutional preference.

Uses of opioids

Opioids are used in labour, preoperatively, intra-operatively, postoperatively and in intensive care for analgesia, sedation and reduction of anxiety. Administration may be intramuscular, intravenous, epidural, **intrathecal**, buccal, oral or transdermal, depending on the setting. Opioids are able to reduce the hyperventilation induced by pain and maintain carbon dioxide at near normal concentrations (Clyburn and Rosen, 1993). Some low-dose opioid preparations, usually containing codeine, are sold as over the counter preparations for controlling the symptoms of cough or diarrhoea, but are not recommended.

Analgesia

Intramuscular opioids provide greater pain relief in labour than either no treatment or injection of sterile water, but the differences on visual analogue scales are not large (Tsui et al., 2004). Nevertheless, many women report that pain relief in labour from pethidine is inadequate (Ranta et al., 1995), and when opioids are discontinued, there is frequently a rebound increase in pain sensitivity. When administered epidurally or intrathecally, opioids provide rapid and effective analgesia. Although 6–30 hours of analgesia are provided by this route, the adverse effects may be troublesome, particularly urinary retention, sedation, nausea, itching, hypotension and, occasionally, respiratory arrest (Chrubasik et al., 1992). Opioids may be administered intravenously in association with general anaesthesia, postoperatively or if epidural or intrathecal injections are **contraindicated**.

Anaesthesia, sedation and reduction of anxiety

The benefits of opioids can be attributed to both their analgesic and anxiolytic actions. The release of adrenaline/epinephrine and noradrenaline/norepinephrine due to pain and anxiety decrease uterine blood flow. This is reversed by opioids, to the benefit of the fetus (Hollmen, 1993). Opioids also reduce the hypertension and tachycardia associated with intubation (McAtamney et al., 1998).

How the body handles opioids

Opioids are rapidly transferred across the placenta: changes are detected by fetal scalp electrodes within 7 minutes of intramuscular administration of pethidine. Transfer is more rapid and complete for the more lipophilic (fat-soluble) compounds, such as diamorphine, fentanyl and fentanyl derivatives. The concentration of fentanyl in maternal plasma and its subsequent transfer into the umbilical vein increases (0.03–0.38 nanograms/ml) as the epidural dose administered increases between 25 and 275 micrograms (Fernando et al., 1997). At doses of 183 micrograms, a small, but variable amount of fentanyl passes into the neonate (Porter et al., 1998). At steady state, opioid concentration will always be higher in the fetal circulation than in the mother, because:

■ The fetus and neonate excrete opioids more slowly than adults, due to the immaturity of their liver enzymes (Chapter 1).

▨ Due to the lower **pH** in the fetus, basic drugs, such as pethidine, are more likely to be **ionized** in the fetus. Therefore, they may become 'trapped', unable to return to the maternal circulation because drugs are only transferred across the placenta in their non-ionized state. The concentration of free fentanyl increases by 4% as pH falls from 7.4 (in mother) to 7.2 (in fetus) (Helbo-Hansen, 1995). In fetuses requiring emergency Caesarean delivery, fetal pH may be lower, which could increase the effective concentration, and sedative effects, of fentanyl. This problem is intensified if the fetus becomes hypoxic, because hypoxia further reduces pH.

▨ There are fewer plasma proteins in the fetal circulation. Therefore, more drug remains unbound and in the free or active state. The fetus has a higher concentration of free or unbound opioids than the mother, and this increases if the fetus becomes acidotic (above).

Practice points

■ If the fetus becomes acidotic due to lack of oxygen, opioids accumulate and their adverse effects are magnified (Connor, 2008). Therefore, blood flow to the placenta and maternal oxygen saturation must be maintained at all times.

■ The blood supply to the placenta is considerably reduced during uterine contractions. Therefore transfer of drug to the fetus may be minimized by intramuscular administration immediately before a contraction (Carson, 1996).

Binding to plasma proteins ranges from 35% for morphine, 58% for pethidine, 85% for fentanyl to 92% for remifentanil. Opioids are metabolized in the liver and excreted via urine and bile. Each opioid has different metabolic pathways.

Intramuscular pethidine (meperidine)

Opioids are not given orally during labour, due to delays in absorption and metabolism. Intramuscular injection is the most convenient alternative. Following a single intramuscular dose of pethidine to the mother, the fetus receives maximum exposure 2–3 hours later; therefore respiratory depression in the neonate is most likely in infants born at this time. If delivery occurs within 1 hour of pethidine administration, relatively little drug is transferred to the fetus. If delivery occurs more than 6 hours after administration, much of the pethidine will have been transferred back to the mother, although the active metabolite norpethidine/normeperidine will remain in the neonatal tissues. This is gradually excreted over several days. During this time, the neonate's behaviour will be suboptimal (irritable and difficult to feed). The amount of norpethidine/normeperidine transferred to the neonate is greater the longer the time between delivery and pethidine administration (Crowell et al., 1994).

Pethidine (meperidine) is metabolized to norpethidine/normeperidine, which causes convulsions in high concentrations. The **half-life** of pethidine is 3 hours in the mother and 4–5 hours in the neonate. The half-life of norpethidine/normeperidine is 20 hours in the mother and 60 hours in the neonate. Therefore, this metabolite takes several days to clear from the neonate, during which time adverse effects on behaviour persist. With multiple doses, it can accumulate in the fetus/neonate and cause respiratory depression and fits that are resistant to, or even exacerbated by, naloxone (Narcan®) administration. Infants of women who abuse pethidine are at particular risk.

Practice points

■ Each institution imposes a maximum dose of pethidine which is never exceeded. The BNF (2009) maximum dose is 400 mg in 24 hours, which will be excessive for most women.

■ Extra help will be needed to ensure that the infant suckles correctly over the first 3–5 days of life. An irritable or jittery infant is unable to suckle the whole areola. Unless corrected, the resulting tissue damage will be painful and may lead to infection. It is better to supplement breastfeeding, preferably by expressed milk in a cup, over the first 2–5 days than to abandon it entirely.

Pethidine passes into breast milk, which compounds early difficulties with feeding (Yerby, 2000).

Epidural and intrathecal opioids

Opioids and local anaesthetics may be administered epidurally or intrathecally or in combination as combined spinal epidural analgesia. Intrathecal opioids afford more rapid analgesia than epidural local anaesthetics; for example fentanyl is effective within 5 minutes, compared to 30 minutes for epidural bupivacaine. The mean time to analgesia is 5.59 minutes (95% **CI**, 6.59–4.48 minutes) shorter with combined spinal epidural than epidural analgesia (Simmons et al., 2007). Local anaesthetics have a longer duration of action than opioids, and opioids alone provide less effective analgesia in second stage (Lindow et al., 2004).

Fentanyl passes into both the colostrum (Steer et al., 1992) and the fetus (Desprats et al., 1991; Bader et al., 1995; Loftus et al., 1995) and is released from binding proteins (albumins) in the first few hours of neonatal life (Porter et al., 1998); therefore, sedation is likely to be marked during this time, which is crucial for the establishment of breastfeeding. The plasma half-life of fentanyl is 3.7 ± 0.4 hours in adults (Brunton et al., 2006) and 5.29 ± 4.4 hours in healthy term neonates (Helbo-Hansen, 1995). Elimination of fentanyl is not always uniform, but may involve transient rebounds, which prolong the depressant effects (Koehntop et al., 1986). This delayed clearance allows accumulation in the central nervous system, which could produce subtle behavioural changes, such as depression of feeding reflexes (Desprats et al., 1991; Steer et al., 1992).

Practice point

■ Neonates may be too sedated to latch correctly until opioids have been eliminated.

Drugs administered intrathecally pass into the fetus to a limited extent; very low concentrations of opioids are found in the systemic circulation or cord blood following spinal opioid administration. Drugs administered epidurally are administered in much larger doses (10–20 times as high) and absorbed into the systemic circulation, making **adverse drug reactions** more likely. For example, the concentration of fentanyl in colostrum is higher following epidural administration of 100–150 micrograms than intravenous administration of 50 micrograms (Goma et al., 2008).

Actions of opioids

Opioids are chemically related to the body's endorphins and enkephalins, which are natural mood changers and analgesics, particularly in times of stress. Opioids act at many sites in the central nervous system, including the spinal cord, the medulla, the midbrain and the cerebral cortex (Figure 4.1). Several classes of opioid receptors exist and different opiate drugs act selectively at different receptors to produce diverse responses. In some situations, the euphoriant or sedative effects of opioids predominate over their analgesic actions (Arner and Meyerson, 1988; Olofsson et al., 1996).

Opioids bind to the cell surface receptors for the endorphins and enkephalins, fitting in like keys into a lock (Chapter 1). This binding triggers changes within the nerve or smooth muscle cells, usually inhibiting their activity and neurotransmitter release. In general, opioids (endogenous and pharmacological) depress the activity of target tissues and have a calming effect. They inhibit the hypothalamus and 'damp down' the level of activity in the autonomic nervous system, partly by reducing the stress response attributable to noradrenaline (norepinephrine).

Several classes of opioid receptor, which are assigned Greek letters, are of pharmacological importance: μ_1 (mu 1), μ_2 (mu 2), δ (delta), κ (kappa), and peripheral opioid receptors. These are summarized in Box 4.1.

Box 4.1 Actions and effects of opioids

Actions of opioid receptors:
- κ (kappa) receptors: analgesia, sedation and dysphoria
- μ_1 (mu 1) receptors: supraspinal analgesia, euphoria and addiction
- μ_2 (mu 2) receptors:
  - depression of vital centres:
    - respiration
    - HR
    - postural BP adjustments
    - thermoregulation
    - cough
  - affect smooth muscle of:
    - uterus – prolonged labour
    - urinary tract – retention of urine
    - gut – constipation, ileus, gastric stasis
    - blood vessels – hypotension
    - eye – pupillary constriction (not seen in pethidine overdose)
- δ (delta) receptors: spinal and supraspinal analgesia

Stimulation of:
- Chemoreceptor trigger zone – nausea and vomiting
- Histamine release
  - bronchospasm in asthmatics
  - vasodilation and hypotension

Inhibition of:
- Substance P release
  - pruritus
  - spinal analgesia
- Neuroendocrine function (Chapter 20)
- Inhibitory neurotransmitters
  - behaviour disturbance
  - muscle spasms
- Immune function (Chapter 20)

Adverse effects of opioids

Central nervous system: higher functions

Opioids act on more than one type of receptor in the cerebral cortex. While sedation is the usual result, central nervous system excitability, including hallucinations and convulsions, sometimes occurs.

Central nervous system depression

Opioids produce drowsiness, mental clouding and sometimes euphoria. These actions may be beneficial in some situations, for example in intensive care, but sedation is disadvantageous to both mother and infant in a normal labour. Sedation is intensified with higher doses and intravenous administration. Opioids may provide sedation rather than analgesia (Olofsson et al., 1996): following administration of opioids, a woman may fall asleep, only to be woken by the pain of contractions (Fairlie et al., 1999). CNS depression/**obtunding** and sedation induced by opioids reduce the mother's ability to cooperate with labour. Administration of >100 micrograms of intraspinal opioids may sedate and depress the respirations of infants (NCC, 2007). Sedation (of mother) may be profound if any degree of thyroid imbalance is present (Ogrin and Schussler, 2005) (Chapter 17).

Practice point

■ A woman who has received opioids may be sedated and less able to 'push' in the second stage, which will prolong labour.

The fetal electroencephalogram is modified soon after intramuscular administration of pethidine to the mother; this effect persists for the first 4 days of life, and corresponds to the neonate's decreased level of arousal and muscle tone (Clyburn and Rosen, 1993). Due to the long half-life (60 hours) of the metabolite (norpethidine/normeperidine), neonatal behaviour is depressed for approximately 3 days after administration of pethidine during labour. During this time, reflexes and thermoregulation are compromised and abnormal reflexes are more likely (Crowell et al., 1994).

Practice point

■ The poor muscle tone of affected infants means that they are less likely to suckle on the whole areola.

Infant feeding

For neonates, exposure to pethidine reduces muscle tone and depresses the central nervous system (Wagner, 1993). This causes delay in the sucking and rooting responses (Nissen et al., 1995). Establishment of breastfeeding appears to be delayed by several hours if opioids are administered 1–5 hours before birth (Crowell et al., 1994): several mothers in this study who had received pethidine discontinued breastfeeding because the infant was not feeding well. If delivery is delayed by more than 8 hours after pethidine administration, there is less impact on feeding behaviour. In one study, infants who failed to suck had higher plasma concentrations of pethidine than those who started to feed, which suggests that failure to feed is a dose-dependent adverse drug reaction (Nissen et al., 1997). Increase in oxytocin in response to suckling declined when intravenous morphine was administered (n = 17) (Lindow et al., 1999). Opioid-induced disruption of oxytocin release at the sensitive period of delivery may also affect maternal personality or 'mothering behaviour' and block longer term maternal adaptations up to 6 months postpartum (Jonas et al., 2008).

Practice point

■ Problems with breastfeeding are more likely to arise if the dose of pethidine is 100 mg, rather than 50 mg (Nissen et al., 1997). The dose of pethidine is subject to institutional preference. Doses usually range from 50–100 mg by subcutaneous or intramuscular injection (BNF, 2009).

Cohort studies indicate that epidural opioids reduce the chances of breastfeeding (Jordan, 2006). This has been confirmed in two randomized controlled trials (Henderson et al., 2003; Beilin et al., 2005), and breastfeeding at discharge is related to the dose of epidural fentanyl (Jordan et al., 2005). Infants with higher concentrations of fentanyl in colostrum were more likely to display suboptimal breastfeeding behaviour (Goma et al., 2008).

Practice point

■ Epidural doses of fentanyl greater than 100 micrograms may make the infant drowsy and depress respirations (NCC, 2007: 113). Therefore, close observation and breastfeeding support are needed until the infant has eliminated the fentanyl; in healthy neonates, this should take 16–27 hours, but can take up to 28–48 hours.

Suboptimal breastfeeding behaviour, such as poor rooting, latching and fixing to the nipple, is linked to increased weight loss at one week, and is associated with epidural or intrathecal analgesia (n = 280) (Dewey et al., 2003).

Practice point

■ Where feeding behaviour is suboptimal, assistance is needed to prevent excessive weight loss and long-term introduction of formula feeding.

The manufacturer of tramadol advises against use during breastfeeding (BNF, 2009).

Central nervous system excitability

Opioids may induce euphoria, dysphoria, tremulousness, restlessness or delirium. Visual disturbances, hallucinations and nightmares may accompany opioid use. Norpethidine/normeperidine (a metabolite of pethidine) may cause neurobehavioural abnormalities such as twitching and convulsions. Although respiratory depression produced by pethidine can be reversed by naloxone, any convulsions and respiratory depression caused by norpethidine/normeperidine are less likely to respond (Clyburn and Rosen, 1993).

Practice point

■ Not all respiratory depression will respond to naloxone, particularly in infants where norpethidine/normeperidine may have accumulated, for example following repeated doses and long delays between administration and birth.

Opioids reduce the availability of the neurotransmitter responsible for inhibiting the nervous system, GABA (gamma amino butyric acid). This can lead to convulsions or muscle spasm, muscle rigidity, agitation, confusion, aggression, abnormal movements, dystonic reactions (Chapter 5) or **myoclonus** (muscle jerks). If the chest wall is affected, respiration will be compromised. This problem is most likely with high doses of pethidine, fentanyl or fentanyl derivatives. Muscle rigidity can usually be relieved with naloxone (Bowdle, 1998).

Central nervous system: brainstem

Opioids inhibit the activity of the vital centres in the brainstem. Therefore, midwives always pay close attention to the vital signs of the mother, fetus and neonate.

Respiratory depression

Opioids act directly on the respiratory centre in the medulla to depress respiration, and also, in rare instances, on the peripheral receptors to induce apnoea (Bowdle, 1998). Opioids reduce the sensitivity of the respiratory centre to carbon dioxide, thus reducing the normal drive to respiration (Gutstein and Akil, 2006). Therefore, respiration fails to increase to meet the high metabolic demands of labour. Rate, depth and regularity of respirations are decreased, reducing alveolar ventilation and oxygenation. This effect is intensified if the woman becomes so sedated that she falls asleep. If the circulation is adequate, respiratory depression is maximal within 90 minutes of intramuscular administration. If the peripheral circulation is 'shut down', as in **shock** or haemorrhage, the absorption and adverse effects of intramuscular drugs may be delayed.

Depression of the carbon dioxide respiratory drive means that the patient's breathing depends on the hypoxic respiratory drive. Administration of a high concentration of oxygen to a patient (adult or neonate) whose respirations are depressed due to opioids can remove the remaining respiratory drive and precipitate a sudden respiratory arrest. This may be difficult to reverse, due to a sharp rise in carbon dioxide concentration (Gutstein and Akil, 2006).

Respiratory depression of the woman during labour may lead to:

- retention of carbon dioxide and respiratory acidosis, in mother and fetus
- hypoxia in mother and fetus, which causes fetal heart rate decelerations.

Under these conditions, fetuses become acidotic, increasing their accumulation of pethidine and metabolites. In a randomized controlled trial of 100 mg intravenous pethidine versus saline (n = 383), acidosis (35/189 versus 5/194), low **Apgar score** and admission to neonatal intensive care were more common in women receiving pethidine. Acidosis was most marked 4–6 hours after intravenous administration (Sosa et al., 2005, 2006).

Practice points

- Maternal respirations are carefully monitored for rate, depth and rhythm.
- A pulse oximeter offers a useful guide as to the degree of oxygen saturation in the mother.
- Fetal monitoring for signs of acidosis is important in prolonged labours.

Following administration of normal doses of intrathecal or epidural opioids, maternal respiratory depression, apnoea and sedation may occur 30 minutes later or be delayed up to 16 hours, presumably due to the gradual spread of the drugs, and last up to 24 hours (Catterall and Mackie, 2006).

Case reports

Epidural or intrathecal opioids may cause sudden, profound maternal respiratory depression.

1 During labour, 1 mg of morphine was administered intrathecally. Apnoea occurred 7 hours later, after birth. It was fortuitous that apnoea did not occur during labour.

2 For a Caesarean section, 100 micrograms of fentanyl were administered extradurally. Profound respiratory depression occurred 100 minutes later.

These cases, cited by Clyburn and Rosen (1993), show the effects of delayed respiratory depression on the mother.

Practice points

- Vital signs, sedation and pain scores are monitored up to 24 hours after administration of intrathecal opioids (12 hours for diamorphine) (Hall, 1996; NCC, 2004).
- If the spinal (intrathecal) anaesthetic has 'worn off', administration of other opioids, for example pethidine intramuscularly, may intensify respiratory depression (Arkoosh, 1991).
- Particular care is needed for obese women, those suffering from sleep apnoea or respiratory disorders, those who have received parenteral opioids, morphine or higher doses (Eltzschig et al., 2003).

In *neonates*, measurements with fetal scalp electrodes indicate that transcutaneous oxygen tensions (levels) fall to 37% of baseline values 7 minutes after the intramuscular administration of 50 mg pethidine but recover within 15 minutes (Clyburn and Rosen, 1993). Depression of the central nervous system (above) reduces the neonate's reflexes, including the respiratory reflexes needed to cope with hypoxia and birth (Wagner, 1993). Studies in neonatal anaesthesia indicate that the neonate's spontaneous respiration may fail if neonatal plasma fentanyl concentration rises above 0.05–0.77 nanograms/ml, and sensitivity of the neonatal respiratory centre shows considerable inter-individual variation (Koehntop et al., 1986).

Respiratory depression in the neonate is potentially lethal; premature infants are particularly at risk. Rapid resuscitation is mandatory, and the need for naloxone should be assessed (below). A review of clinical trials found an association between opioid analgesia and low Apgar scores (Howell, 1994).

Practice point

- If opioids are administered, oxygen, means of ventilation for the neonate and naloxone must always be available.

Bradycardia

Opioids reduce the heart rate by: direct action on the cardiovascular centres in the medulla; decreasing the activity of the sympathetic nervous system; and reducing anxiety. In labour, this may contribute to a fall in BP and a consequent reduction in placental perfusion. The subsequent depression of the fetal heart rate and loss of fetal heart baseline variability may be interpreted as fetal distress, triggering medical interventions (Aronson, 2006).

Some fetal bradycardia on administration of opioid analgesia by any route is normal. This is attributed to the transient release of oxytocin (below), which causes a brief tetanic contraction of the uterus (Eberle and Norris, 1996). However, bradycardia lasting beyond 5–8 minutes may be a sign of metabolic stress (Arkoosh, 1991).

Practice point

- Fetal heart monitoring should be undertaken before and soon after administration of opioids. Changes should be interpreted cautiously. Intermittent monitoring is often the preferred option.

Hypotension

Hypotension may be defined as systolic BP below 100 mmHg or a fall of 20% below baseline (Eggers et al., 2008: 269). Action on the cardiovascular centres in the medulla, the sympathetic nervous system and histamine release may combine to produce a fall in BP. This is exaggerated on standing or sitting up, partly due to inhibition of the baroreceptor reflex (Gutstein and Akil, 2006). Sudden standing may result in dizziness, loss of balance or falls. Bed rest, fluid depletion, alcohol or phenothiazines such as prochlorperazine (Stemetil®) will exacerbate the effects of opioids on BP. Hypotension can impair placental and renal perfusion. Any hypotension is likely to be exaggerated by the uterus and fetal head compressing the maternal aorta and inferior vena cava if the mother adopts the supine position. Compression of the inferior vena cava prevents blood returning to the heart, which is then unable to maintain a **cardiac output.**

Practice points

- The woman should not lie in a supine position.
- The woman will need assistance to get up slowly after administration of opioids (Mayberry et al., 2002).
- Opioids should be used with caution, if at all, in women with decreased blood volume, as the effects of hypovolaemic shock will be aggravated (Gutstein and Akil, 2006).

When opioids are administered epidurally or intrathecally, hypotension is likely to occur within 30 minutes of administration. This may be accompanied by severe fetal bradycardia (Richardson, 2000).

Depression of thermoregulation
Opioids act on the hypothalamus to reduce the thermoregulatory set point. This has been recorded following pethidine administration during labour (Clyburn and Rosen, 1993), and may be hazardous for the neonate, whose thermoregulatory mechanisms rely on the sympathetic nervous system. The vasoconstrictor and shivering responses are depressed in all neonates, and this is accentuated by opioids.

Practice point

- The neonate must be kept warm, preferably by the mother. However, the mother may be sedated following opioid administration, and she should be carefully observed to minimize any danger of 'overlying'.

Cough
Opioids suppress the cough and sigh reflexes and depress the movement of respiratory cilia. This causes accumulation of the mucus secreted by the respiratory tract. Depression of the respiratory cilia is compounded by smoking. These factors increase the risks of pulmonary **atelectasis** and chest infections.

Actions on smooth muscle

Generally, opioids cause relaxation of smooth muscle and contraction of sphincters in the genitourinary and gastrointestinal tracts.

Prolonged labour
Administration of intramuscular pethidine briefly stimulates the hypothalamus to release oxytocin, which causes a brief tetanic uterine contraction (Eberle and Norris, 1996). Stimulation is superseded by decreased release of oxytocin and reduced contractility of uterine smooth muscle from direct action on mu_2/μ_2 opioid receptors and decreased response to oxytocin. These inhibitory actions are also observed following administration of epidural opioids and local anaesthetics

(Rahm et al., 2002) and endogenous opioids (dynorphin) (Carson, 1996; Carter, 2003). Uterine contractions may diminish following the administration of pethidine (Baxi et al., 1988), and the duration of both first and second stages of labour is directly related to the amount of pethidine administered during the first stage of labour (Thompson and Hillier, 1994). In a randomized controlled trial of women (n = 407) with **dystocia**, 100 mg pethidine intravenous had no impact on duration of labour and increased the need for oxytocin (Sosa et al., 2006).

Retention of urine and dysuria

Opioids reduce urine formation by reducing renal perfusion and augmenting the effects of anti-diuretic hormone. They also inhibit the smooth muscle of the bladder. The voiding reflex is inhibited, while the tone of the internal urethral sphincter is increased. Combined with trauma to the urethra during labour, retention of urine is common following birth. A full bladder may inhibit uterine contractions both during labour and postpartum.

Practice points

- Urine output should be monitored during and after labour.
- A full bladder may increase blood loss postpartum.
- Encouraging women to void after delivery may be helpful.

Gastrointestinal tract

The motility of the stomach, small intestine and colon is decreased. Opioids inhibit the propulsive, peristaltic actions of the gut, while increasing segmental, non-propulsive contractions, particularly in the pyloric region of the stomach, the first part of the duodenum and the colon. Gastric stasis may cause oesophageal reflux (heartburn), nausea and vomiting. Opioids contribute to the constipation that commonly follows childbirth. Opioids decrease gastrointestinal secretions, causing a dry mouth. Spasm of the biliary tract, producing pain on the right side of the abdomen, and gastrointestinal obstruction are rare adverse effects of opioids.

Practice points

- Painful abdominal cramps may follow administration of opioids.
- The woman must be positioned so that gastric contents do not enter the airway.
- Prescribers may request nitrates or atropine to manage biliary colic.

Nausea and vomiting

Gastric stasis and stimulation of the chemoreceptor trigger zone (in the medulla) combine to cause nausea; this is experienced by 30–60% of women receiving opioids by intramuscular or intravenous injection. Ambulation and sudden movement stimulate the vestibular apparatus, and contribute to the nausea associated with opioids. Nausea and vomiting are less likely to occur if the patient remains resting. Pain, labour, fear and anxiety also induce gastric stasis, nausea and vomiting. When these physiological effects of labour are combined with the sedative actions of opioids, the dangers of gastric aspiration become very real. Ingestion of food stimulates secretion of gastric acid, which damages the lungs on contact; therefore women who receive opioids are advised not to eat during labour, and may be prescribed acid suppressants (NCC, 2007; Chapter 12).

Bronchospasm

Histamine release causes bronchoconstriction and may occasionally precipitate an attack of asthma (Beischer et al., 1997). Opioids are not administered during an asthma attack since they may worsen symptoms.

Pruritus

As opioids inhibit transmission in the pain fibres, the 'itch sensation' fibres become active. Stimulation of the pain fibres by scratching suppresses the itch sensation. Opioids also act on nerve roots to cause flushing, urticaria (hives or 'nettle rash') and sweating, particularly in the face and upper body, and particularly in labouring women. This is the most common adverse drug reaction when opioids, particularly morphine or high doses, are given by the epidural or intrathecal routes (Herpolsheimer and Schretenthaler, 1994); however, most women neither request nor require treatment (Mayberry et al., 2002). Intrathecal opioids are more likely than epidurals to cause pruritus (Simmons et al., 2007). For some opioids, such as fentanyl, pruritus is more likely with higher doses and if local anaesthetics are not co-administered (Ghodse and Galea, 2008).

Neuroendocrine actions

The secretion of hypothalamic hormones is altered, but this is rarely a problem with short-term administration (Chapter 20):

■ In women with disorders of adrenal or thyroid function, opioids may suppress the release of these hormones (see Cautions below).
■ The release of hormones associated with stress, both those of the sympathetic nervous system and the adrenal cortex, is suppressed. This may be advantageous (above), but may contribute to impaired immune function, particularly with long-term use. Epidural/spinal analgesia containing fentanyl was associated with reduction of the normal stress response and cortisol release in infants, persisting for 2 months (Miller et al., 2005).
■ Opioids may enhance the secretion or activity of antidiuretic hormone. Occasionally, this can cause water retention and **hyponatraemia**, which is a *medical emergency*. This is described in Chapter 6.

Practice point

■ Women should be advised to drink only moderate quantities of plain water. Fluid balance must be checked following delivery.

Immunosuppression

Immunosuppression is associated with long-term opiate use, but a recurrence of *Herpes simplex* infections with the spinal administration of opioids has been reported (Bowdle, 1998); this may be associated with pruritus (Ghodse and Galea, 2008).

Contact dermatitis and urticaria (hives or 'nettle rash') can occur with protracted occupational exposure, and practitioners are advised to wear gloves or avoid direct contact with opioids (Kalant, 2007a).

Dependence

One case control study linked use of opioid analgesia in labour with an increased risk of opiate addiction in adult offspring in later life through a process of imprinting (Jacobson et al., 1990). This work should be interpreted cautiously, since there were more males in the study group than the control group, and males have a greater risk of drug addiction (Clyburn and Rosen, 1993).

Cautions: opioids

Opioids are used with caution, if at all, in the following circumstances:

* *Reduced respiratory reserve*, for example in asthma, obesity, kyphosis (excessive spinal curvature), and diseases of muscles or nerves (for example disseminated sclerosis). Opioids are contraindicated if the partial pressure (or concentration) of carbon dioxide (pCO_2) is raised, as in severe respiratory disease.
* With increasing *age* or *debility* or *malnutrition*, lower doses are needed, since standard doses will produce excessive adverse effects. For example, a 40-year-old may need half the analgesic dose required by a 20-year-old (Twycross, 1994).
* Pre-existing *hypotension* may be dangerously worsened, for example following haemorrhage.
* Excessive *sedation* and coma may result from administration of opioids to women with *hypothyroidism* or *Addison's disease* (Wall, 2002; BNF, 2009).
* Pethidine is one of the opioids most likely to cause convulsions with repeated administration. This may be exacerbated by fluid retention following oxytocin administration.
* The CNS depressant effects of opioids will complicate any *rise in intracranial pressure* (for example following a cerebral vascular accident or an eclamptic seizure) by worsening respiratory depression and obscuring vital signs. Opioid-induced respiratory depression causes carbon dioxide retention, which will exacerbate any rise in intracranial pressure, cerebral ischaemia or seizures.
* Reduced doses of opioids are needed if liver or kidney function is impaired, for example in pre-eclampsia. Pethidine is not recommended for women with poor renal function, due to the risk of accumulation of norpethidine/normeperidine and subsequent convulsions.
* Possibility of *paralytic ileus*, for example women with inflammatory bowel disease.
* Epilepsy increases the risk of myoclonus.
* Known allergy to opioids.

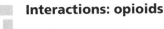

Interactions: opioids

Opioids interact with many drugs, and this section offers only a guide:

- *Enhanced depression of central nervous system and vital centres:* Administration of more than one depressant will intensify any opioid-induced reduction in BP, respiration and conscious levels. Central nervous system depressants include alcohol, antihistamines, barbiturates, anaesthetics (nitrous oxide), benzodiazepines, metoclopramide, phenothiazines (for example prochlorperazine (Stemetil®)), tricyclic antidepressants, and other non-opioid sedatives such as chloral hydrate. While phenothiazines have useful antiemetic actions, they worsen postural hypotension, respiratory depression, sedation, and bradycardia. Fentanyl plus diazepam or midazolam may cause hypotension and profound respiratory depression in adults and neonates (Baxter, 2006).

Case report

This case illustrates the dangers of combining sedative drugs.

A woman with severe pre-eclampsia was induced at 26 weeks' gestation. She received intravenous hydralazine and chlormethiazole, plus 100 mg pethidine intramuscularly for analgesia. An hour later she was deeply sedated, and her airway was obstructed. The sedation was unrelieved and urine output was poor. She died later of adult respiratory distress syndrome (ARDS), probably due to gastric aspiration while unconscious (DH, 1991: 79).

Two potent sedative drugs were administered. Together, these drugs inhibited the vital reflexes. Aspiration of stomach contents is a risk in unconscious or heavily sedated patients. The dose of pethidine seems high for a woman known to have a reduced circulatory volume due to pre-eclampsia.

- *Selective serotonin uptake inhibitors* (SSRIs) or monoamine oxidase inhibitors (MAOIs) (including moclobemide and fluoxetine) and pethidine, pentazocine, dextromethorphan or tramadol may interact to produce hyperpyrexia, accompanied by either hypotension or hypertension, which can be fatal (Bowdle, 1998). (See Serotonin syndrome, Chapter 19.) *These opioids must be avoided for 2 weeks after discontinuation of an MAOI.* This reaction is possible but less well documented with other opioids (*Drugs and Therapy Perspectives*, 1993b).
- *Gastric emptying:* The gastric stasis induced by opioids is reversed by metoclopramide (Maxalon®), cisapride and domperidone.
- *Reduced elimination of opioids:* Cimetidine inhibits liver enzymes, preventing the breakdown of other drugs. This may increase the concentration of pethidine, methadone, fentanyl, alfentanil, or morphine. Apnoea and confusion may result. Isolated reports exist of a similar reaction between morphine and ranitidine (Baxter, 2006). Ritonavir (for HIV/AIDS) also inhibits liver enzymes and may intensify respiratory depression (Aronson, 2006).
- *Increased doses needed:* Anticonvulsants (phenytoin, carbamazepine, phenobarbitone), rifampicin, oestrogens, and tobacco all induce (speed up) liver enzymes. Therefore, some opioids (including pethidine, methadone, morphine, and pentazocine) may be more rapidly eliminated, and more frequent dosing may be required to achieve pain relief (Baxter, 2006).
- *The antidiuretic actions of oxytocin* may be augmented by opioids, increasing the risk of water intoxication (Sweetman et al., 2007).
- *Cyclizine* co-administered with opioids can precipitate pulmonary oedema but only in seriously ill patients (BNF, 2009).

Implications for practice: opioids

Potential problem	Management suggestions
Women	
Respiratory depression, leading to hypoxia. Delayed reactions are possible with regional analgesia	Respirations should be assessed prior to, during and after administration of opioids. If the respiration rate is below 12/min, or the breathing is unduly shallow or irregular, the opioid should be withheld until further assessment
	A pulse oximeter should be used to check oxygenation (Bem et al., 1996). Administration of prochlorperazine will intensify these problems
Respiratory arrest due to loss of carbon dioxide respiratory drive	Avoid administration of high dose oxygen to a patient whose respirations are depressed due to opioids
Chest infection	The detrimental effects of reduced airway clearance can be mitigated by breathing exercises, positioning and turning. Avoid smoking until the opioid has been eliminated
Hypotension	Avoid supine positions
	Monitor lying and sitting BP and pulse. This will also detect dehydration. Observe closely for first 30 minutes of epidural/ intrathecal administration
	Mobilize slowly. Report any dizziness to reduce the likelihood of falls. Administration of prochlorperazine will intensify these problems
	Fluid balance charts: intravenous fluid available to correct hypovolaemia and hypotension
Prolonged labour, decreased uterine contractility	Monitor uterine contractions. Advise women of this before labour
Nausea	Reduce anxiety, fear and pain
	Avoid sudden movements, particularly of the head. Extra care during transfers. Resting decreases nausea
	Nausea may be a symptom of hypotension. Check BP
Sedation	Monitor level of consciousness and drowsiness
	Encourage the mother not to allow sedation to interfere with appropriate 'pushing'
	Advise against use of water bath if drowsy or within 2 hours of opioid administration (NCC, 2007)
	Record mobility
	Ensure that the woman is not left unattended following administration of opioids during labour (CEMACH, 2007: 90)
	Avoid other sedating drugs, for example prochlorperazine
	Seek advice before administration to women with a history of thyroid or adrenal imbalance
Aspiration of gastric contents	Prevent/minimize sedation and nausea
	Adopt the recovery position should nausea and vomiting occur ·
Constipation/constriction of the anal sphincter	Anticipate difficulties with rectal administration of medicines if the sphincter is tight and the rectum is full
Reduced renal perfusion and retention of urine	Urine output should be monitored to exclude oliguria and retention of urine
	Ensure that a full bladder does not impede postpartum contraction of the uterus, and increase blood loss

Potential problem	Management suggestions
Pruritus/itching	Coolant gels, calamine or antihistamines should be available
	For intraspinal administration, substitution of fentanyl may be helpful
Sleep disturbance, shadows in peripheral vision	Offer reassurance and explanation. Avoid dehydration, which increases the risk of these problems (Aronson, 2006)
Myoclonus and muscular rigidity	Administer intravenous injections slowly
	Check oxygenation
	Ensure naloxone is available
	Discuss, with prescriber, possibility of excessive dose
	Ascertain if muscles of chest wall are affected
Scarring at injection site (pethedine)	Document site of injection. Do not reuse that site
Therapeutic failure	Monitor pain
Neonates	
Respiratory depression	Close observation. Extra vigilance if >100 micrograms of epidural opioids have been administered (NCC, 2007)
	Availability of oxygen, ventilatory support and naloxone. Ensure guidelines for naloxone administration are followed. If naloxone is required, a second dose will usually be necessary
	If high doses of pethidine have been administered, be aware that the infant may not respond to naloxone
	Monitor to prevent fetal acidosis
Fetal bradycardia	Monitor fetal HR regularly. Recognize a prolonged, abnormal fetal bradycardia and refer as appropriate
Sedation and/or irritability	When an opioid analgesic has been administered during labour, infants should be left with their mothers and additional assistance given to establish breastfeeding. Support may be needed for several days, until the effects of the opioid have worn off
Hypothermia	Ensure neonate is well wrapped and close to mother

Individual opioids

Although opioids have many adverse effects in common, there are some important differences between individual agents. The main distinguishing features are described below.

Pethidine

Pethidine given by subcutaneous or intramuscular injection causes local irritation, and frequent repetition at one site may lead to severe fibrosis of muscle tissue. *It is recommended that no site is used twice during labour.* Pethidine is the opioid most likely to induce maternal tachycardia and myocardial depression; therefore it is contraindicated in women with heart disease. Myoclonus and muscular rigidity, potential adverse effects of all opioids, are more likely with pethidine than other intramuscular opioids (Cherny, 1996). Pethidine is more likely to cause nausea than either morphine or diamorphine (Olofsson et al., 1996; Elbourne and Wiseman, 2000). A woman who has experienced nausea with morphine may not feel sick with pethidine and *vice versa.* Pethidine has also been used as the sole agent for epidural analgesia since it has both local anaesthetic and opioid properties.

Meptazinol

Meptazinol (Meptid®) produces less sedation and respiratory depression, but more nausea, than either pethidine or morphine (Elbourne and Wiseman, 2000). It is used intrapartum and postoperatively in some centres, but an antiemetic is often necessary. Pain relief has been found to be indistinguishable from that of pethidine (Sheikh and Tunstall, 1986; Osler, 1987; Elbourne and Wiseman, 2000). Duration of action (2–7 hours) is shorter than morphine or pethidine. Unlike pethidine, meptazinol can be metabolized by the neonate (Bushnell and Justins, 1993).

Diamorphine (heroin)

Diamorphine is rapidly metabolized in the liver to 6-monacetylmorphine (6MAM) and then to morphine. Both diamorphine and 6MAM are highly lipid soluble (more so than morphine) and therefore readily cross the blood/brain barrier to achieve rapid symptom relief (Gutstein and Akil, 2006). Diamorphine is eliminated slowly from the fetal central nervous system (Aronson, 2006), and may have a negative impact on breastfeeding (Jordan et al., 2005). Due to its high lipid solubility, enough diamorphine for 24 hours can be placed in a small volume patient-controlled analgesia (PCA) device. Diamorphine is administered by intramuscular injection in labour or by epidural or intrathecal injections, usually in association with urgent or emergency Caesarean delivery, when its rapid onset of action is important. Diamorphine is reported to produce less nausea but more euphoria and central nervous system obtunding than equianalgesic doses of morphine. This may be useful if death *in utero* has occurred. A randomized controlled trial found higher maternal satisfaction and less nausea with intramuscular diamorphine than pethidine (Fairlie et al., 1999). Intrathecal diamorphine may be less analgesic than epidural diamorphine, but causes less nausea (NCC, 2004).

Morphine

The relatively slow onset and association with pruritus have reduced the popularity of morphine in childbirth (Pang and O'Sullivan, 2008). Intraspinal morphine induces pruritus and emesis in the majority of women (Richardson, 2000).

There are case reports of intrathecal morphine or diamorphine worsening pain, due to the unopposed action of a metabolite (morphine-3-glucuronide) in the central nervous system (Twycross, 1994). Nalbuphine may be more effective than naloxone at reversing the adverse effects of epidural morphine following Caesarean delivery.

Fentanyl and derivatives

Fentanyl and its analogues, remifentanil, alfentanil, and sufentanil, are all lipid soluble and short-acting. They have largely superseded morphine in combined spinal epidurals, due to their lower incidence of nausea and pruritus. However, they have the potential to cause respiratory depression in the woman and fetus in the absence of maternal sedation (Herman et al., 1999), which is not always detected by the Apgar score (Reynolds, 1993a). Modified-release preparations are under development.

Fentanyl

This lipid-soluble opioid can be administered by several routes: transdermal, transmucosal, intravenous, epidural, and intrathecal. Since it is 80 times more potent than morphine, relatively small volumes are required. The rapid action of fentanyl (within 5 minutes) and longer duration of action (80–90 minutes) offer a considerable advantage over morphine (Kan and Hughes, 1995). The **lipophilic** properties of fentanyl make it more likely to remain in the spinal cord and less likely to spread to the medulla and cause respiratory depression (Gutstein and Akil, 2006). There is less reliance on the kidneys for elimination, making fentanyl more suitable in pre-eclampsia and for long-term administration, but it may accumulate in the occasional patient (Bem et al., 1996).

Fentanyl may reduce the heart rate of mother and fetus, and even cause asystole if the mother is intubated. Although reductions in BP are usually minor, severe hypotension has been reported. Increases in heart rate and blood pressure occur in a minority of patients (Bowdle, 1998). There-fore low concentrations of 1–2 micrograms per ml and total doses below 100 micrograms are recommended (NCC, 2007).

Fentanyl-induced cough has been reported with intravenous administration (Ghodse and Galea, 2008).

Fentanyl provokes less histamine release than morphine, reducing the incidence of:

- pruritus (66% incidence)
- hypotension
- nausea
- asthma attack.

Fentanyl requirements are increased in women regularly taking anticonvulsants.

Sufentanil (not currently available in UK)

Sufentanil is more potent than fentanyl. Duration of action may vary from 30–300 minutes. Onset of analgesia is within 5 minutes of intrathecal administration (Kan and Hughes, 1995; Harsten et al., 1997). However, the rapid passage into the brain may increase the risks of opioid myoclonus or muscular rigidity (Bowdle, 1998), swallowing difficulties (Richardson, 2000), respi-ratory arrest and profound hypotension (Aronson, 2006). Delayed hypotension and respiratory depression have been reported (Gautier et al., 1997). Itching was reported by 44% of women receiving intrathecal sufentanil (Norris et al., 1994). Sufentanil gives longer duration of both analgesia and pruritus than fentanyl (Gaiser et al., 1998). Effects on the neonate appear to be similar to those of fentanyl (Aronson, 2006).

Alfentanil

Alfentanil has shorter onset and duration of action than sufentanil but is more likely to cause nausea (Scholz et al., 1996; Bowdle, 1998). Neonatal elimination of this drug is delayed, with cases of neonatal hypotonia and respiratory depression reported (Armand et al., 1993). Alfentanil is not recommended before cord clamping, due to the dangers of transfer to the neonate. Breastfeeding is not recommended for 28 hours after administration. Skin contact and inhalation of alfentanil may cause hypersensitivity responses (Sweetman et al., 2007; Hameln Pharmaceuticals, ABPI, 2009).

Remifentanil

Remifentanil has been developed from fentanyl as an ultrashort-acting opioid. It is highly lipid soluble, and so enters the fetus and the brain readily, and rapidly relieves pain. It is rapidly broken down by enzymes in blood and tissues (esterases) in both mother and fetus. (Adult half-life is 10 minutes.) Therefore elimination does not depend on the liver and kidneys, and accumulation and impairment of breastfeeding are less likely. In a small (n = 36) randomized controlled trial, a fall in oxygen saturation to <94% and instrumental or Caesarean delivery were more likely in women receiving intravenous patient-controlled remifentanil than those receiving intramuscular pethi-dine (Thurlow et al., 2002). When compared to epidurals, intravenous remifentanil gave less analgesia, more sedation, and lower oxygen saturation (n = 52) (Volmanen et al., 2008). The rapid actions of remifentanil also predispose to respiratory depression, hypotension, bradycardia and sedation, which may occur suddenly (Aronson, 2006).

■ Intravenous remifentanil for patient controlled analgesia may be useful for women where intraspinal/ regional analgesia is contraindicated or ineffective. However, the risks of hypoxia indicate that women should be given one-to-one care (Pang and O'Sullivan, 2008), and continuous oxygen saturation monitoring is recommended (Harries and Turner, 2008).

Codeine

Codeine is a mild opioid, which is usually avoided, due to its constipating effects (particularly important following episiotomy). In normal doses, it is unlikely to be any more effective than NSAIDs. However, it is sometimes added to paracetamol or NSAIDs to control the pain following an episiotomy. Codeine is metabolized by liver enzymes into morphine, which is responsible for analgesia. However, some 10% of Caucasians lack the necessary enzyme and gain no pain relief from codeine. A further 2% metabolize codeine into morphine very quickly and may experience marked adverse reactions. Should such women be breastfeeding, a high concentration of morphine may pass into the infant, who may become sedated.

■ It is not possible to identify rapid metabolizers by laboratory tests. If breastfeeding women use codeine, infants must be observed for emesis, constipation, sedation and vital signs. Problems are most likely to arise in women who have experienced these adverse effects themselves or who have never taken codeine (MHRA, 2007).

Administration of opioids, including codeine, within 24 hours of intrathecal morphine can induce severe respiratory depression (Harries et al., 2008).

Naloxone

Naloxone (Narcan®) is an opioid antagonist: it reverses many of the actions of other opioids. It may be administered subcutaneously, intramuscularly or intravenously to reverse the respiratory depression of opioids in neonates following maternal intrapartum analgesia, but its use is controversial (Gill and Colvin, 2007). The half-life of naloxone is 1.1 ± 0.6 hours; the duration of action is 1–4 hours (Gutstein and Akil, 2006). These values are much shorter than (approximately half) those of pethidine, meptazinol and morphine. Therefore, following administration of naloxone, close observation of the neonate is required to identify a recurrence of the initial respiratory depression, and *a second dose is usually required*. In adults, administration of naloxone is usually followed by a return of pain. Other adverse effects of naloxone include changes in blood pressure, tachycardia, ventricular fibrillation, and pulmonary oedema (BNF, 2009). Naloxone may exacerbate cerebral injury in neonates (ILCR, 2006).

Naloxone is administered in accordance with published guidelines, ensuring that:

■ opioids have been administered to the mother within 4 hours of birth
■ adequate ventilation is being maintained to restore heart rate and colour
■ the mother has not abused opioids
■ respiratory function continues to be monitored (ILCR, 2006).

■ Any recreational use of opioids should be documented, as this contraindicates naloxone administration.

Summary

Although only 50% of women feel that intramuscular opioids offer adequate pain relief in labour, they are often preferred over no analgesia or nitrous oxide alone (Fairlie et al., 1999). Intramuscular opioids provide greater pain relief than a placebo, but many women remain dissatisfied (Elbourne and Wiseman, 2000). Opioids may be providing sedation rather than analgesia (Olofsson et al., 1996; Reynolds and Crowhurst, 1997). Professionals are more likely than mothers to consider pain relief to be adequate and tend to underestimate the level of pain experienced (Rajan, 1993, 1994). Intraspinal/regional opioids are becoming increasingly popular. The adverse affects of opioids on the mother, the fetus and the neonate are significant and therefore their use should continue to be approached with caution with all routes of administration, as summarized in Implications for practice (above).

II

Local anaesthetics

Local anaesthetics were developed from cocaine, which was first used in dentistry and ophthalmology in the 19th century. Cocaine has been superseded by lidocaine (lignocaine), bupivacaine (Marcain®), prilocaine, and ropivacaine. Prilocaine is primarily used in topical preparations. This chapter focuses on bupivacaine and lidocaine/lignocaine. Ropivacaine is described in Box 4.1.

Uses of local anaesthetics

Local anaesthetics provide short-term pain relief. In midwifery, they may be administered by several routes:

■ *topical or surface*, for example for intravenous cannulation (Chapter 2)
■ *subcutaneous/intradermal* for suturing

Local anaesthetics may be infiltrated directly into tissue, to varying depths, to anaesthetize relatively small areas. The addition of a vasoconstrictor (adrenaline/epinephrine) reduces the peak concentration of local anaesthetic in plasma (Catterall and Mackie, 2006). However, vasoconstrictors carry an inherent danger of ischaemic necrosis. Due to potential cardiotoxicity, the total dose of adrenaline/epinephrine is limited (Chapter 2; BNF, 2009). When intradermal lidocaine/lignocaine is being administered to decrease the pain of perineal trauma or an episiotomy, accidental injection into the presenting part of the neonate may produce serious adverse drug reactions: apnoea; loss of muscle tone; and fixed dilated pupils.

■ *infiltration around a single nerve*, for example a pudendal block for instrumental delivery

A solution of local anaesthetic is injected into or around individual nerves or nerve plexuses. The onset of action is 3 minutes for lidocaine/lignocaine and 15 minutes for bupivacaine. The duration of actions are 2–3 hours and 5–7 hours respectively, affecting motor as well as sensory modalities. A pudendal block may be performed prior to short procedures such as instrumental delivery, suturing or the manual removal of the placenta. This procedure may increase the administrator's risk from transmission of blood-borne infections (Hughes, 1992).

■ *epidural*, on the surface of the dura for labour or Caesarean section, and perineal repair, usually combined with opioids (Figures 2.1 and 2.3)
■ *spinal* (intrathecal), into the cerebrospinal fluid of the subarachnoid (intrathecal) space for labour and Caesarean section, and perineal repair, usually combined with opioids (Figures 2.1 and 2.3).

When urgent Caesarean delivery is necessary, general anaesthesia allows more rapid preparation (by 10–15 minutes) and a lower failure rate than intraspinal or regional analgesia (NCC, 2004).

How the body handles local anaesthetics

Regardless of their route of administration, local anaesthetics pass into the blood stream, whence they are eliminated (Catterall and Mackie, 2006). Local anaesthetics pass from the woman to the fetus, where they may be responsible for adverse drug reactions. As with pethidine, placental transfer and 'trapping' are increased if the fetus becomes acidotic. Local anaesthetics are extensively bound to tissues and alpha 1-acid glycoprotein (a plasma protein) in the circulation of the woman and the fetus. Only the unbound (free) fraction of the drug is responsible for actions and adverse effects. Since the fetus/neonate is relatively deficient in plasma proteins to bind these drugs, the proportion of free drug is higher and adverse effects are more likely.

The elimination of local anaesthetics is important, because any failure to clear these drugs may result in toxicity. Local anaesthetics in the bloodstream are eliminated by metabolism in the liver of the woman, fetus or neonate and the metabolites are eventually excreted by the kidney. In view of this, local anaesthetics should be avoided in patients with liver problems as they may not be able to metabolize them effectively (BNF, 2009).

Lidocaine/lignocaine

Lidocaine has been used for over 50 years, but is now reserved for situations where rapid analgesia is required (Collis et al., 2008). It is metabolized in the liver of the woman, fetus and neonate into active metabolites. Although the duration of action and the half-life of lidocaine/lignocaine are relatively short (82 minutes in the woman and 95 minutes in the neonate), the metabolites continue to be excreted by the neonate for 36–48 hours after birth, depending on the route of administration. These metabolites are responsible for some of the toxic effects of lidocaine (Kuhnert, 1993). With repeated administration, there is a danger of accumulation (Carson, 1996).

Bupivacaine

Bupivacaine (Marcain®) has a longer duration of action than lidocaine/lignocaine (2–3 hours as epidural, or 8 hours as nerve block) and therefore it is used extensively for epidural analgesia in labour. However, in the event of accidental overdose, the effects of bupivacaine will take longer to 'wear off'. The half-life of bupivacaine is 9 hours in the woman and 18 hours in the neonate. Bupivacaine, and its (relatively inert) metabolites, continue to be excreted by the neonate for 36 hours after birth. The continued presence of the drug and its metabolites may induce subtle neurobehavioural changes in the neonate, which may not be clinically significant (Kuhnert, 1993). Bupivacaine is usually administered as 0.065–0.1% solutions, and concentrations above 0.25% are rarely used (NCC, 2007).

To reach their site of action (the sodium channels in the axon membrane, below), local anaesthetics must diffuse through surrounding tissues, the myelin sheath surrounding the axon and the cell membrane itself. Therefore pain relief is not achieved for about 30 minutes with bupivacaine, which is too slow for many emergency Caesarean sections (MCHRC, 2000).

Actions of local anaesthetics

Communication in the nervous system and mechanical activity in muscle depend on the electrical excitability of the cell membranes of those tissues. Nerve impulses depend on the generation of action potentials in the cell membranes of axons of neurones. The main action of local anaesthetics is to reduce the ability of nerves to conduct action potentials and impulses.

At rest, the cell membranes of nerve and muscle are polarized (or charged). When an action potential is triggered, the nerve is depolarized (or discharged) by a rapid influx of sodium ions, followed by repolarization (recharging), due to an efflux of potassium ions. The entire process takes about one millisecond. Local anaesthetics prevent the rapid influx of sodium ions by blocking the fast sodium channels in the nerve cell membranes. This inhibits the formation of action potentials, preventing the transmission of impulses and signals along the axons and therefore blocking normal nerve function. The action of local anaesthetics is reversed when the drug passes into the bloodstream and is excreted.

The effect of a local anaesthetic on any axon depends on both the size and myelination of the axon (Catterall and Mackie, 2006). Small diameter, unmyelinated axons, which transmit pain sensation and impulses of the sympathetic nervous system (SNS), are the most sensitive to local anaesthetics, while larger, myelinated axons responsible for movement and pressure/touch sensation are relatively resistant. The interruption of sensory functions in a nerve due to the action of local anaesthetics progresses in a definite order: the sensation of pain is the first to disappear, followed by cold, warmth, touch and pressure. This means that movement and coarse touch are often preserved during local anaesthesia. When a local anaesthetic is discontinued, sensations and functions return in the reverse order, so that pain may be experienced while movement is inhibited. The interference with the functioning of the SNS is responsible for many of the adverse effects of epidural anaesthesia such as hypotension.

Regional analgesia aims to inhibit pain impulses in the spinal nerves supplying the uterus, T10–L1, while leaving the nerves needed for walking (L2–L5) intact. This is achieved by the administration of low doses and co-administration of an opioid. Further doses of local anaesthetic to the sacral region of the spinal cord may be administered for instrumental delivery (Pang and O'Sullivan, 2008).

Patient controlled epidural analgesia may offer advantages. Addition of background infusions increase dose without improving satisfaction (Pang and O'Sullivan, 2008).

Adverse effects of local anaesthetics

The potential adverse effects of local anaesthetics are the same, regardless of the route of administration. However, when normal doses are used topically and intradermally, problems are rarely encountered. Close observation for adverse effects is needed when local anaesthetics are used *via* the epidural or spinal routes or if a local anaesthetic has been inadvertently injected into a vein.

The adverse effects of local anaesthetics are related to their actions, in particular their ability to inhibit conduction of impulses in excitable tissues. Local anaesthetics block the fast sodium ion channels of *all* the body's conducting tissue, namely: central nervous system, sympathetic nervous system, peripheral nervous system, neuromuscular junctions, skeletal muscle, heart muscle, smooth muscle. Adverse effects arise from disruption of impulse transmission in the:

- central nervous system
- sympathetic nervous system
- cardiovascular system
- smooth muscle: uterus, bladder, gut
- peripheral nervous system.

Central nervous system excitation and inhibition

In the central nervous system (CNS), the sodium ion channels of the inhibitory neurones are blocked more readily than those of the excitatory neurones. Therefore, CNS responses to local anaesthetics pass through several stages from excitation through to inhibition and depression; this is seen following accidental intravascular injection:

- 'ringing in the ears', 'funny taste in the mouth'
- confusion/agitation, blurred vision, shivering
- restlessness, euphoria, chills
- nausea
- tremor
- cardiac arrhythmia
- convulsions
- respiratory or cardiac depression
- coma and death.

Practice point

■ The first signs of local anaesthetic entering the circulation are usually tingling around the mouth or ringing in the ears, and this should be reported immediately (Collis et al., 2008).

In the event of accidental intravenous administration, the initial response to local anaesthetics is usually excitation, restlessness, tremor, cardiac arrhythmia and convulsions (Hughes, 1992; CEMACH, 2007). This paradoxical excitation is followed by central nervous system cardiac and respiratory depression. However, if the systemic administration of lidocaine/lignocaine or bupivacaine is rapid, the excitatory responses may not be seen. Instead, only central nervous system depression and sudden respiratory arrest will be observed.

Practice points

■ Failure to attribute the early signs of toxicity to excessive absorption of local anaesthetic could mean that:
   ■ symptoms may be allowed to progress to more profound stages of CNS depression
   ■ further doses of local anaesthetic could be administered, intensifying the problem (Hughes, 1992).
■ 'Lipid rescue' packs containing lipid emulsions, such as Intralipid®, for intravenous infusion may be urgently requested by doctors attempting to resuscitate women who have received an overdose of local anaesthetics (Association of Anaesthetists, 2007).
■ Nausea caused by local anaesthetics may be attributed to opioid administration or the physiological response to labour and treated with antiemetics. However, nausea, disturbed mood, feelings of faintness or light-headedness may be caused by local anaesthetics, either directly or secondary to anaesthetic-induced hypotension. This possibility should be considered before further doses of local anaesthetic are administered (Brownridge, 1991).

Sympathetic blockade

The consequences of sympathetic blockade are:

■ maternal and neonatal thermoregulation failure and fever
■ loss of neonatal asphyxia reflexes
■ reduced maternal blood pressure.

Local anaesthetics inhibit the functioning of the sympathetic nerves. These control the diameter of the blood vessels, and thus affect an important aspect of blood pressure regulation (the total peripheral resistance). With the activity of the sympathetic nerves impaired, blood vessels dilate, causing both a drop in BP and an inability to vasoconstrict in response to a cold environment. The woman may complain of feeling cold, shiver uncontrollably or, conversely, may develop a fever/pyrexia, particularly nulliparous women or if epidural administration exceeds 5 hours (Leighton and Halpern, 2002). Likewise, the neonate will be vulnerable to the cold (Howell, 1995c; El-Refaey et al., 2000).

Practice point

■ Blankets should be available to provide optimum comfort in labour. The neonate should be maintained in a warm environment, preferably by contact with the mother.

Maternal pyrexia (>38°C or 100.4°F) is associated with administration of epidural analgesia (Anim-Soumuah et al., 2005). This was recorded in 16.6% (120/724) of healthy parturients (n = 1218). These infants are more likely to convulse, develop abnormal heart rates, become hypotonic or require resuscitation. Maternal intrapartum fever may induce an even higher temperature in the fetus (by 0.5–0.9°C); where the neonate is also suffering from an ischaemic insult, this degree of pyrexia may increase the extent of neurological damage (Lieberman et al., 2000).

Practice point

■ While unnecessary antibiotic administration to neonates and new mothers should be avoided (Klein, 2006), it is essential that infection is recognized and treated promptly.

At birth, neonates rely on reflex responses to asphyxia to take a first breath, and this reflex depends on the activity of the sympathetic nervous system. With the use of local anaesthetics, the neonate's reflex responses to delivery may be suppressed, requiring careful assessment and possibly prompt action.

The cardiovascular system: hypotension

The fall in BP that may accompany intraspinal local anaesthetics is due to vasodilation plus simultaneous myocardial depression. However, the relief of pain and distress afforded by effective analgesia may be a contributory factor.

Local anaesthetics inhibit the sympathetic nervous system, which is responsible for keeping the arterioles constricted and the BP and heart rate within normal limits. Thus they have the potential to compromise the cardiovascular system, causing hypotension, bradycardia and even cardiac arrest. Clinically significant maternal hypotension, defined as a fall of 20–30% in pre-anaesthetic systolic BP, or a systolic BP below 100 mmHg, occurs in 5–15% of deliveries with epidural anaesthesia and 5–82% of deliveries with spinal anaesthesia (Hollmen, 1993; Shennan et al., 1995); however, a much lower incidence is reported in clinical trials (Simmons et al., 2007). The frequency of hypotension increases with concentration of bupivacaine (Hess et al., 2006).

The risk of hypotension is greater if the woman is dehydrated, hypovolaemic or suffering from septicaemia/bacteraemia. Therefore, prior to intraspinal administration of local anaesthetics for Caesarean section or if high doses are to be administered, intravenous fluids are infused, for example 20–25 ml/kg crystalloid solution (Hollmen, 1993) or 1 litre of compound lactate solution (Shennan et al., 1995). The infusion of fluids aims to maintain **venous return** and therefore **cardiac output**, thus countering any hypotension (NCC, 2004). Where low doses of local anaesthetics are administered (usually with fentanyl), venous access is secured should intravenous fluids be needed to correct hypotension urgently, but fluids are not routinely infused before analgesia is administered (NCC, 2007).

Case report

A woman was given epidural analgesia 36 hours after a forceps delivery to control perineal pain, despite refusing an intravenous infusion. She was passing little urine, with evidence of dehydration; frusemide had no effect on the urine output. This indicates poor renal perfusion, due to hypotension. Her hands became numb, due to the effects of the local anaesthetics. There were no recordings of: blood pressure, respirations, level of block or pulse oximetry.

She received sedation when she became agitated. Restlessness may have been due either to hypoxia or the drugs administered. Hypoxia was diagnosed on the ECG. Only then was oxygen given. Hypotension developed, leading to cardiac arrest and death (DH, 1996: 93).

This woman died of hypoxia, due to hypotension and poor ventilation. Hypotension was caused by the combination of epidural opiates and local anaesthetics administered without intravenous fluids. With better monitoring and the appropriate use of intravenous fluids, this woman would have lived. However, rapid administration of crystalloid intravenous fluids (such as Ringer's, saline or glucose) may induce a diuresis and fail to prevent a drop in blood pressure (Richardson, 2000).

Practice point

■ Cardiac output and circulating volume are assessed by careful monitoring of urine output, which can act as an 'early warning sign'. Oliguria (low urine output) indicates that renal autoregulation is occurring in an attempt to counteract impending or actual hypotension. It is essential that the midwife responds to any decline in maternal urine output (Chapter 1).

Failure to monitor urine output in women receiving epidural anaesthesia is cited as a contributory factor in maternal deaths (DH, 1998).

Case report

Three hours after the administration of epidural analgesia, an emergency Caesarean section was performed for fetal distress. Prior to section, 0.5% bupivacaine (2 x 10 ml) was administered. Recovery and initial observations taken by the midwife were normal. However, 40 minutes later, the woman was unrousable. Autopsy showed extensive haemorrhage into parametrial tissues (DH, 1994: 91).

The physiological signs of haemorrhage were modified by the blockade of the sensory and sympathetic nervous systems. The inadequacy of vital sign recordings indicated to the assessors that postoperative care was substandard.

Local anaesthetic-induced vasodilation may reduce the ability of blood vessels to constrict in response to haemorrhage. Therefore even a moderate haemorrhage may cause hypotension and blood loss postpartum may be increased (Beischer et al., 1997); a retrospective cohort study identified epidural analgesia and prolonged labour as risk factors for postpartum haemorrhage (n = 13,868) (Magann et al., 2005). However, for Caesarean section, blood loss is greater with general anaesthesia (NCC, 2004).

Practice point

■ It is important that any maternal hypotension is recognized immediately, because *the blood flow to the uterus, and hence fetal oxygenation, declines in direct relation to maternal blood pressure.* By jeopardizing the blood supply to the placenta, hypotension causes fetal acidosis, and depresses the neonate's central nervous system (Roberts et al., 1995).

Hypotension is compounded by aortocaval compression by the infant's head, particularly if the woman is supine or obese, or if the uterus is enlarged due to multiple pregnancy, diabetes or polyhydramnios (Hollmen, 1993). To avoid compression of the vena cava, the woman should remain upright or the uterus must be displaced laterally; a woman receiving local anaesthetics during labour should avoid the supine position, including reclining chairs, and the midwife should regularly ascertain the position of the uterus. If the woman does not wish to remain upright, a lateral position should be adopted, or alternatively, a 20 degree tilt achieved by using a 'wedge'. Operating tables are often titled 15 degrees for Caesarean delivery (NCC, 2004). Aortocaval compression may be less if the woman is upright and ambulant (Al-Mufti et al., 1997). If a woman (inadvertently) lies supine at term, the placental blood flow will decrease by 20–30%, without any change in maternal vital signs. If position is not corrected, supine hypotension syndrome, leading to maternal collapse, may follow. This suggests that practitioners should consider performing vaginal examinations with the woman in a lateral position (Yerby, 2000).

Case report

A woman of 30 weeks' gestation was given a spinal anaesthetic. She was premedicated with 15 mg papaveretum and given 400 ml of Hartman's solution, followed by 1 ml of 0.5% heavy bupivacaine. She noticed her legs becoming weak, which was attributed to bupivacaine, and she was placed in a supine position with the table tilted laterally. Her blood pressure fell rapidly and she was treated with fluids and ephedrine (2 x 15 mg). Further measures taken were the administration of oxygen, atropine, adrenaline/epinephrine, and a further 1,600 ml of fluids. Pulmonary oedema and subsequently death from adult respiratory distress syndrome followed (DH, 1994: 83).

It is likely that the hypotension was due to aortocaval compression, because a small degree of lateral tilt would not prevent this. The interventions that led to this catastrophe followed attempts to correct the hypotension. Pulmonary oedema was caused by the combination of fluids and two vasoconstrictors (that is, adrenaline/epinephrine plus ephedrine).

When 14 healthy labouring women, receiving effective epidural analgesia, 0.25–0.5% bupivacaine, adopted the supine position for 10 minutes, an 18% fall in maternal lower limb digital artery pressure and a, clinically significant, 8% fall in fetal cerebral oxygen delivery occurred (Aldrich et al., 1995). Hence, measuring maternal blood pressure in the arm could allow significant hypotension at the level of the uterus to remain undetected. This suggests that the use of leg cuffs should be considered when regional analgesia is used (Hollmen, 1993).

If placental blood flow is already compromised, for example by pregnancy-induced hypertension, the vulnerable fetus may not be able to withstand the extra stress of low maternal blood pressure; so fetal monitoring is recommended when regional anaesthesia is administered for emergency Caesarean delivery (NCC, 2004). Maternal deaths have occurred when epidural analgesia has been used alone to control hypertension in women with pre-eclampsia or eclampsia (DH, 1994). Thus the use of epidural analgesia in these women requires careful management (Hollmen, 1993).

Practice point

■ Particularly careful BP monitoring is needed on initial administration of regional analgesia and when top-up doses are administered. Measurements every 5 minutes for the first 15 or 30 minutes are recommended (Shennan et al., 1995; NCC, 2007).

Hypotension is more likely with a spinal (intrathecal) than an epidural anaesthetic. High-risk situations include:

■ within the first 30 minutes of administration

- when top-up doses are administered
- aortocaval compression (exacerbated in the supine position)
- hypovolaemia
- when anaesthesia reaches the level of the T4 segment (nipple level) (Box 4.2, below)
- if there are pre-existing cardiac problems such as heart block
- standing may induce postural hypotension.

Clinically significant maternal hypotension, jeopardizing the fetus, may not be manifest as maternal symptoms. If hypotension is not *corrected within 2 minutes*, fetal bradycardia, acidosis and depression will follow (Hughes, 1992; Downing and Ramasubramanian, 1993). Clinically it may be difficult to attribute fetal heart rate abnormalities to the direct action of the local anaesthetics or to maternal hypotension caused by drugs, although fetal acidosis during Caesarean section is a recognized complication of local anaesthetics (Steer, 1995).

Practice points

- If blood pressure falls, the woman should be turned on her left side, her legs elevated (Trendelenburg position) if possible and intravenous fluids administered, according to local protocols. Medical advice must be sought immediately. If blood pressure does not improve within 2–3 minutes, oxygen and vasopressors (ephedrine or phenylephrine) may be required (Box 4.2) (Davis, 1992).
- Following epidural anaesthesia, the functions of the sympathetic nervous system and blood pressure control may return *after* the return of sensation. It is therefore important that BP monitoring is continued during this period.

Bupivacaine has more myocardial depressant action than lidocaine/lignocaine. This is most severe if the parturient is acidotic or hypoxic. The cardiotoxicity threshold is lower in pregnancy; this is attributed to increased progesterone concentrations and increased sensitivity of the **alpha receptors** of the sympathetic nervous system. Cardiac arrests and maternal deaths have been reported. Therefore, low concentrations are used in labour.

Practice point

- If the local anaesthetic has reached the cardiac nerves (which arise from thoracic segments T1–T4), heart rate will be slowed, despite hypotension. This can be identified by heart rate monitoring (Collis et al., 2008).

Bupivacaine is never used for intravenous anaesthesia since bupivacaine-induced cardiotoxicity is difficult to treat (Catterall and Mackie, 2006). Accidental intravenous administration of bupivacaine during epidural anaesthesia in labour has produced cardiovascular collapse (Kuhnert, 1993).

Box 4.2 Vasopressors: ephedrine and phenylephrine

Synthetic compounds acting on the sympathetic nervous system are known as **sympathomimetics**. These include bronchodilators, tocolytics, stimulants (Chapter 20) and vasopressors. To correct hypotension, phenylephrine or ephedrine may be administered by slow intravenous injection. These drugs stimulate **alpha receptors** of the sympathetic nervous system to constrict blood vessels and raise blood pressure; this may reflexively reduce heart rate, most particularly following phenylephrine administration. In contrast, the direct action of ephedrine on the heart is to increase heart rate (via the **beta receptors**). The response in an individual woman cannot be predicted, and heart rate monitoring is essential.

The potential to constrict uterine vessels is minimized if the drug is given slowly or as an infusion. Although this is considered safe for a full-term healthy fetus, a high-risk fetus may not be able to tolerate this vasoconstriction (Hollmen, 1993) and therefore the dose may be reduced (Hughes, 1992).

Several adverse reactions, such as nausea, hypertension, heart rate changes, cardiac dysrhythmia, and chest pain require monitoring. Other potential problems include anxiety, restlessness, headache, breathing difficulties, dizziness, tremor, sweating, retention of urine, hypersalivation, hyperglycaemia and, rarely, glaucoma (BNF, 2009). These are similar to the adverse effects of ritodrine (Chapter 7). Ephedrine may stimulate the fetal heart, causing tachycardia and hypoxia (Eggers et al., 2008). Like adrenaline/epinephrine, vasopressors may interact with oxytocin to cause severe hypertension.

Vasopressor administration is repeated as needed (every 3–4 minutes, up to 30 mg for ephedrine, every 15 minutes for phyenylephrine) (BNF, 2009). Women receiving regional analgesia for Caesarean delivery may be prescribed intravenous infusions of vasopressors. Phenylephrine may be preferred by some consultants (NCC, 2004), particularly if tachycardia would not be tolerated. However, it may cause fetal hypoxia and bradycardia when administered in labour, and several different drug concentrations are available, which should not be confused during administration (Eggers et al., 2008). Women intaking cocaine may not respond to ephedrine, and phenylephrine may be needed (Kuczkowski, 2004).

Intravenous fluids

During regional analgesia, fluids may be infused to maintain maternal blood pressure and prevent a fall in placental blood flow, with subsequent fetal distress (Hofmeyr, 1995). Maternal death has also occurred from circulatory overload during induced labour (DH, 1996: 26), indicating the importance of careful monitoring (Chapter 2).

Practice point

■ To ensure safety, protocols for management of complications (however rare) must be in place, and experienced personnel must be available. The necessary equipment, including facilities for resuscitation and 'rescue drugs' such as ephedrine, must be in place and checked daily (Brownridge, 1991; *Drugs and Therapy Perspectives*, 1996).

Peripheral nervous system

Loss of sensation and motor control

When administered by the intravenous, epidural or spinal routes, local anaesthetics affect the motor neurones as well as the sensory neurones. The recipient may feel weak and numb. Blockade of motor neurones of the lower spinal segments by epidural anaesthesia inhibits movement during labour. Paralysis of the legs, leaving the woman unable to stand or walk, rarely occurs, unless high doses are administered. This is less evident with bupivacaine or ropivacaine rather than lidocaine/lignocaine (Catterall and Mackie, 2006), lower concentrations (0.0625% or 0.125% rather than 0.25% bupivacaine) (Harms et al., 1999), and regimens containing opioids (NCC, 2007).

Practice point

■ Women in labour should be encouraged to mobilize, accompanied and with continuous fetal monitoring, but this does not affect outcomes (NCC, 2007). Walking may not be advisable for women who feel sedated, unsteady or have abnormal sensation in their legs and feet (Mayberry et al., 2002). Motor function and balance are assessed each time a women starts to mobilize (Clyburn et al., 2008).

Laxity of the pelvic floor muscles, due to the action of local anaesthetics, is the mechanism behind malrotation, malposition and **shoulder dystocia** (Thorp et al., 1993; Howell, 1995c; Klein, 2006). Some studies have linked bupivacaine with reduced neonatal muscle tone, suckling and reflex responses. Also, loss of sensation prevents the woman from feeling aware of uterine contractions and the birth process, which may lead to dissatisfaction later (Brownridge, 1991).

Local anaesthetics for labour are intended to anaesthetize the spinal nerves below the 10–12th thoracic segment (T10–T12) (innervation of the uterus); those for Caesarean sections are intended to reach the 4–5th thoracic segments (T4–T5) (Harries et al., 2008). To ensure effective analgesia, doctors assess and document the level of 'block' bilaterally (Box 4.3).

Accidental intrathecal injection is followed by rapid analgesia and sensory and motor block.

Box 4.3 Assessing the block

The spinal cord has a segmental structure: 8 cervical (C) (neck region), 12 thoracic (T), 5 lumbar (L), 5 sacral (S), and 1 coccygeal. Each segment gives rise to a pair of spinal nerves, responsible for control and sensation in the somatic structures (muscles of trunk and limbs) supplied. Each spinal nerve:

- has a dorsal (sensory) root and a ventral (motor) root
- has sensory, motor and sympathetic components
- supplies sensory nerve fibres to a distinct area of skin, called a 'dermatome'. There is some overlap and individual variation in dermatome distribution.

Spinal nerves emerge between the adjacent vertebrae, through the intervertebral foramina. In adults, the segments of the lower spinal cord are not aligned with the vertebrae.

Dermatomes of the trunk run in parallel horizontal bands, but dermatomes of the limbs are less obvious. The extent or level of anaesthesia can be assessed by:

- testing skin sensation (sensory component)
- observing skin warmth/dryness (sympathetic component)
- ability to raise the legs or move (motor component)

with reference to the dermatome chart/map (Figure 4.2). Three skin sensations – light touch, pinprick and temperature – are experienced by different types of nerve fibres, with different sensitivities to local anaesthetics. During regional anaesthesia, these components and sensations are lost at different dermatome levels.

Practice points

- Light touch may be assessed using cotton wool or Von Frey hairs.
- Cold sensation is tested using ethyl chloride spray or ice cubes. Ice cubes also give sensations of touch and wetness, which appear at lower levels than cold sensation (Harries et al., 2008).
- The soles of the feet will be checked for dryness (no sweat) and warmth (vasodilatation) to ensure the sympathetic nerve fibres are blocked at L5 and S1.
- If the sympathetic nerves are blocked at T4, there is a danger that the sympathetic nerves supplying the heart (T1–T4) may be anaesthetized: heart rate and BP may fall.
- If the motor block rises above the 10th thoracic segment (T10), nerves controlling the intercostal muscles will be inhibited, which may cause breathing difficulties.
- If motor block rises into the mid-cervical region (C3–C5), it will affect movement of the diaphragm; this causes difficulty in coughing and speaking and can lead to respiratory arrest. Rise of the block is tested by assessing movements and grip in the hands, which are supplied by T1–C6.

Testing is undertaken after each dose and regularly (Figure 4.2) (Collis et al., 2008).

Respiratory depression

The intercostal muscles may be impaired by high spinal anaesthesia, causing overreliance on the diaphragm. However, at term, the diaphragm is 'splinted' by the uterus, and is less able to increase its movement to compensate for any inadequacies of the intercostal muscles. When these problems are compounded by the risk of medullary paralysis and the respiratory depression associated with opioids, there is a possibility of inadequate ventilation and even arrest.

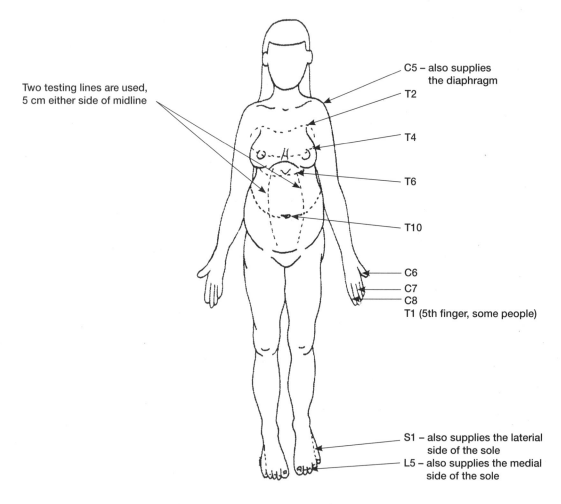

Figure 4.2 Key dermatomes
Source: Harries et al. (2008) © 2008 By permission of Oxford University Press

Practice points

■ Rate and depth of respirations should be monitored and oxygenation checked by pulse oximetry if necessary.

■ Pulse oximetry may not detect mild or moderate ventilatory depression (Herman et al., 1999).

■ If the woman sits up or is supported by pillows, the diaphragm will mobilize more easily and respiratory distress may be relieved. (The diaphragm is supplied by cervical nerves C3–C5, and should not be affected by regional analgesia.)

- The level of the block should be checked by appropriate professionals (Box 4.2).
- Intubation is occasionally needed to counter these problems (NCC, 2004).

Depression of smooth muscle

Uterine, gut and bladder contractions are depressed by local anaesthetics:

- *Inhibition of the bladder* usually reduces the ability to micturate spontaneously and causes retention of urine, but conversely, urinary and faecal incontinence are possible after childbirth, mainly with high-dose local anaesthetics (above 0.25% bupivacaine or equivalent) (NCC, 2007). Epidural analgesia is associated with an increased risk of postpartum urinary retention (Olofsson et al., 1997); the incidence is lower with combined spinal epidural (Simmons et al., 2007). It is important not to underestimate the potential problems, short and long term, arising from repeated urinary catheterization (Mander, 1994). However, after 6 hours of epidural administration, some authors recommended catheterization (Pang and O'Sullivan, 2008).

Practice points

- Since bladder sensation may be absent or diminished, the woman should be encouraged to micturate before initiation of the epidural and every 2–3 hours.
- Bladder distension should not be allowed to occur, as a distended bladder interferes with contractions of the uterus during and after delivery, increasing the risk of postpartum haemorrhage.

- *Postpartum incontinence* is associated with instrumental delivery, large infants, parity and obesity; any effect of epidural analgesia is likely to be secondary to prolonged second stage (Leighton and Halpern, 2002). Perineal trauma is more likely to be attributed to instrumental delivery rather than epidural analgesia *per se* (Lierberman and O'Donoghue, 2002).
- *Nausea and vomiting* associated with regional analgesia may be secondary to hypotension or a direct effect of the inhibition of the smooth muscle of the gut. Antiemetics are often administered to women undergoing Caesarean delivery.

Effects on the uterus

Local anaesthetics prolong labour by:

- relaxing the pelvic floor muscles
- diminishing the 'bearing down' reflexes
- decreasing expulsive efforts
- direct action on the uterine muscle reducing the muscle tone
- diminishing the pulsatile release of oxytocin from the posterior pituitary gland
- interfering with the reflex surge of oxytocin release that occurs between full cervical dilation and crowning of the fetal head; this reflex depends on communication within the spinal cord (Figure 6.1)
- exerting a weak anti-inflammatory action on the collagen fibres of the cervix (Leighton and Halpern, 2002)
- reducing intrauterine release of prostaglandins.

Effects on labour

When epidurals, with or without opioids, are administered:

- the first stage of labour may be more likely to be prolonged (the mean differences between epidural anaesthesia and parenteral opioids was 42 minutes (Halpern et al., 1998)), particularly if oxytocin is not administered (Alexander et al., 2002). However, this is not supported by all reviewers (NCC, 2007)

▨ the second stage of labour is prolonged by 14 (Halpern et al., 1998) or 15 minutes (Anim-Somuah et al., 2005); this may be further prolonged by delayed pushing (Roberts et al., 2004)
▨ cervical dilatation is slower
▨ oxytocin is more likely to be used
▨ fetal malposition is more common (Anim-Somuah et al., 2005)
▨ Caesarean section for fetal distress is more likely (n = 4,421, **RR** (relative risk) 1.42, 95% CI, 0.99–2.03; Note: this does not reach conventional statistical significance) (Anim-Somuah et al., 2005), and the overall rate of Caesarean delivery is doubled if epidurals are administered when the cervix is less than 4 cm dilated (**OR**, odds ratio) 2.59, 95% CI, 1.29–5.23) (Klein, 2006)
▨ instrumental deliveries are more common (n = 4,168, RR 1.66, 95% CI, 1.41–1.94) (Anim-Somuah et al., 2005), mainly in infants in the occiput-posterior position, that is, where malposition has occurred (NCC, 2007). Reviewers suggest that delayed pushing may reduce the numbers of mid-pelvic forceps deliveries in hospitals where this procedure is common (Thorp et al., 1993; Howell, 1995c; Halpern et al., 1998; McRae-Bergeron et al., 1998; Roberts et al., 2004).

Although studies offer no consensus (Dewan and Cohen, 1994; Fung, 2000), in a large study (n = 1,250), the combined use of oxytocin, induction and epidural analgesia appeared to be additive in bringing about a higher rate of instrumental and operative deliveries (Carli et al., 1993). Both opioids and local anaesthetics affect uterine muscle and oxytocin release. In a cohort study involving 1,561 nulliparous parturients, the risk of Caesarean section increased threefold with the use of combined spinal epidural analgesia and 4.7fold with the use of continuous infusion epidurals (Traynor et al., 2000).

The incidence of Caesarean section is increased if:

▨ two or more bolus doses of bupivacaine are administered (Hess et al., 2000)
▨ epidural analgesia is administered prior to either cervical dilatation >5cm (Thorp et al., 1993; Klein, 2006) or engagement of the fetal head (Traynor et al., 2000)
▨ oxytocin is administered as low-dose, rather than high-dose (4–12 milliunits per minute) regimens (Kotaska et al., 2006).

Where epidural analgesia was administered later, when cervical dilation was more than 4 cm, there was no statistically significant increase in Caesarean delivery (Klein, 2006), particularly in hospitals where rates of Caesarean were low (4–5%) (Sharma et al., 1997).

Some authors have suggested that epidural analgesia be discontinued in the second stage of labour, due to increased incidence of malrotation of the presenting part, necessitating assisted vaginal delivery (Howell and Chalmers, 1992). This increases pain, which may have adverse psychological and physiological consequences, including hyperventilation and alkalosis, and is not recommended in current guidelines (NCC, 2007).

Practice point

■ Women should be advised that although epidural analgesia is more likely to be effective than other methods of analgesia, its effects on the physiology of labour reduce the chances of a 'normal' vaginal delivery, particularly in nulliparous women (Howell, 1995c; Lierberman and O'Donoghue, 2002; NCC, 2007).

Reduction in the muscle tone of the uterus may impair the contraction of the uterus after birth and contribute to the increase the risk of haemorrhage (Campbell and Lees, 2000; Magann et al., 2005; above).

Hypersensitivity reactions

Rarely, individuals are hypersensitive to local anaesthetics or their preservatives and some cross-sensitivities occur. The clinical manifestations of hypersensitivity include:

- dermatitis
- asthma
- **anaphylaxis**
- **methaemoglobinaemia**.

Both prilocaine, contained in EMLA® cream, and lidocaine/lignocaine may induce methaemo-globinaemia in rare, genetically susceptible individuals. Methaemoglobin is an oxidized form of haemoglobin that is unable to transport oxygen and is normally converted back to haemo-globin by various enzymes. Genetic deficiencies of these enzymes can be magnified by certain drugs, with disastrous consequences. Methaemoglobinaemia presents as cyanosis, accompa-nied by headache, weakness and breathlessness.

Effects on the neonate

Occasionally, local anaesthetics can be transferred from mother to neonate. Possible adverse effects include respiratory, cardiovascular and central nervous system depression, together with fits.

Case report

A healthy woman received local anaesthetic cream for an episiotomy. A well infant with high Apgar scores was delivered, but within minutes he suddenly stopped breathing, and developed a slow heart rate and poor muscle tone. During transfer to neonatal intensive care, he had several fits. The only abnormalities identified were high levels of lidocaine and prilocaine in blood and urine. Acute intoxication with local anaesthetic was diagnosed. Seizures were treated in intensive care for 5 days, and neurodevelopmental outcomes were normal at 12 months.

In this case, and a similar case where a healthy woman received an injection of local anaesthetic for vacuum extraction, the only source of the local anaesthetic was the mother's perineum (Pignotti et al., 2005).

Practice point

- In these cases, close monitoring, retention of neonatal urine samples and early transfer to neonatal intensive care were essential.

Older studies have linked epidural anaesthesia with neonatal depression and neurobehav-ioural abnormalities at 24 hours postpartum (Catterall and Mackie, 2006). Epidural local anaes-thetics may have subtle neurobehavioural effects on the neonate, which are undetectable at 18 months (Howell and Chalmers, 1992; Kuhnert, 1993). Halpern et al. (1999) suggest that any neurobehavioural adverse effects are no impediment to breastfeeding, providing effective support is offered.

The use of epidural analgesia increases the risk of neonatal hypoglycaemia, tachypnoea and a disturbance of lipid metabolism (Howell and Chalmers, 1992). Fetal acidaemia, without obvious clinical sequelae, was more likely when regional, particularly spinal, rather than general anaes-thesia was used for Caesarean section (Roberts et al., 1995). Neonates are less likely to have low Apgar scores at 5 minutes or to require naloxone after epidural analgesia than after intramuscular opioids (Halpern et al., 1998).

Box 4.4 Ropivacaine and levobupivacaine

Ropivacaine was developed to provide long-lasting local anaesthesia without the cardiotoxicity of bupi-vacaine to which it is chemically related. While some authors consider these two agents to be equally effective (Muir et al., 1997; Irestedt et al., 1998; NCC, 2007), others have found that ropivacaine is less potent (Capogna et al., 1999; Fischer et al., 2000). Suggestions that ropivacaine might provide a less intense motor blockade than bupivacaine that could reduce the rate of instrumental deliveries (Cederholm, 1997) and improve ambu-lation and micturition were not supported by meta-analysis (NCC, 2007: 134). In one study (n = 60), ropivacaine was found to have fewer neurobehavioural effects on neonates than bupivacaine (Stienstra et al., 1995; Writer et al., 1998). However, onset of action and termination of motor blockade following delivery may be slower than with bupivacaine (McCrae et al., 1995).

Levobupivacaine, a form of bupivacaine, has less effect on heart muscle but the same effect on other nerves as bupivacaine, and may be safer (Pang and O'Sullivan, 2008), but there is little evidence of clinically important differences (NCC, 2007). Levobupivacaine caused less motor block than bupivacaine in one trial (n = 102) (Atienzar et al., 2008). It may be preferred for large bolus doses (Collis et al., 2008).

Cautions and contraindications: local anaesthetics

- Local anaesthetics should not be used in individuals where a previous allergy has occurred to any chemically related anaesthetic or other constituent of the preparation.
- Hypovolaemia must be corrected before intraspinal administration (BNF, 2009).
- Administration of local anaesthetics is not advised if the woman has had a recent haemor-rhage or sepsis, as the cardiovascular responses to blood loss or septicaemia will be compro-mised (CEMACH, 2007).
- Topical local anaesthetics should be applied cautiously, if at all, to inflamed areas.
- Cautious use of local anaesthetics is indicated for women with:
  - ❱ heart block or impaired cardiac conduction
  - ❱ hypovolaemia and other forms of shock
  - ❱ maternal bradycardia
  - ❱ **porphyria**
  - ❱ epilepsy
  - ❱ respiratory impairment
  - ❱ liver or kidney disease
  - ❱ hyperthyroidism
  - ❱ family history of malignant hyperthermia
  - ❱ myasthenia gravis.

Interactions: local anaesthetics

The unwanted effects of local anaesthetics may be enhanced by the co-administration of antiarrhythmics, opioids and other central nervous system depressants, including alcohol and prochlorperazine:

- Regular use of alcohol increases the risk of therapeutic failure.

- Calcium channel blockers (nifedipine (for tocolysis) and verapamil) enhance the cardiotoxicity of bupivacaine and increase the risk of hypotension (Baxter, 2006).
- Beta blockers, cimetidine and ranitidine interfere with the hepatic clearance of bupivacaine. This increases the risk of toxicity, but the clinical importance is uncertain (Kuhnert, 1993).
- Benzodiazepines may affect the elimination of local anaesthetics. Increased bupivacaine (but not lidocaine/lignocaine) concentrations have been reported in patients taking diazepam.
- Tricyclic antidepressants and phenothiazines (for example prochlorperazine) increase the risk of heart block, particularly if adrenaline/epinephrine is used.
- Ropivacaine elimination may be affected by some quinolone antibiotics (Baxter, 2006).

Implications for practice: local anaesthetics

Problem	Management suggestions
Topical applications (EMLA®)	
Contact dermatitis	Coolants available. Wear gloves
Epidural or spinal anaesthesia	
Maternal	
Hypotension	Advise the woman to remain upright and mobile in whatever position is comfortable, and avoid supine positions, including reclining chairs
	Secure intravenous access for all women and ensure intravenous fluids are available and clearly labelled, if needed
	Prehydration with intravenous fluids prior to Caesarean delivery or if high doses are employed
	Monitor BP, HR and rhythm, pre-therapy (not during a contraction) and every 5 minutes for 20 minutes, then every 30 minutes. Report systolic BP below 100 mmHg
	Monitor urine output. Consider protocols for catheterization
	Assess skin and oxygen saturation with pulse oximeter (continuously during Caesarean delivery)
	ECG during induction of regional anaesthesia, if indicated
	During emergency Caesarean delivery, monitor fetal HR until skin incision begins
	Ensure vasopressor agents available, for example ephedrine
	Check history and ECG for heart block
	Check history for liver disease, malignant hyperthermia
	Ensure no signs of **shock** present
	Use test dose
Respiratory depression	Report difficulty with breathing, coughing or speaking. Sensation will be monitored (Box 4.2)
Loss of uterine contractility	Monitor
	Advise of possibility of prolonged second stage and increased incidence of instrumental deliveries
Urine retention/incontinence	Monitor output and specific gravity
	Avoid overdistension of the bladder
Emesis	Check BP, minimize hypotension
	Prophylactic antiemetics may be prescribed in association with Caesarean delivery

Reduced mobility	Record mobility and discuss any need for prophylactic anticoagulants. Discuss with the multidisciplinary team the need to leave the catheter *in situ after* delivery
Risk of fits	Diazepam available
Intoxication, loss of consciousness	Ensure protocols are available should accidental overdose or administration by inappropriate routes occur
Loss of thermoregulation	Prevent shivering. Blankets should be available
	Monitor maternal temperature and pre-empt non-infectious fever/pyrexia
	Report temperature ≥38°C and investigate for sepsis
	Monitor infant for convulsions
Hypersensitivity	Be aware of cross-sensitivity between local anaesthetics
Methaemoglobinaemia	Recognize cyanosis. Have oxygen ready
	Methylene blue antidote should be available (rarely needed)
Therapeutic failure	Monitor pain and satisfaction. Report abnormal requests for additional analgesia promptly
	If analgesia is not achieved within 30 minutes, the anaesthetist should be recalled (NCC, 2007)
	If a Caesarean delivery is to be performed, the anaesthetist should be informed of the efficacy (or otherwise) of the epidural
Fetal/neonatal	
Depression of fetal HR	Monitor continuously for the first 20–30 minutes after initial and 10–30 minutes after subsequent doses or for the duration of the epidural. Liaise with medical staff
Respiratory depression	Prepare to assist neonate to establish respirations
	Be prepared to arrange transfer to neonatal intensive care facilities
Impaired suckling reflexes	Give extra assistance to initiate breastfeeding
Spinal/intrathecal anaesthesia	
Respiratory depression	Monitor rate and depth of respirations regularly
	Ensure resuscitation equipment is available

Summary: pain relief in labour

All pharmacological methods of pain relief may have adverse effects that may be detrimental to the mother, fetus, neonate, progress of labour or breastfeeding. All available options, non-pharmacological and pharmacological, should be discussed with the woman, while taking into account her medical and obstetric history (Findley and Chamberlain, 1999). Information given should include adverse drug reactions. Nondisclosure of serious risks is not acceptable to women (Pattee et al., 1997). There may be advantages in selecting analgesia that permits ambulation and mobility during labour, as this, by itself, may shorten labour and reduce the need for analgesia (de Jong et al., 1997; Al-Mufti et al., 1997; Larimore and Cline, 2000). Mobility is hindered by either sedation or motor blockade of the legs.

Regional analgesia offers more effective and satisfactory pain relief than other methods of obstetric analgesia, particularly intramuscular opioids (Anim-Somuah et al., 2005; NCC, 2007); these benefits persist 24 hours after birth (Sheiner et al., 2000). Epidurals are associated with a failure rate of up to 23%, which is improved by resiting (Howell and Chalmers, 1992; Le Coq et al., 1998; Collis et al., 2008). The addition of opioids to regional analgesia offers some advantages, but many adverse effects of opioids remain (Box 4.5 below). Of the neonatal outcomes examined, only acid-base status and naloxone administration were improved (Reynolds et al., 2002; Anim-Somuah et al., 2005). Epidural and combined spinal epidural anaesthesia for Caesarean section carry a lower mortality rate than general anaesthesia (Reynolds, 1993b; DH, 1998).

While intraspinal or regional local anaesthetics and opioids offer the most effective analgesia available (NCC, 2007), the benefits of epidural anaesthesia are tempered not only by adverse effects on mother, infant and initiation of breastfeeding, but also by increases in:

- the duration of the second stage of labour
- the need for oxytocin augmentation
- the incidence of malposition
- the incidence of instrumental deliveries
- and, in some circumstances, Caesarean delivery.

The problems associated with instrumental deliveries, such as vaginal lacerations, should be considered when evaluating epidural analgesia (Okojie and Cook, 1999), and the impact of delayed pushing requires further investigation (Roberts et al., 2004). Carli et al. (1993). Thorp et al. (1993) suggest that epidural anaesthesia may be contributing to the current 'epidemic' of instrumental deliveries and Caesarean sections in primagravidae. However, rising rates of Caesarean section may be attributed to many factors, including fear of the complications of instrumental delivery (Drife, 1996).

Interpretation of studies in this area can be confusing, because:

- variables such as posture and fluid management are not always accounted for
- individual differences exist between patients and midwives
- some observational studies do not compare equivalent groups of parturients
- dystocia may cause painful and protracted labour, and may therefore be the cause, not the effect, of epidural administration (Hess et al., 2000).

Some randomized controlled trials are compromised by: a third or more women crossing over from non-epidural arm to epidural arm and *vice versa*; the atypical nature of the women volunteering to be randomized; low numbers (Lierberman and O'Donoghue, 2002). Women with the highest risks of prolonged labour and complications may require the most invasive analgesic regimens, which complicates any assessment of the risks of adverse reactions (Traynor et al., 2000). Considering the widespread use of regional analgesia during labour, and the potential for adverse reactions, the absence of large randomized controlled trials assessing important outcomes, such as infant feeding and long-term development, is surprising and should be rectified.

Dissatisfaction with childbirth may be linked to the experience of pain (Waldenstrom, 1999). However, successful epidural analgesia is not necessarily associated with high maternal satisfaction and perception of control (Eltzschig et al., 2003; Anim-Somuah et al., 2005). It is not always necessary to achieve complete analgesia during normal childbirth. Many women will be satisfied if the pain is made 'tolerable'. While this reduces the amount of drug administered, the greater risk of analgesic failure requires closer supervision and more frequent dosage adjustments. Where complete analgesia is achieved, it is important that serious pathology, such as genital tract sepsis, is not overlooked (CEMACH, 2007).

Box 4.5 Opioids and regional analgesia

Advantages of including opioids in regional analgesia regimens include:

- opioids do not block the sympathetic nervous system, but hypotension remains a problem
- no motor blockade, therefore movement and ambulation are unaffected
- minimal effect on other sensory systems
- control of shivering induced by local anaesthetics (Sweetman et al., 2007).

  Some of the problems associated with intramuscular opioids, such as constipation, are diminished. However, many opioid **side effects** remain, particularly those shared by local anaesthetics (Kan and Hughes, 1995):

- pruritus/itching, which is more troublesome at higher doses (Lyons et al., 1997)
- nausea and vomiting
- respiratory depression or even arrest
- hypotension
- fetal heart rate changes, mainly bradycardia
- need for neonatal resuscitation
- breastfeeding difficulties
- sedation, slurred speech
- retention of urine.

Sources: Arkoosh (1991); Armand et al. (1993); Norris et al. (1994)

Pain relief in pregnancy and the puerperium: NSAIDs and paracetamol

Paracetamol and NSAIDs reduce pain, inflammation and fever. However, some pains can often be managed using non-pharmacological measures, such as immobilization or warmth.

NSAIDs

NSAIDs include the traditional agents, such as aspirin, ibuprofen, diclofenac, naproxen, piroxicam, indometacin and the newer cyclo-oxygenase-2 (COX-2) inhibitors, such as celecoxib and etoricoxib. NSAIDs should be used under medical supervision during pregnancy. Indications include:

- *Postpartum pain relief:* Following perineal repair, paracetamol or NSAIDs (usually diclofenac) may be offered, providing there are no contraindications. Rectal administration is commonly advised (NCC, 2007: 23), but see Chapter 2.
- *Postoperative analgesia:* Patient-controlled opioid analgesia is recommended following Caesarean delivery. Provided there are no contraindications, paracetamol or NSAIDs may be administered following Caesarean delivery to reduce the need for opioids (NCC, 2004). These are much less sedative than opioids, and are less likely to interfere with breastfeeding.
- *Pre-eclampsia and women at high risk of thrombosis:* Low-dose aspirin (50–150 mg/day) from 12–20 weeks may be prescribed to reduce the risk of pre-eclampsia, preterm (<34 weeks) delivery and neonatal death (Duley et al., 2007) (Box 9.3) or prevention of cardiovascular and cerebro-vascular thrombosis.

In analgesic doses (up to 4 mg/day) in the third trimester, aspirin is associated with reduction in fetal urine output and olighydramnios (BNF, 2009).

Other indications for NSAIDs include pain in: musculoskeletal disorders, including rheumatoid arthritis; injury; migraine; headaches; dysmenorrhoea; and toothache.

Administration

Most NSAIDs are taken orally, with or after meals, accompanied by a full glass of water or milk, and recipients should remain upright for 30 minutes after ingestion. Slow-release preparations offer few advantages and are more likely to damage the lower gastrointestinal tract. Orodispersible or liquid preparations may offer more rapid pain relief.

NSAIDs (such as Ibugel® (ibuprofen gel)) or counterirritants applied *topically* retain the potential for systemic adverse effects, and the same cautions apply as for the oral preparations.

Suppositories may be absorbed erratically and/or cause rectal irritation, ulceration or stenosis (Chapter 2).

Intravenous and *intramuscular* preparations are available. Diclofenac may be administered by intravenous infusion (not bolus) or intramuscular injection deep into the gluteal muscle for up to 2 days, using alternate sides. Patients report that this is very painful.

NSAIDs reduce pain and fever rapidly (within 1 hour), but take up to 3 weeks to reduce inflammation. Duration of analgesia varies between drugs and patients. Many NSAIDs have short half-lives, necessitating frequent dosing; for example diclofenac has a half-life of 1.1 hours, and many people need thrice-daily dosing for adequate analgesia. The exception is piroxicam, which has a half-life of 50 hours: this drug can accumulate with regular use.

Actions of NSAIDs

NSAIDs reduce inflammation, pain, fever and clotting, mainly by inhibiting the formation of prostaglandins, which are important mediators of pain and inflammation in the tissues and temperature control in the hypothalamus. Prostaglandins are formed when cell membranes are disturbed, for example by invading microorganisms, tissue damage, allergy, or other conditions. An important enzyme in this process is cyclo-oxygenase. The key action of NSAIDs is to block this enzyme and reduce the synthesis of prostaglandins. Thus, NSAIDs reduce the build-up of prostaglandins, and prevent pain and inflammation. However, NSAIDs and paracetamol do not block the pain mediators that are already formed in the tissues, so they are less effective at relieving pain than they are at preventing it.

Practice point

■ When pain is anticipated, for example after delivery, doses should be administered at regular intervals. How often the drug is administered depends on guidelines for each drug and the patient's needs: for example, some patients may find that ibuprofen 3 times a day is adequate, whereas others on the same regimen will experience 'break-through' pain before the next dose and require 4 doses each day.

NSAIDs also interfere with related compounds responsible for:

■ clotting (thromboxanes)
■ blood supply to vital organs, including gut and kidney (prostacyclins).

NSAIDs in pregnancy

Prostaglandins play a key role in uterine contraction (Figure 6.1). Reduction of prostaglandin synthesis by administration of NSAIDs, mainly indometicin, has been shown to reduce the incidence of delivery before 37 weeks when compared to placebo and other tocolytics. However, concerns have been expressed regarding the increased incidence of premature closure of the ductus arteriosus, pulmonary hypertension and necrotizing enterocolitis in neonates, and blood loss and oligohydramnios in women (King et al., 2005). Regular use of NSAIDs in analgesic doses in pregnancy is associated with increased risks of bleeding, miscarriage, prolonged and delayed labour, and intrauterine growth retardation. Use in the third trimester may affect the fetal heart, lungs or kidneys. Any NSAID may cause premature closure of the ductus arteriosis, which can lead to pulmonary hypertension and lung damage; most manufacturers advise avoid (BNF, 2009). NSAIDs in early pregnancy may be associated with: an increased risk of congenital anomalies of the respiratory system and cardiac septa (Ofori et al., 2006); and gastroschisis (Siega-Riz et al., 2009; Werler et al., 2009), but further exploration of larger databases is needed.

Breastfeeding

NSAIDs (including topical use) increase risks of bleeding. Aspirin has been linked to Reye's syndrome and jaundice, and is not advised. Paracetamol is considered safe. Manufacturers of ibuprofen advise avoid.

Adverse effects of NSAIDs

Without prostaglandins, several systems are compromised:

- *Bleeding:* NSAIDs reduce the synthesis of thromboxanes and the activity of the platelets, thereby inhibiting clotting. The risk of bleeding is related to the dose administered. Low-dose aspirin for the prevention of pre-eclampsia increased the risk of postpartum haemorrhage >500 ml, but not of neonatal bleeding (Askie et al., 2007).
- *Disruption of lining of gastrointestinal tract:* Prostaglandins are important in maintaining the integrity and blood supply to the lining of the gut.
- *Renal impairment:* Prostaglandins are important in maintaining the blood flow into the renal tubules, and the **glomerular filtration rate**, particularly during periods of dehydration and hypotension. Any reduction in blood flow into the kidneys may lead to retention of fluid and electrolytes and rise in blood pressure. This, in turn, can precipitate heart failure (Slordal and Spigset, 2006). With long-term use, NSAIDs can also damage the kidneys and cause renal failure (Gooch et al., 2007).
- *Cardiovascular disease:* In addition to hypertension and heart failure, NSAIDs inhibit the production of prostacyclin by the blood vessels' endothelial cells, and cause the vessels to narrow (Garret and Fitzgerald, 2004).
- *Poor healing:* Prostaglandins are integral to the natural healing processes and play a part in bone formation and turnover. NSAIDs may disrupt the formation of new blood vessels, important in healing.
- *Neurological effects:* NSAIDs act in the central nervous system to normalize body temperature. They also cause release of noradrenaline (norepinephrine), which may be responsible for the confusion sometimes observed.
- *Hypersensitivity responses:* When the enzyme cyclo-oxygenase is inhibited, the prostaglandin metabolic pathway is diverted to form the inflammatory mediators responsible for allergy and asthma. Over 20% adults are vulnerable to aspirin-induced asthma, and over 90% of these are also sensitive to other NSAIDs. Patients are usually unaware of this problem (Jenkins et al., 2004).

Implications for practice: NSAIDs

Although there are some differences between the NSAIDs, the risks of adverse reactions are very similar at higher doses. Adverse effects may occur with all routes of administration.

Potential problem	Management suggestions
Bleeding tendencies, particularly if other anticoagulants or corticosteroids are co-prescribed	Extra vigilance for blood loss throughout pregnancy and following birth (see Chapter 8 for long-term monitoring of bleeding tendencies)
	Discuss with prescriber any possible need for discontinuation before birth or surgery
Headache	Avoid non-prescription NSAIDs containing caffeine. Caffeine or caffeine withdrawal may cause headaches
Damage to inner ear	Advise patient to discontinue NSAID should tinnitus occur. This may be a warning sign that the delicate nerve cells of the inner ear are being damaged
Bronchospasm/worsening asthma	Avoid NSAIDs in people with asthma, if possible. Enquire if the woman's asthma has been worsened by NSAIDs on previous occasions
	Monitor airways 2–3 times each day to detect early signs of problems
	Prompt response to worsening asthma, difficulty breathing or a 'closing of the throat'
Anaphylactic-like reaction, with bronchospasm and cardiovascular collapse (very rare)	Ensure allergies to aspirin or other NSAIDs are documented
With long-term use, also consider	
Delayed delivery	NSAIDs are not usually administered during labour
Renal impairment	In women at risk of pre-eclmapsia, consider urinalysis for albuminuria/microalbuminuria, **serum** creatinine before and during therapy
Fluid retention	Monitor weight
	Ask patient to observe ankles and fingers and report swelling (see beta blockers)
	Assess cardiac insufficiency and breathlessness
	Avoid regular use of preparations containing sodium, including effervescent formulations, for example Brufen® granules contain 200 mg sodium/sachet (max. 4 tablets/day), Tylex® effervescent tablets contain 300 mg sodium (max. 8 tablets/day) (BNF, 2009). (Recommended sodium intake is 2.4 g/day)
Hypertension/antagonism of antihypertensive therapy	Monitor BP pre-therapy and regularly for patients using long-term NSAIDs or paracetamol
Potassium retention	Avoid potassium supplements, including those purchased in non-prescription medicines
Impaired healing	Monitor wounds, for example episiotomy. Consider using paracetamol alone if possible
Liver impairment (particularly diclofenac)	Liver function tests within 8 weeks of initiation of long-term therapy

Cautions and contraindications: NSAIDs

- *Known hypersensitivity* to aspirin, any NSAID, tartrazine or any component of an injection. A life-threatening reaction could ensue. Allergy to sulfonamides may indicate allergy to celecoxib.
- Asthma, hypertension, heart failure, epilepsy, psychotic disturbances or parkinsonism may be worsened (particularly indometacin).
- *High risk of bleeding*, for example, pre-eclampsia, liver disorders, thrombocytopenia, vitamin K or C deficiency, peptic ulceration, high blood pressure (risk of haemorrhagic stroke). African Americans have a higher incidence of gastrointestinal bleeding. Platelet count should be checked before administration after delivery.
- *Poor renal function/pre-eclampsia* where renal function has not been assessed as normal: low doses may be prescribed in mild renal failure, but NSAIDs (including topical applications) are contraindicated in moderate/severe renal failure or if urine output is low (Collis et al., 2008).
- *Heart failure, hypertension* and fluid retention may be worsened. NSAIDs are contraindicated in severe heart failure.
- *Inflammatory bowel disease* may progress without recognition (particularly enteric-coated NSAIDs), due to 'masking' of symptoms, long term.
- Eight to 12 days after medical termination of pregnancy with misoprostol and mifepristone.
- Aspirin is avoided in:
  - breastfeeding, children <16 (implicated in Reye's syndrome)
  - people with gout
  - people with **G6PD** deficiency.
- **Porphyria** attacks may be precipated by diclofenac.

Interactions: NSAIDs

- Adverse effects of NSAIDs may be accentuated:
  - *Bleeding* is increased by vasodilators (for example calcium channel blockers, nitrates, alcohol), anticoagulants, SSRIs, and some herbal remedies, such as feverfew, *Ginkgo biloba*, and Siberian ginseng. Intravenous diclofenac should not be co-administered with any heparins. Long-term paracetamol enhances the actions of warfarin.
  - *Gastrointestinal adverse effects* are increased by co-administration of more than one NSAID, alcohol, oral anticoagulants, corticosteroids or SSRIs.
  - *Renal problems* are intensified by diuretics, ACE inhibitors, ciclosporin, vancomycin, and tacrolimus.
- Antihypertensive effects of ACE inhibitors, calcium channel blockers, beta blockers and thiazide diuretics are reduced.
- Increased risk of hypoglycaemia with oral hypoglycaemics.
- NSAIDs may increase myoclonus associated with opioids.
- NSAIDs cause accumulation of: lithium, digoxin, quinolones, and methotrexate. Aspirin does not interact with lithium and digoxin.
- Absorption of NSAIDs is increased by metoclopramide and reduced by cholestyramine, opioids, atropine, antipsychotics, or tricyclic antidepressants. The effectiveness of aspirin may change if the pH of urine alters, for example due to antacid ingestion.
- Other drugs interacting with NSAIDs include: sodium valproate, phenytoin, thyroxine, moclobemide, zidovudine, ritonavir, baclofen, oral hypoglycaemics, and some antibiotics (ceftriaxone, chloramphenicol, sulphonamides, rifampicin, and quinolones). Oral contraceptives reduce the effectiveness of paracetamol.

Paracetamol

Paracetamol (acetaminophen in the USA) is usually the analgesic of first choice, as it may offer adequate pain relief and is associated with fewer adverse reactions. It has been used for many years without evidence of **teratogenicity**. Paracetamol has similar actions to the NSAIDs, but is not anti-inflammatory. It is used for control of fever, particularly patients with epilepsy or fever >40°C.

Adverse effects from paracetamol are unusual but include rashes, blood disorders, and, with long-term use, increased incidence of asthma, rhinitis, headache and possibly hypoglycaemia, hypertension and renal failure. Hypersensitivity occurs rarely (Aronson, 2006). High doses of paracetamol during pregnancy may slightly increase the risk of asthma in children (Shaheen et al., 2002).

The main problem with paracetamol is risk of liver, kidney or pancreas damage to both women and fetus following overdose, or even when the dose is only some 2–3 times that recommended. There are some reports of toxicity with long-term use at high prescribed doses. A few patients overusing alcohol and taking paracetamol within the prescribed range (below 4 g/day) have developed liver failure (Baxter, 2006; Aronson, 2006).

Practice points

■ The maximum paracetamol dose of 4 g (8 tablets) per day should never be exceeded, as pregnancy renders the liver vulnerable to injury. In pregnancy, it is advisable to use the lowest possible dose for the shortest possible time.

■ Many over the counter analgesics contain multiple ingredients, such as caffeine or phenylephrine, and these are best avoided. A daily caffeine intake of over 300 mg, from all sources has, in observational studies, been associated with adverse outcomes and low birth weight (Peters and Schaefer, 2007) (Chapter 20).

Paracetamol dose restrictions are advised for:

▪ children
▪ people with liver or kidney disease
▪ those who overuse alcohol and go without food
▪ patients who are HIV positive
▪ co-administration of drugs affecting the liver, for example tricyclic antidepressants, antiepileptics, rifampicin, isoniazid and barbiturates
▪ co-administration of metoclopramide, which increases absorption of paracetamol.

Box 4.6 Migraine

Since migraine symptoms remit in a significant number of pregnant women, prophylaxis may not be necessary during pregnancy. The safety of most preventive regimens, such as beta blockers, serotonin antagonists, and antiepileptics, is not established (Goadsby et al., 2008). Paracetamol is recommended for migraine in pregnancy (Campbell and Lees, 2000). Soluble or liquid preparations may offer a more rapid action (Chapter 1). If paracetamol is ineffective, women should seek advice regarding antiemetics and analgesics; some authors recommend prochlorperazine as a 'rescue' therapy during pregnancy but not breastfeeding (Goadsby et al., 2008). Triptans, such as sumatriptan, vasoconstrict and provide relief from acute attacks when analgesics have failed; however, vasoconstriction may raise blood pressure or affect the coronary arteries. Manufacturers advise against use in pregnancy, and more data are needed to confirm safety. Breastfeeding is not recommended for 12 hours after administration (BNF, 2009).

Further reading

■ Bryant, H. and Yerby, M. (2004) Pain relief during labour, in Henderson, C. and MacDonald, S. (eds) *Mayes' Midwifery: A Textbook for Midwives*, 13th edn. Baillière Tindall, Edinburgh; Chapter 27.

■ Clyburn, P., Collis, R., Harries S. and Davies, S. (eds) (2008) *Obstetric Anaesthesia*. Oxford University Press, Oxford.

■ Jordan, S. (2008) *The Prescription Drug Guide for Nurses*. Open University Press/McGraw-Hill, Maidenhead; see Chapter 20 for long-term administration of NSAIDS.

■ MacDonald, S. and Magill-Cuerden, J. (eds) (2010) *Mayes Midwifery: A Textbook for Midwives*, 14th edn. Elsevier, Edinburgh.

■ Yerby, M. and Page, L. (eds) (2000) *Pain in Childbearing*. Baillière Tindall, Edinburgh.

CHAPTER 5

Antiemetics

Sue Jordan

This chapter discusses metoclopramide, phenothiazines (prochlorperazine) and antihistamines. Brief mention is made of other antiemetics, ondansetron, pyridoxine and cannabinoids.

Chapter contents

- Physiology of nausea and vomiting
- Emesis in early pregnancy
- Pharmacological management of emesis
- Dopamine (D_2) antagonists (metoclopramide and prochlorperazine)
- Antihistamines (cyclizine, promethazine)
- Other antiemetics (antimuscarinics, serotonin antagonists, pyridoxine, cannabinoids)

In midwifery, emesis is encountered in early pregnancy, labour and the postoperative period. It is not only distressing, but may lead to serious physiological consequences. The term 'hyperemesis gravidarum' is applied when vomiting results in fluid, electrolyte or nutritional deficiencies (Friedman and Isselbacher, 1991).

Physiology of nausea and vomiting

Vomiting is usually, but not always, associated with nausea. Nausea is the conscious recognition of subconscious excitation of the vomiting centre or an area close to it in the medulla (Guyton, 1996). Vomiting is a complex series of movements that rids the gut of its contents when any part of it is irritated or distended. The sensory and motor components of the vomiting reflex are governed by the autonomic nervous system. This brings about the emotion of 'feeling sick'.

Causes of vomiting

Many stimuli act directly on the vomiting centre or the chemoreceptor trigger zone (CTZ). The CTZ lies outside the **blood/brain barrier** in the medulla, close to, but distinct from, the vomiting centre. The vomiting centre receives inputs from: the higher centres of the brain, the CTZ, the vestibular apparatus of the inner ear, and the whole body *via* the autonomic nervous system.

Nausea and vomiting depend on the interaction of many factors, including drugs administered, emotional state, pain, tissue damage, motion or changes in homeostasis (Box 5.1). In labour, gastric stasis, pain and pressure on the stomach combine to cause emesis.

Description of vomiting

Vomiting is usually accompanied by secretion of saliva, sweating, pallor, drop in blood pressure, tachycardia and irregular respirations, as well as subjective feelings. Gastric stasis usually precedes vomiting. To remove the gut contents, the lower oesophagus and upper stomach relax, while the duodenum and lower stomach contract. The stomach is squeezed between the diaphragm and the abdominal wall. A deep breath is taken, and the glottis and the back of the nostrils are closed. However, there may be no time for deep inspiration if the urge to vomit is overwhelming.

Practice points

■ If reflexes are dulled by sedation, there is a risk of aspiration of vomit. Adult respiratory distress syndrome has followed aspiration of vomit in some maternal deaths (DH, 1994). Therefore, labouring women who receive opioids should not eat.

■ Fainting may occur if blood pressure drops; therefore, a woman likely to vomit should not be left unattended, for example after administration of opioids (Torrance and Jordan, 1996).

Box 5.1 Causes of vomiting (with some examples)

The vomiting centre is affected by:
- The *chemoreceptor trigger zone*, which detects:
  ◗ circulating chemicals such as oestrogens, alcohol, nicotine, opioids, anaesthetics, ergometrine, thyroid hormones, stimulants (adrenaline/epinephrine, cold cures, **beta$_2$ agonists**, (for example salbutamol, tocolytics), and theophylline), iron tablets, digoxin, NSAIDs, SSRIs, antibiotics, valproate, anti-Parkinson agents, anaesthetics, **antimuscarinics**, chemotherapy, herbal remedies, such as black cohosh, garlic, *Ginkgo biloba*, milk thistle, and valerian, and recreational drugs, such as alcohol, amphetamines, cocaine and LSD
  ◗ electrolyte imbalance (low sodium, including Addison's disease)
  ◗ withdrawal from regular use of alcohol
  ◗ products of tissue damage released into the circulation on injury.
- The *vestibular nucleus*, which detects: motion, including ambulation and sudden movements, for example after labour or an operation.
- *Higher centres*, which detect: tastes, smells, sights, emotion, pain, fear, anxiety, anticipation.
- The *autonomic nervous system*, which detects:
  ◗ irritation to gut, throat or peritoneum such as gastric stasis or distension (for example migraine, pain and labour), liver disease, some foods, alcohol, NSAIDs, obstruction of the gastrointestinal tract, and constipation
  ◗ physiological disturbances such as changes in blood pressure, **pH**, blood gases, blood glucose, pain, **shock**, ketoacidosis, uraemia, organ damage (for example pancreas), infections, urinary tract infections, and intercurrent illness (for example asthma or gallstones)
  ◗ raised intracranial pressure, for example pre-eclampsia/eclampsia, thromboses or dural puncture.

Practice point

■ A urine specimen to test for the presence of ketones and urinary tract infections will be helpful in establishing the cause of emesis. A venous blood sample may be requested to assess the less common causes of emesis.

Consequences of vomiting

It is important that emesis is managed effectively because of the potentially serious consequences:

- dehydration and, consequently, increased risk of thromboses
- electrolyte imbalance (sodium and potassium loss) and, consequently, weakness
- pH imbalance
- ketone formation
- loss of oral medication
- risk of aspiration of vomit and acute respiratory distress syndrome
- risk of hypotension, reduced placental blood flow, syncope, shock, and circulatory collapse
- psychological distress
- hyperemesis gravidarum may result in vitamin deficiency or, rarely, liver failure
- risk of trauma to gastrointestinal tract (Mallory-Weiss tear)
- malnutrition and dental caries (long term)
- women with prolonged severe emesis are more likely to develop depression (Sheehan, 2007).

Practice points

- Frequent drinking is essential to avoid dehydration. Sports drinks or clear soup may be preferred over water.
- If the woman is unable to tolerate oral fluids, admission to hospital must be considered (Sheehan, 2007).
- There is a danger that the symptoms of acute illness may be dangerously masked by the use of antiemetics, impeding the diagnosis of serious pathology, such as rising intracranial pressure in severe pre-eclampsia.
- Vitamin B_1 (thiamine) may be prescribed for women with hyperemesis gravidarum to prevent brain damage (Wernicke's encephalopathy) (Kametas and Nelson-Piercy, 2007).

Emesis in early pregnancy

In early pregnancy, nausea and vomiting are very common, and may even have a physiological role in encouraging the woman to eat more (Huxley, 2000). In pregnancies where there is no nausea, the risk of spontaneous abortion or premature labour is higher (Beischer et al., 1997). Non-pharmacological approaches to the problem are usually preferable to the use of drugs. Women may benefit from the assurance that the problem rarely persists beyond 12–20 weeks of pregnancy. It may be helpful to consider:

- Specific causes of nausea, such as iron tablets, urinary tract infection, thyroid disorders, anxiety (Box 5.1), and multiple or molar pregnancy.
- Rest and intake of bland carbohydrate, such as a biscuit or cereal, may be effective. Lying down may relieve nausea.
- Cold or salty food may be more palatable than hot food. Cooking may worsen emesis (Sheehan, 2007).
- Small, frequent, bland meals and snacks are advised (Chamberlain, 1975). Hypoglycaemia may aggravate emesis, and it is inadvisable to miss meals.
- Distension of the stomach will be reduced if fruit and liquids are taken separately from meals.
- Women are advised to avoid: sudden movements; eating late at night; eating spicy, fatty, greasy or acidic food; and swallowing food without chewing thoroughly (Rogers, 1995).

- Peppermint after a meal relaxes the lower oesophagus and reduces gastric distension, which may relieve nausea after meals. However, peppermint may worsen constipation or induce heartburn, particularly if used before lying down.
- Intake of herbal teas should be limited since their effects on pregnancy are uncertain, for example fennel is contraindicated in pregnancy (see Rogers, 1995).
- A ginger biscuit may be helpful, but the rise in blood glucose associated with too many biscuits could worsen nausea. Some authorities recommend powdered ginger root (below) (Kametas and Nelson-Piercy, 2007).
- Self-administered acupressure has been shown to reduce nausea but not vomiting when compared to placebo (Howden, 1995), and is recommended in guidelines (NCC, 2008b).

Pharmacological management of emesis

A wide variety of drugs may be prescribed as antiemetics, both in labour and in hyperemesis gravidarum. The pattern of use varies between centres. The diversity of drugs used for emesis may be explained by the complexity of the neural pathways affecting the vomiting centre. If vomiting is severe, single agents are not always completely effective. The neurotransmitters involved in vomiting can be modified by the actions of drugs, including dopamine, acetylcholine, histamine, serotonin, benzodiazepines (as endozapines), and cannabinoids.

The antiemetics commonly prescribed in childbirth fall into two main groups:

- the dopamine (D_2) **antagonists**/blockers, such as metoclopramide and prochlorperazine
- the histamine (H_1) antagonists, such as cyclizine, promethazine, and cinnarizine.

For each drug, **adverse effects** depend on the neurotransmitters affected. For example, all histamine (H_1) antagonists can cause sedation, and all dopamine (D_2) antagonists can cause movement disorders. Some drugs such as promethazine (Avomine® and Phenergan®) and prochlorperazine (Stemetil®) are both histamine and dopamine antagonists; while they have the antiemetic actions of both drug groups, they also have the adverse effects of both groups. Table 5.1 aims to clarify this complicated situation.

Table 5.1 Summary of actions and adverse effects expected with commonly administered antiemetics

Drug	Dopamine antagonism (causes movement disorders)	Histamine antagonism (causes sedation)	Antimuscarinic properties (for example drying of secretions; Table 5.2)
Promethazine	+	+	
Prochlorperazine	++	+	+
Chlorpromazine	++	++	++
Metoclopramide	++	+	–
Haloperidol	+++	little	very little
Cyclizine	–	+	+

Key: – No appreciable action; + action important; ++ action prominent; +++ action very prominent.

Most antiemetics can affect gastrointestinal motility and may worsen heartburn, haemorrhoids, or diverticular disease.

Dopamine (D₂) antagonists (mainly metoclopramide and prochlorperazine)

D$_2$ antagonists include metoclopramide (Maxalon®), haloperidol, domperidone and the phenothiazines such as chlorpromazine and prochlorperazine. The actions, adverse effects, cautions and **contraindications** of phenothiazines (prochlorperazine and chlorpromazine) are based on antagonism to dopamine, histamine, sympathetic nervous system (**alpha₁ receptors**), and parasympathetic nervous system (muscarinic **receptors**). Promethazine is a phenothiazine, but its predominant actions are those of antihistamines; it is therefore considered under the antihistamines. Metoclopramide is a substituted benzamide, not a phenothiazine. It is therefore free of antimuscarinic adverse effects such as constipation. Its antiemetic properties are due to actions on both dopamine and serotonin receptors.

Uses of D₂ antagonist antiemetics

D$_2$ antagonist antiemetics are prescribed to counter emesis in a variety of circumstances:

- to counteract the emetogenic effects of opioids and ergotamine
- to counteract the emesis of labour itself, although this is rarely necessary
- prior to anaesthesia
- postoperative emesis
- Ménière's disease, radiation sickness and cytotoxic therapy
- any situation with gastric stasis, for example labour, migraine, pain, and gastric paresis due to diabetes.
- metoclopramide has been used in hyperemesis gravidarum; however, the manufacturer advises 'use only when compelling reasons' (Amdipharm, ABPI, 2008).

D$_2$ antagonists are ineffective in motion sickness. Therefore they offer little protection to the mobilizing woman who has used opioids. Phenothiazines are important in the management of mental illness, usually in higher doses than prescribed for emesis (Chapter 19).

How the body handles phenothiazines, for example prochlorperazine

Prochlorperazine acts within 5–10 minutes of intramuscular injection, and antiemetic actions last for 3–5 hours. Absorption following buccal administration is more rapid (Chapter 1). All phenothiazines cross the placenta, and, if administered at term, may cause movement disorders in the neonate (below). Prochlorperazine is eliminated by metabolism in the liver, with a **half-life** of 4–8 hours. All phenothiazines are highly protein bound, and pass into breast milk in small amounts, and drowsiness of infants has been reported. Animal studies indicate that phenothiazines, in pregnancy or when breastfeeding, may affect the infant's nervous system (sanofi-aventis, ABPI, 2009), particularly with long-term use.

Phenothiazines are eliminated in a complex way, with considerable individual variation; for example, the half-life of chlorpromazine varies from 2–37 hours. This means that, with repeated doses, the drugs will build up in some people, but not in others. There is also a diurnal variation in plasma concentration (Mitchelson, 1992a).

How the body handles metoclopramide

The onset of action of metoclopramide is within 10–15 minutes of injection and 30–60 minutes of oral ingestion. This drug is eliminated rather quickly from the body (half-life 4–6 hours), and antiemetic actions last for 1–2 hours, which necessitates frequent dosing (Pasricha, 2006). Therefore metoclopramide is most effective if given by continuous intravenous infusion (BNF, 2009).

■ The rapid elimination after a single dose is useful if the mother wishes to breastfeed. Although the amount of drug in breast milk is likely to be small, manufacturers advise against breastfeeding (BNF, 2009).

Actions of D$_2$ antagonists

Drugs that block the action of dopamine (D$_2$ antagonists) relieve vomiting by their actions in the gut wall, vomiting centre and chemoreceptor trigger zone. By inhibiting the actions of dopamine, drugs in this group have the potential to:

■ reduce emesis and increase appetite
■ alter gastrointestinal motility
■ depress the central nervous system
■ disturb posture and movement
■ disturb the cardiovascular system
■ trigger **SIADH** (syndrome inappropriate ADH) and water retention
■ increase prolactin production (Chapter 19)
■ suppress the symptoms of schizophrenia and schizo-affective disorders (Chapter 19).

Adverse effects of D$_2$ antagonists (mainly metoclopramide and prochlorperazine)

Gastrointestinal tract

In addition to central antiemetic actions, these drugs increase gastric emptying. This prokinetic action on the stomach and intestine counteracts the gastric stasis induced by progesterone, pain, labour, migraine or opioids. Bowel distension and laxity of the lower oesophageal sphincter induced by progesterone are also reversed. Diarrhoea is a recognized adverse effect of metoclopramide. If stimulation of gastrointestinal motility would be dangerous, for example if the gastrointestinal tract is obstructed or traumatized, metoclopramide is contraindicated (Amdipharm, ABPI, 2009). Intestinal hurry interferes with absorption from the gut, not only of food, but also of other drugs (Interactions, below).

Central nervous system depression

Dopamine antagonists, particularly phenothiazines (prochlorperazine), usually cause sedation or, with long-term administration, depressed mood and blunting of emotions. They also depress the functions of the brainstem such as thermoregulation, thirst, respiration, and the cough reflex. There is an increased risk of seizures in women with epilepsy.

■ The mother may feel cold until the drug has been eliminated. Extra care should be taken to protect the neonate from hypothermia.
■ Depression of the respiratory centres impedes the establishment of normal respirations in the neonate and increases the chances of a postoperative chest infection in the mother, particularly if she is dehydrated. Apgar scores may be low (sanofi-aventis, ABPI, 2009).
■ If mother and infant are sedated, they are less able to initiate effective breastfeeding. For women receiving prochlorperazine, this problem could persist for up to 24 hours. These effects are compounded by co-administration of opioids.
■ D$_2$ antagonists increase the likelihood of fits. They are used with caution in people with epilepsy (BNF, 2009).

Posture and movement disorders

These serious adverse reactions are rare at normal doses but are more likely with higher doses and in young people. Posture and movement disorders (including extrapyramidal side effects) are associated with all the D_2 antagonists due to their actions on the basal ganglia:

- acute dystonia – abnormal muscle tone and spasms
- pseudoparkinsonism
- akathisia – restlessness and involuntary movements
- tardive dyskinesia – involuntary movements of the face or limbs – can occur only with prolonged administration
- neuroleptic malignant syndrome (Chapter 19).

Acute dystonic reactions

Oculogyric crises (spasms of the muscles controlling the eyeballs), torticollis (spasm and twisting of the neck muscles), severe swelling of the tongue, or facial grimacing usually occur within the first 48 hours of use. These very dramatic and distressing adverse effects are rare but occur more commonly in people under 20 when higher doses are used (particularly metoclopramide in doses over 0.5 mg per kg), or if viral infection is present. Bsat et al. (2003) report that 1 of 54 women randomized to metoclopramide 10 mg every 6 hours experienced an acute dystonic reaction, which resolved within 6–8 hours. Acute dystonic reactions may be mistaken for hysteria; however, unlike hysteria, they involve the tongue (Rascol et al., 1995; Aronson, 2006).

Practice points

- During an acute dystonic reaction, it is important that the patient is not left alone, not only because these reactions are terrifying to experience but also because the airway may be jeopardized (Baldessarini and Tarazi, 2006).
- An antidote is administered as quickly as possible; this is usually procyclidine 5 mg intramuscularly or intravenously, repeated if necessary 20 minutes later. Relief may not be obtained for up to 30 minutes (BNF, 2009).
- If dopamine antagonists are likely to be administered, the midwife should seek a specific history of adverse reactions to these drugs.
- Because of the risks of acute dystonia, the BNF (2009) imposes restrictions on the use of metoclopramide in those under 20 years of age. Prochlorperazine is not restricted in this way.

Prochlorperazine given intramuscularly or intravenously for emesis in an emergency department was associated with dystonia in 9/229, 3.9% recipients; 5 of these cases were only apparent on 2-week follow-up (Olsen et al., 2000). This high incidence of dystonic reactions has led to recommendations to use with caution in childbirth in the USA (Brunton, 1996).

Parkinsonian side effects

Masklike faces, swallowing or speech difficulties, bradykinesia (paucity of movement), tremor and rigidity may develop gradually over the first few days or weeks of administration. This reaction may be mistaken for signs of depression in a woman suffering from hyperemesis. If only one side of the body is affected, it is important that the possibility of a stroke is excluded.

Neonates whose mothers have received prochlorperazine may display excitability and tremor (sanofi-aventis, ABPI, 2009).

Akathisia

Akathisia presents as restlessness, inability to keep still, anxiety, agitation, insomnia or confusion. Drowsiness or restlessness occur in 20% of recipients of D_2 antagonists (Mitchelson, 1992a), and akathisia in 36/229 (16%) within 2 weeks of use for emesis (Olsen et al., 2000). If these drugs are rapidly administered intravenously, feelings of anxiety and agitation are particularly likely (Spencer, 1993a).

Practice point

■ It is important that these adverse reactions are recognized and explained to women, rather than attributed to psychological factors.

With continuous use in the last 3 months of pregnancy, D_2 antagonists can cause prolonged movement disorders or swallowing difficulties in neonates (Cox and Nicholls, 1996). This may occur in women with mental health problems or those suffering from hyperemesis.

Neuroleptic malignant syndrome

Neuroleptic malignant syndrome is usually associated with antipsychotic medication and has been reported with metoclopramide and prochlorperazine (Blair and Dauner, 1992). This rare but serious adverse effect is described in Chapter 19.

Cardiovascular adverse effects

D_2 antagonists are associated with **cardiac dysrhythmias**, particularly when given rapidly by the intravenous route (Spencer, 1993b). Cardiac dysrhythmias are particularly likely in women who are potassium depleted, for example due to prolonged vomiting or co-administration of corticosteroids, ritodrine or diuretics. Cardiac dysrhythmias may also occur as a result of drug interactions.

Practice points

■ An intravenous injection of metoclopramide should be given over at least 1–2 minutes (BNF, 2009).
■ With prolonged administration of antiemetics, signs of dysrhythmia may be detected by monitoring the pulse and ECG.

Metoclopramide may cause tachycardia and elevation of blood pressure, which should be monitored. It has the potential to alter the release of aldosterone, affecting salt/water and potassium balance, complicating any fluid and electrolyte disturbance (Spencer, 1993b).

Phenothiazines (for example prochlorperazine) inhibit the vasoconstrictor actions of noradrenaline (norepinephrine) on the peripheral blood vessels. The resultant vasodilation reduces blood pressure, makes the patient feel the cold and may cause orthostatic hypotension. In young women, this inability to adjust the peripheral blood vessels may cause dizziness on sudden standing. Hypotension may decrease placental blood flow: if phenothiazines are prescribed during pregnancy, close fetal monitoring is required. In labour, blood pressure must be closely observed, particularly if intraspinal analagesia or opioids are co-administered.

Practice point

■ To prevent falls, advice on standing slowly should be given and orthostatic hypotension should be assessed.

Syndrome inappropriate ADH (SIADH)

SIADH is a rare adverse effect of several drugs (including phenothaizines, opioids and anaesthetics). The clinical picture is of water intoxication (Chapter 6).

Antimuscarinic adverse effects

Phenothiazines (including prochlorperazine), antihistamines, and antimuscarinics may cause antimuscarinic (anticholinergic) adverse effects. These drugs block the actions of acetylcholine, a key neurotransmitter of the parasympathetic nervous system. Antimuscarinic medications inhibit the mucus-secreting glands, which moisten all the epithelial linings of the body, such as the linings of the digestive, respiratory and genitourinary tracts, and the conjunctiva. Long-term disruption of the central nervous system muscarinic receptors can cause confusion, irritability, insomnia, tremor, or hallucinations (Table 5.2).

Table 5.2 Antimuscarinic effects (prochlorperazine and promethazine)

Potential problem	Patient care
Short term, for example in labour	
Dry mouth, thirst	Dental hygiene, mouth care. Offer ice cubes to alleviate dryness
Stuffy nose	Provide tissues
Raised HR	Monitor pulse
Hypotension	Monitor BP and fluid balance. Ensure rehydration after vomiting
Drowsiness	Advise regarding driving and co-administration of alcohol
Confusion, insomnia, agitation	Ask women how they are feeling. Seek alternative antiemetic if problems are suspected
Photophobia	Advise that bright lights or sunlight may cause discomfort because the pupil cannot constrict as normal
Glaucoma	Avoid if the woman has acute angle glaucoma; cautious use with relevant family history, or other types of glaucoma
Blurred vision	Likely to subside on discontinuation or >2 weeks' use
Retention of urine, dysuria	Assess output
Medium term, for example postoperative	
Drying and thickening of respiratory tract secretions	Breathing exercises
Chest infection	Advise cessation of smoking
Ear infection	
Raised HR	Monitor, be alert for signs of myocardial ischaemia
Longer term, for example emesis in pregnancy	
Dry eyes	Artificial tears if needed, protect eyes from wind. Advise contact lens wearers of potential problems
Constipation, ileus	Monitor output and bowel sounds
Confusion, insomnia, hallucinations	Avoid driving, operating machinery
Dry skin	Skin care using emollients if needed

Potential problem	Patient care
Reduced ability to sweat	Avoid raised temperatures, for example fever, high environmental temperatures
Reduced libido	
Gastric stasis and emesis, leading to therapeutic failure	Monitor therapeutic effects

Hypersensitivity responses

Hypersensitivity responses such as rash, periorbital oedema, and **methaemoglobinaemia**, usually in infants, have been reported with metoclopramide (Pasricha, 2006). All phenothiazines have been implicated in rare cases of hepatitis, agranulocytosis and liver dysfunction (BNF, 2009).

Cautions: D₂ antagonists

- Due to the dangers of acute dystonic reactions, administration of metoclopramide to people under 20 is restricted to premedication, intubation, intractable vomiting of known cause and vomiting associated with cancer therapies. The daily dose should not exceed 500 micrograms per kg body weight per day, or 5 mg 3 times per day in those under 20 and weighing under 60 kg (pre-pregnancy body weight is normally taken) (BNF, 2009).

- Use in *pregnancy* is restricted to second-line treatment, particularly in the first trimester: metoclopramide has been linked with neural tube defects in experimental animals (McLaughlin and Thompson, 1995; Pfaffenrath and Rehm, 1998); preterm birth was more likely in women taking metoclopramide in one study (Goldstein and Berkovitch, 2007); and manufacturers advise avoid without compelling reasons (BNF, 2009). Congenital anomalies in humans have not been reported in association with metoclopramide, but authorities consider that there is insufficient evidence of safety for use in initial management (NCC, 2008b). Metoclopramide and prochlorperazine are second-line treatments (BNF, 2009). Older reviews found intramuscular metoclopramide to be the most effective drug for women hospitalized with hyperemesis gravidarum (*Drugs and Therapy Perspectives*, 1993). There is no evidence that prochlorperazine is associated with fetal malformations (Goadsby et al., 2008).

- D₂ antagonists enter breast milk and are not usually advised during lactation (Pangle, 2000; Amdipharm, ABPI, 2009).

- D₂ antagonists complicate the management of some conditions, such as diabetes, epilepsy and allergy.

- Metoclopramide should be avoided if ileus or gastrointestinal obstruction is suspected.

- All these drugs require healthy liver and kidneys for elimination. Therefore regimens may need adjustment if these organs are impaired, for example in pre-eclampsia. Renal elimination is reduced in dehydration, which intensifies the drugs' adverse effects.

- Masking of emesis is dangerous when raised intracranial pressure is suspected, for example severe pre-eclampsia.

- Cross-allergy with procainamide (Spencer, 1993b).

Other cautions are listed in Appendix I.

Interactions: D$_2$ antagonists

A wide variety of drugs interact. Some drug combinations will require modification of dosage:

- *Movement disorders:* When two or more D$_2$ antagonists are co-administered, the risk of movement disorders increases. Therefore women taking antipsychotic medication, lithium, methyldopa, SSRI antidepressants or (rarely) antihistamines may experience serious central nervous system adverse effects if metoclopramide or prochlorperazine are also administered. A young woman experienced an acute dystonic reaction and respiratory obstruction when metoclopramide was administered after prochlorperazine (Baxter, 2006).
- *Increased sedation:* When two or more sedatives are co-administered, their effects are magnified. D$_2$ antagonists increase the central nervous system depression of all sedatives including alcohol, opioids, barbiturates, antihistamines, benzodiazepines, and anaesthetics. The combination of meperidine (pethidine) and phenothiazines (including prochlorperazine) increases the risk of respiratory depression, sedation, central nervous system toxicity, and hypotension (Baxter, 2006).
- *Loss of effect:* The relief of gastric stasis by D$_2$ antagonists is counteracted by opioids.
- *Lowering seizure threshold:* The protective effects of anticonvulsants may be reduced.
- *Potentiation of muscle relaxants:* This could result in prolonged apnoea (BNF, 2009).
- *SSRI antidepressants – metoclopramide only:* Metoclopramide may cause accumulation of serotonin, resulting in pyrexia and confusion (Chapter 19, Serotonin syndrome) (Amdipharm, ABPI, 2009).
- Due to its effects on gut transit time, metoclopramide increases the oral absorption and peak plasma concentrations of some drugs, including alcohol, aspirin, and paracetamol (Baxter, 2006).
- *Risk of hypotension – phenothiazines only:* Hypotension is more likely with antihypertensives, diuretics, opioids, anaesthetics, and tricyclic antidepressants.
- *Risk of cardiac dysrhythmias:* Drugs used in mental illness or cardiac dysrhythmias, some antimalarials (including quinine), and potassium or magnesium depletion increase the likelihood of cardiac dysrhythmias (Chapter 19).

Antihistamines

The term 'antihistamines' refers to H$_1$ receptor antagonists, which are divided into:

- *Sedating antihistamines*, for example cinnarizine, meclozine, cyclizine, promethazine, and chlorpheniramine. Promethazine hydrochloride is available as Phenergan®. Promethazine teoclate is marketed as Avomine®. These drugs are sometimes used to relieve the symptoms of emesis in early pregnancy, during labour or post-anaesthesia.
- *Non-sedating antihistamines*, for example cetirizine and loratadine. Sedation is less pronounced but still important with the 'non-sedating' antihistamines. They are used to relieve the symptoms of allergic disorders, such as hay fever and urticaria. These are not included in this book, since manufacturers advise to avoid in pregnancy and lactation, in view of embryo toxicity in animal studies at high doses (BNF, 2009).

Antihistamines are available in a variety of over the counter products.

Uses of antihistamines

- Antiemetics, in association with opioids, anaesthesia, or motion sickness.

- Emergency management of **anaphylaxis** and angioedema after adrenaline/epinephrine administration (BNF, 2009).
- Symptom relief for allergies, including drug allergies, pruritus, urticaria, insect stings, hay fever, and atopic dermatitis. Administration before release of histamine is important, for example at the start of the hay fever season.
- Premedication and sedation, for example promethazine and trimeprazine/alimemazine.
- Insomnia may be managed by over the counter preparations, for example promethazine.
- Relief of coughs and colds from over the counter preparations, for example diphenhydramine (Benylin for Chesty Coughs Original®).

How the body handles antihistamines

Antihistamines work within 15–60 minutes of oral administration, are maximally absorbed within 1–2 hours and last 3–6 hours. Intranasal, intraocular and topical preparations are used to control the symptoms of hay fever or rashes. Antihistamines cross the blood/brain barrier and the placenta and pass into breast milk. They are eliminated by the liver and the kidneys.

Role of histamine

Histamine is found in most tissues, particularly lungs, skin, brain and gut. Histamine is involved in central nervous system activity, gastric acid secretion and smooth muscle contraction. It is also an important chemical mediator in anaphylaxis, allergy and inflammation. Several histamine receptor types have been extensively studied. Drugs acting on H_1 and H_2 receptors are widely used. The H_2 receptor antagonists (such as ranitidine and cimetidine) are discussed in Chapter 12.

Actions of histamine via H_1 receptors

- smooth muscle contraction, in lungs, gut and uterus
- vasodilation
- inflammation. Intradermal histamine causes reddening, weals and flare due to vasodilation of the microvasculature and increased permeability of venules
- itch
- sneezing
- central nervous system regulation and maintaining a state of awareness or arousal; histamine-containing neurones are found in all parts of the central nervous system, including the cerebral cortex and the spinal cord.

Adverse effects of antihistamines

The sedating antihistamines cause adverse effects related to antagonism (blocking) of both histamine and muscarinic receptors (Table 5.2). These problems are shared with the phenothiazine antiemetics such as prochlorperazine.

Central nervous system

Both stimulation and depression of the central nervous system are possible adverse effects of H_1 antagonists. The usual effects are sedation, somnolence, diminished alertness, delayed reaction times, confusion, fatigue, depression, weakness or heaviness of the hands and impaired coordination, including diplopia. All these make driving hazardous.

Practice points

■ Cyclizine is not recommended for use in labour by the manufacturers because it may cause respiratory depression in the neonate (Amdipharm, ABPI, 2009).
■ Administration of an antiemetic, such as promethazine or prochlorperazine in labour, could make the neonate too drowsy to initiate breastfeeding efficiently. Careful observation to ensure that the infant latches completely is recommended.
■ If a nursing mother takes antihistamines, the breastfed infant may become sedated, fail to feed and fail to gain weight adequately. Sedation may also impair fluid and nutrient intake in adults.
■ Drowsiness is compounded by co-administration of other sedatives, including alcohol and opioids.

Although sedation is the usual response, the occasional patient will become restless, nervous and insomniac on the conventional dose (Skidgel and Erdos, 2006). Convulsions are possible, especially in neonates and children, and caution is advised with women with epilepsy (BNF, 2009). Other manifestations of central nervous system excitation include: dizziness, headache, tinnitus, euphoria, tremor, and irritability. Some antihistamines, for example promethazine, are structurally related to the phenothiazines and can cause posture and movement disorders (above).

Cardiovascular system

Histamine is a potent vasodilator. This effect is reversed by antihistamines. This action is life-saving in anaphylaxis and angioedema. However, antihistamines can act on the H_1 receptors to cause vasodilation, leading to hypotension, orthostatic hypotension, sweating and headache.

Gut and liver disturbance

Some people experience loss of appetite, abdominal pain, constipation, diarrhoea, nausea or vomiting when taking antihistamines long term. Soreness of mouth and tongue are occasional problems, which can be alleviated by taking the drugs with milk or food (Lucas, 1992). Occasionally, appetite increase and weight gain may occur (Skidgel and Erdos, 2006).

Antimuscarinic adverse effects

All the drugs that antagonize histamine have antimuscarinic (anticholinergic) properties. While these enhance the antiemetic actions, they add further adverse effects, summarized in Table 5.2.

Drying of the respiratory tract may facilitate the formation of mucus 'plugs', which may impede air flow and allow the development of infection or worsen asthma.

Practice points

■ Asthmatic women receiving antihistamines long term should be monitored.
■ If the patient is dehydrated, the drying and discomfort of the mucous membranes will be intensified.

Hypersensitivity responses (rare) include rash, contact dermatitis from topical applications, urine discolouration, photosensitivity, bronchospasm, and, rarely, anaphylaxis. Bone marrow depression is very rare.

Overdose may present as fits, involuntary movements, ataxia, excitement, hallucinations and coma, with fixed dilated pupils. Unintentional overdose by toddlers can be life-threatening, and is not uncommon. Other, rarer, adverse reactions are listed in Appendix I.

Cautions: antihistamines

- As with all drugs, previous hypersensitivity contraindicates use.
- Most manufacturers advise avoiding antihistamines during breastfeeding, due to their sedative properties. Antihistamines may sedate or irritate breastfed infants, and, if use is essential, close observation is needed (Lawrence and Schaefer, 2007). Repeated doses may cause lethargy and failure to feed.
- Abrupt discontinuation of antihistamines after regular use can cause withdrawal symptoms, such as confusion, nervousness, movement problems, muscle spasms, and excitability (Aronson, 2006). There is a report of a neonate exposed *in utero* being affected (van Tonningen, 2007a).
- Use in pregnancy should be on specialist advice, when the potential benefits have been weighed against the known but small risks.

Interactions: antihistamines

The adverse effects of antihistamines are compounded by drugs with similar actions:

- Administration of other sedatives, such as alcohol or opioids, will greatly enhance sedation.
- Concurrent use of another drug with antimuscarinic actions, such as phenothiazines or tricyclic antidepressants, will produce significant drying of the mouth, tachycardia and other adverse effects.
- If antihistamines are combined with drugs that damage the vestibulocochlear (auditory) nerve, such as furosemide (frusemide), gentamicin, or salicylates, any damage to this nerve will be masked and therefore remain undetected, increasing the risk of irreversible damage.
- Antihistamines interfere with skin testing for allergy. Therefore, they should be withdrawn for 1 week before testing.

Other antiemetics

Antimuscarinics, serotonin antagonists, pyridoxine (vitamin B_6), ginger, cannabinoids, benzodiazepines, and corticosteroids (particularly dexamethasone) are also useful antiemetics in some circumstances. In hyperemesis gravidarum, short courses of dexamethasone, prednisolone or oral methylprednisolone are sometimes prescribed to good effect (Safari et al., 1998; Sheehan, 2007). Adrenocorticotropic hormone is ineffective (Jewell and Young, 2000). Corticosteroids are considered in Chapters 7 and 15 and benzodiazepines in Chapters 18 and 19.

Antimuscarinic drugs

Antimuscarinics, such as atropine and hyoscine (scopolamine), are generally second choice antiemetics after antihistamines. Hyoscine hydrobromide (Kwells®) is an important over the counter drug for motion sickness, but it is very sedating. The adverse effect profile of antimuscarinics is as described for antihistamines.

Serotonin antagonists

Serotonin (5-hydroxytryptamine, 5HT) is a neurotransmitter found throughout the brain, where it has many different receptors and actions, and in other body systems (SSRIs, Chapter 19). The receptors involved in vomiting are mainly the $5HT_3$ receptors, but other classes ($5HT_4$) are involved. These are found in the vomiting centre, the chemoreceptor trigger zone and the gut wall; when stimulated, they cause emesis.

Antagonists of serotonin (5HT$_3$), such as ondansetron (Zofran®) and granisetron (Kytril®), are effective antiemetics. The half-life of ondansetron is between 3–5.5 hours. In midwifery, ondansetron is most likely to be used postoperatively, particularly when other, cheaper drugs have failed, or prior to Caesarean delivery if the woman has a history of emesis or migraine. Oral dispersible forms, which allow (rapid) buccal absorption, are available. Granisetron was found to be more effective than metoclopramide or droperidol in reducing nausea and vomiting following spinal anaesthesia for Caesarean section (Fujii et al., 1998).

Practice point

■ Intravenous ondansetron may be urgently required by doctors managing women with severe postoperative emesis.

Although ondansetron is generally well tolerated, there are occasional adverse effects, such as: headache, flushing, sedation, dry mouth, shivering, hypotension, retention of urine, sleep disorders, gastrointestinal disturbances, abdominal pain, and, rarely, hypersensitivity reactions, visual disturbances, jaundice, oedema, cardiac dysrhythmias, or fits. In women of reproductive age, adverse effects following postpartum administration are usually confined to mild headache, drowsiness and dryness of mouth.

Increased incidence of hypospadias was reported following first trimester administration, suggesting a need for fetal ultrasound (Goldstein and Berkovitch, 2007). No information is available in the BNF (2009) on the use of these drugs in pregnancy and breastfeeding, but the manufacturers advise against use unless potential benefits outweigh the risks. Ondansetron passes into breast milk (GlaxoSmithKline, ABPI, 2009), and careful observation of the breastfed infant is recommended.

Pyridoxine

Pyridoxine (vitamin B$_6$) has been used as an antiemetic for 40 years and may be effective in early pregnancy (Mitchelson, 1992b; Mazzotta and Magee, 2000; Sheehan, 2007). It reduces nausea, but not vomiting (Kametas and Nelson-Piercy, 2007). In a double-blind, placebo controlled trial of 342 women attending antenatal clinic, pyridoxine 30–200 mg per day reduced nausea over 5 days, and no adverse effects were reported (Vutyavanich et al., 1995). Doses used ranged from 10 to 100 mg daily, which is above the daily vitamin requirement (2 mg/day) and the recommended safety limits, 10 mg/day (NCC, 2008b), but lower than the dose (200 mg/day) associated with peripheral neuropathy (numbness, paraesthaesia and unsteady gait) (BNF, 2009).

The recommended dose should not be exceeded. Sale of products administering a daily dose of more than 10 mg of pyridoxine is restricted. The BNF (2009) includes premenstrual syndrome, but not pregnancy sickness, under the indications for pyridoxine at 50–100 mg/day. Pyridoxine was one ingredient of Debendox® (dicyclomine, doxylamine and pyridoxine), which was prescribed for emesis in early pregnancy, until it was suddenly withdrawn by the manufacturers in 1983 on suspicion of causing congenital abnormalities (Howden, 1995).

Ginger

Ginger increases gastric motility, and reduces postoperative emesis (Chaiyakunapruk et al., 2006). A randomized controlled trial (n = 123) in Thailand indicated that 750 mg ginger preparation before meals 3 times each day for 4 days was more effective than pyridoxine in preventing emesis in pregnancy. The adverse effects reported were heartburn, sedation and one case of cardiac dysrhythmia (Chittumma et al., 2007). To date, there are no indications that ginger causes congenital anomalies, but there may be theoretical reasons to prefer ginger root to other preparations (Goldstein and Berkovitch, 2007).

Cannabinoids

Cannabis is used by disseminated sclerosis sufferers to reduce pain and emesis (Chapter 20). Nabilone was developed to incorporate the antiemetic effects of cannabis, without the euphoriant actions. All cannabinoids may cause sedation, dry mouth, sleep disturbance, hallucinations, psychosis, dizziness and loss of orientation. Nabilone is likely to be superseded by dronabinol, which has a lower incidence of these adverse reactions. Manufacturers of nabilone advise against use in pregnancy and lactation (BNF, 2009).

Implications for practice: antiemetics

Vomiting is potentially dangerous to mother and fetus. No one should be left alone while vomiting.

Ideally, no antiemetics should be administered to pregnant or lactating women. Non-pharmacological measures should be employed to minimize emesis; if these fail, specialist advice should be sought.

If antiemetics are administered, the midwife must undertake to monitor the client, according to the drug prescribed.

Monitoring for all D_2 antagonists (metochlopramide and prochlorperazine)

Potential problem	Management suggestions
Acute dystonic reaction	Procyclidine and management protocols should be available
Movement disorders/signs of restlessness	Monitor, be prepared to withhold further doses
CNS depression, sedation	Monitor all intake, respirations, sedation in mother and neonate
	Protect neonate from hypothermia
	Provide extra help with breastfeeding
	Avoid other sedatives, for example alcohol, opioids
Hypo- or hypertension	Monitor BP, stand up gradually
Cardiac dysrhythmias	Monitor for palpitations
Drug accumulation	Monitor for dehydration, check urine output
Breast tenderness	Advise client
Risk of seizures	Avoid dopamine antagonists in women with epilepsy
Withdrawal reaction	Following prolonged administration, taper dose over several weeks, observe neonate for signs of restlessness

If a phenothiazine is administered, the monitoring described under antihistamines and antimuscarinics should be added (Table 5.2).

Effects of antiemetics on the fetus

Since midwives are often asked for advice on emesis in early pregnancy, the available evidence is summarized:

■ Antihistamines are considered the safest antiemetics in early pregnancy (Mazzotta and Magee, 2000; NCC, 2008b), but they are often ineffective. Since these drugs have been widely used in the past, it is likely that the risk to the fetus is low when treatment is limited to one or two doses. Studies involving over 200,000 women indicate no additional risk of major congenital malformations (Diav-Citrin et al., 2003; Aronson, 2006; Bartfai et al., 2008), and epidemiological evidence suggests that treating pregnancy-associated emesis may reduce preterm birth and low birth weight (Goldstein and Berkovitch, 2007). Meclozine was shown to confer benefit (Källén and Mottet, 2003). Also, stress is linked to fetal malformations (Hansen et al., 2000), and hyperemesis gravidarum is linked to cleft palate (McBride, 1969).

- Promethazine teoclate (Avomine®), promethazine hydrochloride (Phenergan®), and cyclizine are not recommended in pregnancy by the manufacturers. If used in the last 2 weeks, the neonate may show signs of irritability (Manx Healthcare, sanofi-aventis, Amdipharm, ABPI, 2009).
- Due to risks of premature labour, dimenhydrinate and diphenhydramine are not recommended during the third trimester (Goldstein and Berkovitch, 2007).
- Used in the last trimester, particularly the last 2 weeks, antihistamines have been linked with increased incidence of retrolental fibroplasia in premature infants (Rayburn and Conover 1993; Pangle, 2000), but this is not confirmed in more recent work (Goldstein and Berkovitch, 2007).
- Some over the counter antiemetics and analgesics contain appreciable amounts of caffeine, which, in daily doses over 300 mg, has, in observational studies, been associated with adverse outcomes and low birth weight. This is equivalent to some 3–6 cups of instant coffee per day (Peters and Schaefer, 2007) (Chapter 20).

Practice point

- If any antiemetic is used in pregnancy, it is important that a specialist is consulted if symptoms do not settle within 24–48 hours (BNF, 2009).

Conclusion

Further large-scale cohort studies are needed to establish the true efficacy and incidence of adverse effects of antiemetics in early pregnancy (Mazzotta and Magee, 2000; Jewell and Young, 2000). No consensus exists on the management of emesis in labour. The widespread, prophylactic use of sedating drugs such as prochlorperazine, often in combination with opioids, may impede the mother's participation in labour. The prolonged action of prochlorperazine means that both mother and infant may be sedated at a time when breastfeeding should be initiated. Some US authors advise against the intramuscular administration of prochlorperazine, due to the high incidence of adverse effects (Brunton, 1996). The shorter half-life of metoclopramide makes this drug a more acceptable alternative, but it is not recommended for women under 20 years of age, due to potentially serious adverse reactions. Many adverse effects of antiemetics are subtle, and easily overlooked or attributed to co-administered analgesics. Acupressure may offer a non-pharmacological alternative (NCC, 2004, 2007). Not all women will experience emesis following opioid administration. The 'normal' vomiting of unmedicated labour is usually transient, and less distressing than the adverse effects of antiemetics. Therefore, the value of prophylactic antiemetics in unmedicated labour is uncertain.

Further reading

- Goldstein, L. and Berkovitch, M. (2007) Antiemetics, in Schaefer, C., Peters, P.W. and Miller, R.K. (eds) *Drugs during Pregnancy and Lactation: Treatment Options and Risk Assessment*, 2nd edn. Elsevier, Oxford.
- Jordan, S. (2008) *The Prescription Drug Guide for Nurses*. Open University Press/McGraw-Hill, Maidenhead; Chapter 12.
- Mazzotta, P. and Magee, L. (2000) A risk-benefit assessment of pharmacological and non-pharmacological treatments for nausea and vomiting of pregnancy. *Drugs*, 59: 781–800.

CHAPTER 6

Drugs Increasing Uterine Contractility: Uterotonics (Oxytocics)

Sue Jordan

This chapter considers the drugs commonly used for induction and augmentation of labour and prevention and treatment of postpartum haemorrhage (PPH).

Chapter contents

- Uterine contractility
- Uterotonics (oxytocics)
- Prostaglandins
- Oxytocin
- Newer drugs
- Summary: induction/augmentation of labour
- Ergometrine
- Summary: third stage of labour and postpartum haemorrhage

Uterine contractility

The smooth muscle of the uterus has considerable spontaneous activity, which can be modified by drugs. Smooth muscle contractions are triggered by waves of electrical excitation that rapidly spread from cell to cell. Electrical activity is initiated by 'spike' potentials arising spontaneously in 'pacemaker' areas throughout the myometrium. The force of uterine contraction depends on the number of gap junctions and the frequency and duration of the electrical activity in pacemaker areas. The responsiveness of the uterus varies with the period of gestation, the degree of uterine stretch and the region of the myometrium. Electrical activity, and therefore contractility, is influenced by:

- *Oxytocin:* Fetal and maternal oxytocin play an important facilitative role in childbirth; secretion of both increases during labour. The number of oxytocin receptors in the uterus increases over 100 times during pregnancy.
- *Sympathetic nervous system:* Stimulation of **alpha$_1$ receptors** excites the uterus, while stimulation of beta$_2$ receptors inhibits contractions. If a woman experiences fear or anxiety, endogenous adrenaline/epinephrine may reduce uterine contractions, and postpone or prolong labour. This is more likely if women are exposed to unfamiliar staff, surroundings and technologies (Niven, 1992).

■ *Steroid hormones:* Progesterone plays a role in maintaining the pregnancy by reducing uterine contractility. The falling concentration of progesterone, coupled with the rising concentration of oestrogen towards term, is generally considered to be responsible for the corresponding increase in oxytocin sensitivity.

■ *Relaxin* reduces oxytocin release and inhibits uterine activity throughout pregnancy.

■ *Endothelin-1* induces uterine contractility at term.

■ *Prostaglandins* and related substances, such as platelet-activating factor, are important regulators of childbirth. Production of prostaglandins by fetal membranes increases in the last month of pregnancy. The release of prostaglandins is stimulated by vaginal examination and membrane rupture (Kelsey and Prevost, 1994).

■ *Serotonin* is an important neurotransmitter in all smooth muscle. It increases uterine contractility. Its action is mimicked by the ergot alkaloids, for example ergometrine and lysergic acid derivatives (LSD).

■ *Uterine stretch* increases the number of oxytocin receptors and contractility.

■ *Mechanical stimulation* of the fetal membranes or the cervix can induce labour (Ganong, 2005; Rang et al., 2007).

Uterotonics (oxytocics)

Uterotonics or **oxytocics** are used for induction and augmentation of labour, prevention and treatment of postpartum haemorrhage (PPH), control of bleeding due to incomplete abortion, and active management of the third stage of labour (Table 6.1). The uterotonics used in the UK are prostaglandins, oxytocin, ergometrine, mifepristone and carbetocin, a synthetic analogue of oxytocin. Syntometrine® is a combination of oxytocin and ergometrine.

Table 6.1 Uterotonics in childbirth

Use	Drugs	Route
Induction and augmentation of labour	Oxytocin	Intravenous (5 units/day)
	Prostaglandins (dinoprostone and misoprostol)	Dinoprostone: *per vaginam* Misoprostol: oral or vaginal administration
Prevention of PPH in third stage of labour	Oxytocin	Intravenous or intramuscular (5 or 10 units)
	Ergometrine (ergonovine)	Intravenous or intramuscular (500 micrograms)
	Syntometrine® (oxytocin + ergometrine)	Intramuscular (5 units + 500 micrograms)
Management of PPH	Oxytocin	Intravenous injection followed by infusion if needed
	Ergometrine	Intravenous or intramuscular
	Syntometrine® (oxytocin + ergometrine)	Intramuscular (5 units + 500 micrograms)
	Prostaglandins (carboprost and misoprostol)	Carboprost: intramuscular injection Misoprostol: oral or vaginal administration

Note: Misoprostol is not licensed for these indications in the UK.

Prostaglandins

The prostaglandins are a group of chemically related compounds made *in vivo* from the phospholipids of cell membranes in many tissues. They are important as 'local hormones' or paracrines.

Endogenous prostaglandins in childbirth

The process of parturition has two essential components:

1 *Cervical ripening (prostaglandins):* The formation of prostaglandins by the amnion increases towards the end of pregnancy, raising the concentration of prostaglandins in amniotic fluid, umbilical cord blood and maternal blood. These prostaglandins may be important in the initiation of labour. Uterine sensitivity to prostaglandins increases progressively throughout pregnancy.
2 *Uterine contractions (oxytocin and prostaglandins):* During the last month of pregnancy, the cervix normally 'ripens' under the influence of PGE_2 (prostaglandin E_2), which increases the production of enzymes that break down and loosen cervical collagen.

Four types of endogenous prostaglandins play a role in parturition. The letters assigned to them denote the chemical structure of the ring part of the molecule:

- PGE_1 – ripens the cervix
- PGE_2 – causes uterine contractions from late second trimester onwards and ripens the cervix
- PGI_2 – ensures blood flow from mother to fetus and maintains a patent ductus arteriosus
- PGF_2 – causes uterine contractions at all times (unlike oxytocin). It is also important in menstruation, when it causes vasoconstriction and uterine contraction.

Synthetic prostaglandins prescribed in childbirth

In the UK, the prostaglandins commonly used in midwifery are:

- *Dinoprostone* (PGE_2) for cervical priming and induction of labour, is usually administered vaginally. An overview of studies suggests that the time between induction and delivery is shortened by the use of prostaglandins (Dawood, 1995). The intravenous route is rarely used and is not indicated for induction of labour (NCC, 2008b).
- *Carboprost* (15 methyl PGF_2, a synthetic derivative) is given by deep intramuscular injection to manage PPH. This is usually given after other agents have failed to stop a haemorrhage, but may be the drug of choice if the woman is hypertensive (Gulmezoglu, 2000).
- *Gemeprost* (an analogue of PGE_1) is administered vaginally to assist with uterine evacuation.
- *Misoprostol* (an analogue of PGE_1) has been administered orally, sublingually, buccally and vaginally for induction and augmentation of labour and prevention and management of PPH (Hofmeyr et al., 1998; Amant et al., 1999; Lumbiganon et al., 1999; Souza et al., 2008; Catling, 2008). It is prescribed for the termination of pregnancy (Orioli and Castilla, 2000), following intrauterine death and, occasionally, for management of PPH (NCC, 2008b). Comparison with oxytocin (by randomized controlled trial, n = 150) indicated that misoprostol was associated with faster induction of labour and greater blood loss (ElSedeek et al., 2009). Neither oral, sublingual nor intravaginal misoprostol is currently licensed for use in pregnancy in the UK (BNF, 2009) and uncertainty persists regarding optimum dose, route of administration and safety (Hofmeyr and Gulmezoglu, 2000; Hofmeyr et al., 2000).

Prostaglandins, like oxytocin, increase uterine contractions. They also facilitate oxytocin in the induction of labour, thereby reducing the amount of oxytocin required (Darroca et al., 1996; Kelly et al., 2003). There would seem to be no advantage gained by using repeated applications of prostagandins for induction of labour (Nuutila and Kajanoja, 1996; Rix et al., 1996); lower doses are as effective as higher doses (Kelly et al., 2003). A randomized controlled trial (n = 5,041) found that vaginal PGE$_2$ gel was not associated with an increased rate of Caesarean section (Hannah et al., 1996), and this is supported by a systematic review (Kelly et al., 2003). However, women with a previous Caesarean undergoing induction are more likely to deliver by Caesarean (McDonagh et al., 2005).

How the body handles prostaglandins

Endogenous prostaglandins are largely inactivated at their site of action. Exogenous prostaglandins may pass into the systemic (general) circulation *via* the venous plexuses surrounding the vagina and cervix. Metabolites remain in the circulation for several hours (duration depends on dose), and are transferred to the fetus (Bygdeman, 2003). Vaginal or cervical administration of prostaglandin pessaries or gels reduces but does not abolish systemic absorption and **adverse effects**. Prostaglandins are eliminated by the lungs, liver and kidneys.

Misoprostol – peak plasma concentration is seen within 1 hour of oral administration, but onset of peak uterine activity occurs 5–7 hours later (Ngai et al., 2000). When administered as prophylaxis in the third stage, some authors consider this too slow to prevent early blood loss (Amant et al., 1999), but others disagree (El-Refaey et al., 2000). Adverse effects persist 6–12 hours after oral administration (Lumbiganon et al., 2002).

Dinoprostone acts within about 10 minutes of vaginal insertion. The rate of absorption through the walls of the vagina differs between tablets and gels, with gels being absorbed more rapidly than tablets.

Practice points

■ Manufacturers (Ferring Pharmaceuticals, ABPI, 2009) suggest that following vaginal administration, the woman should remain lying down for 20–30 minutes to improve absorption.
■ Prostaglandin slow-release pessaries or inserts, unlike tablets, can be removed if problems occur and require fewer vaginal examinations (McEwan, 2007). No other differences are reported (n = 200) (Rabl et al., 2002).

Intracervical administration is invasive and no longer recommended for induction of labour, because inadvertent insertion into the extra-amniotic space may cause uterine hyperstimulation (NCC, 2008b). Intravaginal administration is more likely to be effective in bringing about vaginal delivery within 24 hours (Boulvain et al., 2008).

Practice points

■ The doses of the various dinoprostone preparations are related to the formulation and site of administration. For example, if vaginal gel is given by the intracervical route, this could result in dangerous overdose (Sweetman et al., 2007).
■ Different formulations also have different storage requirements and different **bioavailabilities**. Tablets, pessaries and gels are not **bioequivalent** and are not interchangeable.

Actions and adverse effects of prostaglandins

Prostaglandins act on distinct prostaglandin receptors, affecting most systems:

■ smooth muscle contraction – gut, uterus, blood vessels and bronchioles
■ vasodilation and hypotension

- pyrexia
- inflammation
- sensitization to pain
- central nervous system (tremor is a rare adverse effect)
- release of pituitary hormones, renin and adrenal steroids
- inhibition of autonomic nervous system responses
- increase in intraocular pressure
- diuresis plus loss of electrolytes.

Problems are most likely to occur when high doses are used, as in the control of postpartum haemorrhage or evacuation of the uterus, rather than in induction of labour (see Implications for practice below).

Smooth muscle contraction

Intensified uterine contractions

Uterine contractions may become abnormal and too intense, leading to pain, hypertonus and tetany, fetal compromise and **acidosis**, amniotic fluid embolism, placental abruption or rupture of the uterus or cervix, with or without previous Caesarean delivery (BNF, 2009); these problems are intensified if misoprostol is substituted for dinoprostone (Hofmeyr et al., 2000; NCC, 2008b). Women who are administered prostaglandins are more likely to receive epidural analgesia (Kelly et al., 2003). Lower doses and, possibly, gel formulations of dinoprostone present less risk (NCC, 2008b).

The fetal problems are similar to those produced by oxytocin: heart beat coupling, low **Apgar scores**, and risk of fetal death. Reviewers indicated that fetal heart rate changes associated with hyperstimulation are four times more likely than with placebo (RR 4.14, 95% CI, 1.93–8.90) (Kelly et al., 2003).

Uterine hyperstimulation occurred in 3% of women following insertion of vaginal prostaglandins (Blair et al., 1998) and in 8–10% of women following intracervical prostaglandins. Uterine rupture, typically through the lower posterior wall, may occur at any stage of gestation. To prevent this, tocolytics may be administered should uterine hyperstimulation occur (Dawood, 1995). Particular care is required if oxytocin and prostaglandins are administered sequentially.

Case reports

Reports on Confidential Enquiries into Maternal Deaths in the United Kingdom illustrate the danger of uterine rupture following administration of prostaglandins.

1 Labour was induced by prostaglandins at 42 weeks in a woman aged over 35, who had had 4 previous deliveries. After delivery, the woman died of postpartum haemorrhage, due to rupture of the uterus (DH, 1996: 41).
2 A grand multiparous woman was booked into a GP maternity unit. Post-term, labour was induced with prostaglandin pessaries. Following vaginal delivery, the woman became unable to breathe and collapsed. Rupture of the lower uterine segment was found at autopsy (DH, 1996: 84).
3 Labour was induced in an older parous woman with a history of precipitous labour with two 3 mg prostin pessaries. She became hypotensive, due to uterine rupture and postpartum haemorrhage (CEMACH, 2007: 83).

Practice points

■ Use of prostaglandins in grand multiparous women is hazardous and repeated doses may not be advisable in parous women, because the uterus is already weakened by previous deliveries and is more likely to rupture (CEMACH, 2007).
■ Administration of prostaglandins is hazardous if there are no facilities on site to manage emergencies such as rupture of the uterus.

Misoprostol, administered vaginally, has been associated with uterine rupture in women with no previous Caesarean sections (Hofmeyr and Gulmezoglu, 2000).

Practice points

■ Uterine contractility and fetal heart rate should be monitored regularly initially, and when contractions begin, with continuous electronic monitoring. If contractions are normal, intermittent auscultation can replace electronic monitoring (NCC, 2008b). Women should be informed that this will be necessary.
■ The woman should not be left alone for at least 20–30 minutes after vaginal administration (Chamberlain and Zander, 1999).

Pelvic haematoma may arise from violent contractions. If this is extensive, clotting factors will be depleted, leading to coagulation failure and bleeding. The incidence of disseminated intravascular coagulopathy (DIVC), a very serious bleeding complication, is estimated to be 5 in 10,000 deliveries, and is increased some sixfold by administration of prostaglandins, mainly as gels. Risks are increased in post-term pregnancies and older women (de Abajo et al., 2004) (see Case report under Oxytocin, below).

Practice points

■ Close observation for signs of bleeding is important to detect early signs of this very serious condition.
■ Removal of vaginal inserts usually reverses hyperstimulation, but this option is not available with tablets (Rabl et al., 2002).

Increased contractility of the gastrointestinal tract
Increased gastrointestinal contractility causes diarrhoea, nausea, vomiting, bile reflux, abdominal cramps, hiccups, or a choking sensation. These problems are less likely with vaginal administration than with other routes (Mahmood et al., 1995). The incidence of vomiting, diarrhoea and fever following insertion of intravaginal dinoprostone was reported as 0.2% (Sweetman et al., 2007). Oral misoprostol for postpartum haemorrhage prophylaxis was associated with diarrhoea in 5% of women (Lumbiganon et al., 2002).

When prostaglandins are used as abortifacents, the incidence of emesis (60%) and diarrhoea (20%) is high; antiemetic and antidiarrhoeal agents are often needed and may be prescribed prophylactically (Olsen and D'Oria, 1992). Such problems currently preclude the use of prostaglandins for the routine prophylactic management of the third stage of labour (Gulmezoglu, 2000). Prostaglandins may stimulate the fetal bowel, causing meconium release into the amniotic fluid, which may not be related to fetal distress.

Constriction of the bronchioles
Constriction of the bronchioles may induce wheezing, cough and asthma; women with asthma are particularly sensitive to PGF_2 (similar to carboprost – Hemabate®) (Campbell and Halushka, 1996).

Vasoconstriction

Vasoconstriction caused by PGF_2 and 15 methyl PGF_2 (carboprost) may result in hypertension up to 2 hours after injection. Hypertension is more likely in pre-eclamptic/eclamptic patients. Occasionally, carboprost (PGF_2) may cause an increase in pulmonary artery pressure, which alters the perfusion of the lungs, resulting in pulmonary oedema, dyspnoea and reduced **partial pressure** of oxygen and increased partial pressure of carbon dioxide (Hayashi, 1990). Coronary artery spasm, associated with myocardial infarction (Gulmezoglu, 2000), and a fatal myocardial infarction in a high-risk woman have been reported (Sweetman et al., 2007).

Practice point

■ Women receiving carboprost should be monitored for hypoxia, using a pulse oximeter, and administered oxygen if necessary. Problems are more likely if there is pre-existing heart or lung disease (Upjohn, 1990).

Vasodilation

In contrast, PGE_2 (dinoprostone) causes vasodilation, which usually occurs within 30 minutes of administration (Dawood, 1995). The consequences of vasodilation are:

■ sweating, flushing and dizziness
■ cranial vasodilation causing headache
■ reduction in blood pressure (BP), resulting in increased heart rate and contractility, which may induce cardiac dysrhythmias (Sweetman et al., 2007)
■ cases of cardiovascular collapse have been recorded (CEMACH, 2005).

Practice point

■ Women receiving prostaglandins should have regular BP monitoring.

Pyrexia and shivering

During infection, prostaglandins act on the hypothalamus to induce fever. Pyrexia may appear within minutes or hours after prostaglandin administration and may be accompanied by shivering, chills and **leucocytosis**. Distressing shivering in 42% of women (n = 200) detracted from the use of oral misoprostol for postpartum haemorrhage prophylaxis (Amant et al., 1999). Following administration of oral misoprostol for prophylactic management of the third stage, some women shiver for 20–30 minutes, during which time they are unable to hold or feed their infants (El-Refaey et al., 2000).

A pyrexia of more than 1°C occurred in 34% of women receiving oral misoprostol for prevention of postpartum haemorrhage (Amant et al., 1999), and is also associated with intramuscular carboprost. Problems are more likely at higher doses (Gülmezoglu et al., 2007). These effects are usually transient and disappear within hours of the last administration (Upjohn, 1990).

Practice point

■ This pyrexia should not be mistaken for a sign of infection. However, it is important not to overlook the possibility of infection.

The inflammatory response and pain

Prostaglandins are part of the normal response to tissue damage, producing pain, heat and inflammation and therefore may cause pain and redness at the injection or administration site. Vaginal administration is associated with localized pain and irritation; any fever and raised white cell count are likely to be transient.

Local infection may follow intra- or extra-amniotic administration (Sweetman et al., 2007), and vaginal application may introduce ascending infection if membranes are ruptured (Tan and Hannah, 2000).

Backache is reported as an adverse effect of prostaglandins. The increase in pain from uterine contractions would appear to be related to the dose of dinoprostone (Tan and Tay, 1999).

Practice point

■ Contractions associated with induced labour may be more painful than natural contractions. Women should be advised of this and the opportunity to labour in water should be offered (NCC, 2008b).

Pelvic inflammatory disease, particularly endometriosis, may be worsened by prostaglandin administration.

Central nervous system

Tremor or seizures may be due to pyrexia or direct stimulant effects of prostaglandins on the central nervous system.

Endocrine effects

PGE_2 has been administered to suppress lactation (England et al., 1988). It is purported to act as a dopamine agonist in the anterior pituitary and suppress prolactin secretion (Caminiti et al., 1980), but this is contentious (Tulundi et al., 1985). A small reduction in breastfeeding has been observed in association with antepartum prostaglandin administration (Jordan et al., 2009b).

Loss of fluids and electrolytes

Loss of fluids and electrolytes is attributed to impairment of renal tubular reabsorption. It may cause cramps and contribute to hypotension.

Raised intraocular pressure

Prostaglandins may cause eye pain or even precipitate acute glaucoma.

Practice point

■ Prostaglandins should be used cautiously, if at all, in women with a history (or strong family history) of glaucoma (BNF, 2009).

Hypersensitivity responses

Healthcare professionals should avoid skin contact with prostaglandins to avoid possible contact dermatitis (Aronson, 2006).

Contraindications and cautions: prostaglandins

Prostaglandin induction is **contraindicated** in the presence of ruptured membranes (BNF, 2009). Prostaglandins are used cautiously, if at all, in any of the following conditions likely to impede vaginal delivery or predispose to uterine rupture:

- previous uterine surgery
- major cephalopelvic disproportion
- *placenta praevia* or unexplained vaginal bleeding
- malpresentation – particularly transverse lie
- fetal distress
- severe fetal growth restriction
- grand multiparity (4+)
- multiple pregnancy
- history of difficult or traumatic delivery or hypertonic uterine contractions
- polyhydramnios or oligohydramnios
- untreated pelvic infection.

If the fetus is already compromised, prostaglandin administration is likely to worsen the situation. Many existing maternal diseases may be acutely exacerbated by administration of prostaglandins. These include cardiac disease, pulmonary disorders, asthma, hypo- or hypertension, epilepsy, glaucoma, pre-eclampsia or raised intraocular pressure, acute pelvic inflammatory disease, and active genital herpes. In addition, women with liver or kidney insufficiency will be unable to eliminate prostaglandins as rapidly as normal.

Prostaglandin induction increases the risk of uterine rupture and perinatal death in women with previous Caesarean deliveries (Smith et al., 2004). Contrary to manufacturers' advice, the NICE guideline (NCC, 2008b: 10) sanctions induction of labour in women with previous Caesarean or ruptured membranes, with signed informed consent.

Practice point

- Administration of prostaglandins is governed by some restrictions, for example manufacturers advise the administration of only two doses (2 x 3 mg) of dinoprostone as Prostin E2® vaginal tablets (Pharmacia, ABPI, 2009).

Storage

Parenteral prostaglandin preparations should always be kept in a refrigerator. Many of these products have short shelf lives. The exact requirements differ for the various preparations and midwives should consult the manufacturer's data sheet for each preparation. Misoprostol tablets can be stored without a refrigerator and have long shelf lives.

Interactions: prostaglandins

- *Oxytocin:* if two uterine stimulants are administered concurrently, hyperstimulation may occur. Therefore, oxytocin is usually not given until 6–12 hours after the last dose of prostaglandin (Kelsey and Prevost, 1994); the minimum interval is 6 hours (BNF, 2009).

Case report

A woman had labour induced with prostaglandins because of post-maturity. This was later augmented with oxytocin. Fetal distress developed, and delivery was by forceps. The patient collapsed quickly due to haemorrhage from a tear in the lower uterine segment (DH, 1966: 63).

   The combination of prostaglandins plus oxytocin may overstimulate the uterus, which may lead to rupture. Therefore this drug combination requires careful surveillance.

- *Aspirin* and other NSAIDs antagonize the production of prostaglandins, thus delaying or prolonging labour. Paracetamol does not interact.
- *Alcohol* antagonizes the action of dinoprostone.

Implications for practice: prostaglandins

In the event of emergencies, appropriate 'rescue therapies' and staff must be available.

Potential problem	Management suggestions
Dysfunctional uterine contractility	Before administration, check for disproportion and fetal distress
	Avoid prostaglandin induction if there is any risk of uterine rupture, for example when tone is increased or if the fetus is already stressed. Particular care if the woman has undergone a previous Caesarean delivery
	Monitor uterine contractions and fetal heart, particularly for the first hour after insertion. Do not leave unattended
	Limit administration, *both dose and duration*, as advised by manufacturers for different preparations
	Ensure tocolytic therapy is available (Chapter 7)
	Ensure facilities are available for prompt delivery, in the event of uterine hypertonus
	Allow 6 hours between dinoprostone insertion and oxytocin administration (BNF, 2009)
Cord prolapse, secondary to uncoordinated contractions	Ensure engagement has been carefully assessed and the head is not dislodged during vaginal examinations
Respiratory distress, asthma	Monitor breathing patterns, shortness of breath or chest tightness. Avoid in women with asthma, if possible
Fever	Monitor temperature, assess whether infection present. Sponge to prevent hyperthermia, if necessary
Shivering	Offer blankets. Be prepared to assist mother to hold and feed neonate for up to 30 minutes, particularly after misoprostol administration
Cardiovascular collapse	Monitor BP and HR. Hypotension is a danger with dinoprostone. Particular care following repeated doses
Worsening of pelvic inflammatory disease	Before administration, check for history of pelvic inflammatory disease
Parenteral preparations are chemically unstable, and may become inactivated over time	Check storage instructions, shelf life and temperature of the refrigerator used for storage on a regular basis

II

Therapeutic failure	Bishop score should be reassessed 6 hours after vaginal application of gel or tablets or 24 hours after vaginal pessary insertion (NCC, 2008b). Facilities for emergency Caesarean delivery should be available

Summary

When compared to oxytocin for induction of labour, dinoprostone intravaginal gel is equally effective and less likely to cause postpartum haemorrhage and neonatal jaundice. It is also less invasive, and allows ambulation, and is therefore more popular with women. While prostaglandins administered topically are usually safe, they are not without adverse effects. Women should be informed of these. Prostaglandins reduce the need for oxytocin administration. Their ability to influence the outcomes of labour, including rates of failed induction, Caesarean section or instrumental deliveries, remains a subject for further large-scale investigation (Dawood, 1995). Prostaglandins are associated with more adverse effects and are less effective than oxytocin and/or ergometrine when administered to prevent postpartum haemorrhage (Gülmezoglu et al., 2007), and are not recommended for routine use in current guidelines (NCC, 2007).

Oxytocin

The role of oxytocin in normal labour is shown in Figure 6.1.

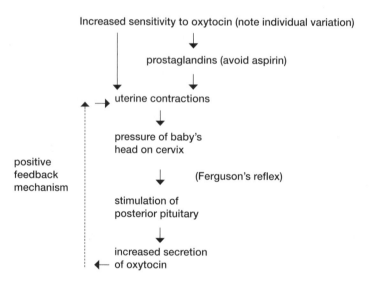

The onset of normal labour depends on a positive feedback mechanism, whereby an initial change is intensified until completion of the process. To summarize, the pressure of the baby's head on the cervix causes the release of oxytocin, which stimulates uterine contractions and further increases the pressure on the cervix, intensifying the release of oxytocin. This feedback loop repeats until the baby is delivered. The positive feedback controls of labour culminate in a surge of oxytocin release.

Figure 6.1 Diagram to indicate the role of oxytocin in normal labour
Source: Adapted from Ganong, 1999

Practice point

■ Ferguson's reflex may be impaired if epidural analgesia is administered (Parker and Schimmer, 2006).

Actions of oxytocin

Oxytocin, in association with other factors, plays a pivotal role in labour, milk ejection and mother–infant bonding. Oxytocin acts on oxytocic receptors to cause:

■ uterine contraction at term by direct action on smooth muscle and increased prostaglandin production
■ constriction of umbilical blood vessels
■ contraction of myoepithelial cells (milk ejection reflex)
■ bonding, including affectionate touch, vocalizations, gaze, frequent checking of infants (Feldman et al., 2007), and social bonding (Leng et al., 2008)
■ attenuation of the stress response, in conjunction with prolactin and endogenous opioids (Slattery and Neumann, 2008).

Oxytocin acts on antidiuretic hormone (ADH) receptors to cause:

■ a sudden increase or decrease in blood pressure (particularly diastolic) due to vasodilation
■ water retention.

(Oxytocin and antidiuretic hormone have very similar structures, which explains the overlap in functions.)

Other actions of oxytocin include:

■ uterine (Fallopian) tube contraction to assist sperm transport
■ male sexual behaviour (Leng et al., 2005)
■ luteolysis (involution of the corpus luteum)
■ other neurotransmitter roles in the central nervous system, including mood regulation postpartum and social learning (Wahl, 2004)
■ suppression of food-seeking behaviour and appetite in mothers (Leng et al., 2008)
■ promotion of feeding and opioid activation in infant animals (Uvnäs-Moberg et al., 1998).

Oxytocin is synthesized in the hypothalamus, the gonads, the placenta and the uterus. From 32 weeks' gestation onwards, oxytocin concentrations, and therefore uterine activity, are higher during the night (Hirst et al., 1993).

The release of endogenous oxytocin is increased by:

■ labour
■ cervical, vaginal or breast stimulation
■ circulating oestrogens
■ increased plasma **osmolality**/concentration
■ low circulating fluid volume
■ stress.

Stress in labour can initiate precipitate labour, known as the 'fetal ejection reflex'. Stress caused by an infant crying will stimulate milk production.

The release of oxytocin is suppressed by:

■ alcohol (alcohol may impair the establishment of breastfeeding)
■ decreased plasma osmolality (concentration)

- high circulating fluid volume (Parker and Schimmer, 2006)
- stress, due to blood loss, Caesarean delivery, pain or prolonged labour, may reduce secretion of endogenous oxytocin and, hence, breastfeeding (Dewey, 2001)
- relaxin, in conjunction with endogenous opioids
- opioids, including morphine and dynorphin (Lindow et al., 1999, 2005), epidurals containing opioids and local anaesthetics (Rahm et al., 2002)
- endogenous cannabinoids
- depletion following bursts of secretion (Cassoni et al., 2006, Rossoni et al., 2008).

Practice points

- Rapid infusion of intravenous fluids may temporarily reduce uterine contractility (Mayberry et al., 2002).
- The requirement for oxytocin during labour shows individual variation.

The endogenous release of oxytocin is pulsatile. Infusions or bolus doses do not follow this pattern. Overexposure to oxytocin may decrease or desensitize oxytocin receptors, leaving the tissues unresponsive to the hormone (Gimpl and Fahrenholz, 2001; Plested and Bernal, 2001).

Practice point

- Women who have received high doses of oxytocin may experience decreased uterine contractility (Robinson et al., 2003), but the impact on lactation is unknown.

Pulsatile administration of oxytocin may allow a reduction in total dose, but has not, to date, shown any benefits (NCC, 2007).

Synthetic oxytocin

Oxytocin (Syntocinon®) is manufactured to reproduce the structure and actions of the natural hormone. The secretion of endogenous oxytocin is *not* suppressed by a negative feedback mechanism. This means that artificial syntocinon will not suppress the release of endogenous oxytocin.

Practice point

- There is a danger that the combined actions of natural oxytocin and artificially administered oxytocin can easily lead to *overstimulation of the uterus*. In view of this, the midwife must be alert for the onset of active labour during oxytocin infusion, as the combined effects of two sources of oxytocin may lead to uterine hyperstimulation and a potentially dangerous situation (Shyken and Petrie, 1995) (see Uterine rupture below).

Indications for synthetic oxytocin

Indications for oxytocin administration include:

- prevention of postpartum haemorrhage by intramuscular injection (alone or combined with ergometrine), slow intravenous injection or intravenous infusion for high-risk women, or following Caesarean delivery (CEMACH, 2005).
- augmentation or stimulation of delayed labour by intravenous infusion, to shorten the first stage (NCC, 2007). Early administration of oxytocin to nulliparous women in early active labour with primary dysfunctional labour shortened duration of labour but had no impact on

incidence of Caesarean delivery; instrumental vaginal deliveries were less common, but the difference did not quite reach statistical significance (47/208 versus 62/204, OR 0.67, 0.4–1.0) (Hinshaw et al., 2008).

■ treatment of postpartum haemorrhage by slow intravenous injection or infusion.
■ incomplete, inevitable or missed abortion (BNF, 2009).
■ management of retained placenta by injection into umbilical vein (NCC, 2007).

Carbetocin is licensed for the prevention of uterine atony following Caesarean delivery. It has many of the properties of oxytocin, but a longer **half-life** and duration of action.

How the body handles synthetic oxytocin

Oxytocin may be administered intramuscularly, intravenously, sublingually or intranasally. Infusion pumps are recommended for intravenous infusions (BNF, 2009). Following intramuscular injection, oxytocin acts within 3–7 minutes and lasts 30–60 minutes. It acts within 1–4 minutes of intravenous administration; increased uterine contractions begin almost immediately, stabilize within 15–60 minutes of commencing intravenous infusion and last for 20 minutes after discontinuation. Oxytocin is removed by enzymes in the liver, spleen, ovaries and placenta. Estimates of half-life range from 1–20 minutes, although pharmacological data indicate a value of 15 minutes (Gonser, 1995). The assumption that oxytocin does not cross the placenta and the fetal blood/brain barrier has been questioned (Graves, 1996; Wahl, 2004).

Practice points

■ Uterine action should be monitored during infusion and for 20 minutes after discontinuation.
■ If dosages are adjusted too frequently, within less than 40–60 minutes, it will not be possible to assess the effect of the infusion, as fewer than 3–5 half-lives will have elapsed (Gonser, 1995; Shyken and Petrie, 1995; Clayworth, 2000) (Chapter 1).

Sublingual and intranasal oxytocin for establishment and augmentation of breastfeeding conferred little benefit in clinical trials (Renfrew et al., 2000,; Fewtrell et al., 2006) (see Breast-feeding, below).

Adverse effects of oxytocin

When synthetic oxytocin is administered, its physiological actions may be intensified, leading to potentially dangerous adverse effects (see Implications for practice). The adverse effects can be grouped:

■ overstimulation of the uterus
■ contraction of umbilical blood vessels
■ antidiuretic actions and fluid retention
■ actions on blood vessels (constriction and dilation) and changes in blood pressure
■ postpartum haemorrhage
■ nausea
■ breastfeeding
■ hypersensitivity responses.

Overstimulation of the uterus

During the last 9 weeks of pregnancy, the responsiveness of uterine muscle to oxytocin increases eightfold (Parker and Schimmer, 2006). When oxytocin is administered, both the frequency and force of smooth muscle contractions are increased, intensifying the pain of labour (Olah and Gee, 1996), more so than prostaglandins (NCC, 2008b). Women report that contractions induced by oxytocin are more painful than those of spontaneous labour (Bramadat, 1994; Fraser et al., 1998). Augmentation of labour with oxytocin carries an inherent risk of uterine hyperstimulation: since some individuals are hypersensitive to oxytocin, infusion always entails some danger of a tetanic or spasmodic uterine contraction, however low the dose.

Practice points

- Following induction or augmentation, uterine action and the fetal heart rate must be continuously monitored (NCC, 2007), and constant attendance is recommended (Chamberlain and Zander, 1999, Gibb and Arulkumaran, 1997).
- If signs of fetal distress or uterine hyperstimulation appear, the oxytocin infusion should be discontinued immediately (BNF, 2009) and medical advice sought. Hyperstimulation should resolve within minutes (Parker and Schimmer, 2006).

Oxytocin administration impairs the application of the fetal head to the cervix (Allman et al., 1996). If the cervix has neither softened nor dilated, labour cannot progress and in these circumstances, violent, prolonged and forceful uterine contractions may have serious consequences:

- *Trauma to neonate and mother:* If the baby is forced through an incompletely dilated cervix, maternal soft tissues may be extensively lacerated.
- *Uterine rupture:* Uterine rupture is less likely in nulliparous women, but has occurred (DH, 1996). Oxytocin is used cautiously in women with a high risk of uterine rupture, for example those with lower segment uterine scars (BNF, 2009).

Case report

A grand multipara was managed by artificial rupture of membranes combined with low-dose oxytocin at 37 weeks' gestation, resulting in a spontaneous vaginal delivery. A laparotomy was undertaken to ascertain the cause of persistent postpartum haemorrhage, and longitudinal lateral rupture of the uterus was revealed. Despite resuscitative measures, the woman died (DH, 1994).

This woman was high risk, due to her age and parity. Grand multiparity is listed as a contraindication to oxytocin use (Alliance Pharmaceuticals, ABPI, 2008).

Practice point

- Guidelines recommend that oxytocin should not be started in the second stage of labour in parous women (NCC, 2007: 240).

- *Postpartum haemorrhage:* Postpartum haemorrhage following induction is more likely with oxytocin than dinoprostone (NCC, 2008b).
- *Pelvic haematoma:* This may arise from violent contractions. If this is extensive, clotting factors will be depleted, leading to coagulation failure and bleeding.
- *Risk of disseminated intravascular coagulopathy (DIVC):* This is increased some eightfold by administration of oxytocin for induction (de Abajo et al., 2004).
- *Placental abruption:* This has been attributed to violent uterine contractions and implicated in maternal death (DH, 1991).

Case report

This case illustrates the need to be alert to the possibility of placental abruption progressing to disseminated intravascular coagulation when oxytocin is administered.

Syntocinon was infused for 21.5 hours before birth. Towards the end of labour, clotting studies became abnormal. A blood loss of 300 ml was recorded at birth. Twenty minutes after birth, the patient collapsed with an unrecordable BP. Death followed the next day, despite intensive treatment (DH, 1991: 37).

Clotting factors were consumed in the placental bed, leaving the woman unable to coagulate and vulnerable to bleeding. Prolonged infusion requires careful monitoring due to the risks involved.

- *Amniotic fluid embolism:* This may be precipitated by tumultuous labour, particularly if the amniotic fluid is stained with meconium or death *in utero* has occurred. In the *Report on Confidential Enquiries into Maternal Deaths* (DH, 1991), 6 out of 9 deaths from amniotic fluid embolism were associated with either prostaglandin or oxytocin administration.
- *Fetal hypoxia:* During uterine contractions, blood vessels are compressed, impairing delivery of oxygen to the uterus, placenta and fetus. Normally, oxygenation is restored during relaxation, preventing accumulation of lactic acid. However, if the uterus is overstimulated and relaxation too brief, fetal hypoxia and acidosis will follow. Uterine tetany or spasm may reduce uterine blood flow to a point where the fetus is asphyxiated, with the possibility of intracranial haemorrhage or death. Therefore, fetal heart rate should be monitored continuously to detect early signs of fetal distress. Higher doses of oxytocin have been associated with increased incidence of assisted deliveries for fetal bradycardia and Apgar scores below 7 (Shyken and Petrie, 1995). Studies in the developing world highlight the increased risk of fetal intracranial haemorrhage associated with oxytocin infusion where facilities for fetal and uterine monitoring are suboptimal (Ellis et al., 2000).

Constriction of umbilical blood vessels

If this physiologically protective mechanism is activated prematurely, the fetus will become starved of oxygen. Fetal hypoxia may lead to bradycardia, cardiac dysrhythmia and even death (Sweetman et al., 2007). Any pre-existing fetal distress is likely to be worsened by oxytocin infusion.

Antidiuretic hormone actions and SIADH

The main action of antidiuretic hormones is to conserve water by acting (mainly) on the collecting ducts of the renal tubules (*via* the V_2 receptors). Due to structural similarities, oxytocin also causes water retention, resulting in:

- reduced urine output
- increased osmolality/concentration (and specific gravity) of urine
- plasma dilution
- **hyponatraemia**.

When synthetic oxytocin is administered, particularly in high doses, the actions of antidiuretic hormone are mimicked. In the absence of careful monitoring, this may produce dangerous water retention and intoxication.

Any water retained passes, by **osmosis**, from plasma into tissue fluids, and thence into the cells, which then swell:

- Water retention may increase the volume of tissue fluid. This causes dependent oedema, raised jugular venous pressure and even pulmonary oedema, which impairs breathing and oxygenation.

■ If water retention causes cells in vital organs to swell, water intoxication may follow. *Most cases of water intoxication are not preceded by signs of fluid retention and present as seizures or loss of consciousness* (Sweetman et al., 2007). Water intoxication is more likely if **hypotonic** infusions, such as glucose (dextrose), are administered (BNF, 2009). If water intoxication occurs:

■ cells of the cardiac conduction system may be disturbed, giving dangerous cardiac dysrhythmias, particularly premature beats, which the woman may experience as 'palpitations'. Cardiac dysrhythmias reduce cardiac output, thus jeopardizing the blood supply to the placenta

■ cells in the brain swell. Initially, the woman becomes confused, drowsy, disorientated, uncoordinated and 'loses touch with reality' – convulsions may follow. Headache and vomiting may be the presenting features; these problems could be attributed to other drugs or mistaken for pre-eclampsia.

Practice point

■ It is important that the midwife recognizes the early signs of water intoxication, because cerebral dysfunction may progress to twitches, fits and eventually brain damage and death (Fraser and Arieff, 1990).

Neonatal hyponatraemia and convulsions following maternal water retention have been reported (Aronson, 2006).

The danger is greatest with administration of prolonged high doses of oxytocin, accompanied by infusions of large volumes of electrolyte-free or hypotonic fluids such as 5% glucose (BNF, 2009). In reported cases of water intoxication, more than 3.5 litres of fluid had been infused (Sweetman et al., 2007).

Case report

Despite deteriorating pre-eclampsia, a planned emergency Caesarean section was cancelled because the fetus died *in utero*. Induction of labour lasted 26 hours. Circulatory overload and death from adult respiratory distress syndrome followed (DH, 1996).

Practice points

■ Prolonged infusions should contain electrolytes (BNF, 2009).
■ Early recognition of water intoxication is important because no specific antidote exists.
■ During oxytocin infusions, it is important that:
■ accurate fluid balance records are kept
■ urine output is monitored and specific gravity checked
■ intake by mouth is restricted and monitored
■ no more than 3 litres of fluid are administered (Sweetman et al., 2007)
■ lung bases are checked for pulmonary oedema (Stock, 1992)
■ furosemide (frusemide) should be available, as this may be required to induce diuresis in an emergency
■ electrolytes should be monitored with prolonged infusions (BNF, 2009).

Neonatal jaundice

When oxytocin crosses the placenta, it causes fluid retention in the fetus. Water retention causes red cells to swell, leading to a dose-dependent increase in red cell fragility, **haemolysis** and hyperbilirubinaemia (n = 12,461; n = 90) (Friedman et al., 1978; Buchan, 1979; Aronson, 2006). It is thought that the glucose injection used to mix oxytocin may have aggravated this problem in the past (Sweetman et al., 2007).

Actions on blood vessels

Oxytocin may either raise or lower blood pressure, depending on the circumstances of infusion and individual responsiveness.

Vasoconstriction

Oxytocin acts on the antidiuretic hormone (V_{1A}) receptors in the blood vessels to produce vasoconstriction. This may lead to a sudden, severe rise in BP, to above 200/120 mmHg, which could produce either a hypertensive crisis or a subarachnoid haemorrhage, and maternal deaths have occurred (Sweetman et al., 2007).

Case report

A multigravida was admitted with a BP of 185/105 mmHg, oedema, 3+ proteinuria, headache, epigastric tenderness, hyper-reflexia and vomiting. Over the telephone, the consultant advised induction. Within 2.5 hours, a fit had occurred. Following an emergency Caesarean section, a second fit occurred and disseminated intravascular coagulation developed. The patient remained in the labour ward, where she was overtransfused, and eventually died of adult respiratory distress syndrome (DH, 1996: 28).

The effects of oxytocin on fluid balance can be serious, even fatal, particularly if pre-eclampsia/eclampsia is present.

Practice points

- The hazards of oxytocin administration are increased when a degree of vasoconstriction is already present, as in pre-eclampsia, renal impairment and heart failure.
- Close monitoring of blood pressure is essential. The midwife should be alert to warning signs such as severe headache, visual disturbances and epistaxis (Stock, 1992).
- If vasopressors (such as adrenaline/epinephrine or ephedrine) have been administered with local or regional anaesthesia, particularly caudal block, the likelihood of a hypertensive crisis is increased (BNF, 2009).

Hypotension and transient vasodilation

Oxytocin may lower, rather than raise blood pressure, with the potential for equally catastrophic results, including cardiac arrest (Shyken and Petrie, 1995). The administration of large amounts of oxytocin may produce a sudden but marked vasodilation, with a consequent fall in BP, particularly the diastolic, headache, flushing, and feeling of warmth. Venous return and cardiac output may be reduced, provoking a reflex tachycardia in an attempt to restore BP. However, if the woman is hypovolaemic following delivery or the heart muscle is depressed, this response will be ineffective and blood pressure can plummet.

Vasodilation increases the risk of postpartum haemorrhage or blood loss during Caesarean delivery. Rapid administration of 10 units of oxytocin is associated with a fall of 10 mmHg in mean arterial BP. Low blood pressure may result in insufficient oxygenation of heart muscle: ECG changes associated with hypoxia, sometimes in association with heart muscle necrosis, may be observed during Caesarean deliveries (Aronson, 2006).

- The increased blood flow to the limbs and head may cause sweating, headache, dizziness or tinnitus. These effects are more pronounced if the woman is anaesthetized or hypovolaemic (Parker and Schimmer, 2006). For these reasons, the BNF (2009) advises against rapid intravenous injection.
- Particular care is needed if 10 units of oxytocin are infused for management of postpartum haemorrhage or during Caesarean delivery. For prevention of postpartum haemorrhage, the licensed dose is currently 5 units by slow intravenous injection (BNF, 2009).

Postpartum haemorrhage (PPH)

Protracted administration of oxytocin, particularly at high doses, may exhaust and desensitize the uterine muscle, leaving it unable to contract and unresponsive to oxytocin (Chapter 1). This increases the risk of PPH. Observation studies have linked induction of labour with increased incidence of PPH (Gilbert et al., 1987; Bais et al., 2004; Magann et al., 2005).

Practice point

- Extra vigilance is needed for loss of uterine contractility and signs of haemorrhage. Should PPH occur in a woman who has received prolonged administration of oxytocin, further administration of oxytocin will be ineffective, and ergometrine, prostaglandins or other agents will be needed urgently (McEwan, 2007).

Nausea, vomiting and abdominal pain

Emesis may be due to either contraction of the smooth muscle of the gut or direct action on the chemoreceptor trigger zone and vomiting centre in the medulla. Oxytocin may cause a metallic taste (Aronson, 2006).

Practice point

- It is important not to dismiss the nausea caused by hypotension, water intoxication or other causes of raised intracranial pressure as an adverse effect of oxytocin.

Breastfeeding

Induction of labour by any method, including administration of oxytocin, is associated with increased numbers of women abandoning intentions to breastfeed (Ounsted et al., 1978; Out et al., 1988; Rajan 1994; Leng et al., 1999). Oxytocin infusion reduces the chances of breastfeeding within 4 hours of birth and increases the chances of artificial feeding (Wiklund et al., 2009). Oxytocin is essential for initiation of breastfeeding and milk ejection, which requires intermittent contraction of the myoepithelial cells surrounding the alveoli. These rhythmic contractions and therefore initiation of breastfeeding depend on pulsatile secretion of oxytocin from the posterior pituitary (Nissen et al., 1997; Winberg, 2005). There would appear to be little information regarding the administration of oxytocin on the possible disruption of pulsatile oxytocin release (Nissen et al., 1996; Carter, 2003). During stress, including blood loss, prolonged labour or Caesarean delivery, pulsatile secretion is replaced by continuous secretion, which has less effect on the myoepithelial cells (Russell et al., 2001; Dewey, 2001). Whether administration of oxytocin could mimic or augment the stress response, and abolish the pulsed secretions and subsequent contractions of the myoepithelial cells necessary for the initiation of lactation (Russell et al.,

2001), or desensitize cells to oxytocin (Plested and Bernal, 2001; Robinson et al., 2003) requires further research. Administration of oxytocin during active management of third stage of labour was associated with reduced breastfeeding rates in a retrospective cohort (n = 48,366) (Jordan et al., 2009b).

Anaphylactoid reactions

Hypersensitivity responses, including anaphylaxis have been reported.

Cautions and contraindications: oxytocin

- Oxytocin is contraindicated if the uterus is already contracting vigorously, or if there is a mechanical obstruction to delivery such as *placenta praevia* or cephalopelvic disproportion. Commencing oxytocin infusion during the second stage of labour in parous women is associated with a high risk of uterine hyperstimulation, and is not recommended in current guidelines (NCC, 2007).
- If the cervix is unfavourable, cervical ripening should be performed prior to the administration of oxytocin (Shyken and Petrie, 1995).
- The potential disruption to fluid balance and blood pressure makes oxytocin less suitable for women with: pre-eclampsia, cardiovascular disease, increased risk of disseminated intravascular coagulopathy (including those who are post-mature), age over 34 years.
- Oxytocin infusions are contraindicated in women who are at risk from vaginal delivery, for example those with malpresentation or placental abruption or at high risk of uterine rupture, including those with previous Caesareans. Persistence with oxytocin infusion in the face of uterine resistance and inertia is contraindicated (BNF, 2009).
- Constriction of the umbilical vessels by exogenous oxytocin is likely to intensify any fetal distress.
- Overadministration of oxytocin may cause the uterus to become non-responsive, due to receptor down regulation (Chapter 1).
- *Starved uterus.* Muscle contraction requires both glucose and oxygen. If either of these is not supplied to the contacting muscle, due to starvation or inadequate blood supply, the response to oxytocin will be inadequate, and dose increments will be ineffective. This situation is most likely to arise in prolonged labour or if the woman has vomited more than once (Clayworth, 2000).
- Women with pre-existing ECG abnormalities may be vulnerable to cardiac dysrhythmias associated with hypotension.

Storage

Storage of oxytocin ampoules should be between 2–8°C, for example, in a refrigerator. If stored at higher temperatures, up to 30°C, the shelf life is reduced to 3 months (Alliance Pharmaceuticals, ABPI, 2009).

Drug interactions: oxytocin

- *Prostaglandins, oestrogens:* if more than one agent promoting uterine contractility is administered, uterine overstimulation is more likely to occur.

Case report

Labour was induced at 42 weeks with prostaglandin pessaries followed by an oxytocin infusion. The oxytocin constricted the umbilical arteries, causing fetal distress in the second stage, necessitating forceps delivery, and augmented uterine contractions to such an extent that the uterus ruptured, resulting in an amniotic fluid embolism. The woman collapsed after delivery and died 24 hours later (DH, 1996).

In this case, the combination of oxytocin with prostaglandins induced vigorous contractions, leading to a uterine tear. The BNF (2009: 436) advises careful monitoring with this drug combination.

- If oxytocin is administered with another vasoconstricting agent, there is a danger of a catastrophic rise in blood pressure, leading to a cerebrovascular accident. This may occur if adrenaline (epinephrine) is added to a local anaesthetic, for example with a caudal block, or if ephedrine is administered to correct hypotension induced by epidural anaesthesia.
- *Inhalational anaesthetics* may further lower blood pressure or induce cardiac dysrhythmias.
- *Blood, plasma or metabisulphite* will inactivate oxytocin if infused in the same intravenous giving set (Alliance Pharmaceuticals, ABPI, 2009).
- *Opioids* have antidiuretic effects, which may contribute to water intoxication (Sweetman et al., 2007).
- *Ergometrine* and oxytocin act synergistically and are often co-prescribed in the management of the third stage of labour.

Implications for practice: oxytocin infusions

- It is essential to gain informed consent from the woman and document the reasons for induction or augmentation of labour. Fetal maturity and presentation must be documented to avoid iatrogenic prematurity and malpresentations (Kulb, 1990).
- Because of the inherent dangers and the intensive monitoring required, it is important that anyone receiving an infusion of oxytocin is never left alone (Parker and Schimmer, 2006).
- Protocols should be in place to terminate the infusion if uterine hyperstimulation, precipitous labour, abnormal vaginal bleeding, water intoxication, alterations in BP or fetal asphyxia occur (Kulb, 1990).
- It is prudent to use Y-tubing for infusions, since the port not in use will afford intravenous access should any emergency arise.

Potential problem	Management suggestions
BP increased or decreased	Monitor every 15 minutes. Administer by infusion, particularly if the woman may be hypovolaemic. If intravenous injection is essential, it must be administered slowly (CEMACH, 2007)
HR	Monitor every 15 minutes
Overstimulation of uterus	Monitor contractions. Discontinue oxytocin if frequency > every 2 minutes (4–5 contractions in 10 minutes) and duration > 1 minute or >50 mm Hg
	Uterine resting tone should be below 20 mm Hg
	Oxygen and a tocolytic should be available

Overstimulation of uterus	Avoid if there is a risk of uterine rupture
	Avoid concurrent use of prostaglandins
	Be prepared to decrease or discontinue oxytocin infusion when the active phase of labour begins (Daniel-Spiegel et al., 2004)
Painful contractions	Epidural analgesia is likely to be required from early labour
Fetal asphyxia	Monitor fetal HR. If abnormalities develop, seek medical advice and check rate of contractions. Be prepared to reduce or discontinued administration
	Avoid maternal supine position
Water retention	Fluid balance, restrict fluid intake (maximum 3 litre in 24 hours)
	Check lung bases, respiration rate and oedema of dependent parts
	Check jugular venous pressure and distension
	Avoid in women with pre-eclampsia
	Administer in electrolytes, such as 0.9% sodium chloride (Sweetman et al., 2007)
Water intoxication	Check level of consciousness and/or confusion. Monitor for cardiac dysrhythmia, ECG if necessary
PPH	Monitor loss of tone in uterine muscle and vital signs. Ensure ergometrine, carboprost and, if local protocols permit, misoprostol are available for urgent administration
Disseminated intravascular coagulation	Check for any evidence of bleeding into the uterus or pelvis after delivery. Clotting factors should be checked if there is any uncertainty
Unresponsive uterus	Avoid prolonged labour with inadequate oxygenation and food/energy supply. Discuss possibility of tolerance with prescriber

Newer drugs

Mifepristone (RU 486) is a progesterone antagonist. It prevents progesterone exerting a calming effect on the uterus, thereby increasing uterine contractility. Together with misoprostol, it is administered for medical termination of early pregnancy. Mifepristone is rapidly absorbed following oral administration, and, with a half-life of 20–40 hours, remains effective for some 24 hours. There have been suggestions that mifepristone may be suitable for induction of labour following fetal death or at term. However, mifepristone may damage fetal kidneys, and is not suitable where live birth is anticipated (NCC, 2008b). Relaxation of smooth muscle of the genitourinary tract may increase the risks of vaginal bleeding. Mifepristone antagonizes corticosteroids and androgens, and is not suitable if corticosteroids are co-administered (Loose and Stancel, 2006).

Drugs acting on the cervix

The cervix acts as a mechanical and biological barrier between the fetus and the environment and its pathogenic microorganisms. Extensive changes occur during childbirth – softening, ripening, dilation and repair. Cervical remodelling and ripening precede uterine contractions by several weeks. This breakdown and rearrangement of collagen fibres depends on the activation of prostaglandins and enzymes that break down connective tissue; similar changes are seen during infection and inflammation (Facchinetti et al., 2005). Several drugs, in addition to prostaglandins, are being investigated for their potential to improve the 'favourability' of the cervix.

The large molecules forming the **ground substance** of connective tissue, such as hyalurinic acid, may be broken down by hyaluronidase (this is also administered in some cases of drug extravasation; Chapter 2). However, administration by cervical injection is considered unacceptable (NCC, 2008b).

Nitric oxide is an important mediator in a number of physiological processes, such as vasodilation, and is released locally during cervical ripening. Nitric oxide donors, such as glyceryl trinitrate and isosorbide mononitrate, widely used for angina and hypertension, have been investigated for induction of labour. When administered vaginally, they tend to be less effective than prostaglandins and produce less uterine hyperstimulation. However, adverse effects related to vasodilation, including headache and blood loss, and gastrointestinal stasis, such as nausea, may preclude prescription.

Oestrogens and corticosteroids have not been shown to be effective (NCC, 2008b).

Summary: induction and augmentation of labour

Although prolonged labour is commonly assumed to be deleterious (Nkata, 1996), the outcome may not be improved by uterotonics. In many nulliparous women, the reasons underlying delay in progress in labour are unclear, and may be due to causes other than failure of the myometrium to contract (Olah and Gee, 1996). Where both mother and fetus are well, there are wide variations in the normal duration and progress of labour (Gennaro et al., 2007). Where membranes have ruptured between 34 and 37 weeks, the risk of infection may be reduced by induction of labour (NCC, 2008b). In a large trial (n = 756), induction at 37 weeks reduced the risks of hypertensive disorders progressing (Koopmans et al., 2009).

In one trial (n = 405), high-dose oxytocin reduced duration of labour by a mean of 1.7 hours (Rogers et al., 1997). High-dose oxytocin can shorten prolonged labours (Blanch et al., 1998; Sadler et al., 2000a), while increasing the risk of uterine hyperstimulation (NCC, 2007). However, in other trials (n = 2000; n = 306), the early use of oxytocin and active management of labour in nulliparae conferred no advantages (Frigoletto et al., 1995; Cammu and Eeckhout, 1996). The available trials suggest that oxytocin does not improve Caesarean section rates, operative vaginal delivery rates or neonatal outcomes (Kelly et al., 2003; Hinshaw et al., 2008); however, it increases pain, uterine hyperstimulation and fetal heart rate declerations (Spencer, 1995; Olah and Gee, 1996; Fraser et al., 1998).

Actively managed labour makes no statistically significant difference to rates of Caesarean or instrumental deliveries in low-risk women (Brown et al., 2008). Non-selective use of amniotomy and oxytocin may offer no benefits over conservative regimens (Thornton, 1996). In one trial (n = 196), the durations of the first and second stages of labour were similar when amniotomy alone was performed compared with amniotomy plus oxytocin infusion (Moldin and Sundell, 1996).

Induction and augmentation of labour are associated with reduced satisfaction with childbirth (Bramadat, 1994), and increased incidence of uterine rupture (Zwart et al., 2009). Concerns over the use and management of induction of labour were a prominent feature of the first *Confidential Enquiry into Stillbirths and Deaths in Infancy* (Neale, 1996), which are echoed in subsequent editions (for example MCHRC, 1997). Further research is needed to clarify:

■ the optimum strategy for induction of labour (Busowski and Parsons, 1995; O'Connor, 1995)
■ protocols for administration and monitoring
■ the contribution of uterotonics to adverse outcomes (Cotter et al., 2001), such as failure to breastfeed (Wiklund et al., 2009; Jordan et al., 2009b) and childhood development (Wahl, 2004).

The risk of failed induction necessitating emergency Caesarean delivery, and the increased risks associated with previous Caesarean deliveries, should be discussed with the woman before induction. Failure is more likely if the woman has a high body mass index (**BMI)** or the fetus is heavy (McEwan, 2007).

Ergometrine

Ergot is a fungus that grows on rye, wheat and other grasses. Since medieval times, ergot poisoning, from eating infected rye bread, has been associated with abortion, mental disturbances and gangrene. Several pharmacologically active substances are derived from ergot; these are known as the ergot alkaloids and include ergometrine (ergonovine in the USA), ergotamine, LSD, methylsergide and bromocriptine (Rang et al., 2007). Historically, ergometrine reduced maternal mortality from postpartum haemorrhage. However, the use of ergot alkaloids for induction and augmentation of labour proved extremely hazardous (van Dongen and de Groot, 1995). In view of this, use prior to delivery of *all* fetuses is now firmly contraindicated.

Ergometrine remains important in the management of acute postpartum or post-abortion haemorrhage. As one of the constituents of Syntometrine®, it is widely used prophylactically for the active management of the third stage of labour.

When Syntometrine® is administered:

- The almost immediate effects of oxytocin are followed by the slightly delayed and more sustained contractions induced by ergometrine.
- Ergometrine acts on the inner region of the myometrium, whereas oxytocin and prostaglandins act on the outer myometrium (de Groot et al., 1998).

Used alone, ergometrine offers less effective prophylaxis than Syntometrine® (NCC, 2007).

Ergometrine may be administered intravenously or intramuscularly (BNF, 2009). Oral preparations are unreliable due to difficulties with storage and bioavailability (de Groot et al., 1998). Onset of action is within 1 minute of intravenous administration, 2–7 minutes with intramuscular administration and up to 10 minutes if given orally. If intramuscular injections are placed in subcutaneous fat, they will not be absorbed adequately (Chapter 2). Half-life is 3 hours. Duration of action is 45 minutes following intravenous administration and 3–8 hours following intramuscular administration. Excretion is *via* the kidneys.

Actions and adverse effects of ergometrine

Like other ergot alkaloids, ergometrine interacts with serotoninergic, dopaminergic and noradrenergic (alpha$_1$) receptors in a complex manner. Actions on alpha$_1$ and serotonin receptors are thought to underlie the uterine and gut contractility brought about by ergometrine.

Contraction of the uterus

Ergometrine has a rapid stimulant effect on the uterus, particularly at term. The resultant contractions are uncoordinated and in rapid succession (de Groot et al., 1998). Ergometrine and related drugs are contraindicated during pregnancy (Aronson, 2006).

Practice point

- There is a danger that the uterus will fail to relax between contractions. Therefore ergometrine is never administered before delivery of *all* fetuses (BNF, 2009).

Contractions may be so painful or cramping that women will require analgesia postpartum, and so powerful that the risk of retained placenta is increased (Begley et al., 1990a). This may be caused by excessive contraction of the lower segment of the uterus hindering placental separation (Yuen et al., 1995). Active management shortens the third stage of labour, but is associated with manual removal of placenta in low-risk women (RR 2.05, 95% CI, 1.20–3.51) (Prendiville et al., 2000).

Practice point

■ Administration prior to delivery of the placenta may result in entrapment, unless the placenta is removed by controlled cord traction as soon as it is perceived to have separated from the uterine wall (Steer and Flint, 1999).

Retention of placental fragments may account for the reported association with increased problems with bleeding in the first 6 weeks postpartum (Begley, 1990a).

Diarrhoea and vomiting

Ergometrine mimics the actions of dopamine, causing nausea and vomiting in 20–32% of parturients, depending on dose administered (Begley, 1990a). Reviewers indicate increased risk of emesis with active management of third stage involving ergometrine combined with oxytocin (Prendiville et al., 2000). Mild or moderate diarrhoea may result from increased contractility of the gastrointestinal tract.

Vasoconstriction

Ergometrine acts on alpha$_1$ (noradrenergic) receptors in arterioles and veins to bring about vasoconstriction and venoconstriction. This raises total peripheral resistance, causing hypertension (diastolic >95 mmHg) in 5% of parturients with intravenous administration (Begley, 1990a), and an increased risk of diastolic BP >100 mmHg) when co-administered with oxytocin (Prendiville et al., 2000). This may lead to:

■ reflex bradycardia and reduced cardiac output
■ a hypertensive crisis and cerebral haemorrhage
■ postpartum eclamptic fits
■ raised central venous pressure
■ coronary artery spasm.

Cerebral vasoconstriction may cause sudden severe headache, tinnitus, dizziness, sweating, confusion, retinal detachment, cerebrovascular accident or seizures.

Case reports

1 Two women given 500 micrograms ergometrine intravenously for active management of the third stage of labour suffered eclamptic seizures within 4 hours of delivery, despite no previous history or record of high blood pressure in pregnancy or labour. The problems were attributed to ergometrine (Begley, 1990a).
2 Administration of Syntometrine® following delivery precipitated eclampsia in one woman, who eventually died (DH, 1996: 29).
Ergometrine raises blood pressure and contracts circulating volume, exacerbating the effects of pre-eclampsia. Ergometrine must be avoided in *all* cases of pre-eclampsia unless there is severe haemorrhage (DH, 1996).

Vasoconstriction may also affect the peripheral circulation, making the hands and feet cold; occasionally the woman may experience numbness, paraesthesia, pain, weakness or even gangrene.

Practice points

To minimize the risks, the midwife should:
- check the temperature and circulation of hands and feet
- monitor blood pressure during and after the third stage of labour
- be alert for symptoms of chest pain or palpitations.

Vasospasm of coronary arteries may cause chest pain, cardiac dysrhythmias and even cardiac arrest.

A thorough assessment of cardiovascular risks is essential before administration of ergometrine for the prophylactic management of the third stage of labour.

Case reports

1   A 27-year-old woman was known to have familial hypercholesterolaemia. She smoked 20 cigarettes per day. After an uncomplicated pregnancy, at 41 weeks she had an unplanned vaginal delivery at home. After birth, the midwife administered an intramuscular injection of oxytocin (5 units) and ergometrine (500 micrograms). Five minutes later, the woman complained of acute chest pain. She was then rushed into hospital, where an acute myocardial infarction was diagnosed and treated (Mousa et al., 2000).

2   A 20-year-old woman sustained a permanent hemiparesis following a heart attack related to post-partum administration of intramuscular ergometrine. The only risk factor was a history of migraine. This catastrophic outcome was related to the failure of staff to recognize and treat the signs and symptoms of coronary artery spasm (Taylor and Cohen, 1985).

3   Two women presented late in labour and were administered routine prophylactic oxytocin (5 units) and ergometrine (500 micrograms) as Syntometrine® intramuscularly, but blood pressure was not assessed. In both cases, BP rose to 210/115 mmHg, with catastrophic consequences (CEMACH, 2007: 76).

Practice points

Because of the dangers of cerebrovascular or cardiovascular accidents and cardiac dysrhythmias, ergometrine is:
- only given intravenously in emergencies (BNF, 2009)
- not used if the woman has pulmonary, hypertensive or cardiovascular disorders (including pre-eclampsia and anaemia)
- not administered unless BP has been checked and shown to be normal (CEMACH, 2007)
- only administered in emergencies to women with a sensitivity to coronary artery spasm such as migraine and Raynaud's phenomenon.

Breastfeeding

Ergot alkaloids act on dopamine receptors to suppress prolactin production and lactation. One drug in this group, bromocriptine, is prescribed to manage galactorrhoea and, occasionally, to suppress lactation postpartum. Intramuscular methylergonovine, 200 micrograms after delivery of the placenta, inhibits the normal postpartum rise in serum prolactin (Weiss et al., 1975). Oral ergometrine, 600 micrograms daily for 7 days, reduces serum prolactin and progressively inhibits lactation, with some individual variation (Canales et al., 1976). Intravenous ergotamine, 500 micrograms,* was associated with a statistically non-significant reduction in serum prolactin concentration 48–72 hours postpartum, after suckling (n = 132) (Begley, 1990b). In this study, use of intravenous ergometrine for active management of the third stage of labour gave a statistically significant increase in the number of women supplementing and ceasing breastfeeding by 1 and 4 weeks postpartum, mainly because lactation was inadequate for the infants' needs (Begley, 1990b, 1990c). Observation data indicated a significant association between formula feeding and ergometrine administration with or without oxytocin (Jordan et al., 2009b).

Note: the dose recommended for intravenous ergotamine administration is 250–500 micrograms. The current recommendation for postpartum haemorrhage prophylaxis with Syntometrine® (500 micrograms ergometrine with 5 units of oxytocin) is intramuscular administration on delivery of the anterior shoulder (BNF, 2009: 435).

Practice point

■ Where ergometrine alone has been administered, usually to control severe postpartum haemorrhage, extra support will be needed to establish and continue breastfeeding, particularly if sedating analgesics and antiemetics have been co-administered. Women who have received ergometrine in any form may benefit from an explanation of any difficulties they may be encountering and time to allow ergometrine to be eliminated.

Effects on the neonate

Ergometrine is linked to hyperthermia, increased muscle tension, respiratory problems and convulsions in neonates (de Groot et al., 1998). Seven cases have been reported where ergometrine or Syntometrine® have been mistaken for intramuscular injections of vitamin K and accidentally administered to neonates. All infants convulsed, and most required cardiorespiratory support in special care units. Feeding was initially problematic. However, most infants recovered within 4 days and no long-term sequelae were reported (Dargaville and Campbell, 1998). The onset of respiratory distress may be delayed, and affected infants should be transferred to neonatal units for observation (Bangh et al., 2005).

Hypersensitivity/hypersusceptability

Pulmonary oedema and dyspnoea are also reported (BNF, 2009). Ergometrine can induce bronchospasm in asthmatic women and should be avoided outside emergency situations (Campbell and Lees, 2000). There are suggestions that puerperal psychosis may be associated with ergometrine administration (de Groot et al., 1998).

Cautions and contraindications: ergometrine

- The vasoconstrictor properties of ergometrine make it unsuitable for women with pre-existing pulmonary, cardiac or vascular disorders including pre-eclampsia, eclampsia, hypertension, migraine, Raynaud's phenomenon.
- If sepsis, renal or hepatic failure are present, sensitivity to ergometrine is increased.
- Porphyria is a relative contraindication.
- Repeated use of ergometrine is only justified in difficult circumstances, due to the risks of **adverse drug reactions**.

Storage

Ergometrine must be stored in a cool (below 10°C), dark place, preferably a refrigerator, and expiry dates checked regularly (Hemeln Pharmaceuticals, ABPI, 2009). Loss of potency after 1 year of storage may be 90% (El-Refaey et al., 2000). Ergometrine tablets are unstable in all conditions, particularly high humidity, and therefore not recommended (de Groot et al., 1998).

Syntometrine® should be stored away from light, between 2–6°C. If stored at higher temperatures, up to 25°C, preparations should be discarded after 2 months (Alliance Pharmaceuticals, ABPI, 2009).

Interactions: ergometrine and ergot alkaloids

- The effectiveness of ergometrine may be compromised if the woman is hypocalcaemic; this can be rectified by the intravenous administration of calcium salts (McKenry et al., 2006).
- Nicotine, beta blockers, beta agonists (for example salbutamol), sumatriptan, ritonavir and related drugs (for HIV/AIDS), clarithromycin, erythromycin and other macrolides, Synercid®, tetracyclines, some antifungal agents, and reboxetine intensify the actions of ergot alkaloids. There are reports of interactions with other antidepressants. The above interactions relate to drugs similar to ergometrine, about which there is very little information.
- Women may be best advised to refrain from using tobacco for 3 hours following administration.
- Halothane (an inhalational anaesthetic) may reduce the efficacy of ergometrine (BNF, 2009).

Implications for practice: ergometrine

Problem	Management suggestions
Hypertension	Monitor BP and HR, take a careful history to exclude cardiovascular disease and pre-eclampsia
	Be alert for warning signs, such as headache or emesis
Abdominal cramps	Assess, discontinue if excessive
Vomiting and diarrhoea	Warn, prior to administration
Chest pain	Take a careful history to exclude pre-existing cardiovascular risk factors
	Recognize association with myocardial infarction. Arrange ECG. Withhold further doses
Signs of peripheral vasoconstriction	Monitor temperature of hands and feet regularly. Withhold further doses
Hypersensitivity	Monitor breathing patterns, BP
	Ensure protocol for anaphylaxis is in place
Difficulties with breastfeeding	Support and reassurance that this will be easier when the effects of ergometrine have worn off
Therapeutic failure	Ensure bladder is empty
	Monitor vaginal blood loss, uterine tone, and venous blood sample for calcium concentrations

Summary: third stage of labour and postpartum haemorrhage

The management of the third stage of labour should be discussed with women, as part of the birth plan. Pharmacological options and associated adverse effect profiles should be discussed with all women so that informed choices can be made (Harris, 2004). Further research is needed, but closely observed expectant management of the third stage of labour is regarded as safe for low-risk women in parts of Europe and the USA (de Groot et al., 1996a, 1996b; Leung et al., 2002; Winter et al., 2007; Euphrates Group, 2005). Some, not all, research suggests that this may not be associated with increased blood loss or incidence of 500 ml or 1 litre haemorrhage (Bais et al., 2004), and may be supported in low-risk women, providing risk factors, including oxytocin use, induction, prolonged first, second or third stage and epidural analgesia (Magann et al., 2005), precipitate labour, operative birth, are absent (NCC, 2007: 183; Jordan et al., 2009b).

The risk of postpartum haemorrhage – blood loss greater than 500 ml and 1 litre and necessitating blood transfusion – is reduced by active management of third stage of labour, including the administration of uterotonics (by about two-thirds), and mean blood loss is reduced by 79 ml; when only low-risk women are considered, the figures are largely unchanged. In a Cochrane Review, 18/1,793 low-risk women in the active management group lost >1 litre of blood compared to 39/1,823 in the expectant management group (Prendiville et al., 2000). The incidence of anaemia (Hb < 10 g/dl) postpartum is also reduced (Nordstrom et al., 1997; Rogers et al., 1998).

In low-risk women, blood loss associated with 'physiological management' of the third stage may depend on the technique employed by the midwife (Begley, 1990a). Although active management shortens the third stage of labour, it is associated with an increase in nausea, vomiting and hypertension (diastolic BP >100 mmHg) and, in low-risk women, with manual removal of placenta (RR 2.05, 95% CI, 1.20–3.51) (Prendiville et al., 2000). When only active management regimens containing oxytocin are compared to expectant management in randomized controlled trials , the risk of postpartum haemorrhage greater than 500 ml is reduced, but the reduction in blood loss greater than 1 litre does not reach statistical significance (RR 0.72, 95% CI, 0.49–1.05, 41/619 women lost >1 litre in the oxytocin groups versus 62/654 in the comparator groups), and there is no difference in the number of women requiring blood transfusion; differences in nausea and manual removal of the placenta are not statistically significant (Cotter et al., 2001).

Choice of uterotonic

Randomized controlled trials (n = 3,497; n = 2,189) of oxytocin alone (intramuscular or intravenous) versus oxytocin plus ergometrine indicate that oxytocin (5 or 10 units) used alone causes less nausea, vomiting, headache, sweating, shortness of breath, chest pain, blood pressure elevation and bradycardia, and is equally effective in preventing blood loss greater than 1 litre and blood transfusion (McDonald et al., 1993; Khan et al., 1995; Soriano et al., 1996; McDonald et al., 2004). The addition of 250 micrograms ergometrine to 20 units of oxytocin for intravenous administration following Caesarean delivery did not affect blood loss in a small trial (n = 40) (Balki et al., 2007). The addition of ergometrine does, however, decrease the risk of blood loss greater than 500 ml (McDonald et al., 2004). The optimum dose of oxytocin requires further study (de Groot et al., 1998).

Due to the differences in the adverse effect profiles of the drugs, several authors (Kelsey and Prevost, 1994; Rogers et al., 1998; de Groot et al., 1998; Steer and Flint, 1999), and current guidelines (NCC, 2007) suggest that oxytocin (10 units) is the prophylactic drug of choice for the prevention of postpartum haemorrhage, and ergometrine should be used only if this is found to be ineffective, or in high-risk cases. However, oxytocin is not currently licensed for intramuscular administration

(BNF, 2009), and many women do not have intravenous access established. Therefore, the BNF (2009) recommends ergometrine 500 micrograms plus 5 units oxytocin by intramuscular injection for the routine management of the third stage. Use of this regimen necessitates the careful exclusion of women who should not receive ergometrine, for example those with hypertension or pre-eclampsia. In contrast, 5 units of oxytocin can be administered following most normal labours (Nordstrom et al., 1997). In view of the possible disruption to the delicate homeostatic balance at the sensitive transition period of parturition, the impact of exogenous oxytocin on infant and maternal behaviour, particularly breastfeeding, needs further research (Carter, 2003).

Some authors have suggested that if refrigeration is not readily available, misoprostol tablets may be an acceptable and effective alternative to traditional uterotonics for the management of the third stage of labour (El-Refaey et al., 2000; Walley et al., 2000). However, using a lower dose of misoprostol than other investigators (400, rather than 600 or 500 micrograms), Cook et al. (1999) found that misoprostol was less effective than the traditional uterotonic agents in reducing blood loss after delivery. The increased incidence of adverse effects, shivering, pyrexia, diarrhoea, nausea and vomiting (Gülmezoglu et al., 2007), and the increased risk of postpartum haemorrhage also militate against use of misoprostol for management of third stage (NCC, 2007).

Haemorrhage

Severe postpartum haemorrhage is a life-threatening emergency for which all units have established protocols. In the event of postpartum haemorrhage, the BNF (2009: 430) recommends oxytocin (5–10 units) by slow intravenous injection, followed, if necessary, by intravenous infusion of 5–30 units in 500 ml of fluid. Ergometrine, either alone or combined with oxytocin, may be added if necessary, providing pre-eclampsia/hypertension can be excluded. Carboprost is generally reserved for severe haemorrhage. In the developing world, misoprostol has not been effective in reducing hysterectomy and mortality rates (Mousa and Alfirevic, 2007). If these measures fail, advice from a haematologist may be needed (NCC, 2007).

Further reading

- Begley, C. (1990) A comparison of 'active' and 'physiological' management of the third stage of labour. *Midwifery*, **6**: 3–17.
- Begley, C. (1990) The effect of ergometrine on breast feeding. *Midwifery*, **6**: 60–72.
- NCC (National Collaborating Centre for Women's and Children's Health) (2007) *Intrapartum Care: Care of Healthy Women and their Babies During Childbirth: Clinical Guideline September 2007*, commissioned by NICE. RCOG Press, London.

CHAPTER 7

Drugs Decreasing Uterine Contractility/Tocolytics

Sue Jordan

This chapter considers the most widely used tocolytic agents. Nifedipine is included in this chapter, as it is now more widely used as a tocolytic than an antihypertensive. Magnesium sulphate has not proved an effective tocolytic (Simhan and Caritis, 2007), and is discussed in Chapter 9.

Chapter contents

- Calcium channel blockers/antagonists (mainly nifedipine)
- Atosiban
- Beta$_2$ adrenoceptor agonists (ritodrine, terbutaline and salbutamol)
- Corticosteroids and tocolysis

There is limited evidence of improved fetal outcomes in association with tocolysis (Steer, 1999; Gyetvai et al., 1999; BNF, 2009). Several classes of drugs have **tocolytic** properties, including, beta$_2$ adrenoceptor agonists (such as ritodrine), calcium channel blockers (such as nifedipine), prostaglandin synthetase inhibitors (such as indomethicin and sulindac), oxytocin antagonists (for example atosiban), alcohol and nitric oxide donors (for example glycerol trinitrate) (Simhan and Caritis, 2007). Current UK practice favours calcium blockers/antagonists (for example nifedipine) or oxytocin antagonists over beta$_2$ adrenoceptor agonists, based on the **adverse effect** profiles (RCOG, 2002; Silberschmidt et al., 2008), with indometacin reserved as second- or third-line treatment due to the risks of bleeding in mother or infant and, if administered after 32 weeks, fetal renal toxicity, particularly pulmonary hypertension (BNF, 2009). Nifedipine and indometacin are not licensed for tocolytic therapy in the UK (BNF, 2009). Maintenance treatment is not recommended outside research settings (RCOG, 2002).

Bed rest and hydration are traditionally the first line of management for premature labour, but tocolytics may have a limited role in delaying premature labour in women of 24–33 weeks' gestation. Infants born earlier have reduced chances of survival. The administration of tocolytics is seen as useful in postponing labour long enough to allow:

- transfer to specialist centres for operative delivery if emergencies arise, such as cord prolapse, breech presentation or partial premature detachment of the placenta

▓ time for administration and action of corticosteroids (at least 48 hours) to hasten fetal lung maturation (BNF, 2009).

Tocolytics may also be administered to manage uterine hypercontractility causing fetal heart rate abnormalities unassociated with oxytocin administration, unlicensed use (NCC, 2007), and external cephalic version to reduce the incidence of breech presentation, where terbutaline may be more effective than nifedipine (Collaris and Tan, 2009).

Calcium channel blockers (mainly nifedipine)

The actions, adverse effects and interactions of nifedipine are described here, although they are equally relevant to the management of hypertension. While the emergency administration of nifedipine is usually for tocolysis, in the UK, prolonged administration is only associated with hypertension, outside clinical trials.

Calcium channel blockers are prescribed for tocolysis and hypertension. Nifedipine is as effective as beta$_2$ agonists (for example ritodrine) in inhibiting premature uterine contractions. Since nifedipine is associated with fewer maternal adverse effects (Lockwood, 1997), longer postponement of delivery and lower incidence of neonatal morbidity (King et al., 2003), nifedipine is now the first-line agent in many units (Simhan and Caritis, 2007). It is more suitable than ritodrine for women with diabetes (van Dijk et al., 1995). No placebo controlled trials of nifedipine for tocolysis were identified (King et al., 2003), and long-term effects on the infant are unknown.

For the control of hypertension in pregnancy, nifedipine (in a modified-release preparation) is usually reserved for those who do not respond to, or cannot tolerate, other preparations (Chapter 9). Due to the variety of preparations on the market, each with its own **bioavailability**, in long-term therapy, it is important that the same brand of nifedipine is prescribed each time (BNF, 2009).

How the body handles nifedipine

Unlike other tocolytics, nifedipine is administered orally (Smith et al., 2000). Nifedipine acts within 30–60 minutes when taken as tablets or capsules. Food increases absorption of nifedipine from tablets but decreases absorption from capsules (Sweetman et al., 2007). The short **half-life** (1.2–3.8 hours) of standard preparations may allow potentially dangerous oscillations of blood pressure when nifedipine is prescribed regularly; therefore, sustained-release preparations are in common use. Nifedipine is extensively metabolized by the liver, so lower doses are prescribed for those with liver disease (for example alcoholism and HELLP syndrome). Some authorities consider sublingual capsules to be unsafe as they can cause severe hypotension, leading to maternal cardiovascular events (Grossman et al., 1996) (Chapter 2).

Nifedipine crosses the placenta and passes into the fetus; however, the incidence of adverse neonatal outcomes is comparable with beta$_2$ agonist tocolytics (Silberschmidt et al., 2008).

Actions and adverse effects of nifedipine

Calcium channel blockers inhibit the passage of calcium ions into smooth and cardiac muscle cells, reducing their contractility (Figure 7.1):

▓ The smooth muscle cells of the walls of the arterioles depend on the entry of calcium ions for their contractility. It is this contractility that maintains blood pressure.
▓ The myocardium, like other smooth muscle, depends on calcium ion influx for its contractility. Nifedipine depresses the action of the heart but less so than other calcium blockers (Robertson and Robertson, 1996).

■ Nifedipine reduces uterine contractility, inhibiting labour and is more likely than hydralazine to prolong pregnancy if it is used as an antihypertensive (Sweetman et al., 2007).

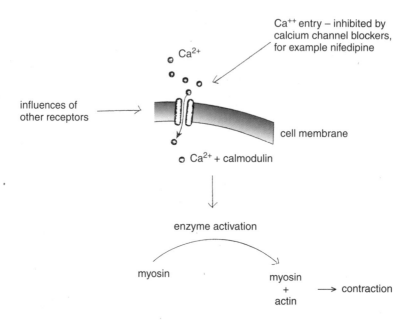

Figure 7.1 The actions of calcium channel blockers on smooth muscle cells

Hypotension and ischaemia

Calcium blockers dilate arterioles, which causes blood pressure to drop. As blood pressure falls, and heart rate increases, the woman may experience chest pain or palpitations due to myocardial ischaemia (Robertson and Robertson, 1996). Myocardial infarction due to hypotension occurred after administration of modified-release nifedipine to a healthy 29-year-old woman at 29 weeks (Aronson, 2006). Hypotension of sufficient severity to warrant Caesarean delivery is more frequently reported by teams whose first choice tocolytic is nifepine. The reduction in placental perfusion associated with hypotension can cause fetal hypoxia, acidosis and, rarely, death (Maggioni et al., 2008).

Practice points

To minimize hypotension during tocolysis:
■ Intravenous fluids may be administered as a 500 ml preload.
■ The woman is asked to assume a left lateral position.
■ BP and heart rate are recorded at least every 15 minutes.
■ Evidence of symptomatic (dizziness, lightheadedness) hypotension is sought regularly.
■ Infusions are adjusted according to signs and symptoms.
■ Strict fluid balance is maintained.
■ Intravenous, rather than sublingual nifedipine is administered.

Symptomatic hypotension may necessitate the use of an alternative tocolytic.

Pulmonary oedema

Pulmonary oedema may be caused by dilution of the plasma due to vasodilation, combined with the infusion of intravenous fluids and loss of protein in the urine (in pre-eclampsia). Pulse oximetry and urine monitoring are indicated during tocolysis (Hill, 1995).

Vasodilation

Whether prescribed for hypertension or tocolysis, nifedipine lowers blood pressure by relaxing arteriolar smooth muscle, bringing about general vasodilation. This may predispose the woman to perioperative or postpartum blood loss (Davis et al., 1997). Vasodilation causes flushing, dizziness, oedema, headache, tinnitus and nausea, causing about 10% of women to discontinue long-term medication. Localized oedema may lead to blurred vision or nasal congestion (stuffiness). Gravitational oedema may develop 10–14 days after starting nifedipine, and must be distinguished from signs of pre-eclampsia. Dilated blood vessels lose more heat from the body; if thermoregulatory mechanisms do not cope, the woman may feel cold.

Practice points

- Blood loss at delivery should be very carefully monitored.
- For ambulatory clients, postural hypotension is a significant problem that must be assessed.

Gastrointestinal problems

Nifedipine relaxes the smooth muscle of the gut, causing nausea, constipation and gastro-oesophageal reflux with heartburn. With long-term use, gingival hyperplasia may occur. This can be avoided with scrupulous attention to dental hygiene.

Central nervous system adverse effects

A variety of central nervous system adverse effects are occasionally reported with nifedipine, including depression, fatigue, somnolence, lethargy, weakness, insomnia, agitation, eye pain, frequent micturition, mood changes, posture and movement disorders (Aronson, 2006).

Hypersensitivity responses

Hypersensitivity responses have occasionally occurred, including rashes, telangiectasia and maternal hepatotoxicity. Liver function tests are probably indicated (Hill, 1995).

Effects on the fetus

Intracellular calcium is important in fetal development and animal testing has raised concern over adverse effects in the fetus. Reduction in blood pressure may be excessive, jeopardizing the blood flow to the placenta and the fetus; this may explain possible associations with intrauterine growth retardation and prematurity (Schondorfer, 2007). Manufacturers state that nifedipine is **contraindicated** in pregnancy before 20 weeks and during breastfeeding, citing embryotoxicity in animal studies (Sibai, 1996; Bayer, ABPI, 2009). However, comparisons with other tocolytic agents in human infants have, to date, not been unfavourable (Hill, 1995). Verapamil has been linked to myocardial hypertrophy in the neonate (Schondorfer, 2007).

Breastfeeding

Manufacturers advise that nifedipine should be avoided during breastfeeding (Bayer, ABPI, 2009), but relatively low doses reach the neonate (BNF, 2009).

Cautions and contraindications: nifedipine

- Particularly close monitoring for signs of pulmonary oedema (below) is required if nifedipine is administered to women with any degree of cardiovascular compromise, including hypertension, intrauterine infection and twin pregnancy (Maggioni et al., 2008).
- Abrupt withdrawal of calcium channel blockers may precipitate a re-emergence of cardiac problems, such as chest pain (Aronson, 2006), and gradual withdrawal may be advised. Contraindications to tocolytic therapy are discussed above.

Storage

Storage should be in airtight containers and away from the light.

Interactions: nifedipine

- Concurrent use of other antihypertensives, particularly magnesium salts and alpha receptor antagonists (for example labetolol), may provoke a profound hypotension (Oates, 1996).
- Alcohol also has hypotensive effects and is best avoided.
- Baxter (2006) suggests that there is potential for profound hypotension should bupivacaine be inadvertently administered into a vein (rather than the epidural space) of a patient receiving nifedipine.
- Care is also needed with vancomycin injections.
- Magnesium sulphate combined with nifedipine may induce a profound neuromuscular blockade (Hill, 1995; Magee et al., 1999), colonic pseudo-obstruction (Aronson, 2006) or cardiac depression and even arrest (Davis et al., 1997). Therefore, some clinicians prefer to avoid nifedipine if there is any chance that the woman will develop eclamptic seizures.

Case report

Where two drugs have the same action, they may dangerously potentiate each other.

A woman of 32 weeks' gestation received nifedipine for premature uterine contractions. However, 12 hours later, contractions returned and intravenous magnesium sulphate was administered for tocolysis. The woman developed jerky movements in the extremities (tetany), difficulty in swallowing, paradoxical respirations and muscle weakness so intense that she was unable to lift her head from the pillow. Magnesium was discontinued, and the woman recovered within the next 25 minutes (Baxter, 2006: 658).

This case illustrates the hazards of drug interactions, particularly in units where certain agents are rarely needed.

- Grapefruit juice, erythromycin, cimetidine, ranitidine, fluoxetine (Prozac®), quinupristin with dalfopristin (Synercid®), and some antifungals and antivirals inhibit the liver enzymes responsible for the elimination of nifedipine, prolonging its action and causing profound hypotension (Dresser et al., 2000; Baxter, 2006). Anecdotal reports suggest that raw grapefruit can have a similar effect.

Implications for practice: calcium blockers

Women receiving tocolytics must be closely monitored both for adverse effects and the failure of tocolysis. If premature labour continues, despite maximum tolerated doses, drugs should be discontinued and preparations made for the care of a premature neonate.

Potential problem	Management suggestions
Short term	
Headaches and flushing	Be prepared to administer paracetamol
	Reassure: this is a normal reaction
Oedema	Monitor weight
	Examine lower legs
	Monitor for signs of heart failure
Pulmonary oedema	Strict fluid balance records
	Observe for shortness of breath, inability to finish sentences
	Listen to lung bases with a high-quality stethoscope
	Ensure diuretics and potassium monitoring available
Hypotension, orthostatic hypotension, dizziness, nausea, sweating, pallor, weakness, even fainting, decreased placental perfusion	Administer injections slowly
	Maintain adequate fluid intake
	Record BP before therapy and regularly thereafter
	Measure BP lying/sitting and standing: a fall in systolic BP >20 mmHg or 10% indicates orthostatic hypotension
	Change position slowly
	Monitor fetus for signs of placental insufficiency
Angina, even myocardial infarction (BP falls so low that coronary perfusion falls, reducing oxygen delivery to heart muscle)	Check for hypotension while patient is symptomatic, if possible
Alteration in HR (bradycardia or tachycardia)	Check pulse before and 30 minutes after administration
	If <60 or >100, consult prescriber
	Administration with food may help
Uterine bleeding	Monitor. Ability to vasoconstrict is inhibited
Additional issues with long-term use	
Headaches and flushing	Administration with food may help
	Anticipate this problem some 30–60 minutes after oral administration (Michel, 2006)
	If problem intensifies during first few weeks of therapy, discuss with prescriber the possibility of increasing duration of action and the need to review regimen
Oedema	Monitor weight
	Examine lower legs for oedema, skin changes and skin breakdown
	When sitting, elevate legs. A daily/afternoon rest in a horizontal position may help
	Encourage regular activity
	Minimize salt intake (to 2.4 g/day)
Hypotension	Avoid prolonged standing, hot showers, exposure to hot environment
	Avoid constipation to prevent straining during defecation (see laxatives)
	Advise that driving may be affected, particularly on starting treatment

Potential problem	Management suggestions
GI disturbances:	
Taste changes	Taste may normalize with continued therapy
Nausea/anorexia	Small regular meals. Monitor weight
Heartburn	Avoid meals before lying down
Constipation	Regular activity, adequate fluids and diet (see laxatives)
GI obstruction/colicky pain	Be aware that some outer membranes from slow-release preparations can obstruct the gut
GI bleeding (rare)	Report black stools or other signs of blood loss

Atosiban

Atosiban is an oxytocin antagonist/blocker that prevents oxytocin reaching its receptors in the myometrium. It may be more effective towards term, when the uterus has more oxytocin receptors.

Atosiban is licensed for intravenous administration for tocolysis, with a number of restrictions, including severe pre-eclampsia, intrauterine infection, *placenta praevia*, ruptured membranes after 30 weeks; its use is restricted to 48 hours (BNF, 2009).

When atosiban is compared to placebo, outcomes are not improved. Comparisons with both placebo and beta agonists link atosiban with an increased risk of low birth weight (Papatsonis et al., 2005), and some authorities have expressed concern over increased mortality among infants whose mothers received atosiban before 28 weeks' gestation (Simhan and Caritis, 2007). Atosiban may also block/antagonize fetal oxytocin, which plays a role in regulating amniotic fluid and development of fetal kidneys and lungs; these mechanisms may account for the lack of clinical benefit seen in randomized controlled trials (Papatsonis et al., 2005).

Maternal adverse effects associated with atosiban include vomiting, hypotension, hot flushes, tachycardia, dizziness, headache, hyperglycaemia, injection site reactions, itching, rash, fever, and insomnia (BNF, 2009). However, US authors report that atosiban is generally well tolerated (Valenzuela et al., 2000). When compared with beta agonists in women without ruptured membranes or other complications, atosiban was equally effective, and there were fewer maternal adverse effects, including dyspnoea, chest pain, palpitations, tachycardia, nausea, vomiting, tremor, and hyperglycaemia (Moutquin et al., 2000).

Beta$_2$ adrenoceptor agonists

This group of **sympathomimetics** includes ritodrine, terbutaline, salbutamol, and adrenaline. Dose restrictions have been imposed following clinical incidents (DH, 1996; BNF, 2009).

How the body handles beta$_2$ adrenoceptor agonists

Administration may be intravenous, intramuscular, subcutaneous or oral.

Practice point

■ A large vein should be used for cannulation to reduce the risk of drug extravasation. If this emergency arises, protocols for extravasation of vasopressors should be followed; these may include administration of normal saline containing phentolamine, which is an alpha$_1$ adrenoceptor antagonist, to counter the vasoconstrictive actions of sympathomimetics (Olsen and D'Oria, 1992).

Intravenous administration of ritodrine is effective within 5 minutes, with peak concentration and adverse effects occurring after 50 minutes (Olsen and D'Oria, 1992). Because of the danger of pulmonary oedema, intravenous administration in minimum volumes of 5% w/v glucose is recommended (DH, 1996; BNF, 2009), and saline is avoided (Lamont, 2000). Dextrose (unlike saline) is distributed into all the body's fluid compartments rather than being confined to the extracellular compartments where a build-up may cause oedema (Chapter 2). Intravenous ritodrine should be administered *via* a controlled infusion device (DH, 1996).

The short-acting beta$_2$ agonists, for example ritodrine, salbutamol, or terbutaline, are effective for about 4 hours. Therefore, if not given by continuous infusion, these drugs must be administered frequently during periods of uterine activity (BNF, 2009). Beta$_2$ adrenoceptor agonists cross the placenta and enter breast milk, thus neonates may experience adverse effects. Beta$_2$ adrenoceptor agonists are eliminated by the liver and kidneys, but due to the complexities of the triphasic half-lives of these drugs, elimination may be delayed and cardiovascular symptoms may recur up to 12 hours after terbutaline discontinuation. Half-life is estimated at 16–20 hours (AstraZeneca, ABPI, 2009).

Actions of beta$_2$ adrenoceptor agonists

These drugs act, like adrenaline, by stimulating the beta$_2$ **receptors** present in the liver, smooth muscle and glands of many organs, including the uterus, lungs and gut. There is also pronounced action on the beta$_1$ receptors, which stimulate the heart, in a manner similar to adrenaline/epinephrine and noradrenaline (norepinephrine). Due to individual differences, doses are adjusted according to response and adverse effect monitoring (see Implications for practice).

Adverse effects of beta$_2$ adrenoceptor agonists

Serious and even fatal **adverse events** have occurred. Perry et al. (1995) found that 0.54% of women receiving continuous intravenous terbutaline infusion experienced serious cardiopulmonary problems (n = 8,709). These were related to the total dose, but dose changes (Holleboom et al., 1996) and individual susceptibility (MacKay and Evans, 1995) were contributory factors. Neonatal cardiovascular and metabolic problems have been reported (Hill, 1995).

Adverse effects follow from stimulation of the beta$_2$ adrenoceptors affecting the:

- cardiovascular system
- renin-angiotensin-aldosterone system
- central nervous system
- smooth muscle of many organs
- mucus-secreting glands
- metabolic processes.

Cardiovascular stimulation

Beta$_2$ adrenoceptor tocolytics are related to the hormones used to drive the cardiovascular system in 'fright, flight or fight' situations. This involves increasing the heart rate, pulse pressure and cardiac contractility *via* beta$_1$ receptors. On administration of tocolytics, maternal heart rate normally rises by 20–40 bpm and neonatal tachycardia also occurs. Fetal heart rate also rises, usually by about 20 bpm, and tachycardia can be serious (Aronson, 2006).

Practice points

■ Careful monitoring is required because an excessive rise in heart rate is associated with myocardial ischaemia, cardiac dysrhythmia, reduced cardiac output and pulmonary oedema (Vesalainen et al., 1999).
■ Patients should be asked to report any palpitations, chest pains or shortness of breath.

In addition to a rise in heart rate, the work of the heart is further increased by the rise in pulse pressure, normally:

■ systolic BP rises about 10 mmHg
■ diastolic BP falls about 10–15 mmHg (MacKay and Evans, 1995).

Vasoconstriction or a sudden rise in blood pressure has the potential to trigger migraine or a cerebrovascular accident (Aronson, 2006). The putative link between maternal blood pressure fluctuations and periventricular-intraventricular haemorrhage in preterm infants requires further investigation (Holleboom et al., 1996).

Practice point

■ The effect of maternal blood pressure changes on uterine blood flow is reduced by placing the woman on her left (or right) side (AstraZeneca, ABPI, 2009).

Vasodilation

Beta$_2$ adrenoceptor agonists relax the vascular smooth muscle and dilate the blood vessels. This reduces the diastolic blood pressure in the mother and blood flow to the placenta. This is most marked if the woman is hypovolaemic. Dilation of blood vessels increases blood flow to peripheral tissues, including the uterus. These drugs are therefore not advised for use where antepartum haemorrhage has occurred (BNF, 2009).

Practice points

■ Increased uterine blood flow increases the tendency to (uterine) bleeding. This is problematic during delivery (Aronson, 2006).
■ Dilation of the peripheral blood vessels increases the blood flow to the skin, causing redness, sweating or a rash. The colour of the skin should be noted before and during therapy.
■ Dilation of the pulmonary vessels affects the ventilation/perfusion imbalance. The increased flow of blood to the lungs may result in a transient fall in pO$_2$.
■ The woman should be advised to get up slowly due to the fall in diastolic blood pressure and the consequent risk of postural hypotension.
■ Increased cerebral blood flow gives rise to a headache, which is a common adverse effect of these drugs.

Activation of the renin-angiotensin-aldosterone system

Beta$_2$ adrenoceptor agonists stimulate the **renin-angiotensin-aldosterone system/axis**. This normally maintains blood pressure, by regulating fluid balance and constricting the arterioles. Combined with the expanded cardiovascular volume of pregnancy, stimulation of the renin-angiotensin system may lead to pulmonary oedema (Lamont, 2000).

Overstimulation of the renin-angiotensin-aldosterone axis may be life-threatening, due to:

■ pulmonary oedema, secondary to acute fluid retention, which may or may not be accompanied by bloating

- fluid retention, bloating and fluid overload or congestive cardiac failure
- hypertension
- **hypokalaemia**.

The precipitous decline in potassium levels is caused by uptake of potassium ions into skeletal muscle due to the stimulation of beta$_2$ adrenoceptors. This results in weakness, cramps, bradycardia and **cardiac dysrhythmias**. Over several hours, potassium is lost from the body by the actions of aldosterone on the renal tubules.

Case report

This case illustrates the need for careful monitoring and rigorous protocols, as outlined in Implications for practice.

A young woman in premature labour at 33 weeks' gestation was given intravenous ritodrine for 3 days, before being converted to oral ritodrine. At this point, she developed a persistent tachycardia and fetal distress. Following Caesarean section, pulmonary oedema developed. This led to lung damage, fibrosis and acute respiratory distress syndrome, which proved fatal.

Ritodrine was the probable cause of pulmonary oedema in this case. The long half-life of ritodrine caused accumulation. When the drug was discontinued, it could not be quickly eliminated. Therefore, vigilance should have been maintained after drug discontinuation (DH, 1996).

Practice points

To prevent pulmonary oedema, it is essential that:

- Accurate fluid balance is maintained; fluid input is restricted to 2.5 l/24 hrs (MacKay and Evans, 1995).
- The lung bases are regularly auscultated.
- Warning signs such as shortness of breath (inability to finish a sentence), dry cough, chest pain and tachycardia are heeded.
- Sodium chloride infusions are avoided, as they remain within the extracellular compartments.
- The maximum infusion rate of the drug is *never* exceeded (DH, 1996).
- Administration is avoided if intrauterine infection is present (BNF, 2009).
- The supine position is avoided (Lamont, 2000).

Due to the potentially serious sequelae, such as acute respiratory distress syndrome, if pulmonary oedema occurs, the tocolytic infusion should be discontinued immediately and diuretics administered (BNF, 2009).

Case reports

1 A young woman in premature labour at 33 weeks' gestation was given intravenous ritodrine in normal saline. Tachycardia and patient anxiety prompted a dose reduction after 36 hours. On transfer to the antenatal ward, the woman became short of breath. This was treated as bronchospasm and worsened. The woman was transferred to ICU. A Caesarean section was performed for fetal distress. The woman developed acute respiratory distress syndrome and died of a myocardial infarction.

The use of normal saline contributed to this death. The absence of fluid balance charts and a written protocol for administration of ritodrine indicated to the assessors that care was suboptimal (DH, 1996).

2 An older woman received ritodrine therapy in an unsuccessful attempt to delay premature labour. Some 24 hours later, she became acutely unwell and breathless, with a dilated heart. She died despite administration of diuretics and heparin.

The role of ritodrine in the development of pulmonary oedema in this woman is uncertain (CEMACH, 2005: 146).

Central nervous system

The effects of beta$_2$ adrenoceptor agonists on the central nervous system are well known: tremor, tension, headache (10–15% with intravenous use), anxiety, nervousness, insomnia, irritability, emotional liability, dizziness, hallucinations, and even paranoia. In addition, retinopathy has been observed in premature infants following use of ritodrine or salbutamol (Sweetman et al., 2007).

Practice point

■ Orientation should be checked before and during therapy.

Smooth muscle inhibition

Inhibition of the smooth muscle of the gastrointestinal tract/gut may cause gastric stasis, leading to loss of appetite, nausea and vomiting. With intravenous use, 10–15% of patients will experience nausea. Gastric reflux may cause heartburn. After 2–3 days of use, the patient may experience constipation and paralytic ileus may occur in the fetus (Olsen and D'Oria, 1992). Inhibition of the smooth muscle of the genitourinary system reduces uterine activity but also depresses bladder and ureteric contractility, possibly causing retention of urine and dysuria.

Practice point

■ An accurate record of fluid output will highlight problems.

Drying of mucus secretions

Beta$_2$ adrenoceptor agonists inhibit mucus secretion, which may cause:

■ dry mouth, which requires frequent water rinses
■ drying of lung secretions, which may lead to chest infections. The risk can be minimized if dehydration is avoided and deep breathing exercises are followed.

Metabolic adverse effects

The administration of beta$_2$ adrenoceptor agonists produces hyperglycaemia. If the woman is diabetic, there is an appreciable risk of ketoacidosis and subsequent fetal loss; diabetes is a contraindication to administration (NCC, 2008a). Hyperglycaemia may stimulate overproduction of fetal insulin, resulting in neonatal hypoglycaemia. Hypocalcaemia in the neonate has been reported (AstraZeneca, ABPI, 2009).

Hypersensitivity

Hypersensitivity responses include:

■ bronchospasm
■ rash in 3–4% of recipients

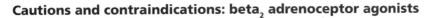

- depletion of white cells after several weeks' administration
- liver enzyme elevations/abnormalities (de Arcos et al., 1996)
- **anaphylaxis**.

Cautions and contraindications: beta$_2$ adrenoceptor agonists

- Beta$_2$ adrenoceptor agonists are considered particularly dangerous for women with cardiac disorders (congenital or acquired), hyperthyroidism or hypertension, including pulmonary hypertension (Lamont, 2000), imminent miscarriage, risk of bleeding or intrauterine infection (AstraZeneca, ABPI, 2009).
- Pre-existing diabetes, hypokalaemia, acute angle glaucoma or migraine may be dangerously worsened.
- Although severe pre-eclampsia precludes tocolytic therapy, mild pre-eclampsia is considered a relative contraindication (BNF, 2009).
- Other tocolytic agents, such as nifedipine, may be acceptable if beta$_2$ adrenoceptor agonists are contraindicated (van Dijk et al., 1995) (above), but may be slower acting (Cararach et al., 2006).

Storage

Storage must be in a cool dry place and away from light (protected by the manufacturer's carton) (AstraZeneca, ABPI, 2009).

Interactions: beta$_2$ adrenoceptor agonists

- Hypokalaemia may be intensified by drugs and conditions that dangerously increase the loss of potassium, such as steroids, theophylline, diuretics, digoxin or hypoxia. If pulmonary oedema occurs, it should be treated with diuretics (BNF, 2009). In this situation, hypokalaemia (involving cardiac dysrhythmias) is a real danger that must be closely monitored.
- The risks of cardiac dysrhythmia, fluid overload and pulmonary oedema may be compounded by co-administration of corticosteroids (Vesalainen et al., 1999).
- The risks of cardiac dysrhythmias and hypertension are increased by addition of other sympathomimetic drugs, such as over the counter cold cures, amphetamines, cocaine, antidepressant medication, ergot alkaloids, and drugs prescribed for asthma or bronchospasm, such as salbutamol or terbutaline (McKenry et al., 2006).

Implications for practice: beta$_2$ adrenoceptor agonists

Potential problem	Management suggestions
MI, tachyarrhythmia, chest pain or heart failure	Monitor maternal pulse/HR at least every 15 minutes
	ECG. Ensure HR remains below 130–140 bpm (BNF, 2009)
	Monitor pulse before each dose; withhold dose or dose incremenation and seek advice if HR >110 or 120
	Monitor fetal HR; this should remain <170–180 bpm
Maternal hypertension, leading to cerebrovascular accident	Monitor BP at least every 15 minutes

II

Maternal hypotension, impairing uterine perfusion	Left lateral position during infusion
Hyperglycaemia, leading to neonatal hypoglycaemia or (rarely) maternal or neonatal ketoacidosis	Four-hourly blood glucose measurements, for example by testing capillary blood. Monitor neonate for hypoglycaemia
Pulmonary oedema, leading to hypoxia and ARDS	Strict fluid balance records. Limit intake to 2.5 l/24 hrs. Observation for shortness of breath, inability to finish sentences. Auscultation of lung bases with a high-quality stethoscope. Body weight before and during therapy. Diuretics and potassium monitoring available
Hypokalaemia, leading to cardiac dysrhythmia, or arrest, and muscle weakness, impairing respiration	Venous blood sample for urea and electrolytes at least every 24 hours. Monitor neonate for hypokalaemia
GI tract stasis	Assess bowel movements. Be prepared for client to feel nauseous and vomit. Maintain adequate fluid intake
Increased uterine bleeding, should Caesarean section be needed	Beta blockers should be available to counter this emergency
Tremors affecting woman or neonate	Offer reassurance and support for neonate
Premature labour, despite tocolytic therapy	Monitor uterus. Facilities for premature delivery should be in place

Corticosteroids and tocolysis

Corticosteroids are an important component of the management of preterm labour. For premature infants born within 7 days of administration, corticosteroids reduce the incidence of neonatal respiratory distress syndrome, intraventricular haemorrhage and neonatal death (NIH Consensus Development Panel, 1995; Crowley, 1999; Roberts and Dalziel, 2006). The overall benefits (if any) of multiple weekly doses over a single injection have been widely discussed. A Cochrane Review indicated a reduction in neonatal lung disease, but no other benefits, when single courses were compared to weekly administrations (Crowther and Harding, 2007). Both dexamethasone and betamethasone are prescribed. Betamethasone is a more potent steroid and associated with more maternal adverse effects (Mulder et al., 1997) but less puerperal sepsis, and is regarded as more effective (Roberts and Dalziel, 2006) and safer for the infant by some authors (Klinger and Koren, 2000). One randomized controlled trial found fewer cases of intraventricular haemorrhage with use of dexamethaone (6/105 versus 17/100) (Elimian et al., 2007), and the Cochrane reviewers favoured dexamethasone (Brownfoot et al., 2008).

Fetal lung maturation

Infants born prior to 34 weeks' gestation have insufficient surfactant in their lungs to breathe effectively. Production of surfactant can be induced by maternal administration of corticosteroids. A single course reduces the incidence of death or respiratory distress syndrome in infants born at 26–35 weeks' gestation, but there are few benefits outside this range (Roberts and Dalziel, 2006).

Administration of corticosteroids

Intramuscular injection may be associated with a lower rate of neonatal intraventricular haemorrhage and sepsis than oral administration (Egerman et al., 1998). Dexamethasone and betamethasone readily cross the placenta. The transfer to the fetus is rapid, and some benefit may be derived even if delivery occurs within 12 hours of administration (Wallace et al., 1997).

Prescribed regimens include 4 doses of 6 mg dexamethasone by intramuscular injection every 12 hours, which should be started 24 hours before birth, if possible. This will remain effective for 7 days (Roberts and Dalziel, 2006).

Practice points

■ Intramuscular injections of dexamethasone may cause excessive bruising if the woman has purpura due to thrombocytopenia (low platelets), for example in association with pre-eclampsia or regular steroid therapy.

■ Care of the injection site is essential, since steroid injections are associated with swelling, tingling, numbness, pain, bruising, sterile abscess and tissue atrophy. Problems are more likely if higher doses are administered (Crowther and Harding, 2007).

■ Each injection site should be used once only and documented, as repeated injections may cause scarring, induration, necrosis and tissue atrophy.

■ Dexamethasone should be administered deeply into the gluteal muscle. The deltoid muscle is too small for steroid injections (McKenry et al., 2006).

■ With intravenous injection, women should be warned to expect a 'tingling' sensation in the perineal area.

Actions and adverse effects of corticosteroids

Dexamethasone and betamethasone act as endogenous corticosteroids. This accounts for their actions and their adverse effects (see Chapter 15, Implications for practice: corticosteroids in pregnancy).

Adverse effects likely to arise immediately include:

■ cardiovascular problems
■ metabolic disturbances – hyperglycaemia
■ central nervous system problems
■ possible increased risk of infection.

Adverse effects likely to arise in the longer term include:

■ anti-inflammatory actions – infection
■ metabolic disturbances
■ adrenal suppression.

The short-term problems are considered here, and long-term problems are considered in Chapter 15 (see also Appendix 1). However, the potential adverse effects of corticosteroids may be encountered in any situation where they are prescribed.

Cardiovascular adverse effects

All steroids increase sodium reabsorption in the kidneys in exchange for potassium or hydrogen ions. This promotes fluid retention, weight gain and hypertension. Cerebral oedema has been reported (BNF, 2009).

Case report

An inpatient of 29 weeks' gestation was treated with labetolol for severe pre-eclampsia. A course of corticosteroids was commenced to hasten fetal maturity. However, after 5 days, BP suddenly rose, precipitating convulsions (DH, 1996: 26).

Administration of corticosteroids to a woman whose circulation was contracted due to severe pre-eclampsia may have been the decisive factor in precipitating hypertension.

■ Women prescribed corticosteroids for any acute condition (premature birth or asthma) should be monitored for fluid retention, hypertension and potassium loss (see Implications for practice: beta$_2$ adrenoceptor agonists).

Corticosteroids promote vasoconstriction during blood loss, and this may account for their protective effect against intraventricular haemorrhage (Roberts and Dalziel, 2006). Hypertension was more common in women receiving a complete course of corticosteroids for fetal lung maturity than in controls (Wallace et al., 1997). Despite this, the benefits of a single course of antenatal corticosteroids are apparent in women with hypertension (Roberts and Dalziel, 2006).

Hypertension and cardiomyopathy can occur in neonates.

Corticosteroids increase the production of erythropoietin, causing polycythaemia, and increase the clotting tendency of the blood.

■ If corticosteroids are administered, it is important to maintain vigilance for thrombosis and mobilize early.

Metabolic disturbances

Corticosteroids reduce uptake of glucose by cells. This causes the plasma glucose concentration to rise, which can lead to diabetes and cataract. Hyperglycaemia is a particular danger in women with diabetes or pre-eclampsia or if beta$_2$ agonists (for example ritodrine) have been administered.

■ Women receiving oral or parenteral steroids (including those receiving tocolytic therapy, particularly repeated courses) should be monitored for hyperglycaemia.
■ Be prepared to increase the dose of insulin for women with diabetes.

A single course of corticosteroids is insufficient to cause bone demineralization (Ogueh et al., 1998), but there is a case report of serious bone damage following 6 courses of antenatal betamethaone (Aronson, 2006).

Maternal (Aronson, 2006) and neonatal adrenal suppression may occur following repeated antenatal courses of corticosteroids, but this is likely to resolve spontaneously (Crowther and Harding, 2007) (Chapter 15).

Administration of dexamethasone, but not hydrocortisone, to neonates for treatment of chronic lung disease has been associated with adrenal suppression (Karemaker et al., 2008).

■ The neonate should be examined for signs of weakness, cardiovascular insufficiency and hypoglycaemia.

Central nervous system adverse effects

Steroids may induce headache, vertigo, insomnia, mood changes or psychoses, or aggravate a pre-existing mental illness (BNF, 2009). There may be euphoria or depression or mood swings, which may resemble postpartum depression. Steroids lower the seizure threshold, causing restlessness or convulsions, especially with intravenous administration.

Practice point

■ Administration to women with epilepsy requires caution.

Infection

Administration of corticosteroids increases the risk of infection in women whose membranes are ruptured (Crowley, 1999; Chapter 14). However, their anti-inflammatory actions may mask the signs and symptoms of infection, complicating diagnosis. The Cochrane Review of antenatal corticosteroids indicated that more women receiving corticosteroids than placebo suffered puerperal sepsis (57/435 versus 44/507). There was no overall increase in chorioamnionitis, but this finding was less convincing for women receiving dexamethasone or with membranes ruptured for longer than 24 hours (Roberts and Dalziel, 2006). Neonatal sepsis, neonatal death, chorioamnionitis and endometritis are associated with repeated courses of corticosteroids (Aronson, 2006). Repeated courses were associated with a higher rate of chorioamnionitis in all women (112/994 versus 89/977, RR 1.23, 0.95–1.59, statistically insignificant), and in women with preterm rupture of membranes, despite antibiotic prophylaxis (39/81 versus 25/80) (Lee et al., 2004; Crowther and Harding, 2007).

Practice points

■ Close monitoring for early signs of infection, including urinary tract infections, in mother and neonate is important.
■ Where intrauterine infection has occurred, infants should be monitored for development of cerebral palsy (Chapter 14) (Lee et al., 2004).
■ Prophylactic corticosteroids may not be advised after 30–32 weeks' gestation for women with premature rupture of membranes (Lee et al., 2004) or after 34 weeks (Montan and Arulkumaran, 2006).

Repeated courses of corticosteroids were associated with increased incidence of Caesarean section (Crowther et al., 2006; Crowther and Harding, 2007).

Effects on the fetus

Corticosteroid-induced depression of the fetal central nervous system may lead to reduced:

■ Fetal heart rate variability (Mulder et al., 1997).
■ Fetal limb, trunk and breathing movements for 48 hours, with full recovery at 96 hours.

However, Doppler flow recordings of umbilical and fetal middle cerebral arteries are unaffected, suggesting that fetal compromise is not associated (Rotmensch et al., 1999).

Practice point

■ Assessments of fetal compromise should take account of corticosteroid administration, to avoid unnecessary interventions (Aronson, 2006). Profound, but transient suppression of fetal movements, heart rate or vasoconstriction following corticosteroid injection may be interpreted as signs of fetal distress (Montan and Arulkumaran, 2006), increasing the risk of Caesarean delivery in mothers prescribed multiple injections (Crowther et al., 2006).

Corticosteroids reduce the production of inflammatory mediators and oxygen radicals, which can damage the developing nervous system. Premature birth is associated with maternal infection, and the ensuing inflammatory processes may damage the fetal brain. In addition, thyroid hormones protect developing tissues from inflammatory cytokines, but very preterm infants often have low levels of thyroid hormones. Very preterm infants may gain some protection from cerebral palsy when their mothers receive injections of corticosteroids (Cowan et al., 2000).

Corticosteroids may inhibit brain cell division and myelination and promote cell destruction; repeated courses of steroids cause neurodevelopmental delay and poor growth in animals, but long-term follow-up of children exposed to repeated injections of corticosteroids *in utero* is needed to identify effects in humans (Brocklehurst et al., 1999; Smith et al., 2000). An observational study in humans suggested that repeated antenatal courses of corticosteroids reduced fetal growth and head circumference (French et al., 1999).

Case report

A paediatrician expressed concern regarding a one-year-old boy in his care, with moderate developmental delay, some spasticity in the legs and a head circumference on the third centile. The boy was born at 20 weeks' gestation following multiple doses of dexamethasone, and no complications of prematurity (Klinger and Koren, 2000).

In Crowther et al.'s (2006) study, reduction in birth weight and head circumference at birth in infants exposed to repeated weekly doses of corticosteroids resolved by the time of hospital discharge; however, only 36% (175/483) of these women received more than 3 courses of relatively low doses of betamethasone, and 42% (201/483) only received 2 courses.

Growth and development

A Cochrane Review indicates that more infants were born small for gestational age following repeated courses of corticosteroids and lower birth weight was more common if women had received 4 or more courses (Crowther and Harding, 2007). A 5-year follow-up of 1,508/2,391 children, 73% of whom had been treated with antenatal corticosteroids, found no differences in the incidence of cerebral or behavioural difficulties (Foix-L'Helias et al., 2008); 2-year follow-up of Crowther et al.'s 2006 study found that a third of children had blood pressure readings above the 95th centile, and the only difference between single and multiple courses was in attention measures (Crowther et al., 2007). The effects of repeated courses of corticosteroids in adult life on diabetes, blood pressure and cardiovascular disease are unknown (Crowther and Harding, 2007).

Interactions: corticosteroids

- *Fluid retention* will be accentuated if steroid therapy is combined with high sodium intake, either orally or by intravenous infusion.
- *Pulmonary oedema* has been associated with co-administration of dexamethasone and ritodrine or other beta$_2$ adrenoceptor agonists, and careful monitoring of fluid balance is needed (Aronson, 2006).
- *Hypokalaemia* is a particular danger if corticosteroids are co-administered with beta$_2$ adrenoceptor agonists (ritodrine), theophylline, aminophylline, digitalis, or diuretics; these drug combinations may be prescribed during tocolytic therapy or management of an acute attack of asthma.

Conclusions: corticosteroids

Authorities state that adverse outcomes are unlikely in association with a single course of dexamethasone for fetal lung maturation (Crowley, 1999; Roberts and Dalziel, 2006). Repeated weekly doses of corticosteroids to women who remained undelivered at 32 weeks' gestation reduced the incidence of respiratory distress syndrome and severe lung disease (Crowther et al., 2006). In contrast, a retrospective analysis of 595 premature infants found increased mortality (13/141 versus 22/454) and early severe lung disease in those receiving three or more courses of corticosteroids (Banks et al., 2002).

Use of multiple courses of corticosteroids is currently widespread. It is not certain that this confers any benefit over a single course (Smith et al., 2000). However, in view of the potential adverse effects of prolonged administration of corticosteroids, and the data from animal studies and randomized controlled trials, this requires further evaluation (Brocklehurst et al., 1999). The effects of antenatal corticosteroids may not be apparent until adolescence; therefore long-term follow-up of all exposed infants, not just those enrolled into clinical trials, is required.

Further reading

- Brownfoot, F.C., Crowther, C.A. and Middleton, P. (2008) Different corticosteroids and regimens for accelerating fetal lung maturation for women at risk of preterm birth. *Cochrane Database of Systematic Reviews*, Issue 4. Art. No.: CD006764. DOI:10.1002/14651858.CD006764.pub2.
- Dodd, J.M., Crowther, C.A., Dare, M.R. and Middleton, P. (2006) Oral betamimetics for maintenance therapy after threatened preterm labour. *Cochrane Database of Systematic Reviews*, Issue 1. Art. No.: CD003927. DOI:10.1002/14651858.CD003927.pub2.
- RCOG (Royal College of Obstetricians and Gynaecologists) (2002) *Tocolytic Drugs for Women in Preterm Labour*. RCOG Press, London.
- Smith, G., Kingdom, J., Penning, D. and Matthews, S. (2000) Antenatal corticosteroids: Is more better? *Lancet*, 355: 251–2.
- Smith, P., Anthony, J. and Johanson, R. (2000) Nifidipine in pregnancy. *British Journal of Obstetrics and Gynaecology*, 107: 299–307.

II

Part III

Disordered Physiology in Childbirth

III

Introduction

This part of the book discusses the management of disorders associated with, but not necessarily exclusive to, pregnancy. In some circumstances, it is the midwife who identifies these conditions and refers the woman to obstetricians. Midwives also play a crucial role in administering appropriate medications in primary, secondary and tertiary care.

Emboldened terms can be found in the Glossary.

CHAPTER 8

Drugs Affecting the Coagulation Process

Sue Jordan

This chapter considers the anticoagulants employed in the management and prophylaxis of thromboembolic disorders. Vitamin K administration, both therapeutic and prophylactic, is also discussed.

Chapter contents

- Haemostasis
- Anticoagulants
- Heparin
- Warfarin
- Vitamin K

III

Aspirin is discussed in Chapter 9; it is not prescribed for thromboprophylaxis in midwifery (Marik and Plante, 2008). Of the oral anticoagulants, only warfarin is considered, since others are seldom prescribed in the UK.

Pulmonary embolism was the cause of 33 maternal deaths between 2003 and 2005, a higher number than in the previous triennium. Maternal deaths represent only a very small proportion of the women who suffer pulmonary emboli (PE) , deep vein thromboses (DVT), cerebral thromboses or arterial occlusion of limbs. Consequently, professionals are urged to assess all women for risk of thromboembolism, maintain a high index of suspicion for thromboembolic disorders, and be prepared to administer prophylactic anticoagulants as soon as possible. There is increasing recognition of the need for anticoagulant therapy in obese women and those with inherited pro-coagulant disorders (thrombophilias) who are at high risk of thromboembolic events (CEMACH, 2007). Therefore midwives are likely to encounter increasing numbers of women prescribed anticoagulants, mainly low molecular weight (LMW) heparin.

Haemostasis

Normally, a delicate balance is maintained between circulating and endothelial anticoagulant and pro-coagulant factors. If this equilibrium is disturbed, a **thrombosis** or blood clot may form. When a blood vessel is damaged, the clotting mechanisms are activated to seal the vessel and minimize blood loss. Initially, the damaged vessel constricts, and a temporary plug of platelets forms, which is then converted into a permanent clot by the activation of fibrinogen. Normally, various anti-clotting mechanisms restrict and prevent clot formation in undamaged vessels. In due course, blood clots are broken down by the fibrinolytic process, and the vessel heals. The three stages of the coagulation process are summarized in Table 8.1.

Table 8.1 Summary of the three stages of haemostasis

Stage	Requirements	Drugs affecting	Antidote to drug
1 Temporary plug	Platelets	Aspirin, possibly heparin	None
2 Fibrin clot	Clotting factors, vitamin K Anti-clotting factors	Warfarin, coumarin Heparin	Vitamin K Protamine sulphate
3 Fibrinolysis	Plasmin, fibrinolytic system	Streptokinase, tissue plasminogen activators (tPA)	Tranexamic acid

The risk of clotting depends on the composition of the blood, the rate of blood flow, and the state of the blood vessel linings (Figure 8.1). The likelihood of thrombosis can be assessed from known risk factors, which include:

- increased plasma concentrations of oestrogens or progesterone, for example ovarian hyperstimulation
- pregnancy – increased concentration of some clotting factors from the onset of pregnancy and decreased fibrinolysis
- childbirth, especially emergency Caesarean section, midcavity instrumental delivery, prolonged labour (>12 hours) and grand multiparity (para 4+)
- puerperium and the first 3 weeks after childbirth (Saha et al., 2009)
- age >35, >30 with operative delivery
- obesity, body mass index (**BMI**) >30 kg/m² or weight >80 kg in early pregnancy
- immobility, bed rest >4 days, long-term paralysis of lower limbs, long-haul travel
- trauma and surgery
- dehydration, for example emesis or hyperemesis
- haemorrhage
- current infection, sepsis (especially staphylococcal toxins), inflammation
- vessel wall compression, for example from delivery table stirrups, pressure of presenting part
- smoking
- stress
- hypertension, pre-eclampsia
- high fat, low fibre diet
- gross varicose veins
- thrombophilia (one of several inherited or acquired pro-coagulant disorders), including antiphospholipid syndrome, lupus anticoagulant, factor V Leiden, deficiency of antithrombin, plasminogen, proteins S or C, a family history of cardiolipin antibody
- personal or family history of thromboembolism – not all inherited conditions are detectable with haematological screening
- diabetes
- raised concentration of platelets or red cells, for example with prolonged use of corticosteroids
- pre-existing disease: respiratory disorders, cardiovascular diseases, arteriosclerosis, sickle cell disease, nephrotic syndrome, inflammatory bowel disease, cancer (Buckley, 1990; Toglia and Weg, 1996; CEMACH, 2007; Tapson, 2008).

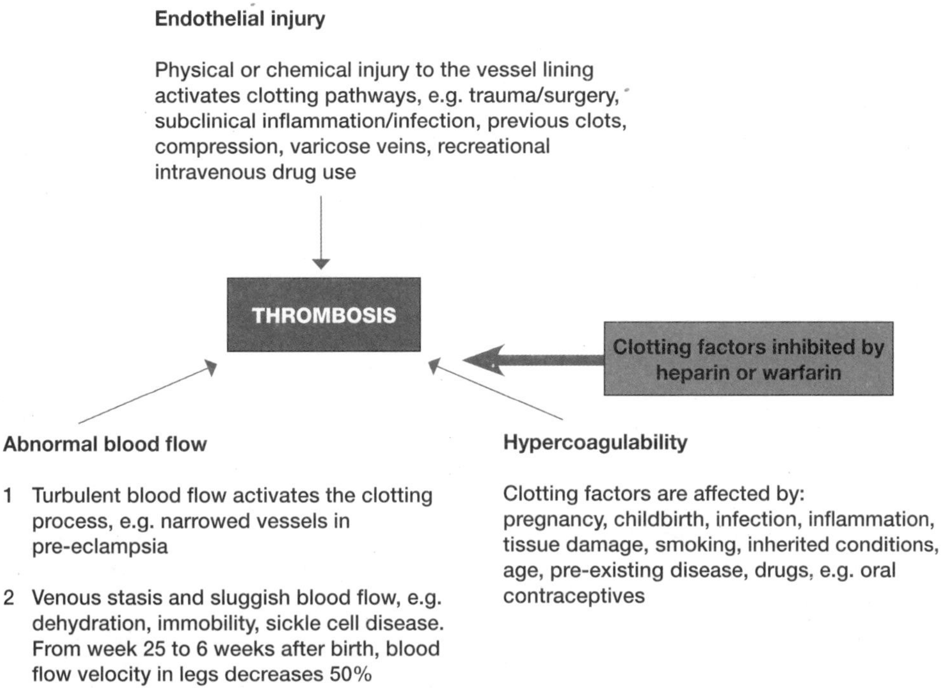

Endothelial injury

Physical or chemical injury to the vessel lining
activates clotting pathways, e.g. trauma/surgery,
subclinical inflammation/infection, previous clots,
compression, varicose veins, recreational
intravenous drug use

THROMBOSIS

Clotting factors inhibited by
heparin or warfarin

Abnormal blood flow

1   Turbulent blood flow activates the clotting
    process, e.g. narrowed vessels in
    pre-eclampsia

2   Venous stasis and sluggish blood flow, e.g.
    dehydration, immobility, sickle cell disease.
    From week 25 to 6 weeks after birth, blood
    flow velocity in legs decreases 50%

Hypercoagulability

Clotting factors are affected by:
pregnancy, childbirth, infection, inflammation,
tissue damage, smoking, inherited conditions,
age, pre-existing disease, drugs, e.g. oral
contraceptives

Figure 8.1 Illustration of the causes of coagulation (Virchow's triad)

III

Case reports

A thorough history should be obtained from every woman to assess the risk factors for thromboembolism,
including past history and family history.

1   An older parous woman did not declare a history of deep vein thrombosis at the booking clinic. She was
    discharged home 3 days after a forceps delivery, but a few days later she was readmitted overnight for
    evacuation of retained products of conception. She suffered headaches and episodes of loss of
    consciousness. A week later she collapsed at home. The problem was diagnosed as a venous thrombosis
    in the cerebral cortex. However, the diagnosis was questioned and no anticoagulants were adminis-
    tered. Death occurred on the 27th day postpartum (DH, 1991: 40).

This case illustrates the importance of history taking and the potential seriousness of headaches.

2   An obese parous woman was booked at home early in pregnancy. There was no record of risk assess-
    ment or referral for the management of obesity. Days later she telephoned her GP complaining of
    breathlessness, and was told to call back if symptoms increased. She died of a pulmonary embolus the
    following day.

The physiological changes of early pregnancy, combined with obesity and associated immobility, precipitated
coagulation. Pulmonary embolus is often preceded by only the mildest symptoms in younger adults (CEMACH,
2007: 60).

Practice point

■ All risk factors for thrombosis should be included when the midwife takes the woman's history, so that
   the prophylactic use of leg stockings and/or anticoagulant therapy can be prescribed (CEMACH, 2007).

Any situation that leads to slow or sluggish blood flow places the woman at risk of a thromboembolic event, including Caesarean section, where prophylactic anticoagulants may be routinely prescribed (NCC, 2004). Onset of coagulation may be rapid, and there should be no delays in seeking medical advice or administering prescribed anticoagulants. Treatment may be commenced on the basis of clinical findings, while investigations are undertaken to establish the diagnosis (RCOG, 2007). Management of a thromboembolic event will be divided into an acute phase of intensive treatment (usually involving heparin), followed by a later preventive phase lasting several months using either heparin or warfarin.

Thrombolytic drugs, such as streptokinase, and recombinant tissue plasminogen activator (rtPA) are used in some clinical situations to break down existing clots, but use in pregnancy is restricted to life-threatening circumstances, and intrapartum administration is particularly hazardous (de Swiet, 1995; Schaefer, 2007a; Tapson, 2008). For further information on thrombolytics, see Galbraith et al. (2007).

Anticoagulants

Neither heparin nor warfarin affect any existing clot but act to prevent the formation of further clots. Following a thromboembolic event, anticoagulants will be prescribed to prevent further clot formation. Heparins, both unfractionated and LMW, may be prescribed in either therapeutic or prophylactic doses. Warfarin is prescribed as prophylaxis.

Case reports

Breathlessness, cough, 'anxiety attack' or chest pain and tachycardia are important features of pulmonary embolism. This can be difficult to recognize because shortness of breath, tachypnoea, swelling and discomfort of the legs are common in late pregnancy (Toglia and Weg, 1996).

1 An obese woman in her thirties was induced at 42 weeks, and had a normal birth. Twelve days after delivery she was readmitted with DVT. A 10-day course of heparin plus support stockings were prescribed. Cough and breathlessness were inadequately monitored and treated. Pulmonary embolism occurred 42 days after delivery (DH, 1994: 46).

2 A woman booked for an elective Caesarean section was admitted with spontaneous rupture of membranes. Following Caesarean section, she developed a low grade pyrexia and a week later was complaining of faintness, giddiness and breathlessness. She died of a massive pulmonary embolism on the tenth day. It would appear that no anticoagulation was administered (DH, 1994: 50).

Guidelines advise early mobilization and good hydration for all women, and support stockings (correctly worn) plus heparin at least until the fifth post-operation day *and until fully mobilized* for the highest risk women, including all women with a BMI >35 (CEMACH, 2007). Investigations into recurrent miscarriage have highlighted the need for heparin prophylaxis in pro-coagulant disorders such as antiphospholipid (Hughes') syndrome (Lima et al., 1996; Rai et al., 1997). A Cochrane Review indicates that unfractionated heparin combined with aspirin has, to date, proved the most effective strategy to reduce pregnancy loss for these women; LMW heparin was less effective (Greaves, 1999; Empson et al., 2005).

Note: antiphospholipid syndrome is defined as thrombosis or recurrent miscarriage plus laboratory evidence of the presence of certain antibodies in the blood, such as lupus anticoagulant (Greaves, 1999: 1348).

Heparin

Synthesized heparins closely resemble natural anticoagulants, which are found on the inner surfaces of capillaries. Two categories of heparin are in general use: standard or unfractionated heparin and LMW heparins, such as enoxaparin, dalteparin, certoparin and tinzaparin. The differences are summarized in Table 8.2. Standard or unfractionated heparins stimulate or catalyse the activity of antithrombin III, an endogenous anticoagulant that binds and inactivates several clotting factors (thrombin, Xa, IXa, XIa and XIIa), thereby preventing the formation of fibrin. However, long-term use of standard heparin will deplete the supply of antithrombin III, decreasing the effectiveness of the therapy (Levy et al., 2000). Measurement of antithrombin III concentration is not usually possible in clinical settings.

Table 8.2 Comparison of standard and LMW heparins

	Standard/unfractionated heparins	**LMW heparins**
Routes of administration	Intravenous or subcutaneous	Subcutaneous
Frequency of administration	Continuous intravenous infusion or subcutaneous every 12 hrs	Subcutaneous every 12 or 24 hrs, depending on preparation
Site of action	Thrombin, Xa, IXa, XIa, XIIa	Only Xa (probably)
Uses	Established DVT and PE	Established DVT and PE
	Prevention of DVT and PE	Prevention of DVT and PE
Advantages	Proven efficacy in severe events, used in highest risk women	Ease of administration
	Dose titration in response to clinical changes with intravenous infusion	Reduced incidence of **adverse effects** (bleeding, osteoporosis, thrombocytopenia)
	Rapid reversal on discontinuation	Reduced need for haematological monitoring

Note: BNF (2009) and RCOG (2007) recommend standard/unfractionated heparin for established PE.

LMW heparins, such as enoxaparin, are widely used in UK maternity units (Khamashta and Mackworth-Young, 1997; Ellison et al., 2000). They inhibit only clotting factor Xa, which may account for their increased **bioavailability** and predictability when compared with standard/unfractionated heparins (Heaton and Pearce, 1995; Geerts et al., 1996). Since the rate of coagulation is limited by factor Xa, LMW heparins are effective prophylaxis when the coagulation process has not been initiated. They have a lower incidence of adverse effects than standard/unfractionated heparin, are equally effective in DVT prevention (Nelson-Piercy et al., 1997; Lensing et al., 1999), and are now preferred for prophylaxis (CEMACH, 2005; RCOG, 2007) and management of all but the most massive thromboembolic events (RCOG, 2007). Unfractionated heparin is an alternative in US guidelines (Bates et al., 2004).

In normal doses, LMW heparins do not inhibit thrombin; therefore their use is not detected by most laboratory tests for coagulation. Formerly, their use in established deep vein thrombosis and pulmonary embolism in pregnancy was accompanied by monitoring the concentration of factor anti-Xa (Thomson et al., 1998; Greer, 1999), but current guidelines recommend this only for women of extremes of body weight (RCOG, 2007) or to calculate dose adjustments as pregnancy progresses (Bates et al., 2004).

How the body handles heparin

Administration of heparin

For prophylaxis, heparin (usually LMW heparin) is given as subcutaneous injections, which may be self-administered (BNF, 2009). In the most acute situations, heparin is given as a loading dose, followed by continuous intravenous infusion (RCOG, 2007); intermittent intravenous injection is no longer recommended.

Doses of standard/unfractionated heparin are prescribed in 'units' and LMW heparins are prescribed in milligrams or 'units' that are not necessarily interchangeable between preparations. Different systems exist in the USA and the UK. United States Pharmacopeia (USP) units are not equivalent to international units (IU), although they are essentially very similar (McKenry et al., 2006, Sweetman et al., 2007). Staff also need to be aware of the dangers of decimal place errors. Heparin sodium is available in three concentrations. Heparin calcium is prescribed less frequently.

Practice points

- If a loading dose is prescribed, it should never be given in less than 1 minute, due to the risks of hypersensitivity responses.
- Heparin flushes designed for maintaining intravenous patency are not suitable for injection.
- Subcutaneous heparins may be injected into rotated sites in the lower abdomen, using a small gauge needle.
- All subcutaneous injections should be 2 inches away from the umbilicus and scar tissue.
- A 'bunching' technique is advised to avoid injecting into underlying muscle.
- To avoid bruising, administration should comprise gentle needle insertion, a 10-second hold and gentle needle withdrawal. Gentle pressure should then be applied to the site for 1–2 minutes (McKenry et al., 2006).
- The use of ice packs pre- and post-injection reduces pain but not bruising (Ross and Soltes, 1995).
- If the subcutaneous injection is too shallow or the site is massaged following administration, bruising is intensified and the action of heparin will be curtailed.
- The pain of subcutaneous injections increases with the volume injected, therefore large doses of heparin should not be given by this route (Jorgensen et al., 1996).
- When heparin is administered in the community, arrangements for safe disposal of needles should be made.

Intravenous unfractionated heparin takes immediate effect, therefore close observation of cannula sites may allow early detection of bleeding. Subcutaneous standard/unfractionated heparin takes effect within 20–60 minutes and is maximally effective 2–3 hours after administration (Lutomski et al., 1995). LMW heparin is maximally effective 3–4 hours after subcutaneous injection.

Initial doses and infusion rates are determined from tables incorporating height and body weight and guidelines (Lutomski et al., 1995; RCOG, 2007). Due to individual differences in response, and the dose-dependent **half-life** of unfractionated standard heparin, ongoing dosage is adjusted according to results of coagulation tests (Majerus and Tollefsen, 2006). Doses may need to be increased as pregnancy progresses and circulating volume increases; this can be assessed by weight changes, calculated in relation to pre-pregnancy body weight or concentrations of active factor Xa in venous blood (Bates et al., 2004).

Practice points

- When checking doses of heparin, it is important to ensure that the dose takes account of pregnancy and the woman's weight.
- To assist prescribers in calculating doses, the drug chart should record the woman's early pregnancy weight.

The response to LMW heparins at any given dose is more predictable, allowing fixed dose administration without laboratory monitoring in many circumstances (Ginsberg, 1996).

Clearance of heparin

Heparin is bound to plasma proteins and inactivated by **macrophages**, the liver and activated platelets. Removal of heparin increases with body weight. Since standard/unfractionated heparin has a short half-life (60–90 minutes at usual doses), intermittent infusion may be unreliable. The risk of bleeding is increased for 2–6 hours after an intravenous injection and 8–12 hours after a subcutaneous injection.

The longer half-life and duration of action of LMW heparins reduce the numbers of injections needed. However, pregnancy increases the clearance of LMW heparins; therefore higher doses and more frequent injections are needed than in non-pregnant women, with many physicians opting for twice-daily administration (Marik and Plante, 2008).

Heparin and LMW heparins neither cross the placenta nor enter breast milk in appreciable amounts, therefore administration during pregnancy and lactation is considered safe for the fetus and neonate (Aronson, 2006). However, use of heparin in pregnancy has been associated with a high incidence of adverse pregnancy outcomes, mainly miscarriage and premature labour (Hall et al., 1980), which may be related to the severity of the underlying disease; more recent reviewers dispute these findings (Toglia and Weg, 1996).

Adverse effects of heparin

The adverse effects and problems arising from short-term heparin use are:

- bleeding
- **thrombocytopenia** (low platelet count)
- hypotension, due to preservative (chlorbutol) in some preparations
- diuresis starting 36–48 hours after initiation of therapy, lasting 36–48 hours after discontinuation
- **hyperkalaemia**, due to aldosterone inhibition
- vasospastic reaction (rare), leading to raised blood pressure, chest pain and parasthesia
- **hypersensitivity** responses.

Further problems may arise with long-term use of heparin, for example in any woman with a history of repeated thromboembolism:

- abnormalities of liver function tests
- decreased renal function
- hair loss – usually reverses on discontinuation
- osteoporosis or osteopenia
- abrupt withdrawal, which may cause rebound coagulation
- heparin resistance.

Bleeding

Bleeding is problematic for up to 3% of patients using all forms of heparin; recent estimates suggest that 2% of women are affected (Aronson, 2006). The importance of this is demonstrated in several studies:

- Hall et al. (1980) cite 14 haemorrhages and 3 deaths in 135 women using heparin during pregnancy
- Sadler et al. (2000b) report anticoagulant-related postpartum haemorrhage following Caesarean section in 4 out of 14 women receiving heparin

■ Ellison et al. (2000) report 1 antepartum and 4 postpartum haemorrhages in 57 pregnancies where low-dose heparin was administered before labour.

Haemorrhage remains a common reason for maternal admission to intensive care and hysterectomy (DH, 1998). Severe bleeding is more likely with: high doses (associated with therapeutic regimens), intravenous administration, an increased **aPTT** (activated partial thromboplastin time), and poor renal function (Aronson, 2006).

Case report

Heparin administration increases the risks of bleeding, necessitating careful monitoring.

A woman with several risk factors for pulmonary embolus complained of severe chest and abdominal pains. A diagnosis of pulmonary embolism was made, and heparin was administered. Later that day she collapsed, and resuscitation was unsuccessful. A retroperitoneal haemorrhage was found at autopsy (DH, 1998: 133).

The exact contribution of heparin to this death is not clear, but it probably intensified the severity of the bleeding.

Practice points

■ It is important to observe for the first signs of bleeding such as bruising, petechiae, haematoma, nosebleeds, bleeding gums or cannulation sites. The peak incidence of problems is on the third day of administration (Aronson, 2006).

■ The recognition of internal bleeding is more difficult but can be identified by symptoms such as abdominal pain or distension, low backache, joint pain or swelling, headache or dizziness. Intra-adrenal haemorrhage is a rare complication.

■ Retroplacental bleeding may only become apparent following a scan. If the woman complains of severe abdominal pain and contractions or shivering and breathlessness, she should be referred immediately to her obstetrician.

■ Checking urine and stools periodically for the presence of blood, both by laboratory tests (multistix and faecal occult blood reagent strips) and observations, will give an early warning of problems. The woman should also be asked to report any increase in bleeding from the gums.

■ To detect any haemorrhage as early as possible, the midwife should monitor vital signs every 4 hours during heparin administration in hospital (McKenry et al., 2006), and be aware that life-threatening haemorrhage may occur without tachycardia and hypotension (Little et al., 1995).

■ Anticoagulants will be withheld and urgently reviewed if bleeding is suspected.

Doctors usually discontinue LMW heparin injections 24 hours prior to planned delivery or at onset of labour to minimize the risks of both bleeding and thromboembolism. Subcutaneous unfractionated heparin is discontinued 12 hours before the induction of labour or insertion of epidural catheters, and intravenous administration 6 hours before (Toglia and Weg, 1996; RCOG, 2007). Some authorities advise shorter intervals (Collis et al., 2008).

Practice point

■ Women self-administering heparin antenatally should be advised to inform all health professionals of this when they make contact to report that they are in labour and to discontinue self-administration until an assessment has been undertaken. Further doses will be prescribed by hospital staff, taking account of physiological changes (CEMACH, 2005).

Wound haematomata are more likely if LMW heparin is administered 2 hours before surgery for Caesarean section. It is suggested that this allows maximum anticoagulation to coincide with recovery of perfusion, some 2 hours after delivery (van Wijk et al., 2002). A prophylactic dose of LMW heparin may be administered 3 hours after Caesarean delivery or more than 4 hours after removal of an epidural catheter (RCOG, 2007). For women without bleeding complications and whose coagulation function is normal, doctors may resume prophylactic LMW heparin injections some 12 hours after delivery or removal of an epidural catheter; where therapeutic doses have been administered, this interval is extended to 24 hours (Marik and Plante, 2008).

Box 8.1 Haematological monitoring for women receiving heparin

Use of full dose standard/unfractionated heparin entails haematological monitoring during therapy, usually aPTT 4–6 hours after the loading dose, 6 hours after a dose change, initially every 6 hours (Majerus and Tollefsen, 2006), and daily (Lensing et al., 1999; McKenry et al., 2006; RCOG, 2007):

- Venous blood samples are taken from the arm not receiving infusions, 30 minutes before the next dose is due.
- Heparin doses are adjusted in the light of laboratory findings, with the aim of maintaining aPTT 1.5–2.5 times the standard value (Majerus and Tollefsen, 2006).

However, aPTT is unreliable during pregnancy, particularly late pregnancy; antifactor Xa concentrations, activated clotting time and plasma heparin concentrations may offer better alternatives (Lutomski et al., 1995; Greer, 1999; RCOG, 2007).

At normal doses, LMW heparins have no effect on haematological indices, therefore routine monitoring is not required with standard regimens (BNF, 2009). However, antifactor Xa may be monitored to guide dosage in women with altered renal function or at the extremes of body weight (Marik and Plante, 2008).

III

Although heparin has a short half-life, the administration of the antidote, protamine sulphate, is occasionally necessary (below).

Thrombocytopenia

Early recognition of thrombocytopenia is important because it is reversible if heparin is discontinued but causes life-threatening or limb-threatening arterial emboli if left unattended (Majerus and Tollefsen, 2006).

Three forms of thrombocytopenia are encountered with heparin administration:

1 The early/mild form occurs in up to 33% of recipients and resolves spontaneously.
2 The severe form is rare and leads to arterial or venous thrombosis.
3 The delayed form occurs up to 14 days after withdrawal of therapy.

In the severe form of thrombocytopenia, antibodies are formed against a heparin-platelet complex. These cause the platelets to aggregate and form a clot, which may be asymptomatic or present as venous or arterial thromboembolism. The clinical manifestations of this include deep vein thrombosis, pulmonary embolism, skin necrosis, occlusion of the circulation to limbs, and thrombosis of mesenteric, coronary or cerebral arteries. The sequestration of the platelets into thrombi reduces the number in circulation, causing thrombocytopenia.

Practice points

■ The BNF (2009) recommends pre-therapy and regular platelet counts for those taking unfractionated heparin for longer than 4 days.

■ If the patient has previously received heparin, thrombocytopenia may arise in less than 5 days, necessitating earlier platelet checks.

The risks of heparin-induced thrombocytopenia, associated thrombotic events and antibodies to heparin are reduced or delayed but not eliminated by the use of LMW heparins (Nelson Piercy, 1997; Lindhoff-Last et al., 2000). Thrombocytopenia and hypersensitivity responses have also been reported following the use of heparin flushes for intravenous infusions (Leo Laboratories, ABPI, 2009).

Practice point

■ Highlight reaction on patient's notes, because further administration of any heparins might be dangerous.

Hypersensitivity responses

All heparin preparations may induce hypersensitivity responses, such as chills, rash, pruritus, urticaria, hair loss, pyrexia, nasal congestion, bronchospasm, lacrimation, diarrhoea and even **anaphylaxis**. Since heparin is derived from animal products, hypersensitivity reactions are relatively common, particularly in atopic individuals. These reactions have been linked to contamination during the manufacturing process (Blossom et al., 2008). Protracted use increases the incidence of rashes.

Practice points

■ Skin allergy may be a sign of thrombocytopenia. If a rash or itching develop, platelet count should be checked.
■ An eczema-like rash may occur around the injection sites, often 3–21 days after starting therapy. Women developing such hypersensitivity responses to one LMW heparin may be changed to another, under close supervision. However, about a third of these women will be allergic to other brands (Marik and Plante, 2008). Such women should be asked to report the earliest signs of a rash promptly.

Abrupt withdrawal

Discontinuation of heparin may lead to rebound coagulation and a rise in plasma lipid concentrations, causing hyperlipidaemia (Majerus and Tollefsen, 2006). Heparin administration is usually followed by oral anticoagulation with warfarin. This prevents rebound coagulation and the formation of deep vein thrombosis or pulmonary emboli.

Heparin resistance

If extensive clotting is present, heparin will be rapidly destroyed and larger doses will be required: this is termed 'heparin resistance' (Lutomski et al., 1995). Also, heparin is neutralized by activated platelets present in arteriosclerosis, which reduce its effect. In very high-risk women, there is considerable risk (4/14) of thromboembolic events if heparin is the sole anticoagulant (Sadler et al., 2000b).

Some individuals have a congenital excess of clotting factor VIII or heparin-binding proteins, which interfere with the haematological monitoring required for heparin administration. If this occurs, heparin concentration monitoring will be necessary (Majerus and Tollefsen, 2006). Heparin resistance and therapeutic failure are summarized in Table 8.3.

Table 8.3 Heparin resistance/therapeutic failure

In some circumstances, heparin may not have its usual efficacy	
Lack of antithrombin	Disseminated intravascular coagulation (DIVC), cirrhosis of liver, nephrotic syndrome, arteriosclerosis, long-term use
Increased clearance of heparin	Pregnancy, obesity, PE, pleurisy, fever, infection, thrombophlebitis, smoking tobacco, extensive surgery (such as abdominal hysterectomy), MI, cancer
Noncompliance	Intermittent administration may not be effective
	Compliance should be monitored in the community
	All doses should be administered without delay, as women can deteriorate very rapidly

Osteoporosis and osteopenia

Bone density is reduced in pregnancy, due to fetal demands for calcium and enhanced bone turnover. This may be compounded by prolonged administration of heparin. Women with diabetes are particularly at risk.

Heparin binds to calcium ions and reduces bone formation. With prolonged administration (>10 weeks), this may induce dose-related osteoporosis and osteopenia. The risk is increased after 3–6 months' use and with doses over 20,000 units/day (Majerus and Tollefsen, 2006). Doses of 10,000 units/day for 19 weeks have led to bone demineralization in pregnant women; 2.2% (4/184) of women receiving heparin during pregnancy and the puerperium sustained osteoporotic fractures (Dahlman, 1993). LMW heparin (40 or 20 mg enoxaprin) has also been associated with loss of bone density in the spine and hip when compared with unmedicated controls (Dahlman et al., 1994; Barbour et al., 1994; Nelson-Piercy et al., 1997, Aronson, 2006). At 3-year follow-up, loss of bone density in the spine was apparent in women managed with unfractionated heparin, but not in those receiving LMW heparin (Bates et al., 2004). Rai et al. (1997) state that bone loss is reversible and equivalent to the loss caused by 6 months' lactation; however, the results of long-term follow-up studies are contradictory (de Swiet, 1995).

Case report

This case illustrates the possibility of compression fractures in women receiving heparin.

A woman had received heparin prophylaxis (5,000 units 3 times per day) during pregnancy and lactation. During the last 2 weeks of pregnancy, she complained of back pain. Six weeks after delivery, she sustained a compression (crush) fracture of the sixth thoracic vertebra, and general osteopenia was noted. Vitamin D concentrations were found to be low (Haram et al., 1993).

In view of these risks, women receiving heparin long term should be given dietary advice and some specialists may prescribe warfarin in the second trimester (Magee and Koren, 2007).

Practice points

- Women receiving any form of heparin during pregnancy should be advised to enhance the calcium, vitamin D and protein content of their diets and take calcium supplements (Ginsberg, 1996; Aronson, 2006).
- Women receiving heparin for recurrent miscarriage and antiphospholipid syndrome during pregnancy should be reviewed regularly, as unduly prolonged treatment increases the risk of osteoporosis (Greaves, 1999).

Effects on the fetus

Although heparin does not cross the placenta, heparin may deprive the fetus of calcium or other nutrients by binding them in the maternal plasma. This could account for the high rates of still-birth and prematurity in early studies of heparin in pregnancy (Hall et al., 1980). In women heparinized for the management of artificial heart valves, the fetal loss rate was 25%, all within the first trimester (Sadler et al., 2000b). Heparin preparations containing benzyl alcohol are considered unsafe for administration during pregnancy: benzyl alcohol toxicity has occurred in neonates, and there is a possibility of placental transfer (BNF, 2009).

Cautions and contraindications: heparin

- Heparin is contraindicated where bleeding would be life-threatening, for example in women with pre-eclampsia, eclampsia and HELLP syndrome, thrombocytopenia, haemorrhagic disorders or active haemorrhage.
- Anticoagulants are not administered to women with severe hypertension, due to increased risk of stroke.

Practice point

■ Blood pressure should be checked before initiating heparin treatment and monitored subsequently. A sustained rise in diastolic BP of 15 mmHg may be considered significant.

- Regional anaesthesia in women who are concurrently receiving anticoagulants is associated with a small but definite risk of spinal haematoma. *The Report on Confidential Enquiries into Maternal Deaths* (CEMACH, 2007: 71) states that on current, non-obstetric evidence, subcutaneous heparin as prophylaxis is not associated with an increased risk of spinal haematoma. However, involvement of a senior anaesthetist is advised (RCOG, 2007). Ellison et al. (2000) experienced no problems during 22 deliveries under epidural and spinal analgesia. Toglia and Weg (1996) advise that safety is increased if aPTT is normal and intravenous heparin has not been administered for 6 hours before the anaesthesia is commenced. Authorities advise against insertion of an epidural catheter for 12 hours after a prophylactic dose of LMW heparin and 24 hours after a therapeutic dose (RCOG, 2007; Marik and Plante, 2008). There were reports of 17 cases of spinal haematoma associated with administration of the first dose of LMW heparin with epidural catheters *in situ* (Aronson, 2006: 1592). Cannula removal should be postponed for 12 hours after the last injection (RCOG, 2007: 10). Risk factors include other drugs affecting coagulation (Aronson, 2006).
- Caesarean section is contraindicated in women who are fully anticoagulated (Marik and Plante, 2008).

Storage

Heparin should be stored in the original package below 25°C, without freezing. Once opened, the product should be used within 28 days (Wockhardt, ABPI, 2009).

Interactions: heparin

- NSAIDs and antiplatelet agents, including aspirin, other salicylates, ibuprofen and diclofenac inhibit the procoagulant action of platelets. If a woman receiving anticoagulants requires simple analgesia, for example for a headache, paracetamol is suitable. Dextrans also interfere with coagulation, increasing the risk of bleeding, particularly from the gastrointestinal tract. Dextran 70 is not recommended for pregnant women (CEMACH, 2007).

- Nicotine accelerates heparin elimination; accordingly, smokers may require higher doses. Nitrates may reduce the effectiveness of heparin (Baxter, 2006).
- Most other drugs react with heparin if given *via* the same intravenous line. Heparin is administered in glucose 5% or sodium chloride 0.9%, preferably using a motorized pump (BNF, 2009).

Laboratory test interactions

Heparin administration can affect the results of several laboratory tests, including calcium concentrations, arterial blood gases, thyroid function tests, and gentamicin concentrations (Aronson, 2006).

Practice points

■ A note of heparin administration placed on patient notes would serve as a reminder to interpret these tests with caution.

■ When sending blood samples to the laboratory, heparin administration should be noted on the form.

Antidote to heparin: protamine sulphate

Protamine sulphate forms an inactive complex with heparin and interacts with platelets and fibrinogen. However, bleeding due to LMW heparins is only partially reversed (Ginsberg, 1996; UCB Pharma, ABPI, 2009). Protamine sulphate must be given by a slow intravenous injection, since rapid administration may cause dangerous hypotension and bradycardia, and the manufacturers' maxmimum dose should never be exceeded (de Swiet, 1995). Following administration, feelings of warmth and flushing are common. Other potential problems with protamine sulphate treatment are:

- bleeding, if given in excess
- urticaria (hives), angioedema or anaphylactic reactions, particularly in women with diabetes and those with an allergy to fish
- pulmonary vasoconstriction
- emesis
- blood pressure and heart rate changes.

Practice point

■ Clotting tests, aPPT and vital signs are closely monitored.

Protamine sulphate acts almost immediately and is active for 1–2 hours; however, its safety in pregnancy and lactation is unknown (UCB Pharma, ABPI, 2009).

Practice point

■ LMW heparins remain active for longer than 2 hours. Specialists should be consulted regarding any need for repeat administration.

Implications for practice: heparin

Potential problem	Management suggestions
Risk of haemorrhage	Observe, (for example catheter sites, drains, and mouth), for signs of bleeding and Caesarean wounds for signs of haematoma
	Check vital signs pre-therapy and every 4 hours, initially. Be prepared to withhold therapy if BP is raised (risk of stroke)
	Inquire about any vaginal blood loss, postpartum bleeding, bruises, petechiae, nosebleeds, oozing cuts
	Advise a medi-alert band with medication clearly written
	Test urine and stools for occult bleeding
	Full clotting screen and full blood count (FBC) before administration (RCOG, 2007)
	Ensure that coagulation and FBC are monitored regularly and that the woman understands the need to attend clinics for this
	Ensure all practitioners are aware that the woman is receiving anticoagulants
Bleeding tendencies	Avoid vigorous nose blowing or teeth cleaning. Use a soft toothbrush
	Avoid razors – electric razors are the least abrasive
	Avoid going 'barefoot'
	Avoid intramuscular injections, catheters, enemas, rectal thermometers if possible
	Apply extra pressure after venepuncture
	Monitor FBC before and during long-term therapy
	Monitor pressure areas in immobile women
Risk of recurrence of thrombosis	Avoid constrictive clothing, leg stirrups
	Mobilize, encourage use of antiembolic stockings
	Measure and compare calf circumferences every 8 hours
	Avoid tobacco
	Assist in turning, coughing and deep breathing every 4 hours
	Check for dyspnoea, pulmonary oedema, cough and haemoptysis at least every 4 hours initially
	Ensure dose is appropriate for body weight and pregnancy
	Arrange follow-up for a minimum of 6 weeks postpartum
	Arrange long-term follow-up to assess risk for future pregnancies, such as tests for thrombophilia
Thrombocytopenia	Monitor platelets pre-therapy, daily or regularly
	Check for purpura or petechiae in dependent areas and under the BP cuff
	Be wary of heparinoids for anticoagulation in women with a history of heparin-induced thrombocytopenia
	Highlight any reaction on the patient's notes, because further administration of any heparins could be dangerous

Potential problem	Management suggestions
Heparin resistance	Inform physician if an infection or thrombophlebitis develops, since the dose of heparin may be increased accordingly
Hyperkalaemia	Potassium concentrations should be monitored on commencement and 7 days later
Diuresis on 2nd day	Advise women that this may persist for 48 hours
Osteoporosis	For those on long-term (1 month plus) heparin, dietary calcium supplementation and review of diet to include fish and milk if possible. Advise on the need for exercise in the long term
Hypersensitivity responses: rashes and itching at administration site, lacrimation, bronchospasm, chills, chest pain, angioedema, anaphylaxis	'Test doses' may be prescribed for patients with allergies Observe for these problems whenever heparin is administered, including cannula 'flushes' Tinzaparin contains sulphites, which may precipitate asthma Ensure reactions are clearly documented
Injection site reactions: irritation, bruising, inflammatory nodules, skin necrosis	Seek alternative therapy at first signs of skin irritation, to avoid progression

Warfarin

Due to the risk of fetal malformations, oral anticoagulants are rarely prescribed during pregnancy but may be used postpartum, following thromboembolic episodes. Warfarin is a more powerful anticoagulant than heparin, and may be used if heparin has been ineffective (Toglia and Weg, 1996). Oral anticoagulants interfere with the action of vitamin K, which is needed for formation of clotting factors II, VII, IX and X, the anti-clotting factors protein S and protein C, and bone formation in the fetus.

How the body handles warfarin

Administration and absorption of warfarin

Following oral administration, coagulation is gradually affected over several days; this is because warfarin interferes with the production of several clotting factors, each with its own half-life. Because thrombin has a half-life of 50–60 hours, warfarin will take 2–4 days to be fully effective. Therefore, heparin is used for 4 days or until the **internal normalized ratio** (INR) has been in the therapeutic range for 2 consecutive days (Ginsberg, 1996).

Practice point

- It is important that warfarin is taken at the same time each day in relation to meals, as absorption is decreased by the presence of food in the gastrointestinal tract.

Elimination of warfarin

There is considerable individual variation in the half-life of warfarin (25–60 hours). Warfarin continues to act 2–5 days after the last dose. Clearance is dependent on hepatic metabolism, which is influenced by age, diseases, such as heart failure and thyroid disorders, genetic factors and many other drugs, including alcohol and tobacco (Chapter 1).

Practice point

■ Ingestion of a high dose of alcohol (a binge) will inhibit the clearance of warfarin, and might precipitate a haemorrhage.

Adverse effects of warfarin

Bleeding

Approximately 10% of those receiving warfarin experience an episode of bleeding; therefore a full blood count, platelets and prothrombin time should be assessed prior to initiation of therapy (McKenry et al., 2006). The risk of bleeding is related to the intensity of therapy and is reduced by regular monitoring of prothrombin time (as INR). The **INR** may not be entirely accurate in some women with antiphospholipid syndrome (Greaves, 1999; Majerus and Tollefsen, 2006); therefore clinical tests of bleeding assume greater importance.

If haemorrhage occurs, vitamin K_1 (phytomenadione; below) may be given by slow intravenous injection, although this will take up to 24 hours to restore coagulation. If major bleeding occurs, a concentrate of clotting factors II, VII, IX and X is needed to cover the immediate danger (BNF, 2009).

Skin necrosis

This occurs, rarely, in extremities or fat-rich areas, typically 3–10 days after initiation. It is attributed to widespread thrombosis of the microvasculature, caused by reduced availability of the anti-clotting factors, proteins C and S. Lesions may spread rapidly and cause disfigurement. Another rare circulatory problem is blue-tinged discolouration of feet 3–8 weeks after initiation of therapy due to cholesterol emboli (Majerus and Tollefsen, 2006).

Warfarin may cause mouth ulcers, gastrointestinal disturbances (diarrhoea and vomiting) and liver damage. Hypersensitivity responses, such as rash, urticaria, fever, nephropathy, reduction in white blood cells, and even **agranulocytosis,** occur rarely.

Effects on the fetus

Risk of fetal damage is appreciable in all trimesters (Hall et al., 1980). Because subcutaneous heparin is less effective than warfarin, warfarin will occasionally be prescribed to women with pre-existing disease; women will need to understand the associated risks, and the importance of close fetal monitoring (de Swiet, 1995; Reuvers, 2007). Malformations are probably dose related, and warfarin has been used without incident in women with artificial heart valves (n = 20).

Warfarin and related drugs interfere with bone formation in the first trimester (weeks 6–12). This results in a high (5–25%), dose-related incidence of cartilage and bone abnormalities, facial deformities and epiphyseal damage. Use during the second and third trimesters is associated with fetal intracranial haemorrhage and subsequent malformation. Warfarin is also associated with a high risk of spontaneous abortion (36%), low birth weight, abdominal and central nervous system malformations (microcephaly, subdural haemorrhage, blindness, spasticity, learning disability), optic atrophy, possibly secondary to intracranial bleeds, and neonatal bleeding. Sadler et al. (2000b) report only 8% live births in women warfarinized for management of artificial heart valves. Other authors suggest that these risks, while substantial, are overestimated (Reuvers, 2007).

Breastfeeding

Although warfarin enters breast milk, breastfeeding may be possible (de Swiet, 1995; CEMACH, 2005). There may be an increased risk of haemorrhage in the neonate, accentuated by deficiency of vitamin K. Some infants are unduly susceptible to bleeding, and some authorities recommend weekly doses of vitamin K for 4 weeks and coagulation tests at 2 weeks (Aronson, 2006; Schaefer, 2007a). These measures are not necessary if heparin is substituted.

Cautions: warfarin

- Use of warfarin within 3 weeks of childbirth risks intrapartum bleeding, either retroplacental or fetal intracerebral (de Swiet, 1995).
- Warfarin is used cautiously, if at all, in people with haemorrhagic tendencies (see heparin).
- Atopic individuals may display hypersensitivity responses.
- Advise patients against abrupt discontinuation of warfarin without medical advice. Supervise gradual withdrawal over 3–4 weeks, with INR monitoring, as necessary.

Interactions: warfarin

- Warfarin interacts with most (approximately 300) other drugs, some foods, and alcohol.
- Co-administration of drugs, such as aspirin, with anticoagulant actions increases the risk of bleeding. Other drugs increase bleeding by decreasing the availability of vitamin K: aminoglycosides, vitamin E, erythromycin, fluoxetine, tetracyclines, mineral oils, colestyramine, thyroid hormones, antibiotics or other agents causing diarrhoea, high doses of ranitidine, and paracetamol (long-term administration).
- The efficacy of warfarin is influenced by the diet. Vitamin K, in cabbage, onions, caffeine or soya products, opposes the action of warfarin. A high fat diet increases the absorption of vitamin K. Large quantities of ice cream (1 litre) have been known to antagonize warfarin (Baxter, 2006).
- Oestrogens (including the oral contraceptive pill), some antiviral agents and tobacco antagonize the actions of anticoagulants and promote clotting.

Practice points

- The dose of warfarin may need to be adjusted if the oral contraceptive pill or other oestrogens are co-prescribed (BNF, 2009).
- Maintain a constant intake of foods and supplements containing vitamins K and C, for example brassicas, onions, lettuce, soya products, mango, and green tea.

Co-ingestion of antacids may discolour urine (red); although harmless, this may provoke anxiety.

Storage

Storage should be in airtight containers, away from heat, light and moisture. Tablet containers should be closed securely.

Implications for practice: warfarin

Potential problem	Management suggestions
Bleeding	See heparin, above
	Ensure prothrombin time/INR is measured regularly
	Advise additional monitoring if liver disease or other illness develop
	Monitor weight and diet, as dose depends on weight
	Ensure that vitamin K_1 and clotting factors are available for intravenous administration
Drug interactions	Advise against use of OTC medications, tobacco or alcohol and casual use of aspirin or vitamin supplements
	Assess diet and advise on the importance of regular food intake
Skin necrosis (0.01–0.1% patients), particularly obese women	Seek reports of painful red areas, particularly 3–5 days into therapy. Urgent medical attention is needed, because lesions spread rapidly
	Ensure vitamin K is available
	Consider screening for inherited clotting abnormalities
Hepatitis (rare)	Report any symptoms of itching
Agranulocytosis (rare)	Report any fever, chills, sore throat
Teratogenicity	Advise of the risks and the need for effective contraception in women using warfarin postpartum
Therapeutic failure	Noncompliance. Women who do not attend for regular blood tests (INR readings) should be contacted urgently

Summary

Thromboembolism occurs in all stages of pregnancy and the puerperium with or without risk factors and in women receiving thromboprohpylaxis (Knight, 2008). The (very real) risks of osteoporosis may be deterring some doctors from prescribing heparin prophylaxis (Nelson-Piercy, 1997).

Vitamin K_1 (phytomenadione)

There are two groups of preparations of vitamin K:

1 Water soluble (menadiol), which is contraindicated in neonates, infants and late pregnancy (BNF, 2009).
2 Fat soluble (phytomenadione), which is discussed here.

Vitamin K is required for bone formation in the fetus and the formation of clotting factors II, VII, IX and X and anti-clotting factors protein C and protein S in the liver. Deficiency of vitamin K may lead to haemorrhage. Vitamin K is obtained from the diet (green vegetables, vegetable oils, eggs, cows' milk) and the gut flora. It is fat soluble, stored in the liver, and may be deficient in any malabsorptive state (for example coeliac disease). Vitamin K deficiency is associated with:

■ neonates whose mothers have received antenatal oral anticoagulants, some antiepileptic drugs or antitubercular drugs
■ neonates, particularly premature infants

- dietary deficiency, including prolonged intravenous feeding
- malabsorption
- disruption to gut flora by antibiotics
- liver disease (including alcohol related), biliary tract disease or surgery.

Haemorrhagic disease of the newborn

Haemorrhagic disease of the newborn (HDN) was first recognized in 1894, when it was distinguished from haemophilia (Lane and Hathaway, 1985). It has since been observed that haemorrhage usually begins on the second or third day of life, commonly from the gastrointestinal tract and is normally self-limiting. Reported incidence in the UK varies from 1:20,000 to 1:1,200, giving an overall prevalence of 1:10,000 (McNinch et al., 1985; McNinch and Tripp, 1991). In most respects, the aetiology of HDN is unknown.

Haemorrhagic disease of the newborn has been subdivided into three categories (Baker, 2006):

1 *Early onset* – at delivery or within 24 hours, in neonates whose mothers have received drugs affecting the metabolism of vitamin K, for example warfarin, carbamazepine, phenytoin, barbiturates, rifampicin, and isoniazid.
2 *Classical* – during the first 2–7 days of life, when bleeding is normally from the umbilicus or gastrointestinal tract, and is usually self-limiting.
3 *Late onset* – 8 days to 12 months, predominantly in breastfed infants. This involves sudden onset of intracranial haemorrhage with serious sequelae (Nishiguchi et al., 1996). Vitamin K deficiency may be precipitated by diarrhoea or malabsorption, for example following prolonged administration of antibiotics. Other risk factors include: birth trauma, chronic diarrhoea, cystic fibrosis, malabsorption syndromes, liver disease, biliary atresia, and alpha-1 antitrypsin deficiency (Sweetman et al., 2007). Many high-risk infants can be identified, and their parents should receive specialist advice regarding vitamin K therapy.

Table 8.4 HDN: comparison of strategies for prophylaxis

Oral vitamin K in neonates
Single-dose vitamin Kmm (mixed micelle) offers protection against classical HDN
Dose may not be complete due to dribbling or spitting
Single dose is not effective against late onset HDN, therefore two or three doses are recommended
Prolonged administration time (first 6 weeks of life) may lead to noncompliance
Is not effective prophylaxis for early onset HDN in high-risk infants
Intramuscular vitamin K in neonates
Pain and swelling at injection site
Risk of kernicterus in premature infants, and those <2,500 g (BNF, 2009)
Risk of hypersensitivity response. Severe local reactions are rare
Greater potential for serious errors or confusion with maternal injections
Fear of possible association with childhood leukaemia

The fetus acquires a store of vitamin K during the last month in utero; however, fetal plasma concentrations are always lower than maternal concentrations, since the placenta acts as a partial barrier, and the efficacy of maternal administration cannot be guaranteed. For the first few days after birth, until the gut flora are established, the healthy neonate has a low intake of vitamin K, particularly if breastfed. In the first few days of life, there is a transient decline in both vitamin K-dependent clotting factors and anti-clotting factors, although the coagulation balance should be maintained in healthy term neonates. Neonatal administration of vitamin K prevents the physiological decline in vitamin K-dependent clotting factors and anti-clotting factors.

Case report

Late haemorrhagic disease of the newborn is extremely rare. A case is reported from Spain following administration of 1 mg vitamin K intramuscularly at birth (Solves et al., 1997).

The infant was healthy and exclusively breastfed until 4 weeks of age. Umbilical bleeding then began, followed by an intracranial haemorrhage 4 days later. Coagulation studies indicated a deficiency of vitamin K-dependent clotting factors, which was corrected on administration of vitamin K.

This case illustrates the importance of all healthcare professionals and parents being alert to the potential severity of bleeding around the umbilicus.

HDN is more likely in infants who are premature, are at high risk (above) or whose mothers use drugs that affect the metabolism of vitamin K (Marcus and Coulston, 1996). Some antiepileptics and antitubercular drugs increase the clearance of vitamin K-dependent clotting factors. If these drugs have been prescribed during late pregnancy, there is an increased risk of neonatal haemorrhage. However, the inefficiency of placental and breast milk transfer of vitamin K means that antenatal prophylaxis to raise maternal levels of vitamin K will be relatively ineffective in elevating the infant's levels.

Practice points

- Some authorities advise women taking carbamazepine, phenytoin, phenobarbital, primidone, rifampicin, and isoniazid to commence oral supplementation with vitamin K 4 weeks before expected delivery (Reuvers, 2007); however, not all authorities consider this necessary (Walker et al., 2009).
- Women with intrahepatic cholestasis of pregnancy should receive oral supplements of vitamin K from 32 weeks (Campbell and Lees, 2000; Kametas and Nelson-Piercy, 2007).
- Women with malabsorption should have prothrombin time assessed at 36 weeks, and, if prolonged, receive intramuscular vitamin K (Kametas and Nelson-Piercy, 2007).
- Intramuscular vitamin K should be given to neonates of women identified above immediately following delivery and repeated if necessary (Sawle, 1995; Marcus and Coulston, 1996).

How the body handles vitamin K

Administration of vitamin K may be oral, intramuscular or intravenous. The route and dose of vitamin K administration to neonates has been the subject of controversy (Table 8.4 above and Implications for practice below). The licensed oral formulation, Konakion MM Paediatric®, appears to offer protection from both classical and late onset HDN (Amedee-Menasme et al., 1992; Isarangkura et al., 1994; Greer et al., 1998). The manufacturer recommends doses at birth and at 4–7 days for all infants, followed by a further dose at 1 month for exclusively breastfed infants (BNF, 2009). For neonates under 2.5 kg, the manufacturer's dosage schedule should be consulted for the necessary dosage reduction (Roche, ABPI, 2009).

Absorption of oral preparations may be too slow or unpredictable to prevent early onset disease in high-risk neonates, who should be given intramuscular vitamin K at birth; however, it is not always possible to identify all 'at-risk' infants (Sweetman et al., 2007). International comparisons indicate that oral regimens are less effective than intramuscular prophylaxis (Cornelissen et al., 1997), and intramuscular administration virtually eliminates the risk of HND (BNF, 2009). Other authorities recommend 1–2 mg oral vitamin K after birth (Reuves, 2007).

Vitamin K$_1$ is rapidly metabolized and excreted *via* the liver and kidneys.

Adverse effects of vitamin K

Vitamin K in the newborn has been associated with **haemolytic** anaemia, hyperbilirubinaemia and **kernicterus**, particularly in premature infants and infants with congenital deficiency of G6PD or vitamin E. These problems are much rarer with phytomenadione than with menadiol (Sweetman et al., 2007). Parenteral vitamin K should be administered cautiously to infants under 2.5 kg, because of the increased risk of kernicterus (BNF, 2009).

Thromboembolic disorders have occurred following vitamin K administration in adults; therefore the prothrombin time is monitored for adults receiving regular vitamin K supplementation (Sweetman et al., 2007). Heparin may be used as a 'rescue' medication in these circumstances.

Hypersensitivity responses, including anaphylaxis, have occurred, very rarely.

Oral vitamin K is generally well tolerated but may cause nausea, headache or flushing. In liver failure, hepatic function will be further depressed (Peschman, 1992).

Intramuscular administration in adults may cause hypertension, bradycardia, chills, sweating, dyspnoea and problems at the injection site. Skin reactions may appear up to 16 days after injection, and may be a form of delayed hypersensitivity (Aronson, 2006).

Practice point

■ Pain and swelling at injection site are not uncommon and should be managed symptomatically.

Intravenous administration is reserved for emergencies, due to the potential severity of the adverse effects and hypersensitivity responses. Administration may be followed by vasodilation and, rarely, cardiovascular collapse or hypersensitivity responses from rashes to anaphylaxis. Accordingly, intravenous injections should always be given very slowly (BNF, 2009). Overdose of vitamin K results in haemolytic anaemia and gastrointestinal tract disturbance.

Childhood malignancy

Extensive reviews have not indicated a significantly increased risk of childhood malignancy associated with administration of intramuscular vitamin K to neonates (Aronson, 2006); effects (if any) are likely to be small and confined to genetically susceptible subpopulations (Sweetman et al., 2007). The relatively low risk of HDN must be offset against any possible increase in the risk of childhood malignancy, which is much more common (Zipursky, 1996). Childhood malignancy was linked to intramuscular, but not oral, vitamin K administration in well-publicized studies (Golding et al., 1990, 1992). The possibility of an association between intramuscular vitamin K administration and acute lymphoblastic leukaemia between the ages of 1 and 6 was confirmed by a case note retrieval study, which simultaneously refuted links with the overall incidence of childhood cancer and leukaemia (Parker et al., 1998). A small additional risk of borderline statistical significance was also found by Passmore et al. (1998a). Other studies did not confirm this association (von Kries et al., 1996; Ansell et al., 1996; Passmore et al., 1998b; McKinney et al., 1998). The research methods used appear to influence the findings in these studies. For example, results may depend on:

▨ whether information on route of administration is obtained from notes or inferred from hospital policies

■ whether matched or unmatched controls are obtained
■ how many of the factors (known and unknown) causing 'clustering' of leukaemia are taken into consideration (Parker et al., 1998).

Vitamin K prophylaxis was introduced randomly without prospective controlled trials. Until long-term results of such trials are available, no firm conclusions can be drawn. The potential human carcinogenicity of vitamin K remains undetermined, but no increase in childhood cancer has been reported since the introduction of vitamin K prophylaxis in the 1960s (Zipursky, 1996).

Interactions: vitamin K

Vitamin K is rendered ineffective by oral anticoagulants but not by heparin. These effects persist for 2–3 weeks after discontinuation of oral anticoagulants (Appendix 1).

Storage

Intramuscular vitamin K and oral vitamin Kmm should be stored in light-resistant containers, below 25°C. Freezing must be avoided and turbid solutions should not be used (Roche, ABPI, 2009). Vitamin K can cause contact dermatitis (Giménez-Arnau et al., 2005), so skin contact is best avoided.

Implications for practice: vitamin K

Due to continuing uncertainty and controversy, parents should be fully informed prior to prophylactic administration.

Potential problem	Management suggestions
Failure of oral administration	Ensure compliance. Repeat dose if medicine is extruded
Pain at injection site	Injection should be given slowly and the area gently compressed on completion of the procedure. The site should not be rubbed as this increases bruising
Concerns over cancer risks	Advise parents of risks and benefits. Offer to discuss the relevant information leaflets
Parent refusal	Document refusal and monitor neonate for signs and symptoms of HDN (particularly bleeding around the umbilicus) for the first 12 months of life

---

Summary

The neonate is born with relatively low concentrations of vitamin K. With breastfeeding, these rise slowly to adult values during the first year of life, thereby putting a small number of infants at risk of HDN. Further research is needed to determine the aetiology of HDN in order to identify those at risk of the disease and explore the possible advantages of physiological concentrations of neonatal vitamin K.

Further reading

■ Bates, S.M., Greer, I.A., Hirsh, J. and Ginsberg, J.S. (2004) Use of antithrombotic agents during pregnancy: the Seventh ACCP Conference on Antithrombotic and Thrombolytic Therapy. *Chest*, **126**(3 Suppl): 627–44.
■ RCOG (Royal College of Obstetricians and Gynaecologists) (2007) *Thrombombolic Disease in Pregnancy and the Puerperium: Acute Management*. Green top guideline no. 28. RCOG Press, London.

CHAPTER 9

Cardiovascular Disorders in Pregnancy

Sue Jordan

This chapter focuses on hypertensive disorders in pregnancy. Cardiac dysrhythmias and cardiac failure are considered briefly. Nifedipine is included under tocolysis, Chapter 7.

Chapter contents

- Blood pressure in pregnancy
- Pre-eclampsia and eclampsia
- Magnesium sulphate
- Pregnancy-induced hypertension and hypertension in pregnancy (methyldopa, beta blockers)
- Drugs used in hypertensive emergencies (hydralazine)
- Other cardiovascular conditions

III

Cardiovascular disorders may arise during pregnancy or predate conception. The commonest cardiovascular abnormality detected in pregnancy is hypertension. Hypertension in pregnancy may be due to:

- pre-existing hypertension, which predisposes to pre-eclampsia and other complications
- pregnancy-induced hypertension, developing in the second half of pregnancy
- pre-eclampsia (Baker, 2006).

These conditions continue to impact on maternal mortality; in the period 2003–5, hypertension accounted for 18 maternal deaths in the UK.

Blood pressure in pregnancy

Normally, blood pressure (BP), systolic and diastolic, falls by 10–15 mmHg during mid-pregnancy, increases towards term, and peaks 3–4 days postpartum. The midwife should explain that observations and any treatment will be continued during this period. For hypertensive women, monitoring for proteinuria and hypertension should continue for 6–12 weeks after delivery (Girling and de Swiet, 1996).

In pregnancy, diastolic BP should normally be below:

- 75 mmHg in the second trimester
- 85 mmHg in the third trimester (Badr and Brenner, 1991)

and systolic BP should be below 140 mmHg (Lumbiganon and Laopaiboon, 2008).

BP measurements are standardized, with instruments that have been validated for use in pregnancy. Automated instruments that have not been validated for use in pregnancy may underestimate systolic BP in pre-eclampsia (CEMACH, 2007). To avoid confusion, clinicians standardize the diastolic measurement using either the K4 (muffled sounds) or the K5 sound (silence) or both (Girling and de Swiet, 1996; Nelson-Piercy, 1996; Helewa et al., 1997; Lumbiganon and Laopaiboon, 2008).

Hypertension in pregnancy is defined as:

- diastolic BP 15 mmHg above the earliest recorded reading on at least 2 occasions or
- systolic BP 30 mmHg above the earliest recorded reading on at least 2 occasions or
- systolic BP reading above 140 mmHg on at least 2 occasions (Baker, 2006) or
- a systolic BP reading above 160 mmHg (CEMACH, 2007) or
- diastolic BP above 90 mmHg on 2 readings 4 hours or more apart (Gallery, 1995) or
- a single diastolic BP reading above 110 mmHg (Redman and Jefferies, 1988; Helewa et al., 1997).

Note: there is no consistency in the literature regarding definitions of either hypertension or pre-eclampsia (Chappell et al., 1999).

The normal fall in diastolic BP makes arterial BP harder to interpret in pregnancy. Pharmacological treatment is likely to be initiated if BP is above 150–160/110 mmHg (Williams et al., 2004).

Practice point

- Hypertension may not be recognized in obese women if a standard cuff is used. The BP cuff should encircle at least 80% of the supported arm. If the mid-arm circumference is more than 49 cm in diameter, a large cuff of 40 cm length should be used (Williams et al., 2004; RCP/BHS, 2006).

Pregnancy renders the mother's cerebral circulation vulnerable to any hypertensive episode, while, simultaneously, the uterine and placental circulations are unable to autoregulate (adjust) to compensate for hypotension and the associated reduced perfusion pressure (Williams, 1991; Williams et al., 2004). Management aims to steer between:

- uncontrolled hypertension, leading to cerebral ischaemia and convulsions or a cerebrovascular accident
- hypotension, jeopardizing the blood supply to the placenta
- possible damage to the infant from any drugs administered.

Practice point

- Anaesthetists should always be informed of any abnormalities in vital signs, as this may influence their selection of medication; for example, intravenous opioids may be needed to prevent a potentially dangerous rise in BP on intubation.

Pre-eclampsia and eclampsia

The definition of pre-eclampsia has changed over time. Most authors use:

■ BP above 140 mmHg systolic or 90 mmHg diastolic plus proteinuria greater than 300 mg in 24 hours (Chappell et al., 1999; Williams et al., 2004; Lumbiganon and Laopaiboon, 2008) or
■ a diastolic BP >90 mmHg on 2 separate days after 20 weeks' gestation plus significant proteinuria, in the absence of pre-pregnancy hypertension (MCHRC, 2000).

Traditionally, estimation of total protein in 24-hour urine collections was considered the safest way to measure proteinuria in hypertensive women, as reliance on 'dipstick urinalysis' may fail to detect significant proteinuria or be contaminated by vaginal discharge (Halligan et al., 1999). However, collecting all urine passed during 24 hours presents practical difficulties, which may lead to inaccuracies. Laboratory measurement of the protein:creatinine ratio in an early morning urine sample is more accurate than dipstick urinalysis (JSC, 2006), and is useful in the assessment of pre-eclampsia (Chappell and Shennan, 2008). Measurement of albumin:creatinine ratio with automated analysers in antenatal clinics offers practical advantages and may be comparable to laboratory measurements of protein:creatinine ratio (Kyle et al., 2008). Doppler assessment identifies poor blood flow in the placental bed and high-risk pregnancies. Clinical signs and symptoms and other laboratory indicators, such as abnormal liver function tests, coagulopathy, raised haematocrit, raised uric acid and **thrombocytopenia**, are of the utmost importance (Badr and Brenner, 1991; Gallery, 1995; DH, 1996).

Note: the normal ranges for the results of liver function tests change during pregnancy (Kametas and Nelson-Piercy, 2007).

Pre-eclampsia and eclampsia may occur any time between 20 weeks' gestation and 6 weeks postpartum. Some 15% of primagravidae are affected. To date, the only effective treatment is removal of the placenta. Risk factors for pre-eclampsia are listed in Box 9.1 and complications are listed in Box 9.2.

III

Box 9.1 Risk factors for pre-eclampsia

Linked to possible immunological reactions:
• First pregnancy or first pregnancy for 10 years
• Rhesus incompatibility
• Renal disease
• Connective tissue disease, for example rheumatoid arthritis
• Donor eggs
Linked to genetic predisposition:
• Sickle cell conditions
• Age <16 or >40
• Prior pre-eclampsia
• Family history of pre-eclampsia
• Trisomy 13 of fetus
Linked to large placenta:
• Multiple pregnancy
• Diabetes
• Molar pregnancy
Linked to atherosclerosis:
• Adverse lipid profile
• Essential hypertension
• Renal disease/urinary tract infection
• Obesity, body mass index >30 kg/m^2
• Insulin resistance
• Raised homocysteine concentrations – associated with low dietary folate
• Some clotting disorders
Source: Brown (1997); Roberts and Hubel (1999); Stevenson and Billington (2007)

Box 9.2 Complications of pre-eclampsia

- Eclampsia – seizures
- Cerebral oedema
- Cerebral haemorrhage
- Retinal haemorrhages, cortical blindness
- Disseminated intravascular coagulation, usually in association with HELLP
- HELLP syndrome (**haemolysis**, elevated liver **enzymes**, low platelets) in 4–12% of severe cases
- Fulminant hepatic failure
- Hepatic infarction, subcapsular haematoma and rupture
- Acute renal failure
- Bilateral renal cortical necrosis
- Haemolytic uraemic syndrome
- Thrombocytopenia – platelets are checked before regional analgesia is administered
- Pulmonary oedema, adult respiratory distress syndrome
- Laryngeal oedema
- Congestive cardiac failure
- Intrauterine growth retardation (IUGR)
- Placental abruption
- Fetal distress, prematurity, intrauterine death

Source: Knox and Olans (1996); Nelson-Piercy (1996); Stevenson and Billington (2007)

The pathophysiological changes underlying pre-eclampsia and eclampsia require further research, which, at present, is hampered by the absence of an animal model for this disease. A variety of mechanisms have been proposed, some of which have led to trials of therapeutic interventions. It would appear that placentation fails, leaving the blood vessels supplying the placenta too narrow to sustain development during the second and third trimesters. The failure of the maternal spiral arteries to dilate (during second wave trophoblast invasion) impairs fetal development and induces placental ischaemia. The placenta responds by releasing **cytokines**, which activate platelets, promote coagulation and damage maternal **endothelial cells**, triggering widespread vasoconstriction and capillary leakage. This reduces the intravascular volume, making the woman vulnerable to both fluid overload and dehydration. As capillaries leak, tissue fluid accumulates, causing oedema. Eventually, deposition of fibrin on the lining of the blood vessels leads to end organ damage, particularly in the kidneys (Knox and Olans, 1996).

Eclamptic seizures are attributed to unremitting vasospasm, raising BP beyond the autoregulatory adjustment capacity of the cerebral blood vessels. This produces oedema, ischaemia, microinfarctions and patches of small haemorrhages in areas of cerebral cortex on the borders of the territories of major arteries, particularly in the occipital cortex. In turn, ischaemia reduces the threshold for seizure activity. This can occur with only a moderately elevated BP.

Case report

It is important that complaints of headache are not dismissed as trivial (Katz et al., 2000).

A patient admitted with severe pre-eclampsia at 29 weeks' gestation complained of a headache. Junior medical staff prescribed co-proxamol over the telephone, failing to appreciate the significance of a rise in BP. Ninety minutes later, she convulsed (DH, 1996: 27).

Detection of pre-eclampsia traditionally depended on the triad of hypertension, proteinuria and oedema. However, rapid deterioration in the presence of only one of these signs has been known (DH, 1996). Any delay in recognition of pre-eclampsia may be fatal to both mother and baby.

Practice points

- Hypertension with proteinuria (>300 mg in 24 hours) indicates the need for urgent (same day) hospital admission (Girling and de Swiet, 1996).
- Important clinical changes include severe headache, visual disturbance, epigastric tenderness (pain below ribs), vomiting, sudden swelling of face, hands or feet, proteinuria, retention of uric acid or sodium, consumptive coagulopathy and hyper-reflexia leading to convulsions (Badr and Brenner, 1991). Other diagnostic indicators include thrombocytopenia, raised uric acid levels and abnormal liver function tests (DH, 1996).

Management of pre-eclampsia and eclampsia

While the underlying causes of pre-eclampsia and eclampsia remain unclear, management will continue to be empirically based. The goals of management remain: prevention of convulsions, control of severe hypertension, and delivery of the fetus and placenta (Chen et al., 1995).

- The initial management of mild or moderate pre-eclampsia may be non-pharmacological. *Rest*, combined with *careful monitoring*, at home or in hospital may be considered. By centrally redistributing the blood flow, bed rest improves the perfusion of the placenta, kidneys, heart, brain and liver and alleviates ischaemia (MacKay and Evans, 1995). The woman should be warned that a diuresis usually follows. A left lateral position may be optimal (Kulb, 1990). When bed rest is prescribed, the risks of thromboembolic disorder should be considered.
- *Controlling BP* protects the mother from the cerebral complications of hypertension but does not influence the disease process underlying pre-eclampsia. There is a danger that signs of disease progression may be masked (Girling and de Swiet, 1996). Antihypertensives reduce BP, but may be ineffective in pre-eclampsia and eclampsia.

Case report

A woman in the third trimester was treated in hospital for pre-eclampsia and discharged taking labetolol. Persistent hypertension necessitated readmission. Hypertension worsened despite oral labetolol, eventually resulting in cerebral haemorrhage (CEMACH, 2007: 74).

It cannot be assumed that antihypertensives will be effective, and close monitoring of vital signs should be maintained.

- *Close monitoring* of urine output and vital signs is essential, before, during and after pharmacological intervention. The density of proteinuria indicates the extent of renal damage. Coagulation may cause necrosis of the renal cortices, which indicates a poor outlook for renal function. Renal failure may follow (Badr and Brenner, 1991).
- *Dietary supplements* have been suggested as prophylaxis, but findings are equivocal. Calcium supplementation did not improve outcomes in hypertensive disorders in pregnancy in a large randomized controlled trial (n = 4,589) (Levine et al., 1997). Calcium intake of 1 g per day reduced the risk of pre-eclampsia, but not severe pre-eclampsia, and increased the risk of HELLP syndrome. Benefits are more likely in women with inadequate dietary intake of calcium (Hofmeyr et al., 2006). Women with low dietary calcium (<600 mg/day) randomized to 1.5 g/day calcium supplements had less severe pre-eclampsia and better pregnancy outcomes than those receiving placebo (n = 8,325) (Villar et al., 2006). Aspirin, fish oils and evening primrose oil alter the composition of endothelial cell membranes. However, they

may be metabolized to produce **free radicals**, which damage, rather than heal, cell membranes (Pipkin et al., 1996) and fish oils may increase the risk of infant brain haemorrhage (Olsen et al., 2000).

▪ *Low-dose aspirin* from 12 weeks' gestation reduces the risk of pre-eclampsia (Duley et al., 2007), but not all authors recommend routine use (Sibai, 1998) (Box 9.3).

Box 9.3 Aspirin and pre-eclampsia

Pre-eclampsia may be characterized by increased endothelial **thromboxane** activity, which implies that aspirin could be an effective therapeutic strategy (Chapter 4, NSAIDs). Accordingly, aspirin has been investigated as prophylaxis in women at high risk of early onset pre-eclampsia (Knight et al., 2000). In a review of 59 trials, low-dose aspirin (around 50–150 mg/day) from 12 weeks reduced (by around 10%) the risk of proteinuric pre-eclampsia, preterm delivery, birth weight <2,500 g and neonatal death in women with gestational hypertension (Duley et al., 2007). However, some large studies indicated that low-dose aspirin (for example 75 mg/day controlled release) had no effects, either beneficial or deleterious (CLASP, 1994; Rotchell et al., 1998; Duley, 1999). Antihypertensive benefits are confined to high-risk women and doses >75 mg/day (Duley et al., 2007).

Further research is needed to establish the safest and most effective dose of aspirin for the prevention of pre-eclampsia. Higher doses increase reduction of pre-eclampsia but doses >75 mg/day do not reduce incidence of preterm delivery or fetal/neonatal death (Duley et al., 2007). Although 60 mg/day aspirin has been widely used, this is only sufficient to inhibit platelet activation and coagulation: it does not prevent other inflammatory processes, which may be more important in pre-eclampsia. This requires 150 mg/day (Pipkin et al., 1996).

Aspirin 50–150 mg/day before 20 weeks' gestation slightly increased the risk for postpartum haemorrhage (RR 1.06, 1.00–1.13) (Askie et al., 2007), but this is not supported in the systematic review (Duley et al., 2007). One randomized controlled trial including 9,000 women indicates that doses below 150 mg/day in the second and third trimesters appear safe (Bates et al., 2004).

High doses of aspirin (3 g or 10 tablets per day) increase the risks of pre-eclampsia and neonatal intracranial haemorrhage in premature infants (Byron, 1995). In the third trimester, it may increase: gestation and labour, blood loss at delivery, minor bleeding complications in neonates, **kernicterus**, and premature closure of the ductus arteriosus, associated with neonatal lung damage (BNF, 2009). There is no evidence that aspirin is teratogenic (Aronson, 2006), and occasional use outside the third trimester is probably not harmful (Pfaffenrath and Rehm, 1998). Aspirin overdose is dangerous to the fetus.

Note: aspirin tablets for analgesia contain a dose of 300 mg.

▪ *Sedatives,* including opioids and prochlorperazine, depress the central nervous system of both mother and fetus, which may interfere with monitoring.

▪ *Diuretics* confer no benefit, and are linked to a disproportionate number of **adverse effects** (Churchill et al., 2007). In pre-eclampsia, the circulating volume is already contracted, and this is compounded by the administration of diuretics, thus jeopardizing the already precarious blood supply to the placenta. In theory, diuretics could dangerously worsen the condition.

▪ *Upper airway oedema* complicates intubation.

▪ *Anticonvulsant prophylaxis* in women who have not suffered a seizure remains controversial. Magnesium sulphate is the preferred anticonvulsant in severe pre-eclampsia (Chien et al., 1996; Duley et al., 2000, 2003). A randomized controlled trial (n = 685) of women with severe pre-eclampsia, defined as symptoms of imminent eclampsia, diastolic BP above 110 mmHg and proteinuria, reported that magnesium prophylaxis reduced the risk of convulsions (Coetzee et al., 1998). The Magpie Trial (2002) (n = 10,110) indicated that magnesium sulphate halves the risk of progression from pre-eclampsia (defined as BP >140/90 and proteinuria) to eclampsia (from 96/5,055, 1.9% to 40/5,055, 0.8%), but the reduction in maternal deaths was not statistically significant, and there was no difference in fetal/neonatal deaths. Long-term follow-up found no differences between the two groups of mothers and children (Magpie Trial Follow-up Study Collaborative Group, 2007a, 2007b). These findings were reflected in the Cochrane Review (Duley et al., 2003). Some obstetricians prescribe magnesium for pre-eclampsia if hyper-reflexia is present (Smith and McEwan, 1997).

■ *Control of convulsions* may involve either magnesium sulphate or diazepam. Since diazepam is familiar to all junior doctors in the UK, and the therapeutic range is relatively wide, it may be given by intravenous injection or rectal solution to rapidly terminate seizures. Any delay in controlling convulsions will be detrimental (Fox and Draycott, 1996).

Magnesium sulphate

This section focuses on magnesium sulphate to control or prevent eclampsia.

Magnesium sulphate has been employed as an anticonvulsant and a **tocolytic** in the USA since 1925 (Robson, 1996). It is currently the drug of choice to prevent further fits in established eclampsia (Eclampsia Trial Collaborative Group, 1995). In this large trial (n = 1,680), magnesium sulphate was more effective than either diazepam or phenytoin in preventing recurrent seizures and was associated with fewer maternal deaths. Subsequently, the role of phenytoin in obstetrics has been very limited. Analysis of trial data indicated that the higher doses used in the intramuscular regimen were more effective in reducing seizures where laboratory monitoring facilities were limited (Graham, 1998).

Administration of magnesium sulphate is not without hazards (DH, 1996), and it is therefore reserved for women who are seriously ill (see Implications for Practice). Most studies indicate that it confers no benefits when administered for preterm labour (Crowther et al., 2002); a large trial (n = 2,241) found no differences in overall outcomes, and more infants in the magnesium group died, but there was a decrease in cerebral palsy among survivors (Rouse et al., 2008).

How the body handles magnesium

Administration of magnesium

Magnesium sulphate may be administered by deep intramuscular injection (into the gluteal region) or intravenously with rapid effect. With the patient placed in the recovery position, seizures may be arrested by an intravenous bolus of magnesium sulphate, administered slowly, for example as 4 g or 16 mmol over 5–15 minutes. (Concentration should not exceed 20%.) An infusion is then administered and continued for 24 hours after the last fit, using a controlled infusion device (BNF, 2009); other regimens have been used successfully (Robson, 1996; Graham, 1998). Bolus doses, depending on patient's weight, should be given slowly, should convulsions recur (BNF, 2009).

Practice points

■ The patient must be carefully monitored for signs of fluid overload, particularly in pre-eclampsia and eclampsia, when intravascular space is contracted.

■ Absorption from intramuscular injections may be slow or unpredictable if circulation has been reduced due to pre-eclampsia or **shock**.

■ Kulb (1990) reports the use of lignocaine to minimize the pain of intramuscular injections, which are repeated every 4 hours for 24 hours after the last fit.

■ Local abscess formation complicates 0.5% of intramuscular administrations (Eclampsia Trial Collaborative Group, 1995). Intravenous administration is usually recommended (Magpie Trial Collaborative Group, 2002).

■ Problems may arise at intravenous or intramuscular injection sites (Duley et al., 2003).

Distribution of magnesium

Magnesium crosses the placenta and affects the fetus in a manner similar to the adult. Magnesium concentrations remain elevated for 24–48 hours after birth (Kulb, 1990). The **blood/brain barrier** may delay the passage of magnesium into the central nervous system; plasma and central nervous system concentrations equalize in approximately 3 hours (Chen et al., 1995). In eclampsia (but not pre-eclampsia), the blood brain/barrier may not be intact, allowing rapid entry in the central nervous system.

Elimination of magnesium

The kidneys are responsible for elimination of magnesium. The elimination **half-life** of magnesium is 4 hours in pregnancy but much longer if the **glomerular filtration rate** falls (Lu and Nightingale, 2000). So the rate of infusion must be in line with renal function, which may change rapidly during the course of the illness. Since pre-eclampsia and eclampsia cause renal impairment, it is important that an accurate measure of renal function (usually serum creatinine) is available for all women likely to require magnesium sulphate in an emergency.

In pre-eclampsia, the glomerular endothelial cells swell. This reduces blood flow into the glomeruli and therefore reduces the glomerular filtration rate, causing serum creatinine to rise above the normal level for pregnancy (70 micromoles/l) to the level for a non-pregnant female (up to 120 micromoles/l). Failure to consider this could result in seriously abnormal serum creatinine values being misinterpreted as 'normal', leading to administration of more magnesium than can be cleared by the patient's kidneys (see Box 1.1).

Practice point

■ During magnesium administration, urine output is closely monitored, as a guide to renal function. Urine output must be at least 25 ml/hour or 100 ml in the 4 hours prior to administration of each dose (Magpie Trial, 2002).

Toxic levels of magnesium can be reached very quickly if the urine output is below normal. If urine output falls and there are no other signs of magnesium toxicity, infusion may be maintained at half the normal rate, combined with serum magnesium concentration monitoring (Duley, 1996; Robson, 1996).

The literature offers no consensus on the need to monitor magnesium concentrations from venous blood samples. Serum magnesium concentration falls during pregnancy. Robson (1996) advises monitoring if seizure prophylaxis fails, urine output falls below 100 ml every 4 hours, signs of toxicity are apparent or staff are inexperienced in administering magnesium. Some units find this helpful (Stevenson and Billington, 2007), while others consider routine monitoring unnecessary (Magpie Trial, 2002; Duley et al., 2003).

Practice points

■ To minimize the effect of cell leakage and obtain an accurate result, blood for magnesium monitoring should be delivered to the laboratory immediately.
■ Current therapy should be noted on the form, particularly calcium gluconate, which may interfere with laboratory tests (Byrne et al., 1986).

Actions of magnesium

Magnesium is vitally important for metabolism, smooth muscle regulation, nerve conduction and impulse transmission. Increased concentrations of magnesium (hypermagnesaemia) depress the activity of all excitable tissue (Box 9.4).

It is thought that magnesium treats eclampsia by relieving the spasm of cerebral blood vessels, which improves cerebral perfusion (Naidu et al., 1996). Magnesium also protects the capillary endothelium from damage by free radicals, which are released in all inflammatory processes. However, eclamptic fits have occurred despite magnesium phrophylaxis and concentrations within the therapeutic range (Katz et al., 2000).

Box 9.4 Actions of magnesium

Hypermagnesaemia depresses the activity of all excitable tissue by:
1 Reduced calcium entry into:
   - *Nerve cells:* Magnesium ions compete with calcium ions for entry into presynaptic nerve terminals. This decreases **neurotransmitter** release at **synapses**. Reduced release of acetylcholine at myoneural junctions causes relaxation of skeletal muscle. Similarly, reduced release of noradrenaline (norepinephrine) from sympathetic nerves supplying vascular smooth muscle causes hypotension.
   - *Cardiac muscle*, causing heart block: Hypermagnesaemia reduces entry of calcium ions into muscle cells, which induces relaxation of smooth muscle and, in high concentrations, heart muscle. The competitive actions between calcium and magnesium mean that calcium is an effective short-term antidote to magnesium toxicity (Rude and Oldham, 1990).
   - *Smooth muscle:* Contraction of all smooth muscle, including blood vessels, uterus and gut, is inhibited. This reverses cerebral vasospasm but induces hypotension.
2 Reduced nerve conduction velocity, that is, slowing nerve impulse transmission.
3 Blocking receptors for excitatory neurotransmitters (glutamiate, NMDA receptors) in the central nervous system. These are activated when oxygen supplies are low; in excess, this causes calcium ion influx and cell death. This may explain the reduction in cerebral palsy among surviving preterm infants (Rouse et al., 2008).

Adverse effects of magnesium

Magnesium sulphate is extremely potent and must be administered cautiously, as its adverse effects are various and hazardous, affecting all systems of the body, and combining to cause problems ranging from generalized discomfort to cardiac arrest (See Implications for practice). Adverse effects may be understood in terms of depression of excitable tissue (Table 9.1) and increasing magnesium concentrates (Table 9.2).

Table 9.1 Summary of actions and adverse effects of magnesium sulphate

Depressant actions of magnesium on:	Potential end point or disaster
Smooth muscle of:	
Blood vessels, especially arterioles	Cardiovascular collapse
Uterus	Tocolysis
Gut	Vomiting, paralytic ileus
Heart	Cardiac arrest, pulmonary oedema
Skeletal muscle	Flaccid paralysis, respiratory arrest
CNS	Somnolence, loss of consciousness
Coagulation	Bleeding
Serum calcium concentration	Hypocalcaemic tetany

Practice points

- Thirst, warmth and flushing are early signs of magnesium toxicity.
- Hypothermia may mask the signs of infection (Hill, 1995).
- The antihypertensive effect of magnesium may not be sustained (Kulb, 1990). Thus it is important that vital signs are monitored regularly throughout administration.

Cardiovascular system
Arterioles

Magnesium relaxes the smooth muscle of arterioles. This reverses the cerebral vasospasm responsible for eclamptic seizures. It also improves blood flow in the maternal uterine artery, which is responsible for some cases of preterm labour. However, smooth muscle of systemic arterioles is also relaxed, inducing flushing, sweating, hypothermia, hypotension and even cardiovascular collapse; 20–65% of women experience flushing (Duley et al., 2003, Rouse et al., 2008).

Heart

Magnesium, in high concentrations, depresses the rate and force of cardiac contractions. This results in bradycardia, widened QRS complexes, heart block, chest pain and eventually cardiac arrest or pulmonary oedema. Cardiac toxicity intensifies with increasing magnesium concentrations, culminating in asystole; however, the concentration of magnesium at which asystole occurs varies among individuals (4–15 mmol/l). Continuous ECG monitoring may reduce the risk of serious **cardiac dysrhythmias.**

Case report

A multiparous woman with signs of pre-eclampsia was admitted to hospital and a magnesium infusion was started. The fetal heart rate decreased, and the woman was transferred to theatre for an emergency Caesarean section. During transfer, the woman complained of nausea and flushing. She suddenly vomited, lost consciousness, stopped breathing and developed ventricular fibrillation. It was then discovered that, during transfer, the magnesium infusion pump had been removed, and the woman had received 1 g of magnesium sulphate per minute for some 10 minutes. After resuscitation, the woman made a full recovery in intensive care. After delivery by emergency section, the neonate was initially flaccid but had an **Apgar score** of 7 at 5 minutes (Morisaki et al., 2000).

If a magnesium infusion is allowed to flow freely, cardiopulmonary arrest can occur without warning signs.

Practice point

- Too rapid administration of magnesium may induce serious dysrhythmia or maternal cardiac arrest (Crowther, 1990).

The fetus may demonstrate decreased heart rate variability and baseline heart rate (Hill, 1995); continuous fetal heart monitoring is essential (Robson, 1996).

Pulmonary oedema is the main cause of death in severe pre-eclampsia (Walker, 2000). Excessive infusion of fluids, and the associated plasma dilution, is the commonest cause of pulmonary oedema (Hill, 1995). Very close observation of input and output must be maintained. High-risk situations include:

- decreased intravascular fluid volume, as in pre-eclampsia and eclampsia

- fluid overload
- administration of corticosteroids – to aid fetal lung maturation
- fluid retention
- decreased renal function
- impaired cardiac function/contractility
- tachycardia
- infection: occult sepsis injures pulmonary capillaries
- prolonged therapy >48 hours
- anaemia.

Bleeding tendency

Alongside the altered coagulation of pre-eclampsia and eclampsia, magnesium sulphate also affects clotting times. Magnesium administration was associated with a higher rate of postpartum haemorrhage in a retrospective cohort study (Szal et al., 1999). Hypermagnesaemia depresses the activity of platelets, increases clotting times and reduces thrombin generation, thereby impairing coagulation (Rude and Oldham, 1990; Assaley et al., 1998). However, disseminated intravascular coagulation may still occur (Crowther, 1990). Therefore venous blood samples are frequently needed for coagulation monitoring.

Skeletal muscle paralysis

Magnesium inhibits contraction of skeletal muscle, depressing deep tendon reflexes and contractility of all muscles, including the muscles of respiration. Muscle weakness and fatigue are early signs of impending toxicity. Flaccid paralysis is possible in mother, fetus or neonate.

Practice point

- Reflexes, such as the patellar reflex (knee jerk), are tested regularly, certainly before each dose, as this may be the first indication of magnesium toxicity. If reflexes are absent, magnesium must be withheld, because respiratory depression is likely to follow (Duley, 1996; Magpie Trial, 2002).

Weakness and gastrointestinal tract stasis combine to cause nausea and anorexia. Reduced protein intake may be compounded by high renal losses.

Respiratory system

Weakness of the respiratory muscles depresses **ventilation** and causes hypoxia (Chapter 4, Opioids). Regular oxygen saturation monitoring will reduce this danger (Stevenson and Billington, 2007). At very high concentrations, magnesium causes apnoea, in mother or neonate, due to a combination of central and peripheral actions (Rude and Oldham, 1990). In the Magpie Trial (2002), respiratory depression was more common in women receiving magnesium. Less than 1% of women experience respiratory depression (Duley et al., 2003). Pritchard et al. (1984) report one maternal death from respiratory arrest.

Practice points

- Respiratory rate and depth are checked regularly, and a minimum value of 16 resps/minute should be recorded before each dose is administered (Magpie Trial, 2002).

■ It is also important to check the neonate for adequate ventilation and to guard against sudden cessation of respiratory movements (Olsen and D'Oria, 1992; Hill, 1995).

Central nervous system

Somnolence, blurred or double vision, nausea, **nystagmus** and slurred speech may be the first signs of a rising magnesium concentration, but these may not be easily detected in an eclamptic patient. Higher concentrations of magnesium lead progressively to confusion and coma (Rude and Oldham, 1990). Therefore regular assessment of conscious level is important.

Kidneys

Magnesium dilates the renal arterioles, which maintain urine output (Crowther, 1990). Since magnesium is osmotically active, its elimination may cause an osmotic diuresis (Hill, 1995). These factors may combine to dehydrate the patient, unless fluid balance is carefully maintained.

Uterus

Magnesium sulphate decreases the amplitude and frequency of uterine contractions, therefore it has been employed as a **tocolytic**. The actions of magnesium oppose those of oxytocin, making vaginal delivery more difficult (Kulb, 1990), and Caesarean section more likely (Chien et al., 1996; Khan and Chien, 1997; Magpie Trial, 2002; Duley et al., 2003). Women receiving magnesium require higher doses of oxytocin (Witlin et al., 1997). A statistically insignificant trend towards longer labour with magnesium therapy has been reported (Szal et al., 1999). However, duration of labour may be more closely associated with analgesia than magnesium therapy (Chapter 4).

Gastrointestinal tract

Nausea and vomiting complicate magnesium therapy in some 15% (166/1,078) of women (Rouse et al., 2008); they result from the combination of actions on the central nervous system and gastrointestinal tract. Constipation becomes clinically significant with long-term parenteral therapy. Paralytic ileus is a rare complication of magnesium therapy (Hill, 1995).

Hypocalcaemia

Short-term administration of magnesium increases the quantity of calcium lost in the urine, and may cause maternal or neonatal hypocalcaemia, tetany and even fits (Lu and Nightingale, 2000), which respond to calcium administration (Baxter, 2006). With long-term therapy, magnesium reduces the secretion of parathyroid hormone, which is responsible for controlling calcium losses in the urine (Rude and Oldham, 1990). This results in increased urinary losses of calcium, and eventually causes bone demineralization in mother and fetus. It is reversible on discontinuation of therapy (Hill, 1995).

Hyperkalaemia

High concentrations of magnesium may impair potassium sequestration and excretion. High concentrations of potassium have been reported in women administering recreational drugs intravenously, who subsequently developed pre-eclampsia and were treated with magnesium (Aronson, 2006).

Emergency measures/'rescue' medications

Both the depressant actions of magnesium and the excitatory actions of potassium are competitively inhibited by calcium. Therefore, calcium gluconate is an effective temporary antidote in magnesium or potassium toxicity. Calcium gluconate is administered intravenously slowly, for example over 3–5 minutes (BNF, 2009). Dialysis provides a more permanent means of correcting magnesium imbalance.

Practice point

■ To facilitate emergency use, a pre-filled syringe containing 10% calcium gluconate (10 ml) is kept by the side of patients receiving magnesium infusions (Smith and McEwan, 1997), as in the Magpie Trial (2002).

Management of eclampsia, severe pre-eclampsia or preterm labour entails infusion of magnesium until the serum concentration is above the normal physiological range, therefore patients should be observed closely for the first signs of these problems (Table 9.2).

Table 9.2 Clinical effects of increasing serum magnesium concentrations

Serum magnesium concentration in mmol/l	Clinical effect
0.75–1.5	Normal physiological range
1.8–3*	Therapeutic range for tocolysis and seizure control, some depression of deep tendon reflexes, for example patellar reflex
2.5–3.5*	Target range for severe pre-eclampsia. Depression of deep tendon reflexes
3.5–5	ECG shows some evidence of heart block, that is, wide QRS complex and prolonged PQ interval; hypotension; somnolence; loss of deep tendon reflexes. *Warning signs of toxicity*
5	Respiratory depression, ECG changes. *Toxicity*
6–7.5	Respiratory paralysis; complete heart block, that is, extreme bradycardia of 15–40 bpm and collapse
12.5 (range 4–15)	Cardiac asystole

Key: * Target range varies among authors.
Source: McKenry et al. (2006: 927); Olsen and D'Oria (1992); Idama and Lindow (1998); Lu and Nightingale (2000)

Neonatal adverse effects of magnesium

Neonates should be monitored for adverse effects of magnesium, particularly respiratory depression, for the first 48 hours. If the mother is ill enough to be receiving magnesium therapy, the neonate is likely to be at high risk. There is no evidence of any association between long-term problems and magnesium therapy (Idama and Lindow, 1998; Riaz et al., 1998; Magpie Trial, 2007b).

Breathing

In one study (n = 64), magnesium administration was associated with poor Apgar score and increased Caesarean section rate for fetal distress (Chen et al., 1995). However, infants born after administration of magnesium were less likely to have a low Apgar score at 1 minute or to be admitted to special care baby units than those whose mothers had received either diazepam or phenytoin (Crowther, 1990; Eclampsia Trial Collaborative Group, 1995). Neonatal depression may not be easily reversed by calcium gluconate administration (Pangle, 2000), and intensive care facilities may be needed.

Unchecked, hypocalcaemia may result in tetany or neonatal convulsions., Therefore monitoring for serum calcium concentration is undertaken and calcium gluconate administered if necessary (Chapter 16).

Breastfeeding

If the neonate is hypermagnesaemic, this may cause drowsiness, blunted reflexes and respiratory depression (Hill, 1995). The neonate may have poor muscle tone (be 'floppy'), cry weakly or demonstrate neurobehavioural impairment (Chen et al., 1995; Riaz et al., 1998). Drowsiness, combined with decreased muscle tone, makes breastfeeding difficult. However, since magnesium will have been eliminated by 24–48 hours, extra support may be sufficient to establish breastfeeding, if the mother is well enough. Breastfeeding is considered safe 24 hours after the last dose of magnesium, as women with normal renal function will have normal serum magnesium concentrations by that time (Idama and Lindow, 1998). Decisions will be taken in the light of postpartum magnesium and renal function measurements.

Cautions and contraindications: magnesium sulphate

- Pre-existing heart block, cardiac disease or myasthenia gravis are likely to be worsened. Caution is advised in renal, hepatic or respiratory impairment.
- Treatment for pre-eclampsia is usually limited to 24 hours (Magpie Trial, 2002).

Interactions: magnesium sulphate

Since magnesium administered to the mother passes into the neonate, it is important that drugs administered to the neonate as well as the mother are checked for potentially dangerous interactions:

- Increased central nervous system depression, leading to confusion and loss of consciousness may occur if sedatives are administered, for example opioids, benzodiazepines, alcohol, phenothiazines (for example prochlorperazine/Stemetil®) and anaesthetics, including nitrous oxide.
- Magnesium potentiates and prolongs the actions of all drugs inhibiting neuromuscular transmission, including muscle relaxants, local anaesthetics (for example epidurals), calcium antagonists (such as nifedipine), and aminoglycoside antibiotics (such as gentamicin). This increases the risks of hypotension, paralytic ileus and respiratory depression or paralysis (Hill, 1995). If a Caesarean section is performed on a woman who has received magnesium sulphate, the dose of muscle relaxants will be adjusted accordingly (Baxter, 2006). Intravenous calcium gluconate is always available at the bedside, should it be needed to assist recovery (BNF, 2009).

Case reports

Drug interactions must be checked before administration to either neonate or mother.
1 A woman with pre-eclampsia had been successfully managed with magnesium sulphate. However, she was noted to have muscle weakness and a serum magnesium concentration above normal limits. When the infant was 12 hours old, she received ampicillin plus gentamicin for a severe infection. After the second dose of gentamicin, the infant stopped breathing; she survived, due to prompt intubation; her condition improved when gentamicin was discontinued (Baxter, 2006: 198).
The additive effects of magnesium plus gentamicin are sufficient to induce neuromuscular blockade. The kidneys of neonates eliminate magnesium very slowly. Therefore, this drug combination is poten-

tially hazardous, and is only safe where facilities exist for artificial ventilation. Where two drugs have the same action, they may dangerously potentiate each other.

2 A woman of 32 weeks' gestation received nifedipine for premature uterine contractions. However, 12 hours later, contractions returned and intravenous magnesium sulphate was administered for tocolysis. The woman developed jerky movements in the extremities (tetany), difficulty in swallowing, paradoxical respirations and muscle weakness so intense that she was unable to lift her head from the pillow. Magnesium was discontinued, and the woman recovered within the next 25 minutes (Baxter, 2006: 658).

This case illustrates the hazards of drug interactions, particularly in units where certain agents are rarely needed.

- Both magnesium and beta$_2$ agonists (such as ritodrine for tocolysis, or salbutamol for asthma) can cause pulmonary oedema. Therefore risks may be increased with co-administration. Although co-administration is reported in some older trials, there is no evidence for efficacy (Dodd et al., 2006).

Implications for practice: magnesium

Magnesium infusions are adjusted in accordance with the results of laboratory and clinical monitoring. The midwife should be prepared to discontinue magnesium therapy and place the patient in the recovery position should signs of toxicity develop (Stevenson and Billington, 2007). In the Eclampsia Trial Collaborative Group (1995) protocol, patellar reflexes and respirations were checked every 15 minutes, more frequently during the first 1–2 hours of an intravenous infusion and before each intramuscular dose (Duley, 1996).

Potential problem	Management suggestions
Hypotension	Vital signs every 15 minutes
	Monitor urine output hourly
Muscle weakness/flaccid paralysis	Deep tendon reflexes, for example patella reflex every 15 or 30 minutes and before each dose
Respiratory depression and apnoea	Monitor respiratory rate and depth every 15 or 30 minutes; 16 resps/min. is the minimum acceptable rate
	Pulse oximetry
	Ensure oxygen is available by mask
	Ensure facilities for intubation and ventilation are in place
	Ensure calcium gluconate is available, for example in a pre-filled syringe at the bedside
	Monitor neonate; apnoea may occur suddenly
	Ensure ventilatory support is available for the neonate, if required
Cardiac dysrhythmia and cardiac arrest	Continuous ECG to detect dysrhythmias
	Calcium gluconate, and a protocol for administration, must be available (see above)
	Expertise to carry out emergency intubation must be available
	Continuous monitoring of fetal HR

III

Potential problem	Management suggestions
Pulmonary oedema	Strict fluid balance records. Monitor HR
	Auscultation of lung bases. Note the development of dyspnoea/ breathlessness
	Monitor protein loss in the urine
CNS depression	Assessment of conscious level of patient
	Special care facilities available for neonate
	Support mother in breastfeeding. This may be difficult for the first 48 hours, while the neonate is eliminating magnesium
Decreased uterine activity	Monitor uterine activity. Ensure facilities for Caesarean section are in place
Impaired coagulation	Haematological monitoring: platelets plus clotting times
	Monitor blood loss at delivery. Facilities for transfusion should be in place
Accumulation of magnesium	Monitor urine output. Record every hour. Minimum level is 25 ml/ hour
	Ensure a measure of renal function, for example creatinine concentration, is available for women who may require magnesium therapy
Nausea and vomiting	Strict fluid balance. Provide support. Monitor plasma proteins
Paralytic ileus	Monitor appetite and intake postpartum
	Monitor stool output until bowel function is restored
Tetany, neonatal convulsions	Ensure availability of calcium gluconate
Hypothermia	Monitor core temperature. Ensure signs of infection are not overlooked. Maintain patient comfort
	Ensure neonate is well protected from the cold
Sweating and flushing	Maintain patient comfort and check for further signs of rising magnesium concentration
Lack of effect, seizures	Convulsions may occur before or after delivery, despite magnesium therapy. Vigilance will need to be maintained
	Monitor serum calcium in mother and neonate

Summary

The use of anticonvulsants in pre-eclampsia, where the risk of convulsions is only 1–2%, remains controversial (Chen et al., 1995; Robson, 1996), and magnesium remains unlicensed for this (BNF, 2009). Women with severe pre-eclampsia are less likely to convulse following administration of magnesium sulphate (Coetzee et al., 1998; Magpie Trial, 2002), but others report no benefit among women with pre-eclampsia prior to labour (Hall et al., 2000). Unfortunately, only 9/53 (17%) of eclamptic seizures can be predicted from the presence of pre-eclampsia, and not all of these will be prevented by administration of magnesium sulphate (Katz et al., 2000). Some 25% of women receiving magnesium suffered adverse effects, compared to 5% receiving placebo (Magpie Trial, 2002); the figures were 77% (833/1,078) versus 12% (140/1,125) in a preterm labour trial (Rouse et al., 2008). Before the use of magnesium sulphate can be extended to lower risk women, it will be important to demonstrate conclusively that it carries no substantial risk to the neonate (Duley and Neilson, 1999).

Pregnancy-induced hypertension and hypertension in pregnancy

The clinical presentation and management of these conditions may be indistinguishable. Hypertension noted during the first trimester is likely to predate pregnancy, but pre-eclampsia cannot be automatically excluded without thorough investigation; this will affect clinical management. Unlike chronic essential hypertension, pregnancy-induced hypertension will have resolved spontaneously by 6 weeks postpartum. Hypertension may be secondary to other, non-pregnancy-related conditions that require investigation, such as renal disease (repeated urinary tract infection), steroid therapy, endocrine disorders or coarctation of the aorta (Nelson-Piercy, 1996).

Note: pre-eclampsia is distinguished from other forms of hypertension by the presence of proteinuria, coagulation disorders, liver dysfunction or contracted circulatory volume (raised haematocrit) (Williams et al., 2004).

Mild, uncomplicated chronic hypertension is a relatively benign condition in pregnancy. However, hypertensive disorders in pregnancy have been associated with superimposed pre-eclampsia, placental abruption, intrauterine growth restriction (IUGR), increased maternal and perinatal morbidity and mortality, and increased long-term risks of renal disorders and hypertension (Nisell et al., 1995; Sibai, 1996). Severe hypertension (>160 mmHg systolic, >105 mmHg diastolic) will require urgent pharmacological intervention to prevent potentially catastrophic maternal cerebrovascular accidents (CEMACH, 2007).

Practice point

- Systolic BP ≥160 mmHg should be reported immediately.

Perinatal outcome is related to both duration and severity of hypertension (Shah and Reed, 1996). However, the effect of hypertension and antihypertensive medications on IUGR is disputed (Plouin et al., 1990; McCowan et al., 1996). Whatever drug is used, reduction in BP may be excessive, jeopardizing the blood flow to the placenta, which lacks autoregulatory capability; this may explain purported associations with IUGR and prematurity (von Dadelszein et al., 2000).

Women with mild or moderate hypertension (140–169/90–109 mmHg) and normal pregnancy-prescribed antihypertensives are less likely to develop severe hypertension, but there are no other clinical benefits. This systematic review of trials involving 4,282 women questioned the benefits of antihypertensives for such women and reported that beta blockers were the most effective agents (Abalos et al., 2007).

A variety of antihypertensive agents are used in pregnancy, including methyldopa, calcium antagonists (nifedipine), hydralazine or labetolol; however, there is little evidence to indicate that any are superior in the management of severe (Duley et al., 2006) or moderate hypertension (Abalos et al., 2007). Other agents are rarely used in pregnancy:

- Other beta blockers (for example atenolol) may cause IUGR, which restricts use to the last trimester (Magee et al, 1999).
- ACEIs (for example captopril or enalopril) and angiotensin receptor blockers (for example valsartan) are implicated in oligohydramnios, hypotension, stillbirth and renal damage, and are therefore **contraindicated** in pregnancy.
- Diuretics reduce circulating volume, thereby jeopardizing placental blood flow and fetal growth. During pregnancy, initiation is reserved for management of pulmonary oedema or heart failure

(Girling and de Swiet, 1996). However, there is little evidence of benefit or long-term harm (Churchill et al., 2007). Prescriptions for diuretics may be continued for women with pre-existing hypertension (Williams et al., 2004), but their well-known adverse effects, including electrolyte imbalance and insulin resistance, may affect the fetus (BNF, 2009). Diuretics increase the concentration of uric acid, which could obfuscate an important clinical sign of pre-eclampsia.

Methyldopa

Due to its long record of safety, including 7-year follow-up studies of infants, methyldopa is often considered the first choice antihypertensive in pregnancy (Sibai, 1996; Nelson-Piercy, 1996; BNF, 2009). Unlike other antihypertensives, methyldopa does not impair renal function and does not reduce cardiac output in young people (Oates, 1996). However, some 60% of women experience sedation or depression, which makes it unpopular during long-term use (Aronson, 2006).

Practice points

- *Methyldopa is taken 1 hour before or 2 hours after meals* to minimize the variability in oral absorption.
- *The woman may opt to take a single dose at bedtime or to divide the dose* in order to minimize dose-related adverse effects, particularly sedation. The long half-life of methyldopa makes this possible. Maximal effects occur at 6–8 hours.
- Follow-up monitoring is essential because:
  - As tolerance develops, over the first 7 days, both the adverse effects and the benefits of the drug may lessen.
  - Any impairment or deterioration in renal function (as in pre-eclampsia) prolongs half-life, necessitating a dose reduction (Hoffman, 2006).

Methyldopa passes into the fetus and reduces BP in neonates, but this is not known to be harmful (Schondorfer, 2007). Methyldopa passes into breast milk, but amounts are considered too small to be harmful (BNF, 2009).

Actions and adverse effects of methyldopa

Methyldopa acts centrally, in the brainstem, to oppose the actions of adrenaline (epinephrine) and noradrenaline (norepinephrine) and dopamine. This causes:

- Inhibition of the sympathetic nervous system, which is normally responsible for controlling BP, regulating the viscera and maintaining a state of 'alertness'. The resultant vasodilatation and bradycardia reduce BP.
- Impairment of the reticular activating system (of the brainstem). This induces sedation, weakness and a reduction in mental energy.

Methyldopa also blocks the dopamine receptors (Hoffman, 2006).

Postural hypotension

Methyldopa impairs BP regulation, particularly on standing (*via* the baroreceptor reflex). As the woman stands, BP may suddenly drop, which leads to sudden dizziness and even falls.

Practice points

- BP should be taken in both a sitting and a standing position.

- Women should be warned to stand up slowly and carefully, particularly during the first week of therapy and in hot weather.
- Women should also be advised to avoid prolonged standing, hot showers or baths, alcohol and strenuous exercise.

Oedema
Prolonged (12 weeks) use of methyldopa may lead to vasodilation with salt and water retention, causing oedema and jeopardizing BP control (Hoffman, 2006). Women should be advised to report any new oedema, as the possibility of pre-eclampsia will need to be investigated.

Sedation
Women prescribed methyldopa should be advised that they will (almost certainly) feel an increased need to sleep, and should be encouraged to do this. Resting will reduce hypertension by redistributing the blood flow. The midwife could advise women to adopt the 'sick role' for the first week, while tolerance is developing, and avoid physical activity, including housework. Driving may be impaired. Sedation will be compounded by alcohol or antihistamine medications, which are best avoided (Nelson-Piercy, 1996) (Chapter 5).

Depression
Since it is likely to cause or intensify depression, methyldopa is avoided postpartum (Nelson-Piercy, 1996) or if the woman is clinically depressed prior to therapy (BNF, 2009). The midwife should be alert for symptoms of depression in women prescribed methyldopa, which will suggest the need to substitute an alternative antihypertensive.

Reduced production of saliva
Methyldopa inflames the salivary glands, reducing production of saliva. Scrupulous oral hygiene should be maintained. The tongue may become inflamed or discoloured. Irritation of the lining of the nose may cause an uncomfortable 'stuffiness'.

Nausea
Emesis and diarrhoea may limit the use of methyldopa in practice.

Tremors
Posture and movement disorders, similar to Parkinson's disease, may occur in susceptible people (particularly those taking antipsychotic medication) and in neonates (Chapter 5). There are occasional reports of methyldopa causing a tremor in neonates whose mothers received methyldopa (Schondorfer, 2007).

Breast discomfort
The reduced activity of dopamine causes the increased production of prolactin, which may cause breast discomfort and a reduction in libido.

Dark urine
A metabolite of methyldopa may darken urine; this is harmless, but women should be aware of this as it may cause alarm.

Liver damage
Hepatotoxicity, with impaired coagulation, has been reported in pregnancy. This potentially serious situation may be avoided by monitoring liver function pre-therapy and 6–12 weeks after initiation of methyldopa (BNF, 2009).

III

Interference with blood tests

Methyldopa may induce the formation of auto-antibodies, which interfere with blood cross-matching (BNF, 2009). Therefore, this must be done before therapy is initiated.

Other immune-mediated adverse effects include: rashes, a 'flu-like syndrome, haemolytic anaemia, thrombocytopenia, leucopenia, myocarditis, and pancreatitis. Therefore, the BNF (2009) advises monitoring FBC and LFTs before and during therapy.

Cautions and contraindications: methyldopa

Pre-existing depression or a history of depression, liver or endocrine disease or blood dyscrasias would make methyldopa an unsuitable antihypertensive.

Interactions: methyldopa

Iron salts interact with methyldopa to reduce the antihypertensive effect. Separation of ingestion by 2 hours only partially reduces this interaction (Baxter, 2006).

Beta blockers (including labetolol)

Beta blockers may be used to manage pregnancy-associated hypertension in the third trimester. They are better tolerated than methyldopa. Beta blockers may be the treatment of choice in controlling hypertension postpartum when, due to its depressive effects, methyldopa is relatively contraindicated (Nelson-Piercy, 1996). However, beta blockers can also induce fatigue and depress mood. Beta blockers cross the placenta. Before the third trimester, beta blockers reduce the fetal blood supply (Sibai, 1996), and are associated with intrauterine growth retardation (IUGR), neonatal bradycardia, hypoglycaemia, and respiratory depression (Aronson, 2006), but early trials did not indicate this (Rubin et al., 1983). Beta blockers are also used to manage thyrotoxicosis, glaucoma (as eye drops), angina, and cardiac dysrhythmias.

Actions of beta blockers

Beta blockers lower BP by reducing heart rate and **cardiac output** and depressing the **renin-angiotensin-aldosterone system**. They act by competing with **beta agonists** (such as adrenaline) for occupation of the beta and beta$_2$ receptors, which control the heart, the liver, the pancreas and the smooth muscle and/or glands of many organs, including blood vessels, uterus, bronchioles and gut.

Adverse effects of beta blockers: both maternal and fetal/neonatal

The adverse effect profile of beta blockers is related to the physiology of the sympathetic nervous system.

Cardiovascular system

Cardiodepressant actions may lead to bradycardia, heart block and even heart failure, precluding use in women with cardiovascular disease. As with all antihypertensive medications, orthostatic hypotension is a potential problem. Beta blockers can block the rise in heart rate and obscure any fall in BP that occurs in association with fluid loss or haemorrhage, thus complicating the timely recognition of serious blood loss. Beta blockers impair the peripheral circulation, making the arms and legs feel uncomfortably cold.

Practice points

■ Vital signs, including orthostatic intolerance, should be assessed regularly (see methyldopa).
■ Increased vigilance for blood loss may allow a haemorrhage to be detected at a relatively early stage.

Case reports describe bradycardia, hypotension, hypoglycaemia, pericardial effusion and myocardial hypertrophy in premature infants born to mothers taking long-term labetolol for hypertension (Aronson, 2006).

Practice points

■ The neonate should be monitored closely for 48 hours to detect and action any transient hypotension, bradycardia and hypothermia (Schondorfer, 2007).
■ Fetal bradycardia may be related to beta blockers prescribed for any reason, including eye drops for glaucoma.

Asthma
Beta blockers prevent the relaxation of the smooth muscle of the bronchioles and cannot be used in women with any history of asthma.

Glucose control
Beta blockers impair the normal sympathetic response to hypoglycaemia, dangerously blocking the warning signs and symptoms of hypoglycaemia. They are less suitable for diabetic women. Infants born to mothers receiving beta blockers should be fed promptly and monitored for hypoglycaemia.

Discomfort
Although generally well tolerated, beta blockers can cause fatigue, nightmares, gastrointestinal upsets, dry eyes or rashes. Psoriasis may be exacerbated.

Withdrawal reaction

Abrupt withdrawal of beta blockers may lead to tremor, headache, sweating, rebound hypertension, and, in susceptible people, myocardial infarction or thyrotoxicosis (BNF, 2009). Thus discontinuation 24–48 hours before planned delivery is controversial (Schondorfer, 2007).

Breastfeeding

Beta blockers pass into breast milk, and acebutol appears in appreciable quantities. The half-life of some agents (for example labetolol) is prolonged in the neonate, increasing the dangers of accumulation (Aronson, 2006). The infant should be carefully monitored, as toxicity cannot be discounted (Schaefer, 2007b; BNF, 2009).

Interaction with adrenaline

Co-administration is very rarely necessary, but see Box 1.2.

Labetolol

Labetolol is a combined alpha and beta blocker. Alpha blockade induces vasodilation. This improves the blood flow to various organs, including the kidneys, and labetolol may be more effective in curtailing the development of proteinuria than methyldopa (Qarmalawi et al., 1995).

III

However, vasodilation also causes postural hypotension (see methyldopa). Labetolol has a faster onset of action than other beta blockers, and may be administered intravenously to control severe hypertension.

Practice points

- During, and for 3 hours after, intravenous administration, the patient should not be allowed into an upright position, due to the risk of profound postural hypotension (BNF, 2009).
- Intensive BP monitoring is required, for example, every 5 minutes for the first 15 minutes, then every 15 minutes during intravenous infusion.
- Atropine, vasopressors and bronchodilators should be available during intravenous administration.

Administration of labetolol is also associated with nasal congestion, a sensation of scalp tingling, headache, dizziness, nightmares and depression. Raynaud's phenomenon may be worsened. Severe liver damage has been reported with both long- and short-term use (BNF, 2009).

Implications for practice: beta blockers

Administration of beta blockers in pregnancy requires careful monitoring.

Potential problem	Management suggestions
Breathing difficulties	Check patient and family history for episodes of bronchospasm or asthma (however long ago) or respiratory conditions. Seek advice before administering if history is positive
	Check lung function before and during therapy by peak flow or spirometry. Seek urgent review if worsening
	In emergencies, high doses of salbutamol may be needed to reverse bronchospasm
Bradycardia and possible heart block; this may reduce the blood supply to the heart muscle and cause angina	Monitor resting HR. Teach patient to monitor pulse. If <50–55 bpm, contact prescriber as dose may need to be decreased
	Ensure atropine is available during intravenous administration
	If heart block is suspected, ECG will be needed
Hypotension/postural hypotension	Ensure the medical team is aware of medication prior to administration of regional anaesthesia or surgery
Heart failure	Ensure a careful record of symptoms is available. Close monitoring on initiation
	Ask patients to report breathing difficulties, difficulty completing sentences, any sudden weight gain or tightness of footwear
Reduced renal blood supply	Pre-therapy and regular review of renal function
Legs become very cold	Maintain a warm environment
Reduced exercise tolerance/capacity, due to reduced cardiac output, blood flow and muscle contractility	Ask patients to monitor their physical exercise and discuss any changes with prescriber

Hypoglycaemia on fasting	Warn patients that severe exercise or prolonged fasting can lead to loss of consciousness due to hypoglycaemia
Impaired recovery from hypoglycaemia	If women with diabetes are prescribed beta blockers, they should monitor frequency and duration of any hypoglycaemic episodes
Hyperglycaemia	Monitor blood glucose pre-therapy and regularly
Dry mouth	Sips of water or ice cubes may help. Attention to dental hygiene is important
Constipation or diarrhoea	Maintain fluid intake, high fibre diet and moderate exercise, if possible. Monitor bowel movements
Nausea	Small frequent meals may help
Fatigue particularly on exertion	Advise patients to be aware that driving may be affected, particularly in the first 3 weeks, and this will be intensified by alcohol
	Report changes in mental functioning
Nightmares/sleep disturbance/insomnia	Patients sometimes benefit from being told that their medication is the likely cause
Depression, lethargy	Discuss with prescriber. Advise against sudden discontinuation of medication

Drugs used in hypertensive emergencies

Rapid control of hypertension may be achieved by intravenous hydralazine or labetolol or oral nifedipine (Girling and de Swiet, 1996). These antihypertensives are also used antenatally, usually for women who cannot tolerate methyldopa. Unlike methyldopa, their use cannot be supported by long-term follow-up studies of infants. Hydralazine is associated with more adverse events (maternal hypotension, Caesarean section, placental abruption and low Apgar score) than either labetolol or nifedipine (Magee et al., 1999).

Hydralazine is a potent vasodilator, capable of achieving rapid reduction of BP when administered intravenously in hypertensive emergencies. Onset of action is within 10–20 minutes and peak effect within 15–30 minutes.

Adverse effects of antihypertensives for emergency use, for example hydralazine

With any drugs in this situation, there is a danger that BP will fall too quickly, risking cardiovascular collapse. Maternal cardiovascular collapse has been reported with sublingual nifedipine (Girling and de Swiet, 1996). If a nifedipine capsule is bitten (or pierced) then swallowed, BP will fall within 5–10 minutes (Smith et al., 2000), and sublingual administration is not advised (Chapter 2).

Rapid changes in vital signs

Parenteral hydralazine rapidly lowers BP, particularly diastolic. As this happens, heart rate suddenly rises (*via* the baroreceptor reflex). This may cause myocardial ischaemia, palpitations or chest pain, particularly if any cardiovascular disease pre-exists, for example in women over 30 who smoke (Robertson and Robertson, 1996). If BP falls too rapidly, this endangers the blood flow to the placenta, and the oxygen supply to the fetus. The woman may sweat profusely and complain of nausea.

Practice points

■ Women receiving parenteral antihypertensives are closely monitored, including vital signs every 5 minutes until stabilized.
■ Fetal distress may complicate administration of hydralazine, and close monitoring is undertaken (Sibai, 1996).

Changes in blood supply

Vasodilation

As blood vessels dilate, the blood supply to the brain, kidneys and skin initially improves. All vasodilators, including hydralazine and nifedipine, cause headache, flushing, nausea, nasal congestion, and tachycardia, which can also affect the fetus. Co-administration of methyldopa may prevent the complications of tachycardia (Nelson-Piercy, 1996) but not the headache and facial flushing (Hopkinson, 1995).

Ischaemia

Generalized vasodilation may divert blood to the skin and prevent an adequate circulation to the brain, retina, heart or kidney, leading to ischaemic injury. Use in those with cardiovascular disease or risk factors or aged over 40 is 'inadvisable' (Oates, 1996; Hoffman, 2006).

Fluid retention and pulmonary oedema

Hydralazine may stimulate the rennin-angiotensin system, causing salt and water retention, which reverses its hypotensive effects, together with potassium loss, possibly associated with muscle cramps. (The ensuing fluid retention should not be mistaken for pre-eclamptic oedema.) The increased cardiac output may cause heart failure (known as high cardiac output cardiac failure) and pulmonary oedema, particularly if intravenous fluids are being administered. There may be an associated proteinuria (Hoffman, 2006).

Practice points

■ Fluid balance should be strictly monitored, and the patient weighed at least daily to detect fluid retention (McKenry et al., 2006).
■ Urine monitoring and pulse oximetry are advised (Hill, 1995).

Hypersensitivity/hypersusceptibility responses

Immunological changes in susceptible individuals can cause vasculitis, lupus-like syndrome and blood disorders (see Aronson, 2006; Hoffman, 2006 for further details).

Cautions: antihypertensives

Because of the dangers of rapid reduction in BP, the intravenous route is reserved for hypertensive crises (BNF, 2009). Any abrupt reduction in BP would be dangerous in certain situations, such as severe pre-eclampsia, cardiogenic shock, heart failure or aortic stenosis.

Hydralazine: maintenance therapy

Hydralazine may, occasionally, be given orally to control hypertension in the antenatal period; it is usually reserved for women who have failed to tolerate other drugs. It is avoided in the first and second trimesters (BNF, 2009).

Practice points

- Hydralazine should be administered with food at the same time each day.
- Women should be warned that abrupt cessation of therapy may lead to a sudden, dangerous rise in BP (McKenry et al., 2006).

Prolonged (6 months plus) therapy with hydralazine has been associated with serious adverse effects, including peripheral neuropathy, tremor, blood disorders and lupus-like syndromes. Vitamin B_6 may minimize these adverse effects. Those with reduced renal function are most at risk. Hydralazine crosses the placenta, and there are reports of neonatal thrombocytopenia following maternal administration (Aronson, 2006).

Implications for practice: antihypertensives

- With all antihypertensives, vital signs will require continuous monitoring to avoid, simultaneously, the dangers of inadequate treatment of hypertension and catastrophic hypotension. Antihypertensives are not always effective in reducing BP.
- Unless fluid balance is accurately recorded and maintained, it will be impossible for the prescriber to avoid pulmonary oedema *and* underperfusion of the placenta and vital organs simultaneously.
- Practitioners may need to distinguish between drug adverse effects and symptoms of disease: for example nausea and headache may be symptoms of impending eclampsia or adverse effects of antihypertensives.
- The midwife should offer the woman reassurance over the 'minor' (non-life-threatening) adverse effects of therapy, such as nasal congestion and flushing. The delivery of such informed care has the potential to make a positive impact in practice.
- Concerns over the putative link between fall in mean arterial pressure and reduction in birth weight suggest that fetal growth should be carefully monitored in women prescribed antihypertensives.
- Where pre-eclampsia is excluded, prescribers may adopt a 'watchful vigilance' regimen in women with BP below 170/110 mmHg (von Dadelszen et al, 2000; de Swiet, 2000). This will involve the midwife in regular monitoring of these at-risk women.
- Women with hypertension in pregnancy or pre-eclampsia are at increased risk of cardiovascular disorders in later life and should be followed up in primary care (Williams et al., 2004).

Other cardiovascular conditions

Cardiac dysrhythmias in pregnancy

Cardiac dysrhythmias may be detected during antenatal examinations. Supraventricular tachycardia is the commonest dysrhythmia in pregnancy. While prompt medical referral is vital, it is important to consider the possible origins of any supraventricular tachycardia:

- unaccustomed exercise
- anxiety
- fever/infection – always consider urinary tract infection
- hypovolaemia/dehydration
- evolving pulmonary embolus – even in apparently healthy women

- use of **sympathomimetics**: over the counter cold cures, amphetamines (including ecstasy), cocaine, asthma medications (salbutamol, terbutaline), and tocolytics (ritodrine)
- antipsychotic or antidepressant medications
- undetected heart valve disease
- undetected cardiac conduction abnormalities, for example Wolff-Parkinson-White syndrome
- undetected thyroid disease
- undetected heart failure
- hypocalcaemia (particularly women with diabetes).

Management of cardiac dysrhythmia in pregnancy requires specialist input. Adenosine has been used to restore sinus rhythm safely in pregnant women. Verapamil is used in young people for prophylaxis of supraventricular tachycardiac, and some specialists will continue this drug during pregnancy. Amiodarone is associated with a variety of long-term adverse effects, including thyroid dysfunction in mother and neonate; it is regarded as a drug of 'last resort' (Hopkinson, 1995; Schondorfer, 2007).

Heart failure in pregnancy

Cardiac output is increased during pregnancy, and further increased during labour. This is achieved by increasing stroke volume. Women with heart failure, congenital heart problems or valve disease are unable to raise stroke volume to meet the demands of pregnancy. Pregnancy carries a recognized risk for a significant number of these women. Most of these women will be receiving specialist medical care prior to pregnancy.

Digoxin

Digoxin is prescribed for atrial fibrillation and cardiac failure. From many years of experience, digoxin is known to be safe in pregnancy, provided digoxin concentrations remain within the therapeutic range (Schondorfer, 2007). Due to changes in drug distribution and elimination (Chapter 1), the dose of digoxin frequently requires adjustment during pregnancy. Also, the signs of digoxin toxicity and therapeutic failure, such as nausea, may be masked by pregnancy. It is important that digitalis toxicity does not occur, as this can be fatal to the fetus (Hopkinson, 1995). Therefore, regular therapeutic drug monitoring is essential, in addition to regular clinical monitoring, including heart rate, BP, ECG, lung bases, renal function, electrolytes, and thyroid function. The midwife should encourage a diet containing plenty of fruit, vegetables and muesli to ensure adequate levels of potassium and magnesium because deficiency of these electrolytes predisposes to digoxin toxicity.

Digoxin crosses the placenta and enters breast milk. The amount of digoxin entering breast milk is small (BNF, 2009). Some infants may be unduly susceptible to digoxin, and the midwife should pay close attention to weight gain in the neonate (Malseed et al., 1995).

Further reading

- Billington, M. and Stevenson, M. (2007) *Critical Care in Childbearing for Midwives.* Blackwell, Oxford.
- De Swiet, M. (2000) Maternal blood pressure and birthweight. *Lancet*, 355: 81–2.
- Idama, T. and Lindow, S. (1998) Magnesium sulphate: a review of clinical pharmacology applied to obstetrics. *British Journal of Obstetrics and Gynaecology*, 105: 260–8.
- Schondorfer, C.W. (2007) Heart and circulatory system drugs and diuretics, in Schaefer, C., Peters, P.W. and Miller, R.K. (eds) *Drugs during Pregnancy and Lactation: Treatment Options and Risk Assessment*, 2nd edn. Elsevier, Oxford.

Part IV

Drugs in Pregnancy

Introduction

This section of the book considers the agents commonly prescribed for or self-administered by women who are otherwise well. Herbal and homeopathic remedies lie outside the scope of this book. Antiemetics are considered in Chapter 5 and analgesics in Chapter 4.

Emboldened terms can be found in the Glossary.

CHAPTER 10

Nutritional Supplements in Pregnancy: Iron and Folic Acid

Sue Jordan
(based on an original chapter by Sue Jordan and Rena McOwat)

This chapter focuses on iron and folic acid, which are frequently prescribed as supplements. Other nutrients are mentioned briefly.

Chapter contents

- Nutrition in pregnancy
- Iron
- Folic acid

Nutrition in pregnancy

The aim of nutrition in pregnancy is to maximize the health of the mother and enhance the development of a healthy infant or infants. There can be no guarantee of a positive outcome with optimal nutrition, but malnutrition can adversely affect the health and development of the fetus. Low birth weight and disease in later life are closely associated with maternal undernutrition (Barker et al., 1990). In the UK, increased dietary intake of iron, zinc, protein and B vitamins during the last trimester proved beneficial for women attending a London teaching hospital (Haste et al., 1991). In California, the incidence of neural tube defects was increased among women who were diagnosed with eating disorders or adopted fasting diets or restricted food intake during the first trimester (Carmichael et al., 2003). In many women, vitamin C intake may also be suboptimal (Coutts, 2000). In less privileged communities, supplements of calories, protein, iron, folic acid, vitamin A, and possibly magnesium, zinc and calcium are needed to optimize the health of women and children (Liljestrand, 1999; Makrides and Crowther, 2000). During pregnancy and lactation, iodine requirements increase from 150 to 250 micrograms/day (Abalovich et al., 2007); however, intake should not exceed 500 micrograms/day.

The overuse of micronutrients may also prove hazardous. Vitamin A in daily doses >10,000 IU was shown to increase the incidence of congenital anomalies, particularly cleft lip, cardiac defects, and central nervous system malformations (Rothman et al., 1995). Vitamin A supplementation, including fish oils, is not recommended in pregnancy, and large doses are not recommended during breastfeeding. High doses of vitamin D may cause hypercalcaemia in mother, neonate and breastfed infants (BNF, 2009). High doses of vitamin E (>14.9 g/day) have been associated with an increased incidence of congenital heart defects (Smedts et al., 2009).

The best possible environment for the developing fetus and its future growth is where the woman is healthy, has sensible eating habits and starts pregnancy with adequate nutrient stores. Most women who are well nourished and active have sufficient stores of minerals and vitamins to meet the increased demands of pregnancy. However, as lifestyles have become more sedentary, calorie intakes have declined. Since dietary iron intake is directly proportional to calorie intake, iron status has declined concomitantly, leaving many young women with inadequate iron stores to meet the demands of pregnancy, particularly if blood loss at delivery is high. Women may be deficient in other essential vitamins and minerals, particularly folic acid. Those at risk include adolescents, women who have several children close together, those with chronic illness such as urinary tract or parasitic infections, pre-pregnancy menorrhagia, malabsorption or malaria, regular users of NSAIDs, women who are anorexic or have a history of eating disorders and those who use appreciable quantities of recreational drugs, tobacco or alcohol. Women with very low incomes may not take in enough calories to meet the energy demands of pregnancy, let alone be able to meet the extra requirements for micronutrients, and therefore some authorities recommend low-dose multivitamin supplements from the pre-conception period. Strict vegetarians are likely to need supplements of vitamins B_{12} and D (van Way, 1999; Coutts, 2000).

Iron

Iron is a mineral required for all body systems. It is essential for haemoglobin synthesis, catecholamine synthesis, heat production and as a component of certain enzymes needed for the production of adenosine triphosphate involved in cell respiration. Iron is stored in the liver, spleen and bone marrow. About 70% of iron in the body is in haemoglobin and 3% is in myoglobin (an intramuscular oxygen store). A deficiency in iron results in anaemia, which reduces the maximum quantity of oxygen the blood can carry. A woman with anaemia is usually very tired, loses her appetite and feels unable to cope. Untreated, anaemia can progress to heart failure. Severe iron deficiency anaemia (haemoglobin below 85 g/l) is associated with premature birth, intrauterine growth retardation and low birth weight (NCC, 2008b). The addition of 60 mg iron to daily folic acid supplementation reduced preterm birth and early neonatal mortality in a randomized controlled trial with women (n = 5,828) in northwest China (Zeng et al., 2008).

Practice points

- Any tiredness, dizziness, tinnitus, anorexia, feeling cold, dry or itching skin, infections, palpitations or breathlessness may be attributable to anaemia, and this should be investigated.
- Shortness of breath and tachycardia should not be attributed to pregnancy itself until possible causes, such as anaemia, have been excluded.
- A full blood count (FBC) and serum ferritin should be measured in women with symptoms of depression, so that iron deficiency may be excluded as a possible cause (Milman, 2008).

In health, the loss of iron from the body is 1–2 mg, daily. This is replaced by the average daily intake of iron, which, in developed countries, is about 15–20 mg. Good dietary sources of iron include meats, eggs, green vegetables (including watercress) and whole grains. Most dietary iron is in the ferric (Fe^{3+}) form. Gastric secretions dissolve the dietary iron, facilitating its reduction to the ferrous (Fe^{2+}) form. This is an important physiological process as iron can only be absorbed in the ferrous form.

Ferric ion (Fe^{+++}) from diet $\xrightarrow{\text{Acid or alcohol in stomach}}$ Ferrous ion (Fe^{++}) $\longrightarrow$ Absorbed into body

Normally, the absorption of iron is carefully regulated so that just enough is absorbed to replace the loss: 3–10% of the daily intake is absorbed. This occurs largely in the proximal duodenum, where the mucosal cells regulate the efficiency of iron absorption.

Practice point

■ Sustained-release preparations may be prescribed if other iron tablets cause **adverse effects,** but they may not release iron until the tablets have passed the duodenum, and therefore may supply no iron (Smith, 1997).

The amount of iron absorbed will depend on a number of factors, such as the content of the diet, the stores of iron in the body, the rate of red cell production and whether or not iron supplements are being taken (Stables, 1999).

If body stores of iron are low, absorption increases up to 30% or even 70% in late pregnancy, when a larger proportion of the iron taken up by the mucosal cells is transported by a carrier mechanism into the plasma. When body stores of iron are high, the mucosal cells transport only a small amount of iron into the plasma. In the plasma, iron binds to the plasma transport protein, transferrin. Most iron is stored within the cells as ferritin. Ferritin is the tissue storage form of iron, and is found in the cells lining the gut, liver, spleen and bone marrow. Serum ferritin measurement provides an index of tissue iron stores, and is considered the most appropriate index for iron status (NCC, 2008b) (see Figure 10.1).

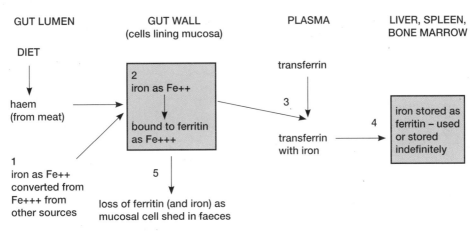

1 iron in diet
2 iron in mucosal cell lining the GI tract: absorbed or shed
3 iron bound to transport protein
4 iron stored
5 iron eliminated

Iron, ferritin and transferrin can all be measured from venous blood samples. Prescription and dose of supplementation should be based on ferritin concentration (Milman, 2008).

Normal values
Ferritin, serum: non-pregnant adult range 15–200 micrograms/litre. Values <30 micrograms/litre indicate iron deficiency. Values below 12 micrograms/litre are taken as indicative of iron deficiency in pregnancy.
Iron, serum: adult range 14–35 micromols/litre males, 11–29 micromols/litre females, 6.6–30.4 micromols/litre in pregnancy.
Transferrin: non-pregnant adult range 1.9–3.75 grams/litre.
Transferrin saturation: all adults: 20–55% <15% indicates iron deficiency.

Figure 10.1 Iron balance

Practice point

■ Ferritin concentrations may not give a reliable estimation of iron stores in women with long-standing inflammation or infections or cancer.

To replenish iron stores, oral iron may need to be continued for several months after an improvement in haemoglobin concentrations (Smith, 1997).

Iron balance is regulated by absorption, but there is no simple mechanism regulating the elimination of iron. Iron elimination is mainly dependent on the shedding of the mucosal cells lining the gut, therefore, overuse of iron can, in susceptible individuals, lead to iron overload (haemosiderosis/ haemochromatosis). In Europe, some 12–13% of women are **heterozygous** and 0.3–0.5% are **homozygous** for haemochromatosis genes: if these women ingest large doses of iron (as tablets), they may develop iron overload, which damages the liver and pancreas (Milman et al., 1999). These genes may also increase susceptibility to iron overload in renal failure (Fernandez, 2000).

Practice points

■ Iron should not be continued longer than six months without medical supervision.
■ A rise in haemoglobin of 20 g/l should be seen within three weeks of starting iron.
■ If there is no response to iron within 3–4 weeks, therapy should be reviewed by physicians.

Iron in pregnancy

Extra iron is needed in pregnancy. Iron requirements for singleton pregnancy are:

■ 200–600 mg to meet the increase in the red cell mass
■ 200–370 mg for the fetus, depending on birth weight
■ 150–200 mg as external loss
■ 30–170 mg for the cord and placenta
■ 90–310 mg to cover blood loss at delivery.

The total iron demands of pregnancy therefore range between 580–1,340 mg, of which 440–1,050 mg will be lost to the mother at delivery (Hillman, 1996). The average net cost is estimated at 630 mg; this can be met from iron stores by the minority of women whose serum ferritin concentration is above 70 micrograms/l (Milman, 2008).

To meet these demands, pregnant women need an average of 3.5–4 mg of iron daily. The requirements increase significantly in the last trimester from an average of 2.5 mg/day in early pregnancy to 6.6 mg/day (Letsky and Warwick, 1994). The iron available from the diet ranges from 0.9 to 1.8 mg/day, depending on the adequacy of the diet. So meeting the demands of pregnancy requires mobilization of iron stores, and an increase in iron absorption. It is estimated that 40% of European women have insufficient iron stores to complete pregnancy and childbirth, and half of these develop anaemia (Milman, 2008); a lack of iron is the principal nutritional deficiency in the USA (Lilley et al., 1996). Although the absorption of iron increases considerably during pregnancy (Barrett et al., 1994), where pregnancies are close together and/or iron stores are low, sufficient iron can only be obtained by supplementation. Only in the most extreme circumstances will the baby be born iron deficient.

Practice points

■ Women with inadequate iron stores need to absorb an extra 2–5 mg of iron per day. This requires a daily supplement of 15–30 mg of iron throughout pregnancy (Hillman, 1996; van Way, 1999), as recommended by some authorities in the USA. Doses of 50–70 mg iron per day from the 20th week are recommended in Scandinavian countries (Milman, 2008).

■ The iron content of beef is around 2 mg/100g, of which 33–66% could be absorbed. To absorb the extra 2–5 mg of iron per day, the woman would need to eat 300–1,500 g of beef per day. Chicken yields less than half this amount of iron. Thus it is unlikely that diet alone can meet the extra demands of pregnancy, and most women will need to draw on their iron stores.

■ Weekly rather than daily supplements may be equally effective (Pena-Rosas and Viteri, 2006).

■ Around 15–30 mg of iron can be obtained from 50–100 mg of dried ferrous sulphate, and 65 mg iron can be obtained from 200 mg dried ferrous sulphate or equivalent (BNF, 2009) (see Table 10.1).

National guidelines vary as to their recommendations for iron supplementation in pregnancy. Routine supplementation is not recommended in the UK (NCC, 2008b).

Lactation also increases the demands for iron; if a mother is iron depleted following childbirth, her infant may require prophylactic iron. Low birth weight infants, particularly those delivered by Caesarean section, may require iron supplements. Anaemia in children has been associated with behavioural and learning difficulties (Hillman, 1996).

Anaemia in pregnancy

Although the daily requirement for iron increases in pregnancy, routine iron supplementation is not usually necessary, if the woman is active, well nourished and eating a balanced diet (NCC, 2008b). If there is evidence of iron deficiency, oral iron supplements may be used, as there is no evidence that they cause any harm to the developing fetus in therapeutic dose. There are relatively few placebo-controlled trials of iron preparations for treatment of anaemia reporting clinical outcomes. Existing trials suggest that oral iron improves haematological indices at the expense of gastrointestinal adverse effects (Reveiz et al., 2007a). Both 30 mg and 60 mg daily iron supplements raised haemoglobin concentrations from below to above 80 g/l in women in rural China (Zeng et al., 2008). Haemoglobin below 80 g/l has been associated with an increased risk of neonatal encephalopathy in developing countries (Ellis et al., 2000). The Cochrane Review of 40 trials in diverse settings indicated that iron supplementation reduces the incidence of mild anaemia (Hb below 110 g/l) at term, but there is less evidence for reduction in moderate (70–110 g/l) and severe (below 70g/l) anaemia (Pena-Rosas and Viteri, 2006).

The diagnosis of anaemia in pregnancy is complicated by the normal changes in haematological indices:

■ *Synthesis of transferrin* (the transport protein) *increases*, reducing the transferrin saturation. Transferring saturation indicates iron availability at the cellular level.

■ *Production of ferritin* (the storage form of iron) *decreases*. Measurements below 12 micrograms/l are taken as indicative of iron deficiency in pregnancy (non-pregnant adult range is 15–200 micrograms/l). Values below 30 micrograms/l indicate low iron status (Milman, 2008), and inadequate iron stores for pregnancy (NCC, 2008b). Low serum ferritin concentrations, particularly in the first trimester, have been linked to increased placental vascularization and size, intrauterine growth retardation and low birth weight (Hindmarsh et al., 2000). However, Barrett et al. (1994) report values as low as 4 micrograms/l in late pregnancy, without clinical evidence of anaemia.

■ *Haemodilution increases*: circulating volume doubles, whereas red cell mass increases by 25%. The concentration of haemoglobin reflects the oxygen-carrying capacity of the blood, not iron stores: women with low iron stores and low serum ferritin concentrations may have adequate haemoglobin concentrations. Haemoglobin values below 110 g/l in the first and third trimesters and 105 g/l in the second trimester are almost always associated with low iron status and are indicative of anaemia (NCC, 2008b; Milman, 2008). However, more stringent criteria should be adopted in women who smoke or live at high altitude (van Way, 1999).

Iron tablets

Dried ferrous sulphate tablets are the most commonly prescribed treatment in the UK, as they are considered to be as effective as other products and cheaper (Table 10.1). Ferrous fumarate tablets contain a similar proportion of iron, and may have a lower incidence of adverse effects. Ferrous gluconate tablets contain less iron, and, consequently, are associated with fewer gastrointestinal adverse effects.

Table 10.1 Comparison of iron formulations

	Iron content %	Dose needed to obtain 60–65 mg iron in an absorbable form
Ferrous sulphate (dried)	30	200 mg
Ferrous sulphate	20	300 mg
Ferrous fumarate	33	200 mg
Ferrous gluconate	11.6	600 mg

Source: BNF (2009)

How the body absorbs iron

Absorption of iron is increased by the presence of acid in the stomach. This can be enhanced by:

- taking with meat or fish, which stimulate gastric acid production
- co-administration with ascorbic acid (vitamin C) 200 mg or orange or tomato juice
- co-administration with alcohol (not advised in pregnancy).

Around 200 mg of vitamin C improves absorption of iron, up to 30%. Vitamin C is water soluble, and rarely accumulates in the body. However, large doses of vitamin C (over 1 g/day) can cause diarrhoea, kidney stones or precipitate a sickle cell crisis in susceptible individuals. The results of urine glucose testing and some forms of uric acid testing may be obscured by large doses of vitamin C.

The relative **achlorhydria** of pregnancy is not reported as an impairment to iron absorption. However, some women with iron deficiency fail to respond to oral iron. The gut is only able to absorb 40–60 mg of iron/day, even in the most severe anaemia, and higher doses may only increase gastrointestinal adverse effects.

Adverse effects of iron therapy

Increasing iron absorption may increase the severity of adverse effects experienced (Smith, 1997).

Gastrointestinal adverse effects

Oral iron supplements may cause nausea, vomiting, stomach cramps, heartburn and constipation (occasionally diarrhoea) (Box 13.1). However, the degree of nausea produced by each preparation depends on the amount of elemental iron absorbed and individual susceptibility. Doses of iron above 60 mg (200 mg dried ferrous sulphate) may produce unacceptable adverse effects in pregnant women, leading to noncompliance (Shatrugna et al., 1999).

Practice point

■ Tablets containing low doses of iron are more likely to be tolerated (and taken) than high doses. If possible, therapy should be commenced with a low dose, especially if the woman expresses concerns over gastrointestinal symptoms. For many women, a low dose will be sufficient.

Taking iron tablets during or immediately after meals reduces the associated nausea but decreases the amount of iron absorbed. Also, many foods interact with iron, if taken within 2 hours (Table 10.2).

Table 10.2 Drugs and foods that reduce the absorption of iron

Substance	Management
Antacids	Separate ingestion by 2 hours
Histamine (H$_2$) antagonists (cimetidine, ranitidine)	Advise clients to manage nausea by adjusting diet
Methyldopa	Separate ingestion by 2 hours
Cholestyramine	Separate ingestion by 6 hours
Calcium supplements	Separate ingestion by 2 hours
Tea, coffee, carbonated drinks	Separate ingestion by 1 hour
Milk, eggs	Separate ingestion by 2 hours
Phytates in bran, corn, beans and cereals	Separate ingestion by 2 hours

Practice points

■ Iron tablets may be better tolerated at bedtime (Engstrom and Sittler, 1994).
■ Doses of iron should be separated by at least 6–8 hours, increased to 12 or 24 hours if adverse effects occur (Smith, 1997).
■ Vomiting and abdominal cramping are both adverse effects and early signs of iron toxicity. They indicate the urgent need to revise (downwards) the dosages of iron.
■ To minimize constipation, advice should be given to:
  ■ drink two litres of fluid each day
  ■ eat fresh fruit and vegetables
  ■ eat plenty of fibre, 2 hours apart from iron tablets
  ■ exercise regularly (see Chapter 13).

Stool and urine discolouration may occur. Women should be warned that stools may be blackened during iron therapy. This may mask any gastrointestinal bleeding.

Micronutrient deficiency

Absorption of zinc and calcium may be decreased by iron tablets. Zinc deficiency has been associated with anaemia, poor absorption of folates, intrauterine growth retardation, preterm delivery, low birth weight and poor wound healing (Long, 1995; Mahmood, 2000). Zinc imbalance is most likely to arise in vegetarians, smokers and heavy drinkers. However, oversupplementation of zinc leads to atherosclerosis and anaemia secondary to copper deficiency (Galbraith et al., 2007).

IV

Iron may increase the need for other micronutrients by stimulating red cell formation, which also increases the body's folic acid requirements. **Macrocytosis** has been reported (Barrett et al., 1994).

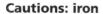

Practice point

■ Folic acid supplements should be continued if iron is prescribed.

Iron excess

Adverse pregnancy outcomes are more likely when maternal haemoglobin falls outside the range 104–132 g/l. Higher concentrations of haemoglobin increase the viscosity of the blood, which may impair the blood flow to the placenta and predispose to coagulation (Long, 1995). There are suggestions that haemoglobin concentration above 13.0 g/dl could predispose to low birth weight (Pena-Rosas and Viteri, 2006). Some 12–13% of women may be vulnerable to iron overload (see above).

Hypersensitivity responses

Rashes developing 2 weeks after initiation of therapy have occasionally been reported (Aronson, 2006).

Cautions: iron

- Risk of iron overload, for example patients receiving blood transfusions.
- Patients with inflammatory bowel disease may develop diarrhoea if administered oral iron.
- **Porphyria** (some forms).
- Pre-existing liver disorders may be exacerbated.

Storage

The storage of iron tablets should be carefully considered, as they are very dangerous (even fatal) in overdose. As little as 2 g of iron (30 dried ferrous sulphate tablets of 200 mg) can be fatal to children. This typically occurs when toddlers ingest their mothers' iron tablets. Urgent referral to intensive care for administration of the antidote (desferrioxamine) can be life saving.

Drug interactions: iron

- Although foods such as orange juice, fish and alcohol help with the absorption of iron, other foods such as eggs and a number of cereal products containing phytates may impair iron absorption. Coffee and tea reduce iron absorption (Barrett et al., 1994). Black tea, which has high concentrations of tannins, is particularly likely to impair iron absorption. Their impact on iron absorption makes tea and coffee unsuitable drinks for infants (Baxter, 2006).
- Co-administration with other minerals, such as calcium or zinc, or some vitamins, including folic acid and vitamin E, reduces absorption of iron. If multivitamin tablets are taken at mealtimes, the amount of iron absorbed from these tablets will be reduced.

Practice point

■ Iron is best administered alone, either at bedtime or between meals (Milman, 2008).

- Iron compounds may interact with antacids in the gastrointestinal tract, forming insoluble compounds and reducing iron absorption. Absorption of thyroid hormones, bisphosphonates, tetracyclines, and fluoroquinolones may be seriously reduced, reducing their clinical benefits. Administration should be separated as widely as possible (by at least 2 hours) (Baxter, 2006; McKenry et al., 2006).
- The antihypertensive effects of methyldopa are antagonized by iron. Administration should be separated by 2 hours. If blood pressure monitoring reveals the recurrence of hypertension, alternative antihypertensives should be considered.

Other formulations of iron

Liquid iron

Liquid iron may be absorbed more readily than tablets, but can stain teeth. This is usually reversible.

Practice points

- Liquid iron should be administered to the back of the throat with an appropriate applicator or (second choice) a straw.
- Liquid iron can be diluted with water or orange juice.
- After each dose, the mouth should be well rinsed with water.
- Stains may be removed with mouthwashes (Galbraith et al., 2007).

Parenteral iron

Parenteral iron is occasionally used for women with gastrointestinal disorders (for example ulcerative colitis), or who are unable to absorb or ingest iron for other reasons. Possible adverse effects include emesis, flushing and dizziness as a result of vasodilatation. Due to the high risks of hypersensitivity responses with iron dextran or iron sucrose, a test dose is mandatory and observation should be maintained for 15 minutes (60 minutes for a first dose of iron dextran). Anaphylactic reactions may be delayed (Box 1.2) (Ostrow and McCoy, 1998; BNF, 2009).

Practice points

- Blood pressure should be monitored following administration of parenteral iron (McKenry et al., 2006).
- Intramuscular iron is not only painful but may cause tissue staining. Therefore administration of iron dextran is into the gluteus maximus, using a Z-track technique (Ostrow and McCoy, 1998).

IV

The high risks of hypersensitivity responses contraindicates administration of iron dextran or iron sucrose to women with allergic disorders, such as asthma and eczema (BNF, 2009).

Summary

One of the aims of antenatal care is to identify women at risk, including those at risk from anaemia. Each woman must be individually assessed, by measurement of serum ferritin and personal history, to differentiate the physiological changes of pregnancy from micronutrient deficiency (Engstrom and Sittler, 1994). Without further research, there is little evidence to suggest that iron therapy is beneficial for women who have no evidence of iron deficiency (Pena-Rosas and Viteri, 2006). Iron supplementation above 70 mg/day (300 mg ferrous sulphate) is rarely necessary for prevention of iron deficiency in pregnancy, and below this dose, adverse effects are unlikely to be troublesome (Milman et al., 1999). Higher doses of iron are used to treat established iron deficiency.

Implications for practice: iron therapy

Potential problems	Management suggestions
Signs and symptoms of anaemia persist despite therapy	Pre-therapy measurements of iron status and activity tolerance
	Administer between meals and warm drinks
	Avoid sustained-release preparations
	Regular evaluation of full blood count, serum iron and ferritin
	An improvement in haemoglobin should be seen after a week
	Inform doctor of any decrease in white cell count, which indicates an adverse reaction
	Consider blood loss, malabsorption syndromes, folic acid or vitamin B_{12} deficiency, sickle cell disease, thalassaemia or other haemoglobinopathies
GI adverse effects	Take in upright position, with full glass of water
	Do not crush the tablets
	Administer with food if nausea is a problem
	Reduce the dose if necessary
	Separate doses by at least 6–8 hours
Dietary inadequacies	Arrange for folic acid supplements to be prescribed
	Consider the diet of the whole family
	Consider the possibility of micronutrient deficiencies such as zinc
Overmedication	Careful assessment of personal and dietary history
	Serum ferritin estimation
	Family history of genetic disorders
Intramuscular iron injections	Discontinue oral iron
	Allow an hour between test dose and full dose administration
	Advise the client to report any unusual symptoms up to 24 hours after iron injections

Folic acid

The only supplement recommended for all pregnant women in the UK is folic acid, which reduces the incidence of neural tube defects by 50–70%, without abolishing the risk (Daly et al., 1997). The administration of folic acid supplements is based on compelling evidence obtained from major studies, including randomized controlled trials (Hibbard and Smithells, 1965; Smithells et al., 1980; Laurence et al., 1981; MRC Vitamin Study Research Group, 1991; Czeizel and Dudas, 1992). The earlier studies provided convincing but not absolutely conclusive evidence of the benefit of folic acid supplementation. The decision to proceed with the larger randomized controlled trials was based partly on the difficulties with randomization in the earlier work. The Medical Research Council study recruited 1,817 women whose previous pregnancies had been complicated by a neural tube defect, and randomized them to receive folic acid (4 mg), vitamin supplements, both or neither. By 1991, neural tube defects had occurred in 27 pregnancies, 6 in the folic acid groups and 21 in the others; this was considered to be sufficient statistical evidence to halt the trial. Czeizel and Dudas (1992) randomized over 4,000 women planning a pregnancy to receive either a mineral or a folic acid supplement (0.8 mg) and found significantly lower rates of neural tube defects in those receiving folic acid (0 versus 6 p = 0.029). The evidence for a protective role in other anomalies, such as cleft palate, congenital heart defects and urinary tract defects is important but less compelling (Werler et al., 1999; Gardiner and Fouron, 2009).

In humans, folic acid is essential for the production of thymidine, a component of DNA. Without folic acid, cell division is impaired, which affects the embryo and the formation of blood cells. During pregnancy, folic acid requirements more than double and remain elevated during lactation (Hillman, 1996). Folic acid is also important in removing the amino acid homocysteine, which is associated with artherosclerosis.

To help prevent the first occurrence of a neural tube defect, all women should be encouraged to take a folic acid supplement of 400 micrograms (0.4 mg) per day from the time they plan to become pregnant (at least 12 weeks pre-conception) until the end of the first trimester (12th week) (BNF, 2009). Starting supplementation before the 7th week offers a significant advantage (Ulrich et al., 1999). Women who have not taken a supplement when they realize they are pregnant should start at once and continue at least until the 12th week (BNF, 2009).

Practice points

- For women who find compliance a problem, a weekly 5 mg folic acid tablet may be an alternative (Mathews et al., 1998).
- To obtain 0.4 mg folic acid from the diet, a woman would have to consume 8 glasses of orange juice, 10 helpings of broccoli, or 3 helpings of Brussels sprouts, lightly cooked (Wald and Bower, 1995).

Higher doses of folic acid, 5 mg, should be substituted for women who are planning pregnancy and:

- have previously given birth to a child with a neural tube defect or
- have a first degree relative with this problem or
- whose partner has a first degree relative with this problem or
- suffer from a malabsorption syndrome or
- have diabetes or
- have sickle cell anaemia or
- are taking antiepileptic medicines (BNF, 2009).

IV

However, a UK database study suggests that folic acid may not reduce the incidence of congenital anomalies in women with epilepsy. Some protection against neural tube defect may be conferred on women prescribed valproate (Morrow et al., 2008).

Folic acid supplementation is associated with higher serum ferritin and haemoglobin concentrations and a reduced risk of anaemia (Hindmarsh et al., 2000).

Adverse effects of folic acid

Adverse effects or hypersensitivity responses associated with folic acid are extremely rare. The most common problem in midwifery is the increased risk of convulsions in women with epilepsy. Such women were excluded from the major trial of folic acid (MRC, 1991).

Seizures

Many women with epilepsy take folic acid supplements with no adverse effects, but there are some reports of an increased incidence and severity of seizures. These may, in some cases, be attributed to interactions with antiepileptic drugs (below). It is not impossible that the neurological effects of undiagnosed vitamin B_{12} deficiency may be exacerbated by folic acid supplements (Aronson, 2006).

Masking vitamin B_{12} deficiency

Vitamin B_{12} deficiency is associated with pernicious anaemia, atrophic gastritis, long-term use of acid suppressant drugs, or bowel surgery for removal of the terminal ileum. Women with these rare conditions should be encouraged to comply with prescribed vitamin B_{12} supplementation, and seek specialist advice regarding any need for dose changes in pregnancy.

If given to people with pernicious anaemia, folic acid supplementation, particularly at the higher dose, may prevent the emergence of the signs and symptoms of this progressive disorder (anaemia and glossitis/sore tongue), allowing the associated neurological degeneration to proceed unrecognized (BNF, 2009). This danger of masking pernicious anaemia, and thereby causing a delay in treatment, is one of the reasons deterring the authorities from fortifying bread and cereals with high doses of folic acid. Pernicious anaemia usually affects women in later life, but does sometimes occur in young women, usually those with a strong family history of the condition.

Practice point

■ Women at high risk of developing pernicious anaemia, or other forms of vitamin B_{12} deficiency, should have serum B_{12} and folic acid concentrations checked as soon as possible to exclude this potentially devastating, but treatable, condition.

Twinning

There have been suggestions from database studies that folic acid supplementation increases the incidence of twin pregnancies, which are associated with increased risks of prematurity and complications: if confirmed, this would reduce the overall benefits of supplementation (Aronson, 2006). For example, a review of the Swedish Medical Birth Registry (n = 6,953 women) indicated that twinning was more likely with folic acid supplementation when other factors, including infertility drugs, were accounted (OR = 1.71, 95% CI, 1.21–2.42) (Källén, 2004a). However, some authorities considered that the impact of assisted conception was not fully accounted for in these studies. Folic acid administration (400 micrograms/day) did not increase multiple births in a Chinese cohort (n = 242,015) (Li et al., 2003).

Suggestions that folic acid may cause nerve damage, malignancy, susceptibility to malaria, or malabsorption of zinc have not been substantiated (Aronson, 2006). Folic acid may cause a harmless yellow discolouration of the urine.

Drug interactions: folic acid

Folic acid is antagonized by several antiepileptics (carbamazepine, phenytoin, barbiturates, primodone, and possibly lamotrigine). These antiepileptics deplete the body of folates, which reduces the elimination of the antiepileptics. When folate stores are replenished by supplementation, the elimination of the antiepileptics increases, reducing the concentration of anticonvulsants, and risking the return of seizures. Women taking antiepileptic therapy should consult their doctors prior to starting folic acid therapy (Baxter, 2006).

Case report

A 26-year-old woman with epilepsy, treated with carbamazepine, was planning pregnancy, and commenced a daily 0.8 mg folic acid supplement for prevention of neural tube defects. Within the next few days, the woman experienced an increase in seizure frequency and her first grand mal fit. The authors attribute the worsening seizure frequency to folic acid supplementation (Guidolin et al., 1998).

Absorption of folic acid may be reduced by magnesium trisilicate or sulphasalzine (Baxter, 2006); therefore, separation of administration by 2 hours would seem advisable. Folic acid also interacts with methotrexate, fluorouracil and some antimalarials.

Folinic acid is derived from folic acid. It is prescribed, as calcium folinate, to alleviate the adverse effects of certain cytotoxic drugs, such as methotrexate.

Implications for practice: folic acid

Potential problems	Management suggestions
Loss of seizure control in women with epilepsy	Ensure women with epilepsy consult medical practitioners prior to starting folic acid
	If possible, women with epilepsy should consult their physicians prior to planning pregnancy
Folic acid taken after conception may not be effective in preventing neural tube defects	Folic acid should be commenced before conception
Need for higher dose of folic acid in women with previous pregnancies complicated by a neural tube defect	Identification of women at risk and pre-conceptual supplementation with the higher dose of folic acid (5 mg/day)

IV

Summary

It has been estimated that folic acid supplementation prevents around 1,000 neural tube defects every year (Wald and Bower, 1995). Pre-conceptual folic acid supplementation by tablets has been recommended for all women in the UK since 1993, as this is the most effective way to increase the availability of folic acid (Cuskelly et al., 1996). Folic acid in food may be destroyed in preparation, and universal food fortification (which is not done in Europe) risks masking the non-neurological signs of pernicious anaemia (Daly et al., 1997). However, offering advice to women in the pre-conceptual period and for the first 4 weeks of pregnancy poses practical difficulties (Mathews et al., 1998).

During the 1980s, the incidence of neural tube defects fell from 45 to 18 per 10,000 births (UK-wide). However, universal folic acid supplements were only recommended in 1993, following the Medical Research Council's trial, published in 1991, indicating that other factors are important in the prevention of neural tube defects. It remains unclear why the recommendation of folic acid supplements has not further reduced the incidence of neural tube defects in the UK (Abramsky et al., 1999).

Further reading

▨ Aronson, J.K. (ed.) (2006) Iron salts and folic acid, in *Meyler's Side Effects of Drugs: The International Encyclopedia of Adverse Drug Reactions and Interactions*. Elsevier, New York; provides further information on parenteral iron.

CHAPTER 11

Management of Gastric Acidity in Pregnancy

Sue Jordan

This chapter considers the available options for reducing gastric acidity, mainly H_2 antagonists and antacids. Other preparations to control gastric acidity (chelates and omeprazole) are mentioned briefly.

Chapter contents

- Causes and management of heartburn in pregnancy
- Antacids
- Chelates and complexes (sucralfate)
- Acid suppressants
- Histamine$_2$ (H_2) antagonists (cimetidine and ranitidine)
- Proton-pump inhibitors (omeprazole)

Causes and management of heartburn in pregnancy

Acid reflux or 'heartburn' during pregnancy is a relatively common problem, affecting 45–85% of women during pregnancy (Broussard and Richter, 1998). The pain of acid reflux could be mistaken for epigastric tenderness, associated with pre-eclampsia; therefore, blood pressure and urine assessments should be undertaken before advice on heartburn is given (NCC, 2007). Heartburn can often be managed by lifestyle adjustments without resort to medications, most of which are available without prescription, over the counter. Gastric reflux is likely to arise for the first time in pregnancy, due to the changes occurring in the upper gastrointestinal (GI) tract, which are maximal around the 36th week. The consequences of this are:

- the lower oesophageal sphincter becomes less competent
- reduced gastric motility and tone
- delayed gastric emptying.

The relaxation of the GI tract during pregnancy is attributed to hormonal changes:

- increase in progesterone
- decrease in motilin (a GI tract hormone)
- increase in enteroglucagon (a GI tract hormone).

IV

These changes increase the dangers of gastric aspiration during anaesthesia. In the past, the aspiration of gastric contents during general anaesthesia was a major cause of avoidable maternal mortality. To lessen these dangers, some anaesthetists administer drugs to reduce gastric acidity (to **pH** >2.5) and volume in all labouring women who are likely to require emergency surgery or receive opioids during labour. Prior to anaesthesia, women may receive:

- metoclopramide to minimize gastric contents (Chapter 5)
- ranitidine
- sodium citrate
- omeprazole (a proton pump inhibitor) (Rowe, 1997; NCC, 2004, 2007).

Women should be warned that they may experience gastric reflux during the later stages of pregnancy and be advised to minimize gastric distension by eating small frequent meals and taking fruit and fluids at different times to meals. Gastric acidity may be reduced by stopping smoking and adjusting the diet (Box 11.1). Stooping or lying flat, peppermint and fatty foods will increase reflux.

Box 11.1 Factors that increase gastric acidity

- Alcohol
- Caffeine
- Hypoglycaemia – missing meals
- High calcium intake, including some antacid preparations
- Adrenaline/epinephrine – released during anger or stress

Practice point

- Isotonic sports drinks are unlikely to increase gastric distension or nausea and may prevent ketosis or starvation during longer labours (Eltzschig et al., 2003).

Disruption of gastric acidity

If drugs are taken to reduce hydrochloric acid secretion or acidity, the normal functions of gastric acid may be disrupted. This is particularly important if the drugs are administered long term:

- Hydrochloric acid is important in reducing the number of bacteria in food (Martinsen et al., 2005). There is no absolute barrier separating the GI tract from the lungs. Fluid from the stomach enters the respiratory tract, *via* the pharynx. Normally, the cilia lining the respiratory tract prevent significant quantities of GI tract secretions reaching the air sacs and alveoli. If GI secretions are not first sterilized by stomach acid, they are more likely to infect the lungs. Women using antacids should take extra care with food hygiene. Nosocomial pneumonia is more common in intensive care patients receiving H_2 antagonists for ulcer prevention: sucralfate is suggested as an alternative (Tryba and Kulka, 1993).
- Hydrochloric acid is important for protein digestion and the normal flow of bile and pancreatic juice.
- Hydrochloric acid is important for the absorption of iron and vitamin B_{12}. With long-term use of drugs for peptic ulceration, iron or vitamin B_{12} deficiency may arise (Aronson, 2006). This is more likely to occur in vegetarians.

Antacids

From long experience, most antacids are considered safe in pregnancy, particularly as they are rarely needed during the crucial phase of organogenesis (18th to 55th days of pregnancy). However, overuse can cause problems such as disruption of gastric acid production (above), and there are isolated reports of serious adverse reactions following heavy use (van Tonningen, 2007b). A variety of antacids is available over the counter for symptom relief, including heartburn and non-ulcer indigestion. Examples include sodium bicarbonate, aluminium hydroxide, magnesium carbonate, sodium citrate, and numerous proprietary preparations. Suspensions may be more effective than tablets. Chewable tablets must be thoroughly masticated and followed by a drink of water. Mixing chewable tablets with water is ineffective.

Antacids provide almost immediate relief of symptoms. On an empty stomach, this lasts for about 30 minutes, but the effects are prolonged by several hours if antacids are taken an hour after food. Most of these compounds are eliminated in the faeces; however, some constituents of antacids are absorbed and excreted by the kidneys (Hoogerwerf and Pasricha, 2006).

Actions and adverse effects of antacids

Antacids decrease the acidity of the stomach, which:

- neutralizes the contents of the stomach
- reduces reflux by increasing the pressure of the lower oesophageal sphincter
- may increase gastric acid secretion, worsening symptoms or increasing the dangers of gastric aspiration.

Magnesium carbonate and *magnesium hydroxide* (found in most over the counter (OTC) preparations including Bisodol® and Andrews Antacid®) neutralize hydrochloric acid for several hours by forming insoluble magnesium chloride.

Magnesium trisilicate (prescribed as tablets or oral powder, Compound BP) also forms colloidal silica. This inactivates pepsin by **adsorption** (taking it onto its surface), and has a more prolonged effect. (Pepsin is the enzyme responsible for digestion of meat. If the lining of the GI tract is ulcerated, pepsin may play a role in mucosal damage.) This preparation may cause kidney stones if used long term (BNF, 2009). All magnesium salts/compounds have a purgative effect (see Chapter 13). Magnesium can accumulate in the body if renal function is poor (Chapter 9). Long-term use of magnesium trisilicate is not advised, due to the risks of respiratory or cardiovascular **adverse effects** and kidney stones (Richter, 2005).

Aluminium hydroxide gel (non-proprietary or as Alu-Cap®) neutralizes hydrochloric acid and forms insoluble aluminium chloride, which adsorbs pepsin. Aluminium compounds cause constipation and delay gastric emptying, therefore they are not usually recommended during pregnancy or breastfeeding. Aluminium binds to phosphates in the gut, reducing their absorption. In women at risk of malnutrition, this can contribute to osteoporosis (Brucker and Faucher, 1997).

Sodium bicarbonate (sodium bicarbonate compound BP and in proprietary products such as Bisodol® and Gaviscon® tablets) acts rapidly to neutralize hydrochloric acid, with the liberation of carbon dioxide. This stimulates gastrin production, which in turn increases gastric acid production and worsens symptoms. Carbon dioxide distends the stomach, promoting belching and worsening reflux (Hoogerwerf and Pasricha, 2006).

IV

Practice point

■ Women should be warned that these preparations may worsen, rather than alleviate, symptoms.

Sodium bicarbonate is absorbed, and is normally excreted by the kidneys. In high doses, sodium bicarbonate can cause oedema, metabolic alkalosis and the formation of kidney stones. Sodium bicarbonate may impede the absorption of B vitamins. It is not recommended in pregnancy (Richter, 2005). Sodium intake from antacids should be limited to avoid fluid retention.

Practice points

■ The sodium content of antacids can be sufficient to raise blood pressure or worsen oedema. If this occurs, antacids without sodium should be substituted, for example Magnesium Trisilicate Tablets BP.
■ Women with borderline pre-eclampsia or at risk of pre-eclampsia should be advised to discontinue antacid preparations.

Sodium citrate is employed prior to general anaesthesia to reduce gastric acidity, and thus reduce the dangers of gastric aspiration. This has the disadvantage that it increases the volume of the gastric contents and reduces the efficacy of metoclopramide (Kennedy and Longnecker, 1996). Sodium citrate reduces gastric acidity within 10 minutes, but may be ineffective after 20 minutes, making it less suitable for elective procedures (Eggers et al., 2008). Citrate ions are metabolized to bicarbonate ions, which affect the pH of the blood. In a small (n = 86) randomized controlled trial to examine the effect of sodium citrate prior to elective Caesarean section, sodium citrate made no difference to either the pH or volume of vomitus, the incidence of nausea or the fluctuations in blood pressure. Despite treatment with sodium citrate, the vomitus was sufficiently acidic to have caused pulmonary damage had it been aspirated (Palmer et al., 1991).

Calcium salts are present in some OTC antacids, such as liquid Gaviscon®, Bisodol® and Settlers®. They are likely to stimulate gastric acid production and worsen symptoms. Prolonged use of calcium-containing antacids can lead to the milk-alkali syndrome, kidney damage or renal stones. There are reports of susceptible individuals developing symptoms of weakness and irritability within days of beginning calcium antacids. It would appear that susceptible individuals absorb a high percentage of ingested calcium, which is deposited in the kidneys, causing long-term damage. The bicarbonate ions ingested with the antacid cannot then be excreted and accumulate, causing alkalosis, with symptoms of weakness, including respiratory depression (Potts, 1991; Hoogerwerf and Pasricha, 2006).

Alginates (contained in Algicon® and Gaviscon®) and simethicone are frequently incorporated into antacids. These reduce flatulence by forming a viscous barrier, which increases the adhesion of gastric contents to the mucosa. Simethicone (for example as Infacol®) is sometimes used for infantile colic, but is no longer recommended (BNF, 2009).

Many *compound preparations* are available. For example, Magnesium Trisilicate Mixture BP also contains sodium bicarbonate, and Gaviscon Advance® tablets contain sodium alginate and potassium bicarbonate. Compounds containing magnesium and aluminium are frequently used because:

■ the constipating and gastric-slowing effects of aluminium are countered by magnesium
■ magnesium provides immediate symptom relief, whereas the effects of aluminium are more sustained.

Practice point

■ All labels of OTC products should be read carefully. It is prudent to avoid preparations containing sodium and calcium salts.

Interactions: antacids

- Absorption of many orally administered drugs, including thyroxine, may be impaired by antacids and enteric coatings may be destroyed (Hoogerwerf and Pasricha, 2006).

Practice point

■ Administration of other drugs, vitamins and minerals should be separated from antacids; an interval of 2–3 hours should be sufficient (Aronson, 2006).

- Antacids increase the excretion of aspirin and aminoglycoside antibiotics, thereby jeopardizing clinical efficacy (Wallace and Amsden, 2002).
- Antacids containing sodium (most antacids) can significantly reduce lithium concentrations, precipitating a relapse of mental illness, and should therefore be avoided in patients prescribed lithium.

Cautions: antacids

- Long-term use of any antacids may cause the formation of kidney stones.
- If any degree of renal insufficiency is present (as in pre-eclampsia, or if there is evidence of repeated urinary tract infection), antacids are best avoided, as they may accumulate and cause toxicity.
- More than 3 months' use of antacids may be associated with birth defects (van Way, 1999).
- Some brands (such as Gaviscon Advance®) contain aspartame, which is harmful to people with phenylketonuria (a genetic condition).

IV

Storage

Storage in the refrigerator may make antacids more palatable. It is important to check expiry dates, as antacids lose their efficacy if stored too long. Liquid formulations must be shaken vigorously before administration.

Chelates and complexes (sucralfate)

Chelates bind to the base of ulcers in the lining of the GI tract and provide physical protection. This allows the natural secretion of bicarbonate to re-establish the normal pH gradient across the gut wall. These drugs must be taken on an empty stomach or they will combine with the protein in food, rather than the gut wall. They should be taken 30–60 minutes before or 2 hours after food. Both liquid and tablet preparations should be administered with water.

Sucralfate consists of sulphated sucrose plus aluminium hydroxide. Sucralfate is only effective if the stomach contents are acid. It is not absorbed, and has few adverse effects, but indigestion, nausea, diarrhoea or constipation, dry mouth, back pain, rash, pruritus, dizziness and sleepiness have been reported. It is **contraindicated** in patients who are seriously ill or have renal failure.

Bezoar (a fibrous mass formed in the stomach from ingested food or hair) formation with GI obstruction has occurred; those with delayed gastric emptying are at risk, and therefore caution is advised in pregnancy and breastfeeding (BNF, 2009). Like other antacids, it interferes with the absorption of other drugs, and administration should be separated by 2–3 hours (Aronson, 2006).

Bismuth chelate is not used in pregnancy since there is a risk of absorption and adverse effects (BNF, 2009).

Acid suppressants

Histamine$_2$ (H$_2$) antagonists

Histamine$_2$ (H$_2$) antagonists (cimetidine, ranitidine, famotidine and nizatidine) are often administered alone or with sodium citrate prior to obstetric anaesthesia to minimize any lung damage caused by the aspiration of gastric contents (CEMACH, 2005). Long-term use during pregnancy and lactation is unusual, and manufacturers advise avoid unless essential (BNF, 2009). They are generally reserved for use in the second and third trimesters where lifestyle changes, antacids and sucralfate have failed (Cappell and Garcia, 1998; Katz and Castel, 1998). One study (Ruigomez et al., 1999) found a statistically insignificant increased risk of congenital anomalies with cimetidine and ranitidine (also omeprazole).

How the body handles H$_2$ antagonists

H$_2$ antagonists are well absorbed orally. They take effect within 1 hour of oral administration, and 30 minutes of intravenous administration, with maximum activity between 1–3 hours. Duration of action varies from 4–12 hours, depending on the drug (Hoogerwerf and Pasricha, 2006). H$_2$ antagonists are eliminated by the liver and kidneys, and are unsuitable for anyone with severe renal or hepatic disease.

The **half-life** of ranitidine is 1.9–2.3 hours; so if ranitidine is administered at the onset of labour, it is likely to be eliminated from the mother before breastfeeding is commenced. Ranitidine crosses the placenta and passes into breast milk. It is not known to be harmful, but manufacturers advise to avoid during pregnancy and breastfeeding without medical advice (GSK, ABPI, 2009).

Actions and adverse effects of H$_2$ antagonists

Histamine, *via* H$_2$ receptors, promotes the secretion of gastrin, which controls gastric motility and secretion. H$_2$ antagonists reduce basal and nocturnal acid output, but have less effect on prandial acid output at standard doses. H$_2$ antagonists are effective and generally well tolerated; with long-term use, the incidence of adverse effects is below 3% (Hoogerwerf and Pasricha, 2006). Adverse effects include:

- *Central nervous system:* Dizziness, somnolence and fatigue may impair the ability to drive. They may also cause headache, hallucinations, confusion and delirium. It is possible that these adverse effects could be mistakenly attributed to an **anaesthetic.**
- *Cardiovascular system:* H$_2$ antagonists administered intravenously can lower or raise heart rate or cause heart block. Therefore intravenous administration is by infusion or slow injection (BNF, 2009).
- *GI disturbances:* Nausea, stomach cramps, constipation or diarrhoea may result from administration of H$_2$ antagonists.
- *Anti-androgen actions:* In long-term use, cimetidine and, to a lesser extent, ranitidine have anti-androgen effects, including breast discomfort and loss of libido, which are reversible on withdrawal. These actions are attributed to an increase in prolactin secretion. Therefore, although there are no reported cases, cimetidine is not advised during pregnancy and lactation (Brucker and Faucher, 1997; BNF, 2009).

Rare adverse effects include: rash, hair loss, hyperthermia, bronchospasm, interstitial nephritis, liver and bone marrow damage.

Interactions: H$_2$ antagonists

- H$_2$ antagonists are not well absorbed in the presence of antacids or metoclopramide, and these drugs should be administered 2 hours apart.
- Blood alcohol concentrations may be raised by concomitant administration of H$_2$ antagonists due to enhanced absorption of alcohol. This exacerbates any problems with driving.
- Smoking reduces ulcer healing and increases the breakdown of H$_2$ antagonists.
- Cimetidine, more than other H$_2$ antagonists, inhibits hepatic metabolism of many drugs. This is the source of numerous drug interactions. Drugs, normally eliminated by hepatic metabolism, will accumulate if taken concurrently with cimetidine. Examples include: opioids (pethidine), antipsychotics (prochlorperazine), warfarin, caffeine, theophylline, many benzodiazepines, nifedipine, tricyclic antidepressants, propranolol, phenytoin, carbamazepine, metronidazole, antiarrhythmics, quinine, and cyclosporin.

Proton pump inhibitors (omeprazole)

Proton pump inhibitors, for example omeprazole, lansoprazole and pantoprazole, inhibit acid formation in the cells lining the stomach. These are the most powerful acid suppressants.

Except for omeprazole, proton pump inhibitors are rarely used in pregnancy due to manufacturers' advice based on teratogenicity in animal studies (BNF, 2009) and concerns in human studies (Ruigomez et al., 1999). Omeprazole has not been associated with increased risk of congenital anomalies (Sweetman et al., 2007). When used as a single dose, omeprazole may be more effective than ranitidine in reducing the pH of gastric contents prior to Caesarean delivery (NCC, 2004). It takes effect within 1 hour of oral administration, and 30 minutes of intravenous administration. Proton pump inhibitors suppress acid secretion for 48 hours, and are administered once daily. They are usually well tolerated, but adverse effects include: emesis, flatulence, diarrhoea, headache, dizziness, fatigue, and, occasionally, raised liver enzymes or hypersensitivity responses, usually rashes.

IV

Implications for practice: antacids and H$_2$ antagonists

Potential problem	Management suggestions
Antacids	
Worsening of symptoms with administration of antacid	Ask clients to monitor frequency of antacid ingestion
	Avoid antacids containing calcium or sodium bicarbonate
	If symptoms increase, suggest non-pharmacological management and seek medical advice
Breathlessness and oedema	Substitute sodium-free products for women with hypertension, heart, liver or kidney problems, however mild
Drug interactions	Separate ingestion/administration by 2 hours
Stool discolouration (whitening)	Women should be advised of this possibility
Kidney stones	Avoid long-term use of antacids

Alkalosis	Minimize use of antacids containing bicarbonate or citrate ions
Unpalatable taste	Chill before taking
H₂ antagonists	
Cardiac conduction disturbances	Observe HR changes during intravenous infusion
	Administer intravenous infusions slowly, never above the manufacturer's recommended rate
Tiredness and confusion	Reassure women that with single doses, these effects will pass within a few hours
Drug interactions with cimetidine	It is more prudent to use ranitidine if any other drugs need to be administered

Conclusion

Ideally, gastric acidity will be managed by non-pharmacological interventions, particularly as uncertainty surrounds the administration of several of the widely used preparations. Antacids are preferred over other preparations. Low-risk women need neither antacids nor H_2-receptor antagonists during labour (NCC, 2007). There are no reports of problems following occasional use of antacids or acid suppressants during breastfeeding (van Tonningen, 2007b).

Further reading

■ Jordan, S. (2008) *The Prescription Drug Guide for Nurses.* Open University Press/McGraw-Hill, Maidenhead; Chapter 2.
■ Van Tonningen, M.R. (2007) Gastrointestinal and antilipidemic agents and spasmolytics, in Schaefer, C., Peters, P.W. and Miller, R.K. (eds) *Drugs during Pregnancy and Lactation: Treatment Options and Risk Assessment*, 2nd edn. Elsevier, Oxford.

CHAPTER 12

Laxatives in Pregnancy and the Puerperium

Sue Jordan and Bronwyn Hegarty

In this chapter, the pharmacological management of constipation associated with pregnancy and the puerperium is outlined.

Chapter contents

- Constipation
- Laxatives

Use of certain laxatives during pregnancy and the puerperium is generally regarded as safe. Bulk-forming laxatives, stool softeners and some osmotic preparations are sometimes administered to women with constipation, where non-pharmacological interventions have failed, or women have pre-existing gastrointestinal or neurological conditions. Opinions vary between practitioners (midwives, nurses, obstetricians, GPs and gastroenterologists) regarding definitions and optimum management of constipation (Brucker and Faucher, 1997; Tytgat et al., 2003; Mahadevan and Kane, 2006; Cox, 2007; Vinod et al., 2007).

IV

Constipation

Normal frequency of bowel movements ranges from 3 motions per day to 1 every 3 days. Some 28% of women report 'constipation' postpartum (n = 2,306) (Yelland et al., 2009). However, clinicians and researchers may use different criteria to define constipation. Simply stated, constipation is present when a person strains to defecate and has infrequent bowel movements with no underlying cause. The feeling of constipation can be subjective, and people often report constipation when they do not conform to clinical criteria used to diagnose constipation (Tytgat et al., 2003). Constipation, as defined by the Rome II diagnostic criteria, is the:

> presence of at least two of the following six features: straining, lumpy or hard stools, sensation of incomplete evacuation, sensation of anorectal obstruction/blockade, manual manoeuvres to facilitate defecation (eg, digital evacuation or support of the pelvic floor), and fewer than three defecations per week (Bradley et al., 2007: 1352).

Some 24% (25/103) of women meet this definition in pregnancy and for the 3 months following delivery (Bradley et al., 2007). This definition does not always match the self-reports of clients: 40–50% of 1,149 participants in a Canadian study who met the Rome II criteria did not feel constipated (Pare et al., 2001). Therefore, some authors suggest making a diagnosis based on self-report rather than standardized criteria (Tytgat et al., 2003), while others disagree (Pare et al., 2001). Although the Rome II criteria are the clinical standards for assessing chronic constipation, they have not been validated for use in pregnancy and the puerperium. Women may feel they are constipated due to 'straining, stools that are excessively hard, unproductive urges, and feelings of incomplete evacuation', even with the passing of a daily bowel motion (Cullen and O'Donoghue, 2007: 808).

Practice point

Simple criteria for diagnosis of constipation in pregnancy are:
- 'low frequency of stools (<3 per week)
- hard stools
- difficulties on evacuation of faeces' (Cullen and O'Donoghue, 2007: 810).

The physiology of small bowel and colonic motility

The smooth muscle of the colon undergoes peristalsis, segmentation and mass action; all gut movements are controlled by several systems, including the enteric nervous system. Factors affecting colonic motility are summarized in Box 12.1, and drugs causing constipation in Box 12.2.

Box 12.1 Controls of intestinal motility

- Autonomic nervous system:
  - Actions of the sympathetic nervous system slow the musculature of the gut and contract both internal and external anal sphincters, particularly in times of stress or anxiety, or if privacy is lacking
  - The parasympathetic nervous system hastens the action of the gut and relaxes the sphincters, for example when the individual is relaxed or extremely fearful
- Higher centres (including the defaecation centre in the medulla) are influenced by stress
- Spinal and local reflexes (mainly parasympathetic nervous system)
- Mobility: colonic motility decreases if people become less mobile for any reason
- Gastrointestinal hormones coordinate the whole gut, for example eating triggers the gastrocolic reflex and motilin stimulates peristalsis
- Stretch of the gastrointestinal (GI) tract stimulates colonic activity, therefore bulky, high-fibre meals promote peristalsis
- Hydration: dehydration hardens faeces and hinders their movement through the intestines
- Irritation of the GI tract, for example by caffeine, toxins or stimulant laxatives, alters intestinal activity
- Circadian rhythm: colonic motility is maximal in the morning, after breakfast. This is upset by any change in routine or inability to heed the feeling to defecate
- Circulating hormones such as thyroid hormones as well as progesterone and oestrogen

---

Practice points

- Including 20–60 g of fibre/day in the diet (Brunton, 1996) and drinking 1 or 2 glasses of fluid with each meal will improve gastrointestinal motility (McQuaid, 1995).

- Stress and tension, for example due to a strange environment such as hospital, can be responsible for constipation. Colonic inertia is more common among women with a history of sexual abuse or psycho-social problems (McQuaid, 1995).
- The gastrocolic reflex is most likely to be active after a high-fibre breakfast (including some caffeine) if taken in a relaxed environment.
- Holistic assessment of all contributing factors and clinical evidence is essential before prescription of laxatives (Cullen and O'Donoghue, 2007).

Box 12.2 Drugs causing constipation

- Opioids (pethidine, codeine)
- Iron tablets
- Antimuscarinics, sedatives
- Sympathomimetics:
  - Amphetamines (including ecstasy), cocaine
  - OTC 'cold cures' (Sudafed®)
  - Salbutamol, terbutaline, and ritodrine
- Antihypertensives: beta blockers and calcium blockers
- Drugs causing dehydration:
  - Diuretics
  - Alcohol
  - Some laxatives, for example lactulose
- Aluminium-containing antacids
- Sucralfate
- Antidiarrhoeal agents
- Stimulant laxatives causing atonic colon (overuse)
- NSAIDs (not aspirin)
- Muscle relaxants given for general anaesthesia

Practice points

- Some drugs, such as iron tablets (Box 12.3), may contribute to constipation.
- Women who use codeine for analgesia or cough suppression are likely to find opioid-induced constipation intolerable in pregnancy (Malseed et al., 1995).
- Clients taking drugs for recreational purposes, such as amphetamines or opioids, may complain of constipation, without disclosing any illegal drug use.

IV

Box 12.3 Iron-induced constipation

There is no consensus on the relationship between iron supplements and constipation in pregnancy (Derbyshire et al., 2006; Bradley et al., 2007). One study (Milman et al., 2006) reported no clinically significant gastrointestinal **adverse effects** when 20–80 mg ferrous iron (as fumarate) was taken between meals (n = 404). In contrast, Ahn et al. (2006) report that vitamin supplements containing 35 mg iron are associated with lower constipation rates than those containing 60 mg iron (n = 135).

Physiological changes in pregnancy and the puerperium

Hormonal and anatomical changes alter the motility of the intestine, slowing activity and transit time, and increasing the risk of faecal impaction (Baron et al., 1993; Cullen and O'Donoghue, 2007; Derbyshire et al., 2007) (Box 12.4). However, most clinical studies in pregnancy are associated with small bowel transit rather than colon motility because the latter is difficult to assess without harming the mother and fetus (Baron et al., 1993).

Box 12.4 Factors predisposing to constipation during pregnancy

Physiological
- Hormone-induced relaxation of the smooth muscle of the gut caused by:
  - an increase in progesterone
  - an increase in relaxin
  - a decrease in motilin, which is produced by the gut wall
  - an increase in enteroglucagon, which is produced by the gut wall (Derbyshire et al., 2007).
- Increased water and salt absorption in the gut caused by:
  - increased transit time, due to relaxation of intestinal smooth muscle (Baron et al., 1993; Cullen and O'Donoghue, 2007)
  - actions of prolactin
  - activation of the **renin-angiotensin-aldosterone axis** by progesterone and oestrogen in pregnancy, which increases absorption of salt and water (Garland, 1985; Cullen and O'Donoghue, 2007).

Structural
- Direct pressure of the uterus and fetus on the bowel (Derbyshire et al., 2007).

Lifestyle
- Reduction or change in food and fluid intake
- Reduction in exercise taken (Derbyshire et al., 2006).

In the puerperium, additional considerations include:

- perineal trauma leading to pain and loss of sensation
- dehydration due to loss of body fluid (sweat and blood) during labour
- poor hydration during labour
- and, possibly, fear and anxiety.

Progesterone concentrations usually remain elevated for several days postpartum, contributing to decreased intestinal motility (Baron et al., 1993: 373). Following the physiological evacuation of the bowel during normal labour, defaecation is usually delayed for several days.

However, the incidence of constipation may be similar in pregnant and non-pregnant women (Bradley et al., 2007; Ponce, et al., 2008).

Management of constipation

If constipation in pregnancy is not resolved, it may inhibit the normal progress of labour by obstructing the birth canal (Bennett and Brown, 1993). Constipation may cause additional problems such as headache, bloating, abdominal pain and appetite impairment (Ganong, 2005). Constipation during pregnancy is initially managed by attention to dietary fibre, fluids, exercise and medication regimens (Prather, 2004; Derbyshire et al., 2006; Cullen and O'Donoghue, 2007; Derbyshire, 2007).

■ Women should be asked if they consider themselves to be constipated, and appropriate lifestyle advice should be offered. Women should be followed up to ascertain the efficacy of the advice and any need for further treatment.

Occasionally, constipation may be a symptom of a serious illness and further investigation will be needed (Box 12.5).

Box 12.5 Constipation may be a symptom of serious pathology

- Dehydration, debility or fever
- Hypokalaemia
- Hypocalcaemia
- Hypothyroidism – *more likely in the postnatal period*
- Gastrointestinal disease – diverticulitis or neoplasm
- Gastrointestinal obstruction or postoperative ileus
- Lesions causing pain on defaecation – perineal damage during parturition, haemorrhoids
- Scleroderma
- Muscle disease/wasting – malnutrition, hyperemesis gravidarum
- Central nervous system disease – multiple sclerosis, depression
- Eating disorders – anorexia
- Autonomic nervous system disease – diabetes
- Liver/gall bladder disease, for example intrahepatic cholestasis of pregnancy
- Laxative abuse and eating disorders
- Substance misuse

Practice point

■ Women with constipation may have other problems requiring attention, such as haemorrhoids, eating disorders or substance misuse, which they are reluctant to disclose.

IV

Dietary interventions, such as increasing fibre and water intake, and other lifestyle changes, such as increasing exercise and heeding sensations of fullness in the rectum immediately, are not always effective, and pharmacological agents may be needed in the short term (1–2 weeks maximum). The aim of treatment is to maintain dietary and other lifestyle adjustments, which will help to prevent constipation in the long term, and alleviate symptoms. When improvement is not achieved with dietary changes or bulk laxatives, short-term use of osmotic or stimulant laxatives can be helpful (Tytgat et al., 2003; Prather, 2004; Mahadevan and Kane, 2006).

Practice point

■ If laxatives are needed, these should be prescribed by healthcare professionals, so that women do not use inappropriate treatments, such as castor oil, which has been associated with premature labour and uterine rupture, or senna, which is excreted in breast milk and may cause diarrhoea in the newborn (Mahadevan, 2007; Vinod et al., 2007).

Laxatives

A laxative is an agent that facilitates evacuation of the bowel (Malseed et al., 1995). Laxatives in pregnancy and the puerperium are recommended for use in particular situations, such as:

■ the presence of constipation where dietary and other lifestyle changes have been unsuccessful
■ client distress due to symptoms of constipation
■ when straining may be harmful, following perineal suturing or trauma, Caesarean section, abdominal surgery, or if the woman has haemorrhoids or cardiac disease
■ with opioids, if use is to continue longer than 4–5 days
■ with oral or intravenous opioids after delivery
■ during immobility from any cause.

Administration of laxatives

Laxatives may be administered orally, as enemas or suppositories. Although less effective than enemas, suppositories are often more acceptable to women and more effective in the puerperium. Suppositories may cause local irritation of the rectum. Rectal stimulation caused by enemas could induce labour; obstetricians favour their use less than gastroenterologists (Vinod et al., 2007), and caution is advised. Current evidence does not suggest that routine administration of enemas during labour confers any benefit (Reveiz et al., 2007b). While the occasional use of laxatives is considered safe, long-term use is associated with complications and bowel damage (Shafik, 1993). Also, laxatives are contraindicated if the GI tract is obstructed (BNF, 2009).

Adverse effects common to all laxatives

All laxatives may cause adverse effects by disrupting: the normal functioning of fluid and electrolyte balance; the colonic flora; and gut motility.

Disruption of fluid and electrolyte balance

The colon is important in the homeostasis of body fluids. Each day, it receives 1–2 litres of isotonic fluid from the ileum, of which it reabsorbs 90%. The colon is capable of absorbing considerable quantities of water and drugs rapidly, although it does this erratically. *Tap water given by enema may be absorbed and cause water intoxication* (Ganong, 2005). Several mechanisms control the movement of ions and water across the wall of the colon. If these mechanisms are disrupted by diarrhoea or laxatives, there is a potential for loss of important fluid and electrolytes. Thus all laxatives:

■ reduce absorption of sodium by inhibiting the Na+/K+ pump, and can cause **hyponatraemia**
■ reduce absorption of water, causing dehydration, which is dangerous in volume-depleted or severely anaemic people
■ increase loss of potassium by increasing the rate and volume of fluid flowing through the colon. Hypokalaemia is an important **side effect** of laxative use, overuse and abuse; it is also a cause of constipation. (Hypokalaemia may arise in association with tocolytic therapy; Chapter 7)
■ increase the loss of magnesium (Nichols, 1993).

These electrolyte changes may be particularly dangerous in pregnancy; any fluid and electrolyte imbalance can alter the distribution of body fluids, which may compromise placental blood flow and fetal wellbeing.

Practice points

- A woman who is complaining of tiredness and constipation may be potassium depleted.
- A venous blood sample to measure the concentrations of electrolytes is helpful in assessing any disturbances potentially caused by regular use of laxatives.
- Dehydration may lead to a fall in blood pressure on standing and feelings of dizziness.

Change in colonic flora

The intestinal flora are established early in life. While these commensal bacteria use some nutrients (vitamin C and choline), they are important sources of vitamin K, some B vitamins and folic acid. Excessive use of laxatives will destroy the resident intestinal flora, and recolonization by other **microorganisms** may produce flatulence and discomfort.

If the colonic mucosa is damaged by overuse of laxatives, commensal bacteria enter the circulation in sufficient numbers to overwhelm the hepatic detoxification mechanisms, and cause serious disease, including **Gram-negative** septicaemia. This is a particular danger if the blood supply to the colon is jeopardized, as in hypovolaemic shock.

Practice point

- Laxatives would not be administered to women who are fluid deficient.

Increased intestinal motility

Some laxatives stimulate the contractions of the intestines, which may cause abdominal cramps, diarrhoea, flatulence and discomfort.

Practice points

- If a laxative (even a single dose) has been effective in evacuating the colon, the woman should be advised not to expect further motions for several days (Brunton, 1996).
- Habitual use of stimulant laxatives may destroy the enteric nerve plexuses, producing an atonic or spastic colon.

There are few randomized controlled trials involving pregnant women (Mahadevan, 2007; Cox, 2007), but laxatives are not usually considered harmful (Prather, 2004).

Types of laxatives

Laxatives can be divided into four main groups (Vinod et al., 2007; Rang et al., 2007). First choice therapy during pregnancy is generally bulk-forming laxatives, with the use of others, such as stool softeners, osmotics and stimulants, restricted to short-term use (Tytgat et al., 2003; Mahadever, 2007; NCC, 2007) (Box 12.6).

Box 12.6 Laxative types

1 *Bulk laxatives* (first-line treatment in pregnancy): bran, methylcellulose (Citrucel®), ispaghula husk (Fybogel® and Regulan®), sterculia (Normacol®), psyllium (Metamucil®)
2 *Faecal softeners and lubricants:* Docusate (Colace®), liquid paraffin (category X), mineral oils, including castor oil (category X),[1] arachis oil enema, glycerol/glycerin suppositories

---

IV

3 *Osmotic laxatives – hyperosmotic:*
   - *PEG (polyethylene glycol) based:* PEG-3350 (MiraLAX®), PEG-4000, PEG solution (GoLYTELY®)
   - *Saline:* Oral sodium phosphate (Fleet Phospho-soda®),[2] sodium phosphate enemas (Carbalax®), sodium citrate enema (Micolette Micro-enema®), magnesium sulphate (Epsom salts), magnesium hydroxide, Cream of Magnesia, saline cathartics
   - *Saccharated osmotics:* Lactulose,[3] glycerol/glycerin suppositories, sorbitol
4 *Stimulant laxatives or purgatives:* Senna (Senokot®), figs, prunes, rhubarb, castor oil (category X), bisacodyl (Dulcolax®), danthron, sodium picosylphate, phenolphthalein, cascara

Notes
1 Mineral oils are contraindicated in pregnancy due to the potential for neonatal coagulopathy and haemorrhage resulting from reduced absorption of vitamin K and other fat-soluble vitamins (Vinod et al., 2007). Category X is the US Food and Drug Administration categorization: drugs to be avoided in pregnancy. Thus castor oil is generally avoided during pregnancy as it can stimulate labour (Vinod et al., 2007).
2 Apart from single use, phospho-soda preparations should be avoided, due to the potential for maternal phosphate overload leading to demineralization of fetal bones and reduced bone development (Vinod et al., 2007).
3 There are no available human studies on the use of lactulose (Mahadeven, 2007: 868), and it is regarded as low efficacy and less tolerable than some other laxatives (Tytgat et al., 2003).

The timing of laxative actions is summarized in Table 12.1.

Table 12.1 Usual timing of action of laxatives

Colon evacuation usually takes:		
1–3 days	**6–8 hours**	**1–3 hours**
Bulk-forming agents	Senna	Magnesium sulphate, Cream of Magnesia
Lactulose	Bisacodyl	Saline cathartics
	Cascara	Castor oil
	Phenolphthalein	Glycerol suppositories

Bulk laxatives

Pregnant women are advised to eat 18–28 g of polysaccharides, such as bran, rye bread, brown rice and pasta, vegetables and fruit, beans and lentils, each day, but most eat less than this (Derbyshire, 2007). If this intake is not feasible or women are noncompliant, substitutes such as bulk laxatives may help.

Bulk laxatives are polysaccharides that are not digested. They attract water by osmosis, which increases their volume and therefore stimulates peristalsis. The more effective bulk laxatives (bran) also work by acting as a substrate for colonic bacteria; these multiply and increase faecal bulk. Bulk laxatives increase the frequency of bowel motions and soften stools during pregnancy (Jewell and Young, 2000), and if women have conditions such as haemorrhoids, colostomy or ileostomy, anal fissure, diverticular disease, irritable bowel syndrome or ulcerative colitis.

Bulk laxatives are safer than other laxatives in pregnancy (Tytgat et al., 2003; Cox, 2007; Vinod et al., 2007). However, an increase in dietary fibre intake to 20–60 g/day is preferable to the use of bulk-forming laxatives, due to the possibility of faecal impaction if inadequate water is consumed, plus adverse effects such as abdominal cramping and bloating (Brucker and Faucher, 1997; Tytgat et al., 2003). Dietary fibres, particularly pectin and lignin, have the added advantage of binding to bile acids, thereby reducing plasma cholesterol (Brunton, 1996).

The disadvantages of bulk laxatives include:

- Bulk laxatives take several days to work and may be ineffective, particularly if the intake of water is not increased and symptoms of constipation (cramping and bloating) are exacerbated. Failure of bulk laxatives is usually associated with weak pelvic floor muscles and the inability to coordinate the pelvic floor muscles (Po and Po, 1992). In some instances, women may discontinue laxatives before they have had time to work, for example flatulence, a common complaint that may subside with continued use, can influence compliance.
- Bran and other fibres containing phytates form complexes with zinc, calcium, iron, magnesium and copper from the diet. This reduces the absorption of micronutrients, which is important if the diet is marginal.
- Additionally, bulk laxatives may coalesce into a hard mass, which will then obstruct the gastrointestinal tract.

Practice point

- It is essential to ensure an adequate fluid intake. Bulk-forming laxatives should be taken with at least 2 glasses of water (Malseed et al., 1995).

Other constituents of laxative preparations that are important to some women include:

- Some laxatives (barley malt extract and Regulan powder®) contain available carbohydrate, which will affect control of diabetes.
- Bran contains gluten and must be avoided in women with coeliac disease.
- Some laxatives (including Fybogel® and Normacol®) contain sodium, which predisposes to fluid retention and oedema.
- Many sugar-free products contain aspartame, which is harmful to people with phenylketonuria (Chapter 1, Drug formulation).

Interactions: bulk laxatives

Bulk-forming laxatives may bind to other drugs (anticoagulants, salicylates, digitalis, and tetracyclines) and minerals, thus impairing absorption.

Practice point

- Laxatives should be administered 2 hours apart from food and other drugs.

Faecal softeners and lubricants

Faecal softeners and lubricants are useful if haemorrhoids, anal sphincter damage and anal fissures are present:

- *Docusate:* Acts as a detergent and as a stimulant; it takes several days to work.
- *Glycerol/glycerine suppositories:* Act quickly within 30 minutes by altering fluid absorption and stimulating the rectal mucosa and underlying smooth muscle (Shafik, 1993).
- *Liquid paraffin:* Interferes with the absorption of fat-soluble vitamins (A, D, K) and some drugs. The oil may leak through the anus. 'Paraffinomas' in the lymph ducts and aspiration pneumonia are very rare **adverse effects**. Liquid paraffin is usually combined with phenolphthalein (Delax®) or methylcellulose (as an emulsion). It is not recommended (BNF, 2009).

Osmotic laxatives

There are several types of osmotic laxatives: PEG (polyethylene glycol) based, magnesium, saline, and lactulose. Osmotic laxatives attract water by osmosis, thus increasing the volume of residue in the gut, and stimulating stretch reflexes. Osmotic laxatives differ in their potency, speed and site of action. Most will act in the upper gastrointestinal tract, but lactulose acts only in the colon, which delays and reduces its potency.

Although the movement of water into the GI tract is beneficial for hydrating the bowel, softening stools and increasing faecal bulk, the overuse of osmotic laxatives may deplete the extracellular fluid volume, leading to dehydration. In some PEG-based laxatives, the additional sodium should be considered (Tytgat et al., 2003).

PEG-based laxatives are regarded as safe during pregnancy as they pass virtually unmetabolized through the gut. PEG-4000 (polyethylene, glycol-balanced electrolyte solution) was reported as effective in treating constipation in pregnant women over 15 days (n = 40) (Neri et al., 2004). Absorption of the compounds is negligible, and no calories are ingested. There are no effects on colonic **microflora**.

Practice point

■ Osmotic laxatives should be taken with a full glass of water and may be added to liquid or food. Once-daily administration is appropriate. Women should be warned that the taste may be unpleasant.

Magnesium salts

A variety of magnesium salts are on sale over the counter, for example magnesium sulphate (Epsom Salts, Andrews Liver Salts®), magnesium hydroxide mixture BP (Cream of Magnesia), and magnesium citrate (Citramag®). They are suitable only for occasional or short-term use (Tytgat et al., 2003; Mahadevan and Kane, 2006). Liquid preparations are more potent than tablets. Chilling and flavouring improves the taste.

Magnesium salts are incompletely absorbed. Their osmotic action distends and stretches the stomach, causing discomfort, abdominal cramps, even triggering the gastrocolic reflex. Flatulence and abdominal cramps may limit use. Passage of a hypertonic solution into the duodenum may trigger vomiting, particularly if taken on an empty stomach. Magnesium salts can act rapidly, within 1–3 hours if taken when the stomach is empty, although lower doses may take 6–8 hours to work. Some magnesium is absorbed from laxatives, which is dangerous in renal and liver failure (Chapter 9).

Phosphate compounds (as enemas)

Phosphate compounds (as enemas) can reduce the plasma calcium concentration (reducing bone mineralization in the fetus), and may irritate the woman's colonic mucosa.

Sodium salts

Sodium salts will worsen fluid retention and heart failure and are not recommended (BNF, 2009). Saline purgatives can cause diarrhoea in neonates, so should be used with caution, particularly if a woman is breastfeeding (Tytgat et al., 2003).

Lactulose

Lactulose is used postpartum both as a treatment and a prophylactic when perineal trauma or haemorrhoids are present. Lactulose is metabolized by colonic bacteria to galactose and fructose, thence to lactic and acetic acids and formate. These attract water into the gut by osmosis, which increases faecal bulk.

Practice point

- Some women may find lactulose unpleasantly sweet (McCartney, 1995).

Lactulose acts within 2–3 days. Tolerance to action and adverse effects develops, thus uncomfortable adverse effects such as cramps and flatulence may dissipate within a few days.

Practice point

- Lactulose can cause nausea, vomiting or loss of fluid and electrolytes (Brunton, 1996).

Lactulose should be used with caution in some circumstances:

- Diabetes mellitus: the sugars in lactulose may cause hyperglycaemia, so careful monitoring is required.
- Seriously ill or malnourished women may not withstand the loss of extracellular fluid and potassium ions.
- Galactosaemia (a rare hereditary condition): galactose is extremely detrimental in galactosaemia and lactulose should be avoided.

Interactions: osmotic laxatives

Diarrhoea, including that induced by laxatives, may prevent the absorption of other drugs. Lactulose is less effective if given with antibiotics, which destroy the colonic flora (McKenry et al., 2006).

Stimulant and irritant purgatives

Stimulant and irritant purgatives are potent laxatives (for example senna) that are widely available. Their role (if any) in pregnancy and the puerperium should be restricted to use as suppositories postpartum. Stimulant laxatives are more effective than bulk laxatives, but they have more adverse effects (Jewell and Young, 2000; NCC, 2007). Stimulant laxatives increase smooth muscle contractions in the gut by stretch and irritation. There is some controversy regarding the actions of stimulant laxatives: they may increase peristalsis in the intestines through irritation of the nerve plexuses (networks) within the walls of the intestines or change fluid and electrolyte transport in the ileum and colon (Brucker and Faucher, 1997).

Practice points

- Short-term use of products such as senna or bisacodyl is regarded as relatively safe during pregnancy (Tytgat et al., 2003; Mahadevan and Kane, 2006; Vinod et al., 2007).
- However, other stimulant laxatives, such as castor oil, are **contraindicated** in pregnancy, due to the risk of uterine contractions and premature labour (van Tonningen, 2007b).
- Women should be cautioned against long-term use of stimulant laxatives, for example senna (Senokot®) (Tytgat et al., 2003; Vinod et al., 2007; Cox, 2007).

All stimulant laxatives reduce the absorption of fluid and electrolytes from the colon, and can cause diarrhoea, abdominal cramps, malabsorption and loss of fluids.

IV

With long-term use, atonic colon, protein loss and **hypokalaemia** are potential problems. Damage to the gut lining may induce protein-losing enteropathy, steatorrhoea and malabsorption of calcium; therefore the use of stimulant laxatives is restricted to 1 week (McKenry et al., 2006).

Stimulant laxatives act within 6–12 hours and they are often taken at bedtime. There is marked individual variation in response. Phenolphthalein, senna, danthron, cascara, aloe, and rhubarb are passed into breast milk, causing diarrhoea in the infant and should be avoided during breastfeeding (Po and Po, 1992):

■ *Glycerol* (glycerin) suppositories act as osmotic laxatives, faecal softeners and mild localized irritants, thus stimulating the rectum and producing a bowel evacuation within 30 minutes of insertion (Shafik, 1993). They are often the first choice laxatives (Vinod et al., 2007).

Practice point

■ Glycerol/glycerin suppositories should be stored in the refrigerator and not handled. If held at body temperature, they will begin to release their contents, and work less effectively (Spencer, 1993a).

■ *Castor oil:* Contraindicated in pregnancy, this powerful laxative acts in 3–6 hours. It is broken down by pancreatic lipase to form ricinoleic acid, which is an irritant to both gut and uterus. It should, therefore, be avoided in pregnancy, including topical applications (Malseed et al., 1995).
■ *Senna, aloe and cascara:* These contain derivatives of anthracene, which are liberated by colonic bacteria and irritate the colon. The ensuing abdominal pain and discomfort are not well tolerated. Anthracene derivatives pass into the bloodstream and appear in urine, saliva and breast milk, therefore they should be avoided during breastfeeding.
■ *Bisacodyl:* This causes rectal irritation; the use of suppositories may cause a burning sensation. If continued over weeks, proctitis and sloughing of the epithelium may result. Bisacodyl is sometimes given as a single dose in pregnancy and the puerperium.

Interactions: stimulant laxatives

Bisacodyl enteric coating is removed by antacids, milk or H_2 antagonists, which causes excessive gastric motility/cramps. To prevent this, administration should be 2 hours apart and chipped tablets avoided.

Laxative abuse

Dependence on laxatives may arise from a desire to lose weight or concern with bowel movements. After using stimulant laxatives or purgatives, no faeces may be passed for several days, which encourages reuse of laxatives. Fluid and electrolyte imbalance may be severe (above).

Implications for practice: laxatives

■ A single dose of a laxative is considered safe after delivery. If a laxative is needed, glycerol/glycerin suppositories may be given (Silverton, 1993).
■ If a laxative is indicated for medical reasons or perineal trauma, use is limited to 1 week. Bulking agents are preferred, and liquid paraffin and stimulant laxatives must be avoided, due to the possibility of excretion in breast milk (Hibbard, 1988; Mahadevan, 2007). If laxatives are used, the midwife should be alert to potential problems associated with their use.

Potential problem	Management suggestions
Dehydration	Take with water, especially bulk laxatives
Intestinal obstruction	Monitor. Limit use to 1–2 weeks
Electrolyte disturbance	Ask the woman to report cramps, weakness, dizziness
Discolouration of urine	Inform woman
Laxative dependence	Maximum 1–2 week use
Passage to breastfed baby	Avoid stimulant laxatives during lactation
Uterine contractions	Avoid certain stimulant laxatives in pregnancy

Conclusion

Constipation is a common problem in pregnancy and the puerperium, although some studies indicate a similar incidence in pregnant and non-pregnant women. Constipation may be due to a variety of illnesses, or fever, therefore serious pathology should be excluded. In antenatal care and the puerperium, it is necessary to check for pyrexia and urinary tract infection as underlying causes of constipation, and the possibility of hypothyroidism should not be overlooked. Constipation can be caused by: poor diet (including lack of fibre), lack of exercise, stress, dehydration, and some drugs. Advice about the prevention and/or alleviation of constipation should be given to all women at antenatal and postnatal visits. Additionally, keeping a record of bowel movements can raise awareness of the problem and may prevent complications, which may reduce the need to administer laxatives.

Further reading

■ Cuervo, L., Rodreguez, M. and Delgado, M. (2000) Enemas during labor. *Cochrane Database Systematic Review* (issue 2). Update software, Oxford.

■ Jordan, S. (2008) *The Prescription Drug Guide for Nurses.* Open University Press/McGraw-Hill, Maidenhead; Chapter 1.

IV

CHAPTER 13

Antimicrobial Agents

Mike Tait and Sue Jordan

This chapter outlines the actions and adverse effects of antimicrobial agents. It also considers the reasons why some courses of antimicrobials are ineffective.

Chapter contents

An **antimicrobial** agent is any substance that inhibits the growth of, or kills, a **microorganism**. This broad definition includes a range of chemicals that have varying degrees of toxicity to humans. Disinfectants such as chlorine and ethylene oxide are strong antimicrobial agents that are toxic to humans but can be used, for example, to prevent growth of bacteria such as *Legionella* in air-conditioning systems (chlorine) or to sterilize heat-sensitive medical equipment (ethylene oxide). Antiseptics such as chlorhexidine and silver nitrate are less toxic to humans and can be used, for example, to inhibit microbial growth on human skin (chlorhexidine) or to prevent blindness in newborn babies caused by *Neisseria gonorrhoeae* infections (silver nitrate). For use inside the body, however, the antimicrobials used must be selectively toxic against microorganisms with as low a toxicity to humans as possible. These include antibiotics such as penicillin, antifungals such as nystatin and fluconazole, and **antivirals** such as aciclovir. Antimicrobials usually exploit the differences between microorganisms and human cells by acting on cell structures or functions that are not shared with human cells.

Pathogenic and beneficial microorganisms

Microorganisms are usually divided into: bacteria, fungi, algae, protozoa, and viruses. Microorganisms that cause disease are called **pathogens**.

Although there are numerous pathogenic microorganisms, there are also many microorganisms living in association with humans that are either harmless or beneficial. For example, the gut is filled with bacteria that aid digestion, produce vitamins and protect against pathogens. *Escherichia coli*, for example, is a normal gut inhabitant that produces vitamin K. Other vitamins produced by gut bacteria include thiamine (vitamin B_1), riboflavin (vitamin B_2) and vitamin B_{12}.

The mixture of microorganisms in the gut – the **microflora** – is not constant. It changes with diet and ageing. Neonates have sterile guts and acquire their intestinal microflora soon after birth. The types of bacteria present depend on whether they are breastfed or bottle fed, and may be influenced by exposure to antibiotics (Chapter 14). As diet changes from milk to solids, the microflora changes.

Pathogenic microorganisms spread from person to person in several ways, both direct and indirect:

- influenza and tuberculosis are spread mainly *via* contaminated air droplets
- *Staphylococcus aureus* can be spread by direct physical contact or indirectly *via* contaminated bedding or surgical instruments
- sexually transmitted diseases are normally spread by direct sexual contact but can be spread by other means. For example, neonates born to mothers with *Neisseria gonorrhoeae* or *Chlamydia* infections can develop acute conjunctivitis caused by contamination of their eyes with these bacteria during birth.

Case report

A pregnant woman had been in contact with a child with chickenpox. She went to the GP with the typical rash, but was only offered symptom relief for the itching. Two days later, she was taken to hospital, very ill, with varicella pneumonia. She died, despite antiviral therapy in hospital. (DH, 1998: 120)

Should infection occur, it must be recognized and treated promptly. Prompt prescription of aciclovir would probably have saved this woman's life.

The barrier defences and the immune system can usually cope with microbial invaders (see Storey and Jordan, 2008, for a review). For example, transient bacterial infections in blood – **bacteraemias** – caused by small cuts are common, and the body normally deals with these without help. Some microbial invaders, however, can evade the body's defences and grow to harmful numbers, or produce toxins that damage body tissues. In this situation, antimicrobials can help to reduce the number of invading cells and allow the body's defence mechanisms to regain control. If, however, there is no appropriate antimicrobial agent, the body must rely on its own defences.

Antimicrobials in pregnancy

Infection is an important cause of preterm birth (Chapter 14). Although antibiotic prophylaxis has not proved useful, prescription of antibiotics to women with preterm prelabour rupture of membranes can delay delivery and may reduce the incidence of infection (Lamont et al., 2001; Kenyon et al., 2003).

Practice point

■ Infection is not always associated with pyrexia or a raised white cell count. However, C reactive protein can be a useful indicator of infection (Storey and Jordan, 2008).

Pregnancy influences the selection of antibiotic. Penicillins and cephalosporins are generally the first choice in pregnancy, as most other drugs have been associated with at least some increased risks of fetal malformation. However, in small studies, the cephalosporin cefuroxime administered in the first or second trimesters has been linked with hip dysplasia, hypospadias or imperforate anus (Aronson, 2006). For some drugs, such as erythromycin, risks are low, and sometimes any risks to the fetus are outweighed by the seriousness of the infection in the mother. For some drugs, such as vancomycin and linezolid, little information is available and manufacturers therefore advise against use by pregnant and breastfeeding women unless absolutely necessary (Table 13.1). Breastfeeding may allow drugs to be passed to the neonate, although any problems with penicillins and cephalosporins are likely to be minor (Midtvedt, 2008). Topical preparations are generally considered safe.

Table 13.1 Antimicrobial agents in pregnancy: some problems and precautions

Drug	Potential problem	Comments
Cefuroxime	Congenital malformations	Best avoided (Aronson, 2006)
Chloramphenicol	Circulatory collapse of the neonate	Avoid in third trimester, when breastfeeding, and for neonates
Chloroquine and proguanil for malaria prophylaxis	Risks of **teratogenesis** are reduced by folate supplements	This is generally considered the safest regimen for areas where drug resistance is low
Co-amoxiclav	Necrotizing enterocolitis when administered in association with premature rupture of membranes	Other antibiotics, such as erythromycin, are preferred (Kenyon et al., 2003)
Dapsone for leprosy and some immunological conditions	Risk of neural tube defects, **haemolysis** and jaundice, associated with **G6PD deficiency**	5 mg folic acid daily should be administered Avoid in 3rd trimester and when breastfeeding
Erythromycin	Possible liver damage to mother Risk of GI upsets	May be the only realistic option if the mother has a history of penicillin **hypersensitivity**
Fluconazole	Congenital anomalies of bone and heart	Highest risk in first trimester, doses >400 mg/day Manufacturer advises avoid
Fluoroquinolones/ quinolones	Bone malformations Haemolysis and jaundice, associated with G6PD deficiency	Avoid (BNF, 2009) Three cases described in Wogelius et al. (2005)
Gentamicin	Risk of hearing loss and renal damage (mother and neonate)	Avoid if possible In severe illness, there may be no suitable alternative Must be monitored
Griseofulvin	Teratogenesis, including conjoined twins reported	Avoid Potential fathers should avoid this drug prior to conception
Iodine, povidone iodine	Neonatal goitre, hypothyroidism	Avoid, including topical preparations, if pregnant or breastfeeding (BNF, 2009)

Drug	Potential problem	Comments
Metronidazole, tinidazole	Hydrocephalus reported Significant amounts in milk	Avoid high doses of metronidazole in pregnancy and lactation Low doses considered safe in second and third trimesters Avoid tinidazole in first trimester
Nitrofurantoin	Haemolysis and jaundice reported in neonates associated with G6PD deficiency	Avoid in third trimester and lactation
Nystatin	Teratogenesis	Absorption from the skin or GI tract is considered too low to present a problem
Penicillins Cephalosporins	**Hypersensitivity**	Widely used Generally considered safe Manufacturer advises avoiding co-amoxiclav
Rifampicin	Teratogenesis Neonatal bleeding	May be the only realistic option for tuberculosis Monitor fetus Extra vitamin K given to neonates
Sulphonamides	Risk of **methaemoglobinaemia** Haemolysis and jaundice, associated with G6PD deficiency	Avoid in third trimester and when breastfeeding
Tetracyclines	Damage to growing bones and teeth Possible liver damage to mother	Avoid in pregnancy and lactation
Trimethoprim	Risk of teratogenesis	Avoid in first trimester If used, folic acid supplementation at normal dose is advised
Vancomycin	Fall in BP during administration	Monitor and ensure resuscitation fluids are available (Garbis et al., 2007)

Antibacterials and their actions

Since the first antibiotics were all antibacterial in their action, the term 'antibiotic' is often restricted to **antibacterial** agents such as penicillin and gentamicin.

Antibiotics are natural products synthesized by certain species of bacteria or fungi. The best known is penicillin, which is produced by some strains of a mould called *Penicillium*. Most antibiotics are produced by microbial fermentation, although some, the 'semisynthetic antibiotics', are chemically modified versions of fermentation products. Some species of bacteria are becoming resistant to the antibiotics that are currently available. Scientists are searching for new natural antibiotics and for ways of creating new synthetic antibiotics, for example by the genetic engineering of antibiotic-producing microorganisms.

Antibiotics are often considered as either broad or narrow spectrum. **Broad-spectrum antibiotics** are effective against both **Gram-positive** and **Gram-negative** bacteria, whereas **narrow-spectrum antibiotics** are effective against fewer species. Gram-positive and Gram-negative bacteria are two major groupings of bacteria that have different cell structures and therefore different antibiotic sensitivities. For example, penicillin is more effective against Gram-positive bacteria, while gentamicin is more effective against Gram-negative bacteria. Gram-positive bacteria include *Staphylococcus*, *Streptococcus*, *Bacillus* and *Clostridium*; Gram-negative bacteria include *Escherichia*, *Salmonella*, *Neisseria* and *Pseudomonas*.

IV

Although thousands of antibiotics have been discovered, only around 100 are used clinically. These can be classified in a number of ways, based on their chemical structures or their targets in the bacterial cell (Table 13.2).

Table 13.2 Some antibacterials and their modes of action

Target in bacterial cell	Chemical group	Mode of action	Examples	Activity
Cell wall	β-lactams	Inhibit cross-linking of peptidoglycan backbone	Benzylpenicillin	Effective against Gram-positive bacteria only
			Ampicillin	Effective against Gram-negative bacteria
			Meticillin	Resistant to β-**lactamases**
			Oxacillin	Resistant to β-lactamases
			Cephalosporin	Broad spectrum
			Clavulanic acid	Inhibits β-lactamases
			Imipenem	Used for severe hospital-acquired infections
			Aztreonam	Effective against Gram-negative aerobes
	Peptide	Inhibit cell wall synthesis	Bacitracin	Effective against Gram-positive bacteria
	Glycopeptide	Inhibit cell wall synthesis	Vancomycin	Effective against Gram-positive bacteria
Protein synthesis	Aminoglycosides	Bind to the smaller subunit of 70S bacterial ribosomes	Streptomycin	Effective against Gram-negative bacteria, serious adverse effects
			Neomycin	Effective against Gram-negative bacteria
			Gentamicin	Effective against Gram-negative bacteria
			Kanamycin	Effective against Gram-negative bacteria
	Tetracyclines	Bind to the smaller subunit of 70S bacterial ribosomes	Tetracycline	Broad spectrum
			Doxycycline	Broad spectrum
	Macrolides	Bind to the larger subunit of 70S bacterial ribosomes	Erythromycin Clarithromycin	Effective against Gram-positive bacteria
	Nitroaromatics	Bind to the larger subunit of 70S bacterial ribosomes	Chloramphenicol	No longer widely used. Toxic to fast-growing human cells
	Lincosamides	Bind to the larger subunit of 70S bacterial ribosomes	Clindamycin Lincomycin	Effective against Gram-positive and anaerobic bacteria
	Streptogramins	Bind to the larger subunit of 70S bacterial ribosomes	Quinupristin/ dalfopristin	Effective against infections caused by multiresistant bacteria

Target in bacterial cell	Chemical group	Mode of action	Examples	Activity
	Oxazolidinones	Bind to the larger subunit of 70S bacterial ribosomes	Linezolid	Effective against infections caused by multiresistant bacteria
DNA synthesis	Quinolones	Inhibit DNA gyrase	Nalidixic acid Ciprofloxacin	Effective against Gram-negative bacteria
RNA synthesis	Ansamycins	Inhibit RNA polymerase enzyme	Rifamycins Rifampicin/ rifampin	Used against tuberculosis infections
Plasma membrane	Polymyxins	Increase permeability of plasma membrane, allowing essential metabolites to leak out	Polymyxin B	Toxic but effective against Gram-negative bacteria, for example *Pseudomonas aeruginosa*

Cell wall inhibitors

The cell wall of most bacterial cells is formed from a **polymer** called **peptidoglycan**. This polymer is unique to bacteria and protects the cell from lysis (bursting), making it a good target for antibiotics. Cell wall inhibitors include: β-lactam antibiotics; glycopeptides; bacitracin; and cycloserine, isoniazid, and ethambutol, which are reserved for the treatment of tuberculosis.

β-lactam antibiotics

The β-lactam antibiotics include penicillins, carbapenems, monobactams, cephalosporins, and clavulanic acid, all of which have a β-lactam ring in their chemical structures. These antibiotics block a key cross-linking reaction in the formation of peptidoglycan. This weakens the wall, causing the cell to lyse (burst) and die. Since these antibiotics only affect newly formed bacterial cell walls, they are only effective against growing bacteria. Benzylpenicillin (penicillin G) is only active against Gram-positive bacteria, although newer semisynthetic penicillins such as ampicillin have a broader spectrum of activity, which includes some Gram-negative bacteria. Other semisynthetic penicillins, such as flucloxacillin, are resistant to penicillin-degrading enzymes (β-lactamases) produced by some bacteria. Augmentin is a combination of amoxicillin with clavulanic acid.

Carbapenems (imipenem with cilastatin and meropenem) and monobactams (aztreonam) are β-lactam antibiotics effective against Gram-negative organisms and anaerobes. They are important in the management of hospital-acquired infections.

Glycopeptides

The glycopeptides, vancomycin and teicoplanin, also inhibit formation of bacterial cell walls, but at a different site. They are effective against staphylococci that are resistant to other drugs, including many strains of **MRSA** (meticillin-resistant *Staphylococcus aureus*). Administration is only advised if potential benefits outweigh risks, and careful monitoring of blood pressure, plasma concentrations and renal function is undertaken (BNF, 2009).

IV

Protein synthesis inhibitors

Macrolides

The macrolides include erythromycin and structurally related antibiotics such as clarithromycin. They are effective against staphylococci and other Gram-positive bacteria. Erythromycin is commonly prescribed for patients allergic to penicillin or other β-lactam antibiotics. It is also used in eye ointments to prevent neonatal acute conjunctivitis caused by *Neisseria* and *Chlamydia*. Use in pregnancy and breastfeeding is considered safe. However, if the neonate is jaundiced, careful observation is needed (Schaefer, 2007c).

Aminoglycosides

The aminoglycosides include gentamicin and structurally related antibiotics such as neomycin. They are effective against Gram-negative bacteria, some of which are associated with serious infections, such as septicaemia. Their action is fairly specific to bacterial cells. Since semisynthetic penicillins and tetracyclines are also available for treating Gram-negative infections, aminoglycosides are now mainly used when the alternatives are ineffective. Absorption by the infant is high during the neonatal period (Schaefer, 2007c).

Practice point

■ If aminoglycosides have been administered during pregnancy or breastfeeding, infants should be tested for renal function and hearing at the earliest possible opportunity (Garbis et al., 2007).

Tetracyclines

The tetracyclines are broad-spectrum antibiotics, inhibiting almost all Gram-positive and Gram-negative bacteria. They are not prescribed in pregnancy and lactation.

Nitroaromatics

The nitroaromatics include chloramphenicol, which is toxic to fast-growing human cells such as those in bone marrow and is only used when no alternatives are available. Its main use is for eye infections, but it is never prescribed in the third trimester (BNF, 2009).

Lincosamides, streptogramin and oxazolidinones

The lincosamide clindamycin is prescribed for peritonitis and osteomyelitis; it is not known to be harmful in pregnancy (BNF, 2009). The streptogramins include Synercid®, a combination of quinupristin and dalfopristin. Like the oxazolidinones (for example linezolid), these are reserved for complicated, hospital-acquired infections with Gram-positive organisms, and are used only if benefits outweigh risks (BNF, 2009).

DNA (deoxyribonucleic acid) inhibitors

Nitroimidazoles

The nitroimidazoles include metronidazole. This is effective against protozoa, such as *Giardia lamblia*, and bacterial vaginosis-related microorganisms, such as *Clostridium spp.* (including *Clostridium difficile*) and *Bacteroides spp.* (Lamont et al., 2001). Metronidazole destroys the structure of DNA, but only in hypoxic environments. Cohort studies indicate that normal doses are probably safe in the second and third trimesters of pregnancy (Donders, 2000), although earlier work in bacteria and rodents, and three case reports of facial defects in infants, raised concerns (Thapa et al., 1998; Alef, 1999). The UK Medicines and Healthcare products Regulatory Agency (MHRA) website contains 15 'yellow card' reports of adverse pregnancy outcomes for 1963–2008 (MHRA, 2009). Women using high oral doses of metronidazole to treat trichomoniasis have a higher incidence of preterm delivery (NCC, 2007). Manufacturers advise against high-dose regimens during pregnancy and breastfeeding (BNF, 2009; Winthrop Pharmaceuticals, ABPI, 2009). There are no reports of **adverse effects** in breastfed infants, although a significant amount of metronidazole (20%) passes into breast milk (Einarson et al., 2000).

Practice point

■ Breastfeeding mothers are advised to take metronidazole after the last feed of the evening (Schaefer, 2007c).

Fluoroquinolones/quinolones

The fluoroquinolones/quinolones (for example ciprofloxacin, nalidixic acid and ofloxacin) inhibit DNA synthesis by blocking the enzyme responsible for uncoiling DNA prior to replication (DNA gyrase). Because this enzyme is structured differently in humans, human DNA is not affected by fluoroquinolones. Fluoroquinolones are effective against Gram-negative organisms (Rang et al., 2007), but are not the treatment of choice in pregnancy (Garbis et al., 2007). Some staphylococci and *Pseudomonas aeruginosa* have developed resistance. Fluoroquinolones have been associated with joint damage in children and pass into breast milk; therefore, they are not considered compatible with breastfeeding (Schaefer, 2007c).

Growth factor analogues

The sulphonamides were the first antibacterial drugs to be used clinically. They are called growth factor analogues because their structure mimics a growth factor required by bacteria.

When bacteria are exposed to a growth factor analogue such as sulphanilamide or trimethoprim, they cannot synthesize folic acid, which is a precursor of DNA. The sulphonamides, including co-trimoxazole (Septrin®), have a broad spectrum of activity. They are selectively toxic to bacterial cells; human cells do not synthesize their own folic acid and use dietary folic acid instead.

Antifungals and their actions

Fungal diseases are often difficult to control because of the lack of suitable drugs. Because of the similarities in cell structure, agents that inhibit fungal cells are likely to affect human cells. Some **antifungals** and their modes of action are shown in Table 13.3.

Fungal pathogens are often opportunistic, growing normally on the surface of the body and affecting the host only when the immune system has been suppressed. HIV/AIDS, transplantation, long-term treatment with broad-spectrum antibacterials or corticosteroids and possibly pregnancy all increase the likelihood of fungal diseases. The infection can be systemic, affecting the whole body, or superficial, as in ringworm and athlete's foot. *Candida albicans*, for example, is a normal constituent of the body microflora that becomes an **opportunistic pathogen** under adverse conditions, causing oral and vaginal thrush (candidiasis) and also systemic infections. *Candida* infections often worsen in pregnancy due to changes in the pH of vaginal secretions. Topical, not oral, treatment is recommended (NCC, 2007).

IV

Table 13.3 Some antifungals and their modes of action

Target in fungal cell	Chemical group	Mode of action	Examples	Activity
Plasma membrane	Polyenes	Bind to ergosterols, increasing membrane permeability and allowing essential metabolites to leak out	Amphotericin B	Broad spectrum; widely used against systemic infections; harmful adverse effects
			Nystatin	Used topically against *Candida* infections; less specific than amphotericin
	Azoles	Inhibit ergosterol synthesis by binding to cytochrome P_{450}	Fluconazole	Broad spectrum; used against systemic infections and cryptococcal meningitis
			Itraconazole Ketoconazole Clotrimazole	Used to treat systemic and skin infections
	Allylamines	Block ergosterol synthesis by inhibiting the enzyme, squalene epoxidase	Terbinafine	Used to treat ringworm
	Thiocarbamates	Block ergosterol synthesis by inhibiting the enzyme squalene epoxidase	Tolnaftate	Used to treat skin infections, for example *Tinea*
Cell division	Aromatic	Inhibits mitosis by binding to growing microtubules	Griseofulvin	Used to treat skin infections
Nucleic acid synthesis	(Fluorinated pyrimidine)	Converted inside cell to 5-fluorouracil, which inhibits DNA and RNA synthesis	5-fluorocytosine	Used to treat *Candida* and *Cryptococcus* infections
Protein synthesis	Glutarimides	Bind to the larger subunit of 80S eukaryotic ribosomes	Cycloheximide	

Amphotericin and nystatin

The polyenes, including amphotericin B and nystatin, bind to ergosterol, which is the principal sterol in fungal plasma membranes. Ergosterol is not found in human cells, therefore these drugs are selectively toxic to fungal cells. Amphotericin B has been used widely against systemic infections, but it has serious adverse effects, including renal damage. Newer formulations, combining amphotericin with cholesterol or other lipids, are less toxic. Nystatin is less selective and more toxic than amphotericin, therefore it is only used topically, mainly for vaginal and oral thrush.

Fluconazole and ketoconazole

The azole antifungals, such as fluconazole, itraconazole, and ketoconazole, are less toxic than amphotericin. They are very important in the management of patients with HIV/AIDS infection. They act by inhibiting the synthesis of ergosterol. The loss of ergosterol destabilizes the fungal plasma membrane and the cell stops growing. Azoles are also used to treat fungal septicaemia in neonates and oral thrush in immunocompromised children. Triazoles, such as fluconazole and itraconazole, are more selective than imidazoles such as ketoconazole and clotrimazole. Ketoconazole can cause liver damage, possibly because it also inhibits sterol synthesis in liver cells. Resistance often develops after long-term treatment with fluconazole. For example, it is estimated that 30% of HIV/AIDS patients in the UK have fluconazole-resistant *C. albicans*. These antifungals interact with many other drugs, including nifedipine and ergometrine.

Terbinafine

Terbinafine (an allylamine) and tolnaftate (a thiocarbamate) damage the plasma membranes of fungal cells. Tolnaftate is used in ointments for dermatophytic fungal infections such as athlete's foot and ringworm.

Griseofulvin

Griseofulvin inhibits cell division. It is used against skin infections, but is given orally and migrates through the bloodstream to the skin. Because of its adverse effects, it is not used for dermatophytic infections that can be treated with topical antifungals. It is a known **teratogen**.

Antivirals and their actions

Viruses are responsible for a range of human diseases, from the common cold to HIV/AIDS. Unlike bacteria and fungi, viruses are not cellular: they are infectious particles that enter a host cell, use it to synthesize copies of themselves, and then release these copies to infect more host cells. To date, **vaccines** have been the most successful way of preventing viral diseases. However, vaccines are ineffective after infection, and are not available for all viral diseases. There are fewer effective antiviral agents than there are antibiotics because it is difficult to inhibit the virus without affecting the human host. Also, viruses replicate rapidly and can reach such high numbers by the time symptoms appear that antiviral drugs may have little effect. Some antivirals that are currently in use or are being tested for use are shown in Table 13.4.

Table 13.4 Some antivirals and their modes of action

Target in virus	Mode of action	Examples	Activity
Penetration of the host cell	May prevent the virus from penetrating host cells	Amantadine, rimantadine	Used against influenza A virus
Nucleic acid synthesis	Inhibition of viral DNA polymerase	Aciclovir (Zovirax®), cidofovir, famciclovir, foscarnet (Foscavir®), ganciclovir, valaciclovir, valganciclovir, vidarabine	Used against herpesviruses including *Herpes simplex*, varicella zoster and cytomegalovirus
	Inhibition of the reverse transcriptase enzyme	Zidovudine (AZT), lamivudine, nevirapine	Inhibit some retroviruses including HIV
	Inhibition of RNA metabolism	Ribavirin	Used against respiratory syncytial and hepatitis C viruses
Assembly and maturation of virus particles	Inhibition of HIV protease enzymes	Saquinavir, ritonavir, indinavir, nelfinavir	Used against HIV
Release of viral particles	Inhibition of neuraminidase enzymes	Zanamivir (Relenza®), oseltamivir (Tamiflu®)	Used against influenza A and B viruses

IV

Agents effective against herpesvirus infections

Aciclovir, famciclovir and valaciclovir are related antivirals that are used to reduce the severity of herpesvirus infections, although they do not cure the disease. Aciclovir is effective against *Herpes simplex* and *Herpes zoster*, varicella (chickenpox) and Epstein-Barr viruses (glandular fever). Aciclovir is activated only within virus-infected cells, where it inhibits the formation of DNA by blocking the enzyme DNA polymerase. This reduces the replication of the virus, but cannot prevent its later reactivation. Topical, oral and intravenous preparations are available. Aciclovir cream (Zovirax®) is suitable for cold sores and labial and genital *Herpes simplex*, but vaginal infections require oral preparations. Aciclovir passes into breast milk. The manufacturers advise caution in pregnancy and breastfeeding, but the amounts absorbed through the skin are likely to be small. Oral administration carries the risk of adverse effects, such as rashes, gastrointestinal disturbance, headache, dizziness and potential upsets to liver, kidney or bone marrow. Another herpesvirus, cytomegalovirus, is associated with immunocompromised patients. Recommended treatments for this include ganciclovir, cidofovir, and foscarnet. These are **contraindicated** during pregnancy and breastfeeding due to their toxicity.

Antiretrovirals

Antiretrovirals are used to treat HIV infections. One of the first to be introduced was zidovudine (AZT). This acts by inhibiting the reverse transcriptase enzyme that is essential for replication of the virus. Other reverse transcriptase inhibitors include abacavir, lamivudine and tenofovir. Another class of antiretrovirals are protease inhibitors such as saquinavir and ritonavir. These act by inhibiting the production of a protease enzyme that is essential for the proper assembly and maturation of new virus particles. Several other antiretrovirals have now been introduced.

Zidovudine slows the progression or decreases the severity of HIV/AIDS, but does not cure it. Intensive combination treatment of mothers and infants is used to reduce infection in babies born to HIV-positive mothers. Zidovudine is more effective against HIV when used in combination with protease inhibitors. Protease inhibitors, however, have many adverse effects and manufacturers advise its use only if potential benefits outweigh risks in pregnant women. Maternal deaths have been attributed to complications of antiretroviral therapy, lactic acidosis and liver failure (CEMACH, 2005).

Transgenerational HIV transmission is not prevented by antiretroviral prophylaxis during lactation (Gray and Saloojee, 2008). Breastfeeding is not advised for HIV-positive women in the UK (BNF, 2009).

Amantadine, oseltamivir, rimantidine and zanamivir

These antivirals are used to treat influenza and are generally well tolerated. They are not recommended during pregnancy due to fetal malformations in animals.

Ribavirin

Ribavirin is used to treat respiratory syncytial virus and hepatitis C infections, but is contraindicated during pregnancy because it is teratogenic in animals.

Antiprotozoals and their actions

Protozoa are unicellular microorganisms. Many species are human parasites, infecting the blood, intestines, urogenital tract and other organs. Examples of medically important protozoa include: *Entamoeba histolytica*, *Giardia lamblia*, *Toxoplasma gondii*, and *Plasmodium spp.*, which cause amoebiasis, giardiasis, toxoplasmosis, and malaria respectively.

Quinine, chloroquine and other antimalarials

Selection of medication for malaria depends on the species of *Plasmodium* involved and whether the drug is being used for prophylaxis or treatment. Some antimalarials may cause birth defects, but there are also risks associated with untreated malaria, including premature birth, miscarriage and stillbirth. In general, pregnant women are advised not to travel to areas where malaria is endemic if possible.

Falciparum malaria is caused by *P. falciparum*. Because this species is now resistant to chloroquine in most parts of the world, the recommended treatment is quinine, Malarone® (proguanil plus atovaquone) or Riamet® (artemether plus lumefantrine). Quinine is often the drug of choice for pregnant women (Lalloo et al., 2007).

Non-falciparum malarias are caused by *P. vivax*, *P. ovale* and *P. malariae*. Chloroquine is the drug of choice, although resistant strains of *P. vivax* have been reported. Primaquine is often used after chloroquine treatment of *P. vivax* and *P. ovale* infections to eradicate parasites remaining in the liver and thus prevent relapses. In pregnant women, however, this follow-up treatment is postponed until after delivery.

Several drugs are used for malaria prophylaxis. These include chloroquine in areas where the endemic species of *Plasmodium* is susceptible. In other areas, a combination of chloroquine with proguanil can be used, although folic acid supplements are required with proguanil during pregnancy. Doxycycline is also used in areas of chloroquine resistance but, like all tetracyclines, is contraindicated during pregnancy due to effects on skeletal development in animals and maternal hepatotoxicity with large parenteral doses (BNF, 2009).

Pyrimethamine

Pyrimethamine is used in combination with sulfadoxine to treat malaria or toxoplasmosis. Generally, *Toxoplasma gondii* infections are self-limiting and do not require treatment. However, if first contracted during pregnancy, the parasite may pass to the fetus, who may subsequently suffer eye or brain damage. In this case, the infection is treated using pyrimethamine in combination with sulfadiazine. Since the latter is a folate antagonist, folic acid supplements are also required. Treatment is also necessary if the patient is immunocompromised or if the eyes are infected.

Antihelminthics and their actions

Helminths are parasitic worms with complex body structures. They include roundworms (nematodes), tapeworms and flukes. The most common helminth infections are caused by the nematodes *Ascaris lumbricoides, Necator americanus, Ancylostoma duodenale*, and *Trichuris trichura* (Haider and Bhutta, 2005). Intestinal helminth infections are associated with haemorrhage, reduced iron absorption, and iron-deficiency anaemia. Treatment during pregnancy reduces the incidence of anaemia-related complications such as premature birth and low birth weight. The four drugs commonly used against helminth infections (albendazole, mebendazole, levamisole, and pyrantel) are thought to have minimal adverse effects. However, data about their use in pregnancy are limited and there have been some reports of more severe adverse reactions. For example, albendazole and mebendazole are reported to be potentially teratogenic in rats and rabbits at high doses (Urbani and Albonico, 2003).

Threadworms

Infection with threadworms (a type of roundworm) during pregnancy is surprisingly common, possibly because pregnant women are often in close contact with young children. The life cycle of the parasite can last up to 6 weeks. Spread of threadworm infection involves anal to oral transmission of the eggs. Thus, with strict adherence to good hygiene, the life cycle of the parasite can be broken, and this represents the safest method of management, particularly in the first trimester of pregnancy.

Practice points

- Women should be advised to wash their hands and scrub their nails thoroughly before each meal and after using the lavatory.
- Infection can be spread *via* clothing. Bed linen should be washed daily.
- A morning shower will remove any eggs laid overnight.

In some women, however, symptoms are intolerable and drug therapy may be necessary. In these circumstances, therapy should be delayed if possible until the end of the first trimester. Piperazine (Pripsen®) has been used over many years without any evidence of hazard. In pregnancy, piperazine must be administered under medical supervision, and manufacturers advise against use in the first trimester (BNF, 2009).

Practice points

- Piperazine may stimulate (sometimes violent) contractions of the gastrointestinal tract, causing vomiting and diarrhoea.
- It is absorbed from the gut and passes into the central nervous system. If the therapeutic dose is exceeded, piperazine can cause incoordination, memory defects and convulsions.
- Hypersensitivity responses have occurred.
- Piperazine is contraindicated in people with epilepsy, renal or liver impairment (BNF, 2009).

Insecticides and their actions

Scabies and lice

Aqueous malathion preparations are the preferred products for managing scabies and head lice during pregnancy. Malathion (an organophosphate) has been available in the UK for longer than other insecticides, for example pyrethroids. Manufacturers have no reports of problems associated with pregnancy and breastfeeding (SSL International, ABPI, 2009). Aqueous preparations, such as Derbac M® and Quellada M®, are preferred to alcoholic preparations, as this avoids exposure to noxious fumes and reduces systemic absorption. Each product should be used strictly in accordance with the instructions provided by the manufacturer.

Practice points

- Malathion should not be applied to broken, infected or hot skin.
- Co-administration with oils or creams will increase absorption and should be avoided.
- Gloves should be worn by pregnant women applying these preparations to others.
- Malathion can cause contact dermatitis (Table 14.1).
- Ingestion or absorption of malathion can cause central nervous system disturbance and convulsions.
- Applications should be no more frequent than once a week or for more than 3 weeks (BNF, 2009).
- Malathion should be left to dry; hairdryers should not be used.

The itching of scabies may persist for some time after eradication and calamine lotion and a sedative antihistamine, for example chlorpheniramine or promethazine (Chapter 5), may be helpful.

How the body handles antimicrobials

Absorption

After oral administration, the plasma concentration peaks 1–4 hours later, depending on the drug. When a more rapid response is required, intramuscular or intravenous injections are administered. Some antibiotics are not absorbed from the gut and are therefore given by injection, for example gentamicin, or applied directly to the infected area, for example neomycin.

Practice point

■ Absorption of antimicrobials is influenced by the motility of the gastrointestinal tract or the presence of food or antacids in the stomach (Baxter, 2006). If these interactions are not considered, the infection may not be eradicated (Table 13.5).

Case report

Infection of the urogenital tract and associated release of inflammatory mediators increases the risk of miscarriage (Chapter 14). If factors affecting drug absorption are not considered, the infection may not be eradicated (Table 13.5).

A young primagravida developed a urinary tract infection, for which her GP prescribed erythromycin 500 mg every 6 hours. However, the patient took the tablets at 8.00 a.m. with breakfast, at 1.00 p.m. with lunch, at 6.00 p.m. with dinner and at 10.00 p.m. with supper. Although her symptoms subsided, some signs of infection remained. Three days later, she was admitted to hospital in premature labour and miscarried.

Had the woman assiduously taken her antibiotics 2 hours away from food, and without a 10-hour dosage interval, it is quite possible that the treatment would have been effective and she would not have miscarried. Therapeutic failure, due to poor compliance/adherence, may occur more often than is commonly realized. Effective patient teaching might have influenced the outcome in this case.

IV

Practice points

■ 'Four times a day' means every 6 hours, not any 4 convenient times. If this is not observed, the concentration of drug in the tissues may fluctuate excessively throughout the 24 hours, causing therapeutic failure (Figure 1.1).

■ Dosage schedules that require administration every 6 hours, away from mealtimes (ampicillin and erythromycin, some formulations), must be carefully planned, as they require patients to adjust their normal routines and interrupt sleep. This is not always practicable in the community and sometimes it may be prudent to seek an alternative prescription (Bootman and Milne, 1996).

Table 13.5 Factors affecting the absorption of antimicrobials

Antibiotic	Problem	Precaution
Tetracyclines	Absorption impaired by iron, zinc, calcium or antacids in the stomach	Take either 1 hour before or 2 hours after ingesting tablets containing these minerals or dairy products
Doxycycline Minocycline	Can cause oesophageal or gastric irritation	Take with food and a full glass of water
Ampicillin Erythromycin Rifampicin	Absorption reduced by food in the stomach	Take 1 hour before or 2 hours after meals
Amoxycillin	Absorption reduced by high fibre diets or laxatives, for example bran or methylcellulose	Dose adjustments may be required
Isoniazid	Histamine-rich foods cause histamine release and unpleasant flushing	Advise client to avoid fish and mature cheese if this reaction is suspected
Most antibiotics	Absorption impaired by antacids, particularly those containing magnesium and aluminium	Take 1 hour before or 2 hours after antacids
Ketoconazole	Only absorbed if the stomach contents are acid	Ketoconazole *must* be taken with food and separated by 2 hours from any antacid medications
Indinavir, didanosine	Gastric acid destroys the drug	Separate from food
Ziduvidane, saquniavir	Food is needed for absorption	Give with food. Sandwiches are suitable outside mealtimes

Severe infections require intravenous administration. Veins should be observed for signs of phlebitis, particularly with penicillins and vancomycin (Chapter 2). Some antimicrobials have 90–100% oral **bioavailability**, which facilitates switching from intravenous to oral administration, for example moxifloxacin, metronidazole, rifampin, doxycycline, and linezolid.

Distribution

Antibiotics are distributed to most tissues. To be effective, the agent must reach the tissues at 2–10 times the minimum inhibitory concentration (MIC). However, lower concentrations may assist white cells in clearing infection. Tissue concentration is affected by:

- Plasma concentration.
- Body compartments. For example, the **blood/brain barrier** or the fibrin wall of an exudate may impede drug penetration.
- Protein concentration too high, for example in exudates or pus. The drug may bind to the protein and not reach the microorganisms.
- Low **pH** inhibits transfer into tissues, for example in abscesses, pleural space, cerebrospinal fluid, urine.
- Low pO_2 inhibits transfer into tissues, for example in abscesses or necrotic tissue (Chambers, 2006). Where the blood supply is poor, antibiotic therapy may not penetrate to the infected tissue. This may occur where an abscess has formed, for example following an episiotomy. It may then be necessary to drain the abscess and apply topical preparations.

Practice point

■ If the meninges are inflamed, antibiotics penetrate into the cerebrospinal fluid. However, as inflammation subsides as the infection resolves, the integrity of the blood/brain barrier will return and the efficacy of the antibiotics will be reduced, risking therapeutic failure. Therefore, continued vigilance for signs of meningitis is important.

Elimination

Route of elimination varies between drugs. Erythromycin, for example, is excreted into bile, and penicillins and gentamicin are excreted into urine.

A venous blood sample to estimate renal function is necessary before administration of certain antibiotics eliminated by the kidney, including tetracyclines (not doxycycline), gentamicin, co-trimoxazole, polymyxins, and vancomycin. Some of these can damage the kidneys, leading to further accumulation and a 'vicious circle'. For example, there is a danger of accumulation of gentamicin if any degree of renal impairment is present or if dehydration occurs. This may lead to dose-related adverse effects, such as hearing loss and kidney damage.

Practice points

■ Taking a full glass of water with oral medications is very important with certain drugs, which can damage the renal tubules if they are allowed to crystallize. Patients taking sulphonamides, including co-trimoxazole (Septrin®), should drink at least 2 litres of fluid each day.
■ Renal elimination of antibiotics is increased in pregnancy, fever, burns or cystic fibrosis, and higher doses may be needed (Quintiliani and Quintiliani, 2008).

Dosage schedules

Dose depends on: nature, cause, site and severity of infection; weight; age; immune and renal function of the patient. Some doses (for example gentamicin and vancomycin) are determined by therapeutic monitoring of venous blood samples, extracted 1 hour before and 1 hour after dosing. The recommended schedule varies with each drug and is different even for very similar drugs.

The ability of antibiotics to kill bacteria is determined by either the drug concentration or the time spent above the minimum inhibitory concentration (MIC):

1 *Concentration-dependent antibiotics* include the aminoglycosides (for example gentamicin), fluoroquinolones (for example ciprofloxacin, moxifloxacin), and metronidazole. For these drugs, duration of exposure is minimally important, and continuous administration is avoided. For example, once-daily aminoglycosides are at least as effective as multiple doses, except during pregnancy or for patients with burns, dialysis, ascites, and enterococcal endocarditis. While the resulting high concentrations do not increase aminoglycoside toxicity, once-daily administration of fluoroquinolones can cause seizures, and excessive doses of most antibiotics can cause *C. difficile and C. albicans* infections.

Practice point

■ The administration schedule for seriously ill women requiring gentamicin will need to take account of the increased drug elimination that occurs in pregnancy.

IV

2 *Time-dependent antibiotics*, for example penicillins (not in meningitis), carbapenems, mono-bactams, erythromycin, linezolid, and vancomycin, need to remain above the MIC for 50% of the dose interval. Doubling the dose to increase the time intervals is inefficient, but continuous administration may be considered (Quintiliani and Quintiliani, 2008).

Therapeutic range

The therapeutic range of a drug is the difference between the minimum effective plasma concentration and the toxic concentration. For some drugs, such as the penicillins, this range is wide and dose-related adverse effects are unusual. For other drugs, such as gentamicin and vancomycin, the therapeutic range is narrow. To ensure effectiveness and minimize adverse effects of such antibiotics, venous blood samples are taken at regular intervals to measure the concentration of drug in plasma.

Adverse effects of antimicrobials

Some antimicrobials that are effective in the laboratory cannot be used clinically, because they are too toxic or are rapidly inactivated. Even when an antimicrobial is approved for clinical use, care is taken to balance likely benefits with possible adverse reactions. Normally, antimicrobials with the least severe adverse effects are used, but if the microorganisms are resistant, potentially more harmful alternatives are prescribed.

The adverse effects of antimicrobials can be grouped as follows:

- allergic and hypersensitivity responses
- direct toxicity of the drugs
- superinfection
- resistance
- therapeutic failure.

The potential toxicity of some antimicrobials are summarized in Table 13.6 and Implications for practice are tabulated below.

Allergy and hypersensitivity

Allergy and hypersensitivity may be delayed or immediate, occurring with the first dose or on subsequent exposures. Hypersensitivity reactions range from a skin rash and itching to fatal **anaphylaxis**. Antibiotics are associated with all four types of hypersensitivity responses (Table 14.1). Some 1–10% of patients are allergic to penicillin. Reactions are more likely with intravenous administration and if the drug is given rapidly, therefore intravenous gentamicin should be administered over a minimum of 3 minutes (BNF, 2009). Cross-allergies occur between similar drugs. For example, 5–15% of people allergic to penicillins are also allergic to cephalosporins (Chapter 1).

Practice point

- After antimicrobial therapy begins, patients need 'watchful vigilance' for signs of 'drug fever', which is a form of hypersensitivity response that should not be confused with recurrent infection (Shuster, 1995; Chambers and Sande, 1996).

Antibiotics administered to pregnant women (Russell and Murch, 2006) or infants may change the neonatal gut microflora, which might affect the regulation of the immune system, allowing allergies to develop (Chapter 14).

Direct toxicity of the drug

Several antibiotics can cause organ damage (Table 13.6). Some of the most serious problems with antimicrobials are the effects on the fetus. Trimethoprim in the first trimester, for example, is potentially teratogenic as it interferes with folic acid metabolism. Most antibiotics can cause gastrointestinal upsets, either due to the irritant actions of the drugs or interference with the normal flora of the gastrointestinal tract.

Table 13.6 Potential toxicity of some antimicrobials and appropriate precautions

Site of toxicity	Antibiotic	Precaution
Brain	Penicillins Cephalosporins Quinolones Aminoglycosides	Avoid intrathecal administration Exercise caution in administering to patients with a history of convulsions and renal failure Avoid co-administration of quinolones and NSAIDs
Peripheral nerves	Aminoglycosides Linezolid (after 10 days' usage)	Monitor pain, numbness, tingling Enquire about sensation in toes Alternative drugs may be needed
Inner ear (hearing and balance)	Gentamicin Vancomycin Erythromycin (rarely)	Avoid use with other drugs affecting the ear, for example furosemide/frusemide Ensure the patient can hear and balance is not affected Mobilize carefully Ask about tinnitus and report to prescriber Administer intravenous therapy slowly
Growing bones and teeth	Tetracyclines	Avoid in pregnant women and children
Liver	Rifampicin Isoniazid Erythromycin (rarely) Tetracyclines Cephalosporins Co-amoxiclav	Undertake liver function tests if use prolonged Avoid in people with a history of alcohol misuse or fatty liver in pregnancy The liver is particularly vulnerable in pregnancy
Pancreas	Co-trimoxazole	Be alert for severe vomiting and pain radiating to the back Glucose and amylase estimations may be helpful
Kidney	Gentamicin Co-trimoxazole Vancomycin Cephalosporins (rarely) Penicillins Tetracyclines Quinolones	Undertake blood tests to assess renal function (Box 1.1) or seek alternative drug if poor renal function is suspected, for example in a woman with a history of UTI Ensure adequate hydration, allowing for losses due to diarrhoea and vomiting
Skin (photosensitivity)	Tetracyclines Aciclovir Quinolones	Avoid prolonged exposure to sunlight. Use high factor, high star sunscreen

IV

Site of toxicity	Antibiotic	Precaution
Bone marrow	Chloramphenicol Co-trimoxazole Linezolid Aminoglycosides Cephalosporins (rarely) Aciclovir	Avoid in patients with history/family history of bone marrow problems or taking other drugs potentially toxic to the marrow (for example carbimazole, carbamazepine, antipsychotics)
		Check FBC pre-therapy, routinely and if sore throat or fever develop
		Linezolid: weekly FBC; vitamin B6 may be prescribed
Lung damage	Nitrofurantoin	Report new onset cough or breathlessness
Tendons	Quinolones	Usually avoided in children and those prescribed corticosteroids
		Pain and soreness over Achilles tendon to be reported immediately
Optic nerve damage	Linezolid	Enquire about changes in vision and colour vision
		Arrange prompt review by ophthalmologist
		Arrange for vision to be monitored if treatment >28 days

Superinfection

Superinfection occurs when antibiotics kill off the normal microflora of the skin or the gastrointestinal tract, allowing resistant and more harmful microorganisms to take their place. Fungi such as *C. albicans* are normally harmless constituents of the skin and gut microflora but can develop into pathogenic forms that cause thrush after antibiotic therapy has weakened their bacterial neighbours, leading to diarrhoea or skin infections. Pseudomembranous colitis occurs after superinfection of the gastrointestinal tract with the bacterium *C. difficile*, which can occur with almost any antibiotic. Superinfection is more likely to occur after administration of broad-spectrum agents, prolonged therapy, low doses, or in immunosuppressed patients.

Practice points

- Minimize use of broad-spectrum antibiotics.
- Specifically enquire about any diarrhoea and vomiting, which may lead to fluid and electrolyte imbalance, particularly in neonates.
- If diarrhoea and vomiting occur, monitor fluid and electrolyte balance and be alert for *C. difficile* infections.
- Monitor for infections due to fungi (for example *Candida*), *Pseudomonas* and enterobacteria.
- Ask women to report any oral or vaginal thrush.
- If aminoglycosides are administered, monitor for worsening of tuberculosis and *Herpes* infections.

Long-term antibiotics may cause nutrient deficiency by inhibiting the vitamin-producing bacteria in the gut. For example, the availability of vitamin K is reduced by gentamicin, tetracyclines and possibly other antibiotics. Care is also needed when drugs are prescribed long term for tuberculosis, as isoniazid requires pyridoxine supplementation (BNF, 2009).

Resistance

Some microorganisms are inherently resistant to certain antimicrobials because of their structure or metabolism. Other microorganisms can *acquire* resistance, often after exposure to the antibiotic (Jordan and Tait, 1999).

Some bacteria produce penicillinase enzymes that destroy penicillins and cephalosporins (the β-lactam antibiotics). Infections with penicillinase-producing staphylococci may respond to flucloxacillin, which is less susceptible to attack by the enzymes, or by augmentin, which is a combination of two antibiotics, amoxicillin and clavulanic acid. MRSA produces an inactivating protein that confers resistance to most other antibiotics.

Resistant mutants can arise spontaneously, often after long-term exposure to an antimicrobial. Bacteria can also acquire resistance by transferring genetic material and information between cells or by absorbing fragments of DNA from ruptured cells. By these methods, resistance can be passed rapidly from cell to cell, making an entire population of bacteria resistant to a range of antibiotics.

Practice points

- Crushing tablets or opening capsules allows growth of resistant microorganisms on the skin or respiratory tract of the administrator.
- Gloves should be worn when opening vials.

Bacteria found in the gastrointestinal tract, *S. aureus* and *P. aeruginosa* can all become resistant by the spread of R (resistance) factors. MRSA, a common source of infection in hospitals all over the world, contains R factors that make it resistant to many antibiotics. Vancomycin and teicoplanin are effective against many MRSA infections, but resistant strains have appeared.

Practice points

The likelihood of resistant strains arising can be reduced by:
- Using short courses of treatment or even single doses, where possible (BNF, 2009).
- Ensuring patients comply with and complete courses of treatment.
- Using high doses to reduce the numbers of bacteria before resistant strains can appear.
- Using two unrelated antibiotics in the expectation that doubly resistant mutants are unlikely to arise, particularly where prolonged therapy is necessary, as for tuberculosis or leprosy.
- Reducing overall usage of antibiotics (Dever et al., 1998).
- Complying with infection control measures (Dennesen et al., 1998).
- Obtaining prompt culture and sensitivity reports if resistance is suspected.

IV

Therapeutic failure

Monitoring vital signs is a key component in diagnosis of sepsis and related therapeutic failure. Not all infections are associated with pyrexia. Immediately genital tract sepsis is suspected, high-dose, broad-spectrum intravenous antibiotics should be commenced (CEMACH, 2007).

Reasons for failure of antimicrobial therapy

The reasons for failure of antimicrobial therapy include:

- wrong drug, dose or route
- drug resistance/tolerance
- inadequate dosage or poor compliance

- serious gastrointestinal upsets, for example erythromycin
- drug not reaching the microorganism, for example intracellular organisms, abscess formation
- superinfection
- undetected microorganisms
- administration problems, for example incompatibilities in intravenous infusions or taking antibiotics with food
- dosage schedule – drug concentration falling below the minimum effective concentration or the minimum time exposure
- foreign body, for example catheters, prostheses, such as artificial heart valves
- pus or haematoma or abscess formation.

Practice points

- Administration of antibiotic prophylaxis for Caesarean delivery does not always prevent infection, therefore recording of vital signs should be maintained until the woman is well (CEMACH, 2007).
- Response to antibiotic therapy should be apparent within 24–48 hours. Should this fail to occur, an urgent review of antimicrobial therapy must be sought. This will be easier if a full history of possible allergies is obtained before microbiologists are consulted.

Cautions and contraindications: antimicrobial agents

- *History of allergy:* Patients allergic to cephalosporins are often allergic to penicillins and *vice versa*. Patients allergic to diuretics or celecoxib or oral hypoglycaemics may be allergic to sulphonamides.

Practice point

- With all drugs, it is important to ask patients if they have suffered previous allergies or hypersensitivity responses. People with a history of atopic or hypersensitivity disorders are particularly at risk.

- *Breastfeeding* allows small amounts of antibacterials to pass from mother to infant. Hypersensitivity responses and adverse effects may occur in the infant. Breastfeeding is not advised in some severe infections.
- *Glandular fever* (Epstein-Barr virus infection), cytomegalovirus infection, AIDS/ HIV or chronic lymphatic leukaemia greatly increase the risk of developing a penicillin-induced rash, particularly ampicillin.
- *Impaired renal function* causes some drugs to accumulate, for example penicillins, tetracyclines, vancomycin, ciprofloxacin, teicoplanin, and gentamicin. Injectable penicillins contain sodium, which may contribute to fluid retention.
- *Impaired liver function* causes some drugs to accumulate, for example metronidazole and rifampicin.
- *Myasthenia gravis:* Aminoglycosides and quinolones exacerbate this condition.
- *Porphyria:* Avoid sulphonamides, cephalosporins, erythromycin, flucloxacillin, rifampicin, and trimethoprin.
- *Penicillins* are not given by the intrathecal route, due to the risk of convulsions.

Interactions: antimicrobials

Antibiotics interact with many other drugs including alcohol, nutrients, oral contraceptives and anticoagulants. Where two or more drugs with the same adverse effects are co-prescribed, the risks are increased. For example, if two drugs with the potential to damage the inner ear are used together, such as gentamicin and furosemide/frusemide, the chances of tinnitus, hearing loss and vertigo are high.

- *Alcohol* is a gastric irritant and likely to exacerbate any gastrointestinal upset caused by other drugs. Some people may suffer an 'antabuse reaction' if they take even a small amount of alcohol with certain antibiotics such as metronidazole and cephamandole. This causes the peripheral blood vessels to dilate, leading to flushing, severe headache and a fall in blood pressure. Fainting, falls and even cardiovascular collapse may follow (Baxter, 2006).

- The *efficacy of the oral contraceptive pill* is reduced by some antimicrobials. A few drugs, such as rifampicin, rifabutin, isoniazid and griseofulvin, render all oral contraceptives ineffective; alternative methods of contraception should be used during treatment and for 4–8 weeks after stopping the drug. Broad-spectrum antibiotics, such as ampicillin, penicillin V, tetracycline, neomycin, sulphonamides, nitrofurantoin and chloramphenicol, interact with combined oral contraceptives and increase the risk of 'pill failure'. By eliminating the normal gastrointestinal tract flora, antibiotics hinder the normal **enterohepatic recycling** of oestrogens, increasing their loss in the faeces and reducing their absorption. Women should be advised to use other methods of contraception during therapy and for 7 days after it ends. If these 7 days run beyond the end of the pill packet, a new packet of oral contraceptives should be started immediately without a break (BNF, 2009).

- *Some drugs alter absorption of antimicrobials from the gut, speed up their breakdown, or alter their activity in other ways.* For example, zidovudine (AZT) concentrations are decreased by clarithromycin, and zidovudine toxicity may be increased when fluconazole or aciclovir are co-administered.

- *Surgery:* Aminoglycosides and vancomycin intensify the action of muscle relaxants such as suxamethonium. All muscle relaxants interact with clindomycin, piperacillin, and polymixins. Use should be highlighted on transfer to the anaesthetic team.

- *Macrolides* cause the accumulation of other drugs, for example digoxin, corticosteroids, anticoagulants, ciclosporin, SSRIs, and some statins. Metronidazole interacts similarly with carbamazepine, ciclosporin, lithium, and tacrolimus.

- *Linezolid is an MAOI:* Patients should avoid Marmite®, mature cheese, alcohol (except spirits), 'cold cures', cocaine, and amphetamines. Prescribers avoid pethidine, antidepressants, triptans, levo-dopa and salbutamol.

- *Carbapenems* reduce the concentration of valproate, frequently resulting in seizures.

- *Cardiac dysrhythmias* are more likely if quinolones are co-administered with several drugs, for example antipsychotics, amiodarone, and some antidepressants.

- *Beta-lactams and metronidazole* may enhance or inhibit anticoagulants.

- *Many antibiotics are incompatible* with other drugs when co-administered in intravenous infusions. For example, if gentamicin is combined with heparin, its antibiotic activity will be lost.

IV

Conclusion

With the appearance of vancomycin-resistant strains of *S. aureus*, this bacterium has now joined *P. aeruginosa*, *Mycobacterium tuberculosis* and *Enterococcus faecalis* in having strains that are resistant to all 100-plus antibiotics available. Perhaps too late, the problem of increasing antibiotic resistance has finally been recognized and serious effort is now expended on minimizing non-essential use of antibacterials. However, despite changes in practice and continuing attempts to find and develop new antibiotics, it is likely that more strains of pathogenic bacteria, resistant to all known antibiotics, will appear.

Antibiotics save lives and cure infections, but they can be overprescribed. Antibiotic prescribing has been extended to non-medical prescribers. Current guidelines and quality indicators for antibiotic prescribing focus on bacterial resistance, and offer no consensus, reflecting tensions between the needs of individual patients and public health priorities. Guidelines take no account of other possible adverse effects, including the possibility that antibiotics may affect the long-term development of the immune system (Jordan et al., 2008).

Withholding therapy from severely ill patients may jeopardize the management of potentially serious or life-threatening infections. Failure to recognize and treat sepsis has led to maternal deaths (CEMACH, 2007), and delayed administration of antibiotics in patients with confirmed bacterial meningitis increases the risk of adverse outcomes (Aronin et al., 1998). Consequently, a selective approach to antibiotic therapy is advocated.

Implications for practice: antimicrobials

Potential problem	Management suggestions
Therapeutic failure	Culture and sensitivity, preferably prior to administration of antimicrobial therapy
	Check drug administration and compliance (Table 13.5)
	Check for foreign bodies and abscesses
	Monitor vital signs during therapy, for example temperature at 6.00 p.m., particularly if the patient is immunocompromised
	If clinical improvement does not occur with 24–48 hours of therapy, an alternative agent may be needed
Teratogenicity	Use penicillins and cephalosporins where possible
	Assess and discuss relative risks and benefits (Table 13.1)
	Use topical preparations if possible, but avoid iodine
	Minimize infection risks, for example discontinue contact lens use during pregnancy and the puerperium
Drug toxicity	Check renal function if there is any risk of impairment
	Administer medication with a full glass of water
	Ensure venous samples for therapeutic drug monitoring are taken immediately before administration of gentamicin or vancomycin
	Monitor for signs of organ damage (Table 13.6)
GI upset	Monitor fluid and electrolyte balance. A venous blood sample may be necessary to check for dehydration or potassium depletion
	Consider nutritional and vitamin deficiencies, particularly if pregnancy-induced vomiting has occurred
	Extra caution is needed in women with diabetes or epilepsy
Hypersensitivity responses	Ensure *all* previous hypersensitivity responses are prominently displayed on the front of the notes
	Check for cross-allergies, particularly before administering cephalosporins, penicillins or sulphonamides

Potential problem	Management suggestions
	Ensure protocols and equipment are in place for management of anaphylaxis
	Administer all injections slowly
Resistance	Culture and sensitivity
	Ensure compliance with the full dose
	Maintain strict asepsis, particularly in hospitals
	Scrupulous attention to hand washing

Further reading

■ Aronson, J.K. (ed.) (2006) *Meyler's Side Effects of Drugs: The International Encyclopedia of Adverse Drug Reactions and Interactions*. Elsevier, New York; see individual drugs, listed alphabetically.

■ Jordan, S. and Tait, M. (1999) Antibiotic therapy. *Nursing Standard*, **13**(45): 49–54.

IV

CHAPTER 14

Drugs and the Immune System

Sue Jordan

This chapter considers the immune system and common immunological problems, such as Rhesus incompatibility and allergy.

Chapter contents

The immune system

The immune system is closely regulated to protect the body from infection and other diseases, including cancers (see Storey and Jordan, 2008, for an overview).

The immune system comprises:

- physical and chemical barriers, such as the skin and linings of the respiratory, digestive and genitourinary tracts
- the white cells, which form:
  - the innate, nonspecific immune system, concerned with inflammation
  - the specific, adaptive immune system, concerned with recognition of individual **antigens** (such as **pathogens**, for example rubella virus, foreign cells and Rhesus antigen), and the subsequent production of matching **antibodies**.

Specific or adaptive immunity

Specific immunity is acquired or 'earned' each time new antigens, including **microorganisms**, are encountered. It depends on the recognition of specific antigens (foreign proteins) by cytotoxic T or B **lymphocytes**, and the subsequent formation of clones of matching antibodies, and requires **T helper lymphocytes**: the two main types are Th1 (for T lymphocytes) and Th2 (for B lymphocytes):

■ *Cytotoxic T cells* respond to foreign cells, including tumour, transplant or virus-infected cells; they carry receptors for recognition of intracellular antigens on their cell membranes.

■ *B cells* divide to form plasma cells, which secrete antibodies into the circulation. There are five classes of antibodies: the first antibodies to be formed are IgM, the most abundant are IgG, IgA are associated with secretions, and IgE with type I allergic responses, including **anaphylaxis**. Antibodies are usually formed actively, but they may be transferred passively. For example, antibodies pass to neonates in colostrum or breast milk, or they can be administered in acute illness, for example antirabies serum.

Antibodies, and T cell membrane-bound antigen receptors, bind antigens by a three-dimensional fit or lock and key mechanism. This neutralizes and agglutinates the antigens and forms antibody/antigen complexes, which activate the inflammatory processes. This may, sometimes, cause serious incidental tissue damage, for example in a transfusion reaction, or a **hypersensitivity** response. Hypersensitivity responses may be associated with diseases or **adverse drug reactions** (Chapter 1; Jordan 2008, Ch. 21).

Practice points

■ Specific antibodies can be measured in venous blood samples. For example, previous exposure to chickenpox can be detected to determine the need to offer immunization to healthcare professionals, and anti-D antibodies can be detected in Rhesus negative women (below).

■ Following occupational exposure to body fluids containing blood-borne viruses (HIV and hepatitis), blood tests are taken to screen for antibodies. If the antibodies are not seen, infection is unlikely (DH, 2006).

Antibodies are destroyed by the **macrophages** of the **reticuloendothelial system**. *Monoclonal antibodies* are medicines engineered to bind with and neutralize specific components of the immune system. They may be administered by specialists to treat an expanding range of conditions, including rheumatoid arthritis, multiple sclerosis, Crohn's disease, other autoimmune diseases, and some cancers unresponsive to other therapies (*Drug and Therapeutics Bulletin*, 2007). If monoclonal antibodies are administered to pregnant women, there is a risk of damage to the fetal immune system, and detailed ultrasound examinations are recommended (van Tonningen, 2007a).

Memory and sensitization. The first time B or T cells encounter an antigen, it takes several days to mount an antibody response. This is too little and too late and the person may succumb to the infection. The first exposure causes the stimulated lymphocyte clone to form memory cells. At second or subsequent exposure to the same antigen, the individual is sensitized and memory cells stimulate production of large numbers of specific, matching antibodies within hours. These rapidly bind and neutralize the pathogen, preventing the development of illness (Abbas and Lichtman, 2004). Once produced, 'the blueprint' for each antibody is remembered by memory cells, which may lie dormant for years in the reticuloendothelial system. Consequently, most people suffer each infectious disease only once. Similarly, where allergies develop, for example to penicillin or a food, the production of IgE antibodies, release of histamine and the inflammatory response intensify with repeated exposures.

Practice point

■ Rashes associated with IgE antibodies are likely to progress to anaphylaxis; therefore, if a patient develops a 'drug rash', blood samples or skin tests may be requested to measure these and predict the outcomes of future exposure (Midtvedt, 2008).

IV

Hypersensitivity or allergic responses

All hypersensitivity responses represent overactivity of the immune system, each with its own time frame (Table 14.1). Most drugs or their metabolites can combine with carrier proteins in the circulation to form 'immunogens', substances that produce an immune response. The resulting antigen/antibody complexes or related inflammatory mediators may damage major organs, including skin, blood vessels, kidneys, bone marrow, liver or pancreas. Delayed hypersensitivity responses, mainly contact dermatitis, may arise from repeated handling of medicines, such as antibiotics, opioids, phenothiazines, and topical antihistamines (see Jordan, 2008, Ch. 21, for further details).

Practice point

■ Gloves should be worn when handling these drugs to prevent contact dermatitis.

Table 14.1 Types of hypersensitivity/hypersusceptibility responses and antibiotics

Type	Response	Drugs involved
I	Anaphylaxis and histamine release Itch and urticaria	Intravenous antibiotics, peanuts, any drug (Box 1.2)
II	Antigen/antibody reactions on surface of blood cells plus complement fixation **Haemolysis, agranulocytosis, thrombocytopenia**	Linezolid, vancomycin, penicillins, methyldopa, cranberry juice
III	Antigen/antibody complexes deposit in tissues, complement activation, cell lysis, tissue destruction Fever, rash, joint pains, renal failure **Stevens-Johnson syndrome**	Antibiotics (cefaclor), lamotrigine, other antiepileptics, iodides, gold salts, penicillamine, microorganisms
IV	Cell-mediated, delayed immunity Contact dermatitis	Handling antibiotics, phenothiazines, opioids, antihistamines
	Agranulocytosis, hepatitis, nephritis, thrombocytopenia, **toxic epidermal necrolysis**	Antiepileptics, antibiotics, microorganisms

Practice points

■ Healthcare professionals should carefully clarify all drug and food allergies, and attach warnings to patients' notes, drug charts or menus.
■ Where a rash is reported, its characteristics should be documented, that is, itching or wheals (urticaria or 'nettle rash').
■ Where an 'allergy' is reported, this should be distinguished from vomiting or diarrhoea (Midtvedt, 2008).
■ Rhesus incompatibility becomes increasingly important on second and subsequent pregnancies.

Blood groups

All individuals carry their own unique antigens on the surfaces of their cells. Therefore, the immune system will recognize the cells of another individual as foreign antigens, and synthesize antibodies to mount a destructive response. The fetus is shielded from attack by the maternal immune system by certain (major histocompatability complex) surface antigens on the trophoblast cells surrounding the embryo.

Blood group is determined by surface antigens on red cells. The most important are those of the ABO and Rhesus systems. The four ABO blood groups are determined by the presence of the A and B antigens on the surface of the red cells and antibodies already present in the plasma. If ABO incompatible blood is accidentally transfused, the donor red cells are recognized and attacked by the recipient's antibodies. As the red cells are split open (haemolysed), releasing their haemoglobin, the patient rapidly becomes unwell, with signs and symptoms of an allergic reaction (fever, chills, change in blood pressure, urticaria, nausea, and respiratory distress). It is not always easy to distinguish ABO incompatibility reactions from other types of transfusion reactions, both mild (allergic reactions and non-haemolytic reactions), and serious (severe allergic reaction, transfusion-related acute lung injury, and bacterial infection of blood).

Practice points

■ If a patient receiving a blood transfusion develops fever, chills, altered vital signs, urticaria, flushing, pain, breathing difficulties, or nausea, it is important to:
   ■ Interrupt the transfusion until a cause of the problems can be ascertained
   ■ Inform the doctor
   ■ Check: temperature, pulse, BP, respiration, and oxygen saturation
   ■ Recheck the patient's identity and the clerical details on the unit for transfusion (Craig et al., 2002).

When blood group is determined, other red cell antibodies, such as Lewis, Duffy, Kell or Kidd, are occasionally detected, typically in grand multiparae. These must be considered when blood transfusions are given.

The antibodies of the ABO system form in the first few months of life, as the neonate is exposed to **Gram-negative** bacteria that colonize the gut (Geha and Rosen, 2008). Therefore, a haemolytic reaction will occur the first time incompatible blood is transfused.

Mother and fetus have different ABO blood groups in 15–20% of pregnancies, but any reaction is usually mild, because the antibodies of the ABO system are usually of the IgM class, which are too large to cross the placenta and attack fetal cells. Occasionally, the mother produces IgG antibodies that cross the placenta and destroy red cells, causing ABO haemolytic disease of the newborn, described below; in severe cases, exchange transfusion will be needed (Koelewijn et al., 2009).

Practice point

■ Close observation for jaundice is needed in the first 72 hours of life, particularly where the mother has blood group O and a sibling had neonatal jaundice (Sarici et al., 2002).

Rhesus incompatibility

The Rhesus or D antigen appears on the surface of red cells early in fetal life. Rhesus incompatibility between mother and fetus, if left untreated, may cause haemolytic disease of the newborn. Before prevention was available, 1% of pregnancies were affected to some degree (Kumar and Regan, 2005).

Rhesus (Rh) positive individuals carry the D antigen on their red cells, and have no Rhesus antibodies in their plasma (Table 14.2).

IV

Table 14.2 The Rhesus system

Blood group	Antigen on red cell	Antibody in plasma	Frequency in UK population
Rh positive	D	None	83%
Rh negative	None	Anti-D, following exposure	17%

Rhesus negative individuals do not have the D antigen, but, on exposure to Rhesus positive cells, can produce anti-D antibodies (of the class IgG), which are able to cross the placenta. This occurs if a Rhesus negative woman receives a transfusion of Rhesus positive blood or becomes pregnant with a Rh positive fetus, and fetal cells enter the maternal circulation.

The first time this occurs, antibody formation by the mother is too little and too late to cause damage, and the first pregnancy is usually unaffected. However, on subsequent exposure in further pregnancies, the woman is sensitized and antibody formation is more efficient. Maternal antibodies cross the placenta and attack the red cells of the fetus, splitting them open, giving rise to haemolytic disease of the newborn. As fetal red cells are destroyed:

- Red cell formation cannot keep up with red cell destruction, and anaemia develops. Intrauterine exchange transfusion can replace lost red cells, and ameliorate the problem.
- If anaemia becomes severe, heart failure, ascites, effusions, and oedema (hydrops foetalis) develop.
- Haemoglobin released into the circulation is broken down into bile pigments. *In utero*, these are removed by the placenta, but they accumulate in the neonate, causing jaundice.
- Bile pigments cross the immature **blood/brain barrier** of the neonate and, if **serum** bilirubin concentration exceeds 120 micromol/litre, damage the rapidly metabolizing areas of the brain, the cerebral cortex, auditory cortex, brainstem, and basal ganglia: this is known as **kernicterus**. Permanent disability is likely.
- Intrauterine death may follow, but, with current management, is now a rare outcome.

Practice point

- Due to the associated risks of brain damage, neonatal jaundice is always reported immediately, so that treatment with phototherapy and, if necessary, exchange transfusion can commence.

The extent of the damage to the fetus varies: the mildest cases are only detected on laboratory screening (Kumar and Regan, 2005).

Most Rhesus incompatibility problems are due to anti-D antibodies, but anti-C, anti-E and anti-Kell antibodies can cause similar problems.

Prevention of haemolytic disease of the newborn

Some 17% of births in England and Wales are to women with Rhesus negative blood group, and about 59% of these infants (10% of total) are Rhesus positive. These 10%, 62,000 per year, are potentially at risk of haemolytic disease of the newborn.

Routine postpartum administration of anti-D (Rh_o) immunoglobulin was adopted throughout the UK in 1969, and the number of fetal deaths due to Rhesus incompatibility fell from 46/100,000 births to 1.6/100,000 (RCOG, 1999). Subsequently, responsive and routine antenatal administration was introduced, and is now subject to NICE guidelines (NICE, 2008). While the evidence from randomized controlled trials has its limitations (Crowther and Middleton, 1997, 1999), the clinical benefits of administration are overwhelming for women planning future pregnancies (NICE, 2008). Meta-analysis of existing UK randomized controlled trials indicates that the addition of routine antenatal administration is likely to prevent sensitization in 1 in 278 women, reducing the numbers of women in England and Wales sensitized and vulnerable to Rhesus incompatibility from 583 to 216 each year (Jones et al., 2004).

Indications for anti-D (Rh$_o$) immunoglobulins

Anti-D (Rh$_o$) immunoglobulins (antibodies) are administered to Rhesus negative women (not infants) to prevent the formation of anti-D antibodies:

- at 28 and 34 weeks' gestation, as prophylaxis, at least 500 units (BNF, 2009) or as a single 1500 unit dose (NICE, 2008)
- following a sensitizing event (below)
- following delivery of a Rhesus positive infant (NICE, 2008).

The anti-D (Rh$_o$) immunoglobulins match, neutralize and destroy the RhD antigens on fetal red cells in the maternal circulation. This ensures that fetal cells do not reach the mother's lymphocytes, thereby pre-empting maternal production of anti-D antibodies, which could cause haemolytic disease of the newborn in subsequent pregnancies.

Practice points

- Following delivery, cord blood is taken and tested for blood group. This is easier if delivery occurs in secondary care facilities.
- Women with Rhesus negative blood group should not be discharged until the need for anti-D (Rh$_o$) immunoglobulin has been assessed and the appropriate dose has been calculated from blood samples and administered.

During pregnancy, small volumes of fetal cells enter the maternal circulation, but they are removed by macrophages before antibodies can be formed. However, larger volumes stimulate antibody production (above), damaging the fetus; this can occur following potentially sensitizing events, such as:

- delivery
- abortion (surgical or medical) at any gestation
- spontaneous miscarriage after 12 weeks, at any gestation if instrumentation has occurred
- threatened miscarriage or repeated bleeding
- hydatidiform mole
- ectopic pregnancy
- amniocentesis
- fetal blood sampling
- chorionic villous sampling and other invasive procedures
- antepartum haemorrhage
- external cephalic version
- intrauterine injury
- trauma, particularly to the abdomen.

Practice points

- Anti-D (Rh$_o$) immunoglobulin is administered following any of these sensitizing events, preferably within 72 hours (RCOG, 1999). Some benefits were shown when administration was delayed by 13 days (Moise, 2002).

IV

■ Early booking is essential to identify women with Rhesus negative blood groups, so that all sensitizing events can be managed effectively.

Anti-D (Rh$_o$) immunoglobulins are also administered following accidental incompatible blood or platelet transfusions. One, WinRho SDF®, is administered as one component of therapy for idiopathic thrombocytopenic purpura, a rare chronic relapsing autoimmune disorder, associated with severe bleeding.

Administration of anti-D (Rh$_o$) immunoglobulin

The dose of immunoglobulin administered depends on the quantity of red cells entering the maternal circulation, local protocols and the manufacturers' guidelines. For example, 500 units of D-Gam® are administered as an initial dose following delivery or other sensitizing events or as antenatal prophylaxis (NICE, 2008). Following delivery or sensitizing events after 20 weeks, the quantity of red cells entering the maternal circulation is estimated from a maternal blood sample taken within 2 hours of birth, using the Kleihauer test, flow cytometry or alternatives. Although not universally available, flow cytometry offers the most accurate method of calculating the dose needed where larger volumes have crossed the placenta (RCOG, 1999).

It is not always possible to predict when high doses of immunoglobulin will be needed, but increased transfer of fetal cells is likely following: Caesarean delivery, manual removal of placenta, intrauterine death, stillbirth, multiple births, traumatic delivery, abdominal trauma in the third trimester, or hydrops foetalis. Low doses are usually reserved for events occurring before 20 weeks' gestation.

Practice point

■ Additional doses of immunoglobulin may be needed when the results of tests become available.

Of the four preparations available, two, D-Gam® and Partobulin SDF®, are administered by intramuscular injection only, and the other two, Rhophylac® and WinRho SDF®, are administered either intravenously or intramuscularly. This reflects their different methods of manufacture: fractionation and exchange column chromatography, respectively. Some preparations, for example D-Gam®, are available in vials in several different strengths and concentrations. Intravenous doses are lower (CSL Behring, ABPI, 2008). Inadvertent intravenous administration of D-Gam® or Partobulin SDF® would place the women at a high risk of an allergic reaction (BPL, 2008).

Following intramuscular administration, antibodies appear in the circulation in about 8 hours, and peak levels occur at 2–3 days. Appearance of antibodies is almost immediate with intravenous injection (CSL Behring, ABPI, 2008). The **half-life** of anti-D (Rh$_o$) immunoglobulin is 24 days for intramuscular administration, indicating a degree of protection for several weeks. Anti-D (Rh$_o$) immunoglobulin can be detected 9–12 months after administration if large doses have been administered (RCOG, 1999).

Practice point

■ Anti-D (Rh$_o$) immunoglobulin given antenatally may be detected in the woman's blood postpartum. This does not indicate that the woman has been sensitized, and anti-D (Rh$_o$) immunoglobulin should be administered according to protocol (RCOG, 1999).

Adverse effects of anti-D (Rh$_o$) immunoglobulin

Excessive doses of immunoglobulin have not been associated with **adverse effects**, whereas underdosing could allow heamolytic disease of the newborn to develop in subsequent pregnancies. However, there have been few long-term studies of women and children receiving anti-D (Rh$_o$) immunoglobulin (Wickham, 2001).

The UK Medicines and Healthcare products Regulatory Agency (MHRA) website (2008) lists 56 reports of 124 adverse reactions, including 16 rashes, 4 cases of anaphylaxis and 3 of haemolysis:

- Anti-D (Rh$_o$) immunoglobulin preparations contain protein, and can, rarely, induce an *allergic* response, including chills, nausea, headaches, rashes (some extensive) or anaphylaxis. Therefore, women are observed for 20 minutes following administration (BPL, 2008).
- In theory, anti-D (Rh$_o$) immunoglobulin could cause destruction of fetal red cells in the maternal circulation, which may account for the rare reports of haemolysis and pyrexia associated with administration.
- Anti-D (Rh$_o$) immunoglobulins can cross the placenta and attack the red cells of the fetus; however, to date, this has not resulted in clinical problems.
- *Platelet* count may increase following administration: therefore, if a woman has a high platelet count, advice should be sought (Zimmerman et al., 1998).
- *Pain* may occur at the injection site. Larger intramuscular doses, particularly those >5 ml, should be divided and administered into different limbs.
- Anti-D (Rh$_o$) immunoglobulin is prepared from pooled plasma donations. Therefore, despite inactivation and removal procedures, there may be risks of transmission of viral or prion disease. This has not occurred in the UK, to date, and the estimated risk is 5 women every 100 years in the UK (NICE, 2002). Since the transmission of hepatitis C occurred in Ireland and Germany (Foster et al., 1995), the method of manufacture has been revised (Jones et al., 2004). However, manufacturers warn of possible hepatitis A or parvovirus B19 contamination.

Practice point

- Following each administration, the name and batch number of the product is registered (BPL, 2008; CSL Behring, ABPI, 2008).

Analysis of fetal DNA would allow antenatal therapy to be targeted towards only those women carrying a Rhesus positive fetus (Finning et al., 2008), removing the risk of infection and other adverse effects from some 40% of Rhesus negative women.

Cautions and contraindications: anti-D (Rh$_o$) immunoglobulins

- Rhesus positive blood group.
- Previous hypersensitivity responses to anti-D (Rh$_o$) immunoglobulin contraindicates further use.
- Some 1 in 600 Caucasians are deficient in IgA immunoglobulins/antibodies, which leaves them vulnerable to chest infections, asthma and diarrhoea. If exposed to IgA, such individuals form antibodies to IgA, leading to serious allergic reactions. Anti-D (Rh$_o$) immunoglobulin preparations contain small amounts of IgA; therefore, manufacturers advise caution in the treatment of such patients.
- If immunoglobulins are administered into subcutaneous tissues, they are less likely to be effective; therefore, administration into the gluteal region is not advised, and one manufacturer recommends injection into the deltoid muscle (BPL, 2008; RCOG, 1999; Chapter 2).

IV

- Intramuscular injections are not advised for women with bleeding disorders or receiving antico-agulants. For such patients, intravenous administration is recommended (CSL Behring, ABPI, 2008). However, for products formulated for intramuscular administration only, manufacturers suggest subcutaneous administration (BPL, 2008).

Following discussions with the woman, in conjunction with the appropriate patient information (NICE, 2002), a decision may be taken not to administer anti-D (Rh_o) immunoglobulin if the woman:

- refuses all blood products
- is certain that she will have no further pregnancies
- has a Rhesus negative partner and is certain that any further pregnancies will be with a partner who is Rhesus negative
- is known to have already been sensitized
- has weak expression of the RhD blood group (D^u) (NICE, 2008).

Practice points

- Such women should be identified on initial booking, and the situation discussed with senior obstetricians.
- The blood of Rhesus negative women should be tested antenatally for the presence of anti-D antibodies, to assess sensitization.

Storage

D-Gam® may be stored in the original container for 1 week at 25°C, or up to 2 years at 2–8°C. Rhophylac® prefilled syringes should be stored away from light. Solutions that have been frozen, are cloudy or contain deposits should not be administered. Products should be brought to room temperature before administration.

Interactions: anti-D (Rh_o) immunoglobulins

- Anti-D (Rh_o) immunoglobulins should not be mixed with other medicines.
- Anti-D (Rh_o) immunoglobulin may reduce the efficacy of live attenuated **vaccines**, such as MMR and rubella vaccinations, for 3 months (BPL, 2008). If MMR is administered, the 2 injections are not given in the same syringe or into the same limb (BNF, 2009). Other live vaccines, such as yellow fever, BCG and oral typhoid, are often indicated for foreign travel; in these circumstances, women should be advised of the reduced protection.
- Administration of anti-D (Rh_o) immunoglobulins interferes with the interpretation of antibody concentrations and blood grouping tests. Laboratory staff should be advised of administration when such samples are dispatched.

Despite improved protocols, haemolytic disease of the newborn still occurs due to Rhesus incompatibility. However, with exchange transfusions and prompt management of jaundice, the prognosis is usually favourable.

The immune system in pregnancy

Pregnancy-induced changes in the immune system do not affect the majority of healthy women, but are important in a number of conditions, such as asthma, eczema, rheumatoid arthritis and other autoimmune conditions.

During pregnancy, the immune system must adapt to tolerate the placenta and fetus, which are analogous to a semi-foreign tissue graft, while maintaining immunity against infections. If immune tolerance mechanisms fail, the fetus will be rejected by activation of inflammatory processes, including coagulation. Modifications of monocyte functions are crucial to achieving the balance between tolerance and defence (Luppi, 2003). Normally, the mother recognizes paternal and fetal tissue as 'foreign' and produces antibodies; these, together with certain major histocompatability complex (MHC) surface antigens, coat the fetus and protect it from her natural killer (NK) cells and immune system. However, women with autoimmune conditions, such as rheumatoid arthritis, systemic lupus erythematosus, and thyroid disease, are more likely to produce antibodies that attack the fetus, increasing the risk of recurrent spontaneous abortion. Based on this theory, some women with recurrent spontaneous abortion have undergone immunotherapy (Pandey et al., 2005).

Practice point

Thyroid function tests are advised for women with:
- recurrent miscarriage or preterm birth
- autoimmune conditions and type I diabetes, when pregnancy is diagnosed (Abalovich et al., 2007).

During pregnancy, the balance between Th1 and Th2 helper cells changes, so that Th2 cells predominate over Th1 cells (Thellin and Heinen, 2003). Increase of Th2 cell activity means that antibody synthesis is increased during pregnancy and, therefore, antibody-related immunity increases and systemic lupus erythematosus is likely to worsen. Suppression of T lymphocyte function reduces the incidence and severity of allergic reactions and autoimmune diseases, such as multiple sclerosis and rheumatoid arthritis. However, these conditions may rebound after delivery and it is important to monitor chronic conditions carefully after childbirth. Suppression of Th1 activity, and the actions of progesterone, reduce immunity to intracellular pathogens, leaving women vulnerable to TB, malaria, toxoplasma, HIV, *Listeria*, and viral infections. This is compounded by increased concentrations of cortisol (Pacheco et al., 2007). The increase in viral infections is partly responsible for increased risk of exacerbation of asthma, particularly non-atopic asthma, during pregnancy (Murphy et al., 2006).

Practice point

- Women with asthma should carefully monitor symptoms during pregnancy, to detect deterioration before oxygen delivery to the fetus is compromised.

Infections or other stressors in pregnancy increase Th1 activity, releasing pro-inflammatory **cytokines**, triggering blood clotting, and activating natural killer cells and neutrophils, which attack the fetus (Thellin and Heinen, 2003). Primary infections of the mother are likely to pass to the fetus from the second trimester onwards. Infection or inflammation trigger ripening of the cervix, and preterm labour. Infection of the placenta (chorioamnionitis) or adjacent tissue, such as the genital tract, Fallopian tubes and bladder,* and subsequent release of cytokines into the fetal circulation, may increase the risk of fetal loss, sepsis or disrupted brain development. At any gestation, this may lead to cerebral palsy, particularly if the fetus is hypoxic (Wu and Colford, 2000; Cowan et al., 2000; Redline, 2004).

Note: the venous drainage of the bladder, vagina and cervix interconnect, allowing spread of microorganisms and inflammatory mediators.

Practice points

Women are advised to:
- avoid unpasteurized dairy products

IV

- minimize exposure to infections and stress
- avoid immunization with live vaccines
- seek prompt treatment for infections, particularly infections of the urogenital tract (Chapel et al., 2006).

Probably the commonest infection in pregnancy is periodontal disease (inflammation of gums leading to destruction of local tissues and tooth decay, associated with proliferation of bacteria, typically Gram-negative anaerobes). Some observation studies indicate that low birth weight and preterm deliveries are more common in women with periodontal disease, and small non-randomized trials involving disadvantaged women have shown a small improvement in outcomes when this is treated (Xiong et al., 2006).

Immunosuppression

The immune system may be compromised by corticosteroids, immunosuppressants, undernutrition, stress, infection, cancer, long-term illness or drug abuse.

Case reports

1 A previously healthy woman who had suffered hyperemesis gravidarum throughout pregnancy contracted a fatal fungal infection, aspergillosis (CEMACH, 2005). Aspergillosis is associated with immunosuppression, induced by the combined effects of malnutrition, caused by vomiting, and the changes in the immune system related to pregnancy (above).

Undernutrition compromises the immune system and predisposes to infection. Where inadequate intake is suspected, information on daily intake (for a weekday and a weekend day) and vomiting should be obtained. A dietician should be consulted if there are concerns.

2 Towards the end of pregnancy and after birth, a woman with a history of anxiety and depression complained of palpitations. Despite a heart rate of 140–170 bpm, she was diagnosed as having panic attacks. After delivery, an antidepressant was prescribed and a referral was made to the community mental health team. She became acutely disturbed and doubly incontinent, and was admitted to a psychiatric hospital, then to intensive care, where sepsis was diagnosed. At postmortem, she was found to have a gangrenous uterus and cardiac dilatation.

The stress associated with mental health problems can make women vulnerable to physical illness, and vital signs should not be overlooked. A heart rate above 100 bpm indicates serious physical illness (CEMACH, 2005: 169).

Allergic conditions in pregnancy

Eczema

Eczema is one of the most common conditions in young women, affecting around 16%. It can occur for the first time in pregnancy or around the areola during breastfeeding. Eczema may improve or worsen in pregnancy and some 10% of affected women experience a serious 'flare' after delivery (Weatherhead et al., 2007).

Eczema or atopic dermatitis is a chronic relapsing form of skin inflammation leading to dry skin and sensitization associated with IgE antibodies and dysfunction of the epidermal barrier (Bieber, 2008). Eczema is worsened by irritants, allergens, and stress.

Eczema and other dry skin conditions, such as pruritic urticarial papules and plaques of pregnancy, disrupt the barrier formed by intact epithelial surfaces and their acid secretions. This exterior defence system excludes microorganisms, and prevents infection by staphylococci and other skin flora (Doan et al., 2005).

Practice points

- To prevent drying of the skin, soap should be avoided and moisturisers should be applied.
- To decrease the risk of infection, dry skin should be promptly treated with emollients. Antihistamines are unlikely to help.

Where possible, eczema and pruritic urticarial papules and plaques of pregnancy are managed with emollients and barrier creams, which are free of important adverse effects. If these fail to control itching, topical corticosteroids are prescribed (also for eczema around the areola) (Matz et al., 2006). If these fail to control the symptoms of eczema, narrowband ultraviolet B is often the second-line treatment. Oral corticosteroids and some topical calcineurin inhibitors or immuno-suppressants may be considered for local application by specialists (Weatherhead et al., 2007).

Topical corticosteroids

Absorption of dermatological preparations is increased during pregnancy and through inflamed skin. Therefore, all the adverse effects associated with oral corticosteroids, including adrenal suppression, can complicate topical therapy during pregnancy for the first time (Hengge et al., 2006). Highly potent topical steroids are not recommended (Weatherhead et al., 2007). Oral corti-costeroids are rarely prescribed for eczema (see Chapter 15, Asthma).

Local reactions to topical corticosteroids are relatively common, and include skin atrophy, striae, rosacea, acne, purpura, hair growth, pigmentation changes, skin infections and delayed wound healing. Repeated application of corticosteroids may reduce their efficacy or engender contact sensitization, which worsens the underlying skin condition.

Scratching causes colonization with *Staphylococcus aureus*, which triggers immunological reac-tions, leaving the skin resistant to corticosteroids and vulnerable to infections.

Practice points

- Eczema-induced itching frequently interferes with sleep, which is particularly important in the puer-perium. Antihistamines are often ineffective at relieving symptoms.
- To explore the possibility of corticosteroid resistance, women should be asked if there is any change in the efficacy of their medicines.
- If topical corticosteroids are not applied regularly and thoroughly, inflammation and itching will inten-sify, and much-needed sleep will be lost. Women may need to be reminded to treat their own eczema, particularly during the puerperium.

The antimicrobial peptides that protect the skin are destroyed by inflammation, which makes it difficult to treat infections associated with eczema (Bieber, 2008).

Practice point

- Prevention of infection with applications of lotions containing antiseptics such as chlorhexidine is advised (Bieber, 2008).

Food allergy

Food allergies, particularly those to nuts and seeds, frequently persist into adulthood. Affected women will make every effort to avoid allergen exposure and ensure that they have adrenaline and rapid-acting antihistamines available at all times (Lack, 2008b).

IV

Hereditary angioedema

Angioedema is the swelling of face, tongue, larynx, limbs, genitalia, trunk and bowels not associated with itching or urticarial rash. It may be acquired (for example in association with ACE inhibitors or NSAIDs) or inherited. Hereditary angioedema is caused by the absence of an enzyme that inhibits the complement system (above); when not held in check, the complement system triggers inflammation and swelling. Stress and oestrogens, including the combined oral contraceptive, may increase the frequency of attacks. To hold the complement system in check, specialists may prescribe androgens, such as danazol. However, these can cause masculinization of the fetus, and are **contraindicated** in pregnancy and lactation. Alternative therapies, such as antifibrinolytic drugs, should be sought as soon as pregnancy is planned (Zuraw, 2008).

Immunosuppressant therapies

Immunosuppressant therapies include azathioprine, ciclosporin, calcineurin inhibitors (for example tacrolimus), and methotrexate; the last is contraindicated in pregnancy and breastfeeding.

Calcineurin inhibitors, such as tacrolimus, pimecrolimus, sirolimus, and ciclosporin, reduce the production of cytotoxic T cells responsible for cell-mediated immunity. In addition to the increased risk of viral infections, these drugs can have serious adverse effects, including kidney, liver or nerve damage; they are not recommended in pregnancy by manufacturers unless clearly necessary, and under specialist supervision. Their use during breastfeeding is contraindicated (BNF, 2009). The absorption of topical preparations is increased during pregnancy and in inflammatory skin conditions. Therefore use of sirolimus or related compounds in the treatment of eczema should be avoided (BNF, 2009).

Women prescribed immunosuppressant therapies are at increased risk of infection, premature delivery and low birth weight. Azothiaprine has been associated with low white cell counts in neonates. In some cases, the risks associated with leaving the underlying condition untreated may be greater than any possible harm to the infant. For example, the incidence of premature birth (46%), low birth weight (31%) and infant mortality (5%) is as high in women awaiting organ transplantation as in those receiving immunosuppressants (van Tonningen, 2007a).

Practice points

■ Although there is no association with congenital anomalies, detailed ultrasound examination is warranted.
■ Regular full blood counts, renal and liver function tests are required.

Development of the immune system

Following delivery, the immune system of the neonate undergoes rapid development. Neonates have no commensal microflora, and acquire this from their mothers and their surroundings. Infants in intensive care may acquire unusual or pathogenic microflora (Posfay-Barbe et al., 2008).

Neonatal immunity depends on breast milk, which contains macrophages, lymphocytes, granulocytes, antibodies, complement and enzymes that destroy bacteria, such as lysozyme. In developing countries, death in the first 6 months of life is 10 times more likely in formula-fed infants (Bahl et al., 2005); for infants born in the UK in 2000, the chances of being hospitalized with a respiratory infection or diarrhoea were reduced by 27% and 53% for every month of exclusive breastfeeding (Quigley et al., 2007). Infants are protected by their mothers' antibodies for the first 2–3 months of life, and are relatively free of bacterial infections during this time (Halken, 2004). Neutrophils and macrophages become fully functional within the first few days of life. However, neonates are vulnerable to viral and intracellular infections, such as cytomegalovirus,

Herpes simplex, *Listeria spp.* and toxoplasma, because natural killer cells and cytotoxic T cells are deficient. Lymphocytes become functional by around 2 months of age, but antibody production does not reach adult levels until age 4. As children are repeatedly exposed to new antigens, their immune systems develop and they become less susceptible to infections. Because of their immunological naivety, infants are very susceptible to respiratory and gastrointestinal infections. When infected children are hospitalized, infections can spread rapidly throughout children's wards, and infection control measures are particularly important (Posfay-Barbe et al., 2008).

Allergic disorders, such as eczema, asthma and hay fever, and drug allergies are associated with **atopy**. Atopy occurs when the regulation of the immune system is upset, and deviates from Th1 towards Th2 helper cells, causing lymphocytes to produce IgE antibodies, rather than IgG antibodies. (IgE antibodies trigger release of histamine and other inflammatory mediators.) At birth, the Th2 cells predominate. Normally, environmental factors, such as exposure to certain bacteria, shift the balance of the immune system away from Th2 cells towards Th1 cells, preventing the development of allergies (Figure 14.1).

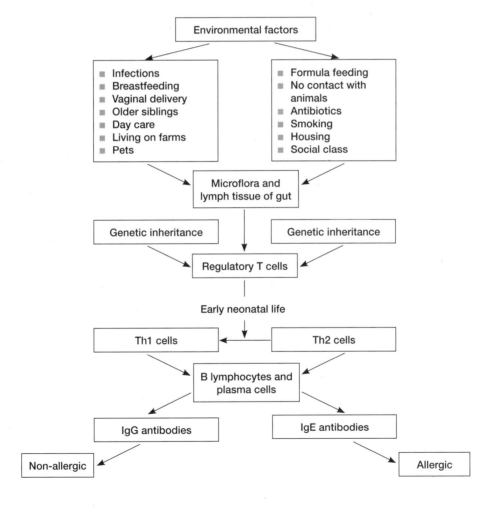

Figure 14.1 Development of the immune system
Source: Storey and Jordan (2008). By kind permission of the RCN Publishing Company

However, this change does not occur in children with atopy (Prescott et al., 1999). Children in rural Eastern Europe have, to date, largely escaped the 'allergy epidemic', which affects around 50% of children in the UK (Austin et al., 1999; Majkowska-Wojciechowska et al., 2007). However, the environmental components responsible for the current epidemic of allergic disorders have not been identified. There are suggestions that antibiotics administered to pregnant women (Bedford et al., 2006) or infants may change the neonatal gut microflora, which might affect the regulation of the immune system, allowing allergies to develop (Jordan et al., 2008).

Practice points

- Antibiotics should only be administered when clinically necessary.
- Any history of atopic disorders should be documented, because of the association with an increased risk of allergic responses to antibiotics.

Conclusion

Modification of the immune system is the basis of a wide range of therapies, from Rhesus immunization to monoclonal antibodies. Immunotherapies are rapidly being developed and prescribed in specialist units for women who would otherwise succumb to disease: how the newest drugs affect human pregnancy is largely unknown. In addition, the functioning of the immune system in pregnancy and neonatal life may guide practice, particularly the selective administration of antibiotics.

Further reading

- Geha, R.S. and Rosen, F.S. (2008) *Case Studies in Immunology: A Clinical Companion*, 5th edn. Garland Science, New York.
- NICE (National Institute for Health and Clinical Excellence) (2002) *Guidance on the Use of Routine Antenatal Anti-D Prophylaxis for Women who are Rhesus D (RhD) Negative* (technology appraisal guidance 41). NICE, London.
- Storey, M. and Jordan, S. (2008) Continuing professional development: an overview of the immune system. *Nursing Standard*, **23**(15/17): 47–56.

Part V

Pregnancy in Women with Pre-existing Disease

V

Introduction

This section describes the medications administered to women with long-term health needs who become pregnant. In the author's opinion, these topics represent the most difficult subjects in medicine. The practitioner needs to be familiar with the disease: how the disease is influenced by pregnancy; how the disease affects the outcome of pregnancy; how the drugs influence the disease; how the drugs influence the outcome of pregnancy and breastfeeding; and how pregnancy affects the actions of the drugs. As if all this were not enough, practitioners need to consider the interactions between the disease, the drugs for the disease and the drugs commonly used in labour. The following chapters are only a guide, and midwives are urged to consult specialists in tertiary referral centres.

We assume that all women affected by a disease prior to conception will be under the care of an obstetrician, and probably also a physician. However, midwives usually play an important role in recognizing and referring medical problems. Also, we hope that the outlines provided will help midwives when advising women in pregnancy, labour and the puerperium.

For most of the drugs described, there is little or no evidence from randomized controlled trials in pregnant and breastfeeding women. Evidence of safety and best practice is largely based on ecological studies, often without long-term follow-up. In general, the manufacturers' literature is cautious, stressing that use of medication in pregnancy and breastfeeding is based on clinical risk/benefit calculations, rather than scientific evidence.

The scope of this book only allows consideration of the commonest diseases in women of child-bearing age.

Further reading

■ Campbell, S. and Lees, C. (2006) Medical diseases complicating pregnancy, in Baker, P.N. (ed.) *Obstetrics by Ten Teachers*, 18th edn. London, Arnold.
■ De Swiet, M. (2002) *Medical Disorders in Obstetric Practice*, 4th edn. Blackwell, Oxford.

Emboldened terms can be found in the Glossary.

CHAPTER 15

Asthma in Pregnancy

Sue Jordan

This chapter describes asthma in pregnancy and the drugs commonly used in the management of asthma. This condition is so common in young people that not all women will be receiving care from a specialist in respiratory medicine. Little information is available on the use of the newest agents, the leukotriene receptor antagonists, in pregnancy.

Chapter contents

- Asthma
- Management of asthma
- Drugs used in asthma
- Bronchodilators (mainly salbutamol)
- Anti-inflammatory agents (mainly corticosteroids)

Asthma

Asthma may affect 20–30% of those born during the 1980s in industrialized countries (Burr et al., 2006), and 7% of pregnant women (Schatz et al., 2004). Asthma is an inflammatory disease affecting the small airways. It is not always reversible, and can be fatal. Bronchoconstriction leads to dyspnoea (breathing difficulties) on expiration and (sometimes) wheezing and cough. Asthma is characterized by inflammation, oedema, eosinophil infiltration and remodelling of the bronchioles. Mucus is produced in excessive amounts, and may form plugs that block the airways. The lining of the bronchioles is shed, also blocking the airways. These changes become permanent in long-standing disease. Narrowing of the airways is intensified at night, following the natural circadian rhythms of hormone secretion.

Defined allergens (such as the house dust mite) are associated with a worsening of symptoms. Strategies for the prevention of asthma include allergen avoidance (including cigarette smoke) in pregnancy and early life, and early treatment with anti-inflammatory agents (Holgate, 1997).

Practice point

- Regular, systematic monitoring of lung function and symptoms forms an important aspect of care for asthmatic women. This will detect any changes that may occur as a result of pregnancy or parturition, and assist compliance.

V

Complications of asthma

Deteriorating asthma is frequently caused by noncompliance with inhaled corticosteroids, which may be due to misplaced concerns that medications are **teratogenic**. For women with severe asthma, there is a risk that the symptoms of asthma will intensify late in the second trimester or postpartum. Mild or moderate asthma may improve during pregnancy but worsen following delivery (Rey and Boulet, 2007).

Hypoxia

Severe, uncontrolled asthma causes chronic or intermittent hypoxia, which adversely affects both mother and baby. Maternal oxygen saturation should never be allowed to fall below 95%, even in an acute attack or in labour (Rey and Boulet, 2007). Hypoxia impairs fetal development, causing intrauterine growth retardation (IUGR), fetal distress and, occasionally, death. Exacerbation of asthma in pregnancy is associated with low birth weight, but there is less evidence of association with preterm birth and pre-eclampsia (Murphy et al., 2005).

Practice points

- Hypoxia causes agitation and confusion: the prompt assessment of oxygen saturation can pre-empt misdiagnosis and the inappropriate administration of sedatives to a patient with asthma.
- Fetal monitoring may be needed during severe exacerbations of asthma (Murphy et al., 2006).
- Asthma exacerbation is more likely in obese women (Hendler et al., 2006), those who gain less weight during pregnancy, those with severe disease, following viral infections, and noncompliance with inhaled corticosteroids (Murphy et al., 2005; Rey and Boulet, 2007). Close observation may minimize these problems.
- Exacerbation of asthma may occur following Caesarean delivery, and close observation is needed to minimize severity (BTS, 2008).

Both high altitude and asthma are associated with *placenta praevia*, suggesting a link to hypoxia (Wen et al., 2001).

Carbon dioxide retention

In a severe asthma attack, carbon dioxide is retained and the work of breathing will be so increased that a build-up of lactic acid occurs.

Acute asthma attack

An asthma attack may be life-threatening to mother and fetus. Nebulized bronchodilators, oxygen, intravenous and oral corticosteroids and, if necessary, ipratropium, magnesium sulphate (unlicensed and undergoing trials) or, rarely, aminophylline are administered, as in non-pregnant women. (Protocols are outlined in the BNF.) An acute attack of asthma is rare during labour; however, should this occur, opioids, prostaglandins and ergometrine should be withheld as they may intensify bronchoconstriction (Nelson-Piercy and Moore-Gillon, 1995). Prostaglandin E2 (dinoprostone) is considered safe by some authorities (BTS, 2008), while others advise caution (Clyburn et al., 2008b). Asthma symptoms manageable with inhaled **beta$_2$ agonists** are relatively common during labour, arising in 18% of women with diagnosed asthma and 46% of women with severe asthma (Schatz, 2003).

Practice points

- Beta$_2$ agonist inhalers, such as salbutamol, should always be available on the labour ward, as women occasionally forget to bring their medicines into hospital.

- Doses of asthma medications should not be omitted, even during labour.
- Placental perfusion should be protected by monitoring blood pressure, placing the woman on her left side, recording fluid balance and administering prescribed intravenous fluids promptly.
- Experienced anaesthetists may be needed if intubation becomes necessary.

Case report

Bronchospasm can complicate labour.

A 26-year-old primipara presented with premature rupture of membranes and breech presentation at 36 weeks, and underwent emergency Caesarean section. No history of asthma was obtained, but examination revealed evidence of **atopic** dermatitis. Spinal anaesthesia was induced using 2 ml of 0.4% tetracaine (a local anaesthetic) in 10% dextrose. Sensory loss extended to T3. The woman began to cough and wheeze and became short of breath. This was treated as an acute attack of asthma. Both mother and infant did well post-section.

It would appear that spinal anaesthesia triggered an asthmatic attack by anaesthetizing the autonomic nervous system supplying the bronchioles rather than by a **hypersensitivity** response (Kawabata, 1996). Spinal anaesthesia can, occasionally, precipitate respiratory difficulties in women with a history of atopic conditions (such as asthma, atopic dermatitis/eczema). However, systemic opioids can also worsen asthma (Beischer et al., 1997).

Pain may increase oxygen consumption and ventilation (Chapter 4), and adequate analgesia is important to reduce physiological and psychological stress. In rare instances, local **anaesthetics** can cause problems.

Asthma and pregnancy

Observation studies suggest that maternal asthma may increase the likelihood of pneumonia, hypertension, preterm birth, admission to neonatal intensive care, congenital anomalies, low birth weight, hypertensive disorders, diabetes, ante- and postpartum haemorrhage, premature rupture of membranes, infections, and Caesarean delivery, but the risks are low and related to the control of the disease (Kramer et al., 1995; Nelson-Piercy and Moore-Gillon, 1995; Schatz, 1999; Munn et al., 1999; Murphy et al., 2005; Rey and Boulet, 2007); some associations, such as diabetes and infections, may not be independent of medications (Wen et al., 2001). Oral corticosteroids or theophylline, prescribed for severe asthma, may be associated with preterm birth and hypertension (Bracken et al., 2003; Murphy et al., 2006).

Management of asthma

The management goal is to control symptoms and avoid complications at all times of the day and night. This is achieved by:

- avoidance of trigger factors (including drugs and viral infections) as far as possible (Box 15.1)
- monitoring and record keeping (Box 15.2)
- pharmacotherapeutic interventions.

The risks from poorly controlled asthma far outweigh any possible teratogenic effects of standard therapies.

Box 15.1 Trigger factors for asthma

An asthma attack may be precipitated by:
- Changes in environmental temperature or humidity
- Exercise
- Worry, stress, or fatigue
- Pollens, fungal spores, the house dust mite, animals
- Smoke and environmental pollutants, for example sulphur dioxide
- Infections
- Hypoxia
- Menstruation
- Thyrotoxicosis
- Industrial irritants, for example laundry detergents, dusty flour or grain
- Certain foods, such as eggs, nuts, chocolate or fish, mainly in children

Drugs causing or exacerbating asthma:
- Hypersensitivity response or anaphylactoid reaction to any drug
- Beta blockers, for example as antihypertensives or as eye drops for glaucoma
- NSAIDs, such as aspirin, salicylates, and diclofenac
- Oestrogens
- Benzodiazepines
- Tobacco, cannabis
- Opioids – fentanyl is possibly the least problematic
- Ergometrine (Syntometrine® rarely causes problems) (BTS, 2008)
- Prostaglandins (carboprost and dinoprostone)
- Antipsychotics
- Tricyclic antidepressants
- Atracurium muscle relaxant – use vecuronium
- Lignocaine
- ACE inhibitors can cause cough and angioedema, which may be mistaken for asthma
- **Hypotonic** or hypertonic solutions when in contact with the airways, for example in nebulizers; therefore normal saline is used as a dilutent in nebulizers
- Preservatives in inhaled drugs, for example lactose
- Tartrazine, for example in fruit squash, coloured fizzy drinks, curry powder and pickles
- Sulphiting agents, for example some wines, shellfish, preservatives on fresh fruit, dried fruits and pickles

Sources: Cochrane and Rees (1989); McFadden (1991); Jordan and White (2001)

Practice point

■ Management of postpartum haemorrhage may be complicated by the possible adverse reactions to prostaglandins and ergot alkaloids, and protocols should be in place to manage this.

Box 15.2 Reasons for monitoring airways

Always monitor airways, because:
- Regular measurements of peak expiratory flow rates (PEFR) are more reliable indicators of disease than subjective symptoms.
- Some causes of exacerbations of disease, for example noncompliance, exposure to dust, menstruation and diet, only become obvious with an asthma diary.

- A change or fall in PEFR will warn of any change in response to therapy and warn of impending 'disasters'.
- 'Nocturnal dips' will indicate loss of control of the disease.
- Inhaler technique needs checking and reinforcing.

Peak expiratory flow rates, lung volumes and ideally FEV_1/FVC ratios (forced expiratory volume in one second/forced vital capacity) are monitored.

Aerosol delivery

Asthma medication is best delivered by inhalation *via* aerosols, and more than 90% of people treated for asthma have no need for other forms of drug delivery. Aerosols reduce the amount of drug in the systemic circulation, and thus reduce both the maternal **adverse effects** and the drug exposure of the fetus and breastfed infant.

Even with optimal inhaler technique, only 2–10% of aerosolized drug reaches the lungs, and the rest is swallowed. This is improved by the use of spacer devices, which also reduce the need for coordination. The type of inhaler device may affect drug absorption by 100%, so careful monitoring is necessary if the type of inhaler is changed. It is important that inhaler technique is checked and discussed (see Jordan, 2008, Ch. 8, for a summary of inhaler technique).

Practice point

■ Spacers should be washed every month with detergent and left to dry in air. Plastic spacers should be replaced every year (BTS, 2008).

Drugs used in asthma

The drugs prescribed will depend on the severity of the disease. The main classes of drugs used in asthma are:

1 *Bronchodilators:*
  - beta adrenoceptor agonists, for example salbutamol, terbutaline
  - antimuscarinic agents, for example ipratropium (rarely used in young adults, but no evidence of harm) (Garbis, 2007)
  - methylxanthines, for example theophylline.
2 *Anti-inflammatories:*
  - chromones, for example cromoglycate and nedocromil
  - corticosteroids and glucocorticoids, for example beclomethasone and prednisolone
  - leukotriene receptor antagonists (not usually recommended in pregnancy) (BNF, 2009).

Extensive clinical experience indicates that inhaled cromoglycate, short-acting $beta_2$ adrenoceptor agonists and corticosteroids are safe in pregnancy (Schatz, 2004; Garbis, 2007).

Bronchodilators

The diameter of the airways is controlled by several factors (see Box 15.3). Bronchodilators relax the smooth muscle of the bronchioles and provide effective 'rescue' medication. In young people, the $beta_2$ adrenoceptor agonists are the most widely used bronchodilators. However, asthma is a chronic inflammatory disease, involving a variety of white cells, platelets and **cytokines**, and therefore only mild forms of asthma are managed by bronchodilators alone. *If a pregnant woman is using 'rescue' inhalations regularly – more than two canisters a month or 10–12 puffs per day – her asthma is probably poorly controlled, necessitating additional therapy and risking hypoxaemia and compromising the fetus* (BTS, 2008).

V

Box 15.3 Control of the airways

1 Normally the smooth muscle of the bronchioles is relaxed by adrenaline (epinephrine) acting on the beta$_2$ receptors, hence the use of beta$_2$ agonists, for example salbutamol
2 Some of the airways are constricted by acetylcholine, hence the use of anticholinergic drugs, for example ipratropium (Atrovent®)
3 There is a third system of nerves not related to the autonomic nervous system, which may be affected by cromoglycate
4 Circadian rhythms: asthma is worst between 2.00 a.m. and dawn

---

Beta$_2$ adrenoceptor agonists

Beta$_2$ adrenoceptor agonists act, like adrenaline/epinephrine, by stimulating the beta$_2$ receptors present in the liver, the smooth muscle and glands of many organs, including the uterus, lungs and gut. They are effective in both asthma and uterine hypercontractility. Aerosol salbutamol or terbutaline are the initial treatment of choice for asthma during pregnancy, provided symptoms can be controlled by inhalation less than twice per week (BNF, 2009). Oral forms of these drugs are rarely used in pregnancy. The pharmacology of the beta$_2$ adrenoceptor agonists is discussed in Chapter 7 and summarized in Appendix 1.

Beta$_2$ adrenoceptor agonists cross the placenta and enter breast milk. There is no evidence that short-acting inhaled beta$_2$ adrenoceptor agonists are harmful to either the fetus or the breastfed neonate. Some fetal abnormalities have been demonstrated in animals using very high doses of these drugs. Oral or intravenous therapy may induce fetal or neonatal tachycardia, neonatal hypoglycaemia and tremor, but this is more likely with the higher doses used for tocolysis (Garbis, 2007). There is little information on long-acting beta$_2$ adrenoceptor agonists in pregnancy and lactation, but manufacturers advise caution (Novartis, Allen and Hanburys, ABPI, 2009). Available data indicate that salmeterol does not cause harm (BTS, 2008).

Uses of beta$_2$ adrenoceptor agonists

The uses of beta$_2$ adrenoceptor agonists include:

- rescue asthma medication
- exercise prophylaxis
- prevention of asthma symptoms in patients also receiving anti-inflammatory prophylaxis (usually salmeterol)
- chronic airways disease, for example cystic fibrosis, and relief of pulmonary oedema
- **tocolysis** (Chapter 7).

Use of inhaled salbutamol or terbutaline to treat symptoms during labour does not prolong labour or delay the onset of labour, probably due to low systemic absorption (Nelson-Piercy and Moore-Gillon, 1995). High doses towards term may delay labour (Garbis, 2007).

An inhaled dose of salbutamol or terbutaline acts within minutes and lasts 3–5 hours. Long-acting preparations, for example salmeterol, formoterol, and fenoterol, last for 12 hours but are not effective rescue medication; they are normally co-prescribed with inhaled corticosteroids. **Tolerance** to beta$_2$ adrenoceptor agonists may develop with repeated exposure (Chapter 1). Administration of corticosteroids may reverse tolerance and restore the effectiveness of beta$_2$ adrenoceptor agonists (Cooper and Panettieri, 2008). Asthma control should be monitored carefully if long-acting beta$_2$ adrenoceptor agonists are prescribed (BNF, 2009).

Practice points

- Sudden withdrawal of therapy causes rebound symptoms. Therefore it is important that asthma therapy is not discontinued (or left behind) should someone suddenly be admitted to hospital.
- Not all asthma responds to bronchodilators. Following administration of beta$_2$ adrenoceptor agonists, vital signs, oxygen saturation and agitation should continue to be monitored (CEMACH, 2007).

Methylxanthines

Theophylline is not recommended during pregnancy by some authorities (Garbis, 2007). However, with regular monitoring of venous blood samples to accommodate the pharmacokinetic changes in pregnancy (Chapter 1), others consider theophyline to be safe (BTS, 2008).

Anti-inflammatory agents

Inflammation causes narrowing of the airways in asthma, both during and between exacerbations/attacks. Many inflammatory mediators, (such as histamine) are involved, therefore effective therapy is directed at the inflammatory processes rather than any single mediator. Anti-inflammatory agents are prescribed to prevent, rather than treat, asthma attacks.

Cromoglycate

Cromoglycate has been widely used in pregnancy without adverse effects, but there is less experience with nedocromil (Garbis, 2007). Although only about 33% of asthmatics respond, this is a useful drug with few adverse effects. Cromoglycate is administered by inhalation, as a preventive therapy, either on a regular basis or prior to exercise. Its mechanism of action is uncertain, but it probably prevents stimulation of irritant receptors and inhibits the inflammatory response. Cromoglycate does not cross the placenta and does not enter breast milk. Inhalation of the dry powder may cause coughing and bronchospasm. Hypersensitivity responses are rare.

Corticosteroids

Corticosteroids have saved lives and revolutionized the management of severe illnesses such as asthma, rheumatoid arthritis, exfoliative dermatitis and Addison's disease. Regular use of inhaled beclomethasone reduces the frequency of severe episodes of asthma in pregnancy (Wendel et al., 1996; Murphy et al., 2006). Due to adverse effects, long-term oral administration is avoided if possible and maintenance doses are kept to a minimum (BNF, 2009; see Implications for practice). However oral corticosteroids, such as prednisolone, are essential in acute, severe asthma.

How the body handles corticosteroids

Topical or inhalational administration reduces, but does not necessarily abolish, systemic adverse effects (CSM, 1998). Inhaled corticosteroids will lead to oral infections such as thrush unless strict oral hygiene is maintained.

Practice points

- Gargling or rinsing with water following corticosteroid inhalation may reduce the risk of oral thrush and systemic absorption.
- Spacer devices may decrease oral candidiasis, but increase cough (Dubus et al., 2001).

Systemic adverse effects are unlikely with inhaled beclomethasone doses below 800 micrograms/day in adults (BTS, 2008).

Corticosteroids are dependent on liver enzymes for elimination. This gives rise to several drug interactions, for example with antivirals, erythromycin, and ephedrine (below). The increase in endogenous cortisol in pregnancy may reduce the elimination of corticosteroids (Pacheco et al., 2007), and women should be referred to prescribers to assess any need for dose reduction. The rapidly declining concentrations of corticosteroid hormones following delivery may necessitate a return to pre-pregnancy doses. Corticosteroids cross the placenta to a variable extent. The risk of intrauterine growth retardation is significant if systemic administration of corticosteroids is prolonged or repeated (BNF, 2009; Chapter 7). Over 80% of orally administered prednisolone is inactivated by the placenta; however, the remaining 10–20% may be sufficient to affect the fetus. Prednisolone passes into breast milk. Doses above 40 mg per day may cause adverse effects in neonates, who should be carefully monitored (CSM, 1998; BNF, 2009). Delaying the feed by 3–4 hours reduces neonatal exposure (Garbis, 2007).

Actions and adverse effects of corticosteroids
The adverse effects of corticosteroids can be summarized under three headings:

1 Adverse effects likely to arise immediately:
   - cardiovascular problems
   - central nervous system problems
   - metabolic disturbances – hyperglycaemia.
2 Adverse effects likely to arise in the longer term:
   - anti-inflammatory actions
   - metabolic disturbances – growth, tissue viability and fat metabolism
   - cardiovascular problems
   - central nervous system problems
   - adrenal suppression (see also Implications for practice and Appendix 1).
3 Possible effects on the fetus – oral and injected corticosteroids (also Chapter 7, Corticosteroids and tocolysis):
   - preterm birth (possibly due to risk of infections)
   - possible growth restriction.

This chapter will only detail problems likely to be more relevant to the long-term administration of corticosteroids. Short-term adverse effects are discussed in Chapter 7, and topical corticosteroids for eczema in Chapter 14. However, the potential adverse effects of corticosteroids may be encountered in any situation where they are prescribed.

Anti-inflammatory actions
All types and stages of the inflammatory response, both appropriate and inappropriate, are depressed, reducing redness, pain, swelling, healing and tissue repair by:

- reduced production and release of inflammatory mediators
- failure of white cells to migrate to site of infection, increasing the risk of infections, including neonatal sepsis
- failure to activate **macrophages**, giving an increased risk of reactivation of TB (tuberculosis), *Herpes simplex*, fungal or viral eye infections
- suppression of immune response and reduced response to **antigens**. Infections are more severe, and the response to immunizations is decreased. Live **vaccines** (MMR, oral polio, BCG, yellow fever and oral typhoid) should not be administered: to anyone with impaired immunity, including those receiving high-dose corticosteroid treatment and within at least 3 months of discontinuation of such therapy (DH, 2006); if contacts are receiving immunosup-

pressive medications such as oral corticosteroids. Spread of malignancies may be enhanced (Aronson, 2006)

■ reduced proliferation of fibroblast collagen formation. This impairs healing and scar tissue formation, and allows rapid spread of infection without signs and symptoms, and impedes healing.

Practice points

■ There is a risk of severe chickenpox, possibly with minimal rash (BNF, 2009).
■ During pregnancy, the risk of infection is higher, and extra vigilance is required to prevent and detect infections (Chapter 14).
■ After childbirth, extra vigilance will be needed to ensure that the perineum heals without infection.
■ Breastfeeding women should be particularly vigilant for signs of mastitis.

Metabolic disturbances
Corticosteroids enhance tissue breakdown and redistribute carbohydrate, fat and protein reserves. The trunk becomes fat, while the limbs become thin. Fats are released into the circulation, and plasma lipids may rise; fat embolus is a rare complication.

Practice points

■ Hyperglycaemia may occur; patients receiving oral corticosteroids, or inhaled corticosteroids over 800 micrograms/day, should be monitored.
■ Corticosteroids encourage the breakdown of glycogen and protein into glucose, and increase appetite and weight. Foods rich in salt or sugar should be avoided to reduce the risks of hypertension and dental caries.

Protein catabolism (breakdown) reduces the collagen content of all tissues, including skin and bones. Long-term use may lead to osteoporosis, muscle wasting, and mineral or vitamin deficiencies. High-dose inhaled corticosteroids have been associated with osteoporosis (Wong et al., 2000).

Thinning of the gut lining may induce peptic ulceration or gastric bleeding, particularly if aspirin, NSAIDs or alcohol are also taken. Problems have occurred in neonates.

Practice point

■ Oral corticosteroids are taken with food to reduce gastric irritation.

Dermatological problems, such as acne, sweating, thinning of skin, facial erythema, petechiae, bruising and hirsuitism, may arise with long-term systemic corticosteroids. On withdrawal of corticosteroids, dermatological conditions, particularly psoriasis, may rebound.

Cardiovascular system
Corticosteroids cause retention of sodium ions and loss of potassium ions. The associated changes in blood pressure and fluid balance are considered in relation to tocolysis.

An independent association between oral corticosteroids and pre-eclampsia was found in one study (n = 1502), not associated with adverse outcomes (Schatz et al., 1997), but not others (Schatz et al., 2004; Garbis, 2007). Associations with hypertension in pregnancy are also reported (BTS, 2008).

Central nervous system

Emotional changes such as moodiness, depression, euphoria, restlessness, insomnia, hallucinations, even suicidal ideation have been associated with corticosteroid use. Patients who resist dosage reduction should be referred to specialists (Schimmer and Parker, 2006). Decreased memory performance has been documented with oral corticosteroids at doses comparable to corticosteroid concentrations observed during severe stress (Newcomer et al., 1999).

Adrenal suppression

Two weeks of systemic corticosteroid therapy (including repeated courses of corticosteroids for fetal lung maturation) is sufficient to disrupt the pituitary/adrenal axis. After 3 weeks' administration, abrupt discontinuation of corticosteroids may cause symptoms and signs of adrenal insufficiency: weakness, depression, fever, muscle and joint pains, runny nose, red eyes, painful, itchy skin nodules, hypoglycaemia, electrolyte imbalance, anorexia, and weight loss. In severe cases, blood pressure falls rapidly and fatalities have occurred (BNF, 2009).

For patients taking oral corticosteroids, labour, severe illness, fever, surgery or trauma may precipitate symptoms of adrenal insufficiency because endogenous corticosteroid production cannot rise to meet the (tenfold) extra demands. This danger may continue for up to a year after cessation of corticosteroid therapy. Corticosteroid administration is increased or reintroduced for these emergencies. Adrenal suppression shows individual variation but occurs with inhaled doses of 1,000–2,000 micrograms/day of beclomethasone (Clark and Lipworth, 1997; BNF, 2009). Fetal and neonatal adrenal suppression may arise if the mother is receiving >10 mg prednisolone per day or equivalent (Ebden and Evans, 1996). In practice, this is rarely a problem (BTS, 2008), but close observation is advisable. Breastfed infants whose mothers are taking more than 40 mg prednisolone per day may show signs of adrenal suppression, and should be monitored (BNF, 2009).

Practice points

- To facilitate emergency admissions, it is important that 'steroid cards' are given to anyone receiving corticosteroids for more than 3 weeks.
- The risk of adrenal suppression is least when oral corticosteroids are given in the morning, as a single dose, before 9.00 a.m. This reduces the disruption to the body's circadian cycle of adrenocorticotropic hormone (ACTH) and corticosteroid secretion.
- To cover the stress of labour, additional corticosteroids may be prescribed for 1–2 days (Rey and Boulet, 2007). Women receiving prednisolone >7.5 mg/day receive parenteral hydrocortisone 6–8 hourly during labour (BTS, 2008).

Effects on the fetus

There is no evidence that inhaled corticosteroids have adverse effects on the fetus (BTS, 2008).

Prolonged treatment with oral or injected corticosteroids has been associated with: preterm birth (Laskin et al., 1997), reduced head circumference (French et al., 1999; Crowther et al., 2006) and low birth weight (CSM, 1998; Crowther et al., 2006; Crowther and Harding, 2007), even when the severity of asthma and demographic variables have been accounted for in the analysis. It is possible that preterm birth could be associated with the increased risk of infection, including subclinical intra-amniotic infection (Chapter 14) (Schatz et al., 2004; Garbis, 2007).

Repeated, but not single, courses of betamethasone were associated with a higher incidence of small for gestational age infants (Crowther and Harding, 2007).

It may not be possible to distinguish between the effects of prescribed corticosteroids and endogenous corticosteroids released as part of the stress response to severe illness or hypoxia. However, an increased risk of oral clefts has been shown in animals and retrospective cohorts (CSM, 1998; Aronson, 2006).

Practice point

■ The effects of oral corticosteroids *are offset by the advantages in severe asthma*, which can be life-threatening (Rey and Boulet, 2007; BTS, 2008).

Interactions: corticosteroids

Corticosteroids antagonize the actions of many drugs (hypoglycaemic agents, anticoagulants, antihypertensives, diuretics, and growth hormone) and intensify the actions of others (oestrogens, anticoagulants, and drugs causing potassium loss or fluid retention). The **bioavailability** of corticosteroids is effectively increased by erythromycin, ketoconazole, itraconazole, ciclosporin, and some antivirals and reduced by carbamazepine, phenytoin, rifampicin, theophylline, and co-administration with antacids, within 2 hours

Leukotriene receptor antagonists

Leutkotrienes are inflammatory mediators formed from cell membranes when tissue damage occurs. They trigger bronchospasm and other signs and symptoms of allergy. The actions of leukotrienes are blocked by leukotriene receptor antagonists, such as montelukast and zafirlukast, which are available as tablets or granules for the treatment of asthma in addition to inhaled corticosteroids if long-acting beta$_2$ agonists have failed (BNF, 2009). Manufacturers advise against use in pregnancy: there are isolated reports of limb defects, but causation has not been attributed (Garbis, 2007). A telephone interview study found serious malformations in 5/96 infants of users; however, the malformations were all different, both here and in other studies, and causation has not been established (Bakhireva et al., 2007).

Implications for practice: asthma in pregnancy

Potential problem	Management suggestions
Undiagnosed asthma causing hypoxia and IUGR	Ask all women in antenatal clinic for any history of asthma or breathing difficulties, particularly at night. Refer for lung function tests to distinguish from 'dyspnoea of pregnancy'
Poor control of asthma, causing waking during the night with coughing and even hypoxia	Records of PEFR and FEV$_1$ should be updated twice daily and checked; any decline in function or 'nocturnal dips' or waking with symptoms of asthma should be referred to the prescriber. Predicted values for PEFR measurements are not altered by pregnancy (Brancazio at al., 1997). Any changes in prescription or inhaler device should be noted
	Record the numbers and types of inhalations used daily and report to prescriber if >two inhalations of salbutamol or terbutaline are being taken per week
	Compliance should be discussed and monitored
	Maintain monitoring during the puerperium and for 6 months after birth.

V

Potential problem	Management suggestions
Rebound symptoms on withdrawal of therapy	Ensure the woman has a spare inhaler, particularly during the puerperium. Ensure inhalers are always available
IUGR, fetal distress	Monitor growth of fetus by serial ultrasound
	Use a pulse oximeter to ensure oxygen saturation remains >95%, including during delivery
Management of labour	Ensure inhalations are maintained
	Monitor lung function to anticipate any problems
	Avoid carboprost and ergometrine if possible. Discuss use of other prostaglandins with obstetricians. Use nitrous oxide as needed. Discuss the potential risks of opioids in relation to benefits during labour. Avoid general anaesthesia if possible. Be aware of case reports of asthma triggered by spinal anaesthesia (above)
	Substitute oxytocin for ergometrine as prophylaxis for the third stage
Advice on breastfeeding	Breastfeeding may help to protect the infant against asthma and eczema
	With the exception of methylxanthines (for example theophylline), asthma medications are no barrier to breastfeeding at normal doses

Implications for practice: corticosteroids in pregnancy

Potential problem	Management suggestions
Increased risk of oral thrush with inhaled corticosteroids	Use a spacer device. Gargle with water after inhalation. Attention to oral hygiene
Exposure to chickenpox	Obtain a history of chickenpox, if possible. If exposed to chickenpox, refer to physicians for prophylactic immunoglobulins. The risks are much greater if the woman is taking oral corticosteroid therapy
	Avoid contact with measles, chickenpox or shingles
Chest infections exacerbating asthma	With oral corticosteroids, a daily temperature at 5–6 p.m. should provide early indication of infection. Refer to doctors if antibiotics should be considered
Poor healing	Anticipate poor healing and contact wound care specialists promptly
	Take swabs if healing delayed
Thrombosis	Mobilize to reduce risks of DVT. Monitor FBC and risk factors for thrombosis
Adrenal suppression if oral corticosteroids are used for longer than 2 weeks	Carry 'steroid cards' in case of emergency admission
	Intravenous corticosteroids may be administered to cover the stress of labour
	Check glucose and electrolytes in neonate
	Observe neonate for appetite, weakness, lethargy, fever

Potential problem	Management suggestions
Corticosteroid adverse effects	Check electrolytes, BP and fluid balance
	Monitor weight and advise on diet
	Check plasma glucose
	Regular exercise may help to prevent or decrease muscle weakness and fatigue
	Foot care to reduce infections
	Eye disease and infections. Extra care with contact lens wearers
Effect on fetus	Monitor fetal growth
	Minimize risk of infection to reduce risk of preterm birth
	Observe neonate for signs of sepsis
	If steroid exposure *in utero* has been appreciable, ensure neonate is seen by appropriate specialists and followed up

Conclusion

Careful monitoring of airways by the multidisciplinary team is essential to pre-empt the exacerbation of asthma, particularly in the third trimester and the puerperium. Women with asthma should be reassured as to the likely outcome of pregnancy, so long as compliance is maintained. However, larger studies are needed to assess the risk of congenital anomalies associated with currently prescribed therapies (Jadad et al., 2000). Use of oral corticosteroids is accompanied by close monitoring of mother and fetus during pregnancy, labour and the puerperium. It is essential that help and surveillance are continued after delivery. This may be the most difficult time for asthmatics. Disturbed sleep and hormonal changes exacerbate asthma, waking the mother and intensifying sleep deprivation.

Further reading

■ Garbis, H. (2007) Antiasthmatic and cough medication, in Schaefer, C., Peters, P.W. and Miller, R.K. (eds) *Drugs during Pregnancy and Lactation: Treatment Options and Risk Assessment*, 2nd edn. Elsevier, Oxford.
■ Jordan. S. (2008) *The Prescription Drug Guide for Nurses.* Open University Press/McGraw-Hill, Maidenhead; Chapter 8, bronchodilators, Chapter 9, corticosteroids.

V

CHAPTER 16

Diabetes Mellitus and Pregnancy

Sue Jordan

Chapter contents

- Diabetes
- Insulin needs in pregnancy
- Insulin
- Labour and diabetes
- Breastfeeding and diabetes
- Oral hypoglycaemics

Diabetes

Diabetes mellitus is a chronic metabolic disorder, arising from insulin deficiency or insulin resistance, complicating up to 2–5% of pregnancies in the UK. Type I (juvenile onset) diabetes is characterized by an absolute deficiency of insulin, due to lack of beta cells in the islets of Langerhans; treatment is replacement therapy. Type II (maturity onset) diabetes is associated with varying degrees of insulin deficiency and insulin resistance; treatment may be by dietary control, oral hypoglycaemic drugs or insulin. To gain adequate control over blood sugar, most pregnant women with diabetes receive insulin.

Gestational diabetes arises when the woman's insulin reserves are insufficient to meet the extra demands of pregnancy. Fifty per cent of affected women develop type II diabetes in later life. Although the woman may be asymptomatic, it is important to detect gestational diabetes, otherwise fetal macrosomia (big baby syndrome) and neonatal hypoglycaemia may not be recognized and managed appropriately. In one trial, perinatal complications (death, **shoulder dystocia**, bone fractures and nerve palsy) were reduced by active management of gestational diabetes in women with plasma glucose 7.8–11.0 mmol/l 2 hours after a 75 g oral glucose tolerance test; however, in the intervention group, more neonates were admitted to neonatal nursery and more women were induced (n = 1,000) (Crowther et al., 2005). The risk of congenital anomalies is directly linked to the degree of hyperglycaemia at diagnosis (Schaefer-Graf et al., 2000). Undetected or unmanaged gestational diabetes is also associated with increased incidence of pre-eclampsia and greater weight gain in pregnancy (Crowther et al., 2005).

Some authorities argue that all pregnant women should be screened for gestational diabetes by glucose tolerance testing (Soares et al., 1997; Jarrett, 1997; Perucchini et al., 1999; van Way, 1999; Dornhorst and Frost, 2000; Greene and Solomon, 2005), but guidelines recommend screening only if one or more risk factors are identified (NCC, 2008a). The benefits of intensive investigation in women with borderline gestational diabetes (fasting plasma glucose 4.8–7.8 mmol/l) require further study (Bancroft et al., 2000).

Practice points

- Urine glucose measurements in adults are not reliable, particularly in pregnancy (NCC, 2008a).
- To screen for diabetes in pregnancy, a 2-hour 75 g oral glucose tolerance test may be arranged. This involves the woman drinking 75 g of glucose, followed by a whole blood glucose measurement 2 hours later. If this value is >6.6 mmol/l, a diagnosis is made.
- Women with gestational diabetes should be followed up and retested for diabetes 6 weeks postpartum and annually (NCC, 2008a).

Control of blood glucose

As the body alternates between the feeding and fasting states, insulin and glucagon are the main hormones keeping plasma glucose concentrations within normal limits. Insulin controls the storage and metabolism of ingested food and conserves the body's energy supplies. Without sufficient insulin, the metabolic pathways are unable to cope with ingested glucose. Directly or indirectly, insulin affects the functioning of every tissue in the body. However, other hormones regulate plasma glucose concentrations, particularly during stress.

Stress causes an increase in blood glucose, due to the release of glucagon, cortisol, growth hormone and adrenaline (epinephrine). Therefore, stressors, such as infection, labour, illness, wounds, trauma or surgery, result in hyperglycaemia. This may be reduced by epidural analgesia in early labour (Clyburn et al., 2008b).

In hypoglycaemia, adrenaline (epinephrine) is rapidly released. This brings about the classic symptoms of hypoglycaemia: sweating, nausea and nightmares, which, together, give 'hypoglycaemic awareness'. However, some people with diabetes lose hypoglycaemic awareness, and do not experience any symptoms when blood glucose falls. If these patients become hypoglycaemic, they develop, without warning, serious problems, including confusion, abnormal behaviour, convulsions, and coma. Because of these dangers, once hypoglycaemic awareness has been lost, the woman cannot receive intensive insulin therapy.

Practice points

- Healthcare professionals should discuss the loss of hypoglycaemic awareness with all women with diabetes and ensure that the family can manage hypoglycaemia.
- Particular vigilance regarding the signs and symptoms of hypoglycaemia are needed at times when hypoglycaemia is likely to occur: early pregnancy; changing insulin regimens; after delivery; and initiation of breastfeeding. Hypoglycaemia is more frequent during pregnancy (Aronson, 2006).

Insulin needs in pregnancy

Perinatal mortality rates and the incidence of pregnancy complications and major congenital anomalies are 2–15 times greater than for non-diabetics, depending on whether care is received in local hospitals or specialist settings and whether pre-pregnancy care is received (Vaughan, 1995; Casson et al., 1997; Kinsley, 2007). Outcomes for women with type II diabetes are likely to be worse than for women with type I; this may be attributed to age, obesity and cardiovascular risk factors (Kinsley, 2007). The higher the plasma glucose concentration at the first measurement in pregnancy, the worse the fetal outcome (Schaefer-Graf et al., 2000).

V

Practice points

■ Control is achieved by regular monitoring of blood glucose (1 hour after each meal and before going to bed), strict attention to diet and dose titration.

■ Women should check urine for ketones if they feel unwell.

■ Early referral to a diabetologist and obstetrician is essential.

■ Ideally, the glycosated haemoglobin A_I (HbA$_{1c}$) should be within the normal adult range (<6.1%) prior to conception to minimize the risk of congenital anomalies (NCC, 2008a).

The complications of diabetes are listed in Box 16.1.

Box 16.1 Complications of diabetes

Hyperglycaemia

1 Hyperglycaemia is not easily recognized without regular measurements of blood glucose. Women with diabetes and their families should be alert for signs and symptoms, such as inability to 'cope', fatigue, failing memory, mood changes and blurred vision. Even moderate hyperglycaemia in pregnancy can jeopardize the outcome.

2 In hyperglycaemia, glucose adheres to various proteins, disrupting them to different degrees. Haemoglobin becomes glycosylated; this is measured as HbA$_{1c}$. This measure is a reflection of the glycaemic control over the preceding 8–12 weeks, and predicts the risk of fetal malformations, particularly cardiac malformations (Vaughan, 1995). Neural tube defects are more common, therefore folate supplements are prescribed at the higher dose pre-pregnancy and screening is undertaken (Chapter 10).

3 Hyperglycaemia affects fetal growth, typically resulting in macrosomia. This, and the increased risk of shoulder dystocia, increases the likelihood of Caesarean section, to over 60% in one series (Hawthorne et al., 1997). Fetal polycythaemia may cause neonatal jaundice when red cells are haemolysed at birth.

4 Hyperglycaemia damages tissues, for example lens of the eye, nerves and joints. Nerve damage (known as diabetic autonomic neuropathy) may cause gastric paresis and hyperemesis or blood pressure instability. Women with long-standing diabetes may have stiff joints, which complicates intubation or epidural insertion (Clyburn et al., 2008b).

5 Microvascular damage occurs, affecting the retina and the kidney. Damage to the kidney causes microalbuminuria and hypertension, both of which should be monitored regularly. For women with elevated **serum** creatinine concentrations (>180 micromol/1), the prognosis is poor, in terms of pregnancy outcome, renal function, life expectancy and eyesight (Box 1.1). Serum creatinine concentrations >120 micromol/1 pre-conception indicate a need for specialist referral. Retinopathy may arise or progress rapidly during pregnancy, therefore regular examinations must be undertaken (by digital imaging) so that treatment can be initiated promptly (NCC, 2008a). Sudden development or progression of retinopathy has been linked to rapidly improved glycaemic control (Pearson, 1993).

6 White blood cells become coated with glucose, making them less able to combat infection and promote healing. Infections, such as urinary tract infection, are a common complication of diabetes, which may explain the increased risk of miscarriage. Prophylactic antibiotics may be administered after Caesarean section (Gillmer, 1996).

Disordered fat metabolism

1 Atheroma is accelerated in diabetics, increasing the risks of cardiovascular, cerebrovascular and peripheral vascular disease at all ages. Lipid profile should be monitored.

2 Blood supply to the extremities is impaired by both atheroma and microvascular damage. Placental insufficiency, polyhydramnios and pre-eclampsia occur more frequently.

Ketoacidosis

Ketoacidosis in pregnancy is an obstetric emergency, with high fetal mortality (Griffith et al., 1996). Pregnancy increases the risks of ketoacidosis. Vomiting may provoke ketosis. If vomiting cannot be prevented, admission to hospital and intensive care is urgently needed (Steel and Johnstone, 1996). The onset of impaired consciousness and confusion is usually gradual. Fetal death from acidosis may occur before the mother is seriously ill. Polyuria and vomiting lead to depletion of circulating fluids and electrolytes, and eventually circulatory collapse.

Note: the first ketone produced in ketosis (beta-hydroxybutyric acid) is not detected by standard Ketostix. Therefore, ketosis can occur and not be detected immediately.

Risks of hypoglycaemia

The fetus is dependent upon glucose not only as an energy source but also for the synthesis of lipids. This extra demand increases the mother's dietary needs by around 200–300 kcal per day (more in thin women). The drain on plasma glucose may lead to hunger in non-diabetic women and to hypoglycaemia in women with diabetes. During the first trimester, fasting plasma glucose concentrations fall by about 12%, partly due to haemodilution; this sometimes reduces insulin requirements (Gillmer, 1996). During the critical period of organ development (days 18–55), hypoglycaemia may cause congenital anomalies (Campbell and Lees, 2000).

Practice point

■ Women with diabetes should be advised against missing meals and being alone at night, when blood sugar is lowest (Steel and Johnstone, 1996).

Risks of hyperglycaemia

In the second and third trimesters, the increased secretion of oestrogens, progesterone, prolactin and human placental lactogen shifts the metabolic pathways to promote the catabolism of fats, rather than glucose. The balance of the metabolic pathways is adjusted during normal pregnancy to promote the deposition of fat stores (3–4 kg) for lactation and to ensure that the fetus receives an adequate supply of glucose as demands rise during the third trimester. From about 24 weeks, maternal tissues develop a resistance to insulin, which inhibits the uptake of glucose from the plasma. As the concentration of glucose in the plasma rises, this helps the fetus to absorb glucose. In those with a genetic predisposition to diabetes, the pancreas is unable to meet the increased demands imposed by raised blood glucose, and gestational diabetes results.

Practice point

■ In women with diabetes, this demand for extra insulin must be met by increasing dosages, usually in increments of 2 units, eventually doubling or tripling the pre-pregnancy dose. Most of the extra insulin will be taken during the day (Steel and Johnstone, 1996). Obesity is likely to further increase insulin requirements.

Normal fetuses do not produce insulin. If maternal glucose concentrations rise, the excess glucose is transferred across the placenta to the fetus. Hyperglycaemia stimulates the fetal pancreas to produce insulin, causing:

- macrosomia, increased risk of shoulder dystocia and brachial plexus injury
- congential anomalies – cardiac and neural tube defects
- delayed production of surfactant and increased risk of respiratory distress syndrome
- neonatal hypoglycaemia
- polycythaemia, leading to excess bilirubin in the neonate.

In all types of diabetes, maternal hyperglycaemia increases the incidence of congenital anomalies affecting all organ systems (Schaefer-Graf et al., 2000).

In contrast, women in whom the predominant complication of diabetes is microvascular disease (retinal and renal disease; Box 16.1) demonstrate placental insufficiency and poor fetal growth rather than macrosomia. In these women, insulin needs in the third trimester are not markedly increased (Pearson, 1993).

Management of diabetes in pregnancy

Ideally, management of diabetes in pregnancy should start with pre-conception care. Good metabolic control maintaining normoglycaemia (fasting glucose 3.5–5.9 mmol/l, 1 hour post-prandial glucose <7.8 mmol/l) over 24 hours is advised, if this can be achieved safely (NCC, 2008a). Poor glycaemic control has been associated with progression of maternal retinopathy (Lauszus et al., 2000), and if control is too strict, hypoglycaemia may prove harmful (Walkin-shaw, 2000); this was associated with three deaths in 2002–4 (CEMACH, 2005). Regular monitoring must be undertaken to adjust for the increased insulin requirements in pregnancy. It is suggested that to achieve this level of control without inducing hypoglycaemic attacks requires daily contact with healthcare professionals specializing in diabetes (Simmons, 1997).

Diet

Calories should be obtained from high-fibre carbohydrates such as rice and pasta, and intake of refined sugars, including sweets, chocolates and soft drinks, restricted. At least 30–35 kcal/kg non-pregnant ideal body weight should be eaten to prevent ketosis. To keep glucose below 6 mmol/l, adherence to this diet should be rigorous in pregnancy. Alcohol is **contraindicated** in all pregnancies but more so in women with diabetes.

It is advisable to ensure adequate intake of calcium and vitamin D, as the concentrations of these are lower in pregnant women with diabetes, and their infants (Kuoppala, 1988).

Drug therapy

For many years, women with diabetes who were planning pregnancy, pregnant or breast-feeding were advised to convert to insulin therapy. However, women with gestational diabetes or type II diabetes or polycystic ovary syndrome may be prescribed oral hypoglycaemic agents, usually metformin (NCC, 2008a).

Insulin

This essential hormone is only produced by the beta cells of the islets of Langerhans of the pancreas. It is secreted into the hepatic portal vein, and therefore acts directly on the liver. This effect is not achieved when insulin is injected into peripheral sites. In health, about 50% of the body's insulin is secreted at a basal rate, and the remainder in response to meals. It is not always possible to achieve this pattern by insulin injections.

How the body handles insulin

Insulin has a short **half-life** of 5 minutes. It does not cross the placenta. Most women administer their own insulin by subcutaneous injection. The amount of insulin absorbed depends upon site and method of administration (Box 16.2); therefore a consistent pattern of rotation must be maintained.

Practice point

■ The abdomen is a good choice for the first injection of the day, because insulin is absorbed most rapidly from here unless the person exercises.

Box 16.2 Factors affecting insulin absorption from subcutaneous injection

- *Injection:* dose, depth, site, volume (slower from large volumes). If injected into muscle, long-acting insulin may be absorbed twice as rapidly as when injected subcutaneously. Cloudy or shaken insulin will not be absorbed properly.
- *Individual:* age (slower with age), condition (slower in type II), amount of subcutaneous fat and insulin antibodies.
- *Blood supply:* skin temperature, physical activity, massage, vasodilatation (for example alcohol and pregnancy), vasoconstriction (for example nicotine and **shock**), position (standing reduces blood flow to legs and abdomen) and tissue hypertrophy. Smoking contracts blood vessels and decreases absorption of insulin.

Actions of insulin

Insulin acts on carbohydrates, fats and proteins to fundamentally alter the directions of the metabolic pathways so that sugars, fats and amino acids are stored and not burnt off. Without insulin, fats, sugars and amino acids cannot enter the cells, and therefore remain in the plasma. Consequently, the cells starve and the plasma concentrations of glucose, cholesterol and fats rise. Subsequently, some nutrients are lost *via* the urine (Box 16.3).

Box 16.3 Actions of insulin

1 *Uptake of glucose by cells* – excluding the brain, red blood cells, intestinal mucosa, renal tubules and placenta. Under the influence of insulin, the cells use glucose as a fuel, instead of fats or proteins. The main **adverse effect** of insulin is hypoglycaemia. During exercise, there is another mechanism whereby glucose is taken into exercising muscle, independent of insulin. Therefore, exercise is particularly important to people with diabetes, as it reduces insulin requirements.
2 *Increased synthesis* of glycogen from glucose in liver and muscle.
3 By removing glucose from the extracellular fluid, insulin reduces *infections*, such as thrush, and promotes wound healing. Gestational diabetes has been associated with an increased risk of wound infection following Caesarean section (Chaim et al., 2000).
4 It is said that diabetes is primarily a deficiency of *fat metabolism.* Insulin:
   ▶ promotes the formation of fatty acids in the liver and fat deposits in adipose tissue
   ▶ inhibits the breakdown of fat
   ▶ maintains low concentrations of free fatty acids, cholesterol and triglycerides in the plasma.
   Therefore, women are at higher risks of thromboembolic events in childbirth and cardiovascular events after age 30.
5 Insulin is important in preserving the *protein* of the body. It has anabolic actions, essential for growth. Unlike the fetus of a non-diabetic woman, the fetus of a diabetic woman produces insulin, promoting growth. Pregnancy in women with diabetes is associated with macrosomia, increasing the rate of Caesarean sections.
6 Insulin causes *potassium ions* to enter the cells. It is therefore important to monitor potassium ion concentration during insulin infusions. Glycosuria leads to loss of potassium and magnesium in the urine, possibly in association with diabetic nephropathy.
7 *Calcium balance:* in some women, mainly those who are poorly controlled, calcium metabolism becomes unstable. Together with low concentrations of magnesium, due to urine losses, this may suppress parathyroid function in neonates (Mehta et al., 1998). Parathyroid imbalance may be responsible for the low calcium and magnesium concentrations seen in some neonates, 24–72 hours after delivery; in extreme cases, this can lead to tetany and convulsions (Tsang et al., 1975).

V

Practice point

■ Neonates should be monitored for calcium and magnesium deficiencies, and excess bilirubin in addition to hypoglycaemia (Campbell and Lees, 2000).

If necessary, calcium gluconate is administered *slowly*, to counter hypocalcaemia or magnesium toxicity. Reported hazards include: skin sloughing, bradycardia, and asystole (Mehta et al., 1998). Careful monitoring is essential.

Type and dose of insulin are determined by specialists, according to: weight, age, growth, fitness, diet, lifestyle, other medications, any insulin antibodies, and treatment response. Insulin pens deliver between 1 and 60 units of insulin.

Unfortunately, the therapeutic range for insulin is narrow: women must steer between disabling hypoglycaemic episodes and hyperglycaemia causing long-term complications (Box 16.1).

Insulin regimens

The four types of insulin available are: fast, short, intermediate and long acting (Table 16.1). Insulin lispro, insulin aspart and insulin glulisine act more rapidly and transiently than short-acting insulin. These preparations allow women to inject themselves shortly before or after eating, rather than 30 minutes before meals. In this way, dose can be adjusted in accordance with food actually eaten, rather than planned, which is particularly important if the woman is feeling nauseous.

Table 16.1 Properties of insulin preparations (some examples)

Insulin type	Onset (minutes)	Peak (hours)	Duration (hours)	Time of injection
Fast acting				
Aspart	5–20	0.5–0.66*\n0.8–1.5**	3–5	Immediately before or soon after meals
Lispro	5–15	0.5–1.17*	3–5	Immediately before or soon after meals
Short acting				
Soluble	30–45	1.5–4	5–8	30–45 minutes before meals
Intermediate				
Isophane (NPH)	60–120	6–12	12–24	Set times of day
Insulin zinc suspension (Lente)	60–120	6–12	12–24	Set times of day
Long acting				
Insulin glargine	120, but may vary considerably	5–24 hours, no peak	18–24+	Once daily, same time

Key: * Type I diabetes; ** type II diabetes.

Sources: Figures compiled from ranges in manufacturers' data sheets (Novo Nordisk, Eli Lilly, sanofi-aventis, ABPI, 2009); Hirsch (2005); Davis (2006: 1625)

Most women with diabetes are prescribed a combination of insulins, in an attempt to replicate the physiological pattern of insulin secretion. In a randomized controlled trial in pregnant women, insulin aspart reduced both postprandial hyperglycaemia and hypoglycaemic episodes when compared to human NPH insulin (n = 322) (Mathiesen et al., 2007). Both insulin aspart and insulin lispro are considered safe for use in pregnancy (NCC, 2008a).

Some people prefer the more convenient insulin pens to traditional syringes: pens may improve compliance, but not disease control (Korytkowski et al., 2003). Insulin glargine is a long-acting insulin, injected once daily; it may reduce nocturnal hypoglycaemia.

Case report

A woman in her second pregnancy with type I diabetes was using isophane insulin. However, she was woken several times with hypoglycaemia, which resolved on injection of glucagon. Problems resolved when insulin glargine was substituted (Aronson, 2006: 1771).

However, due to lack of evidence, current guidelines continue to recommend isophane insulin (NCC, 2008a).

In pregnancy, the need for fast- or short-acting insulin usually increases. The balance between fast/short and intermediate-acting insulins may need to be adjusted, making premixed formulations unsuitable.

Practice points

- Monitoring may indicate that an extra dose of fast/short-acting insulin should be introduced as a separate injection at lunch time, allowing the early morning intermediate insulin to be discontinued.
- After 36 weeks, blood glucose tends to fall, and the evening dose of intermediate insulin may be discontinued or reduced.
- A sudden fall in insulin requirements may indicate serious placental insufficiency.
- Some women with gestational diabetes may need only one injection of intermediate-acting insulin per day, as they have sufficient endogenous hormone to maintain normoglycaemia overnight (Vaughan, 1995).

The 'dawn phenomenon' is morning hyperglycaemia; it occurs in most people, but may complicate diabetes. The timing of the evening insulin dose may need adjusting. The dawn phenomenon must be distinguished from the Somogyi effect, which is nocturnal hypoglycaemia, followed by rebound morning hyperglycaemia. This is treated by increasing the carbohydrate intake at supper time or reducing the insulin dose.

Practice points

- At least 25 g of carbohydrate are needed at supper. Blood glucose measurements at 3 a.m. are suggested to aid diagnosis of the cause of morning hypoglycaemia (Foster, 1991).
- Blood glucose testing before retiring is recommended (NCC, 2008a).

Infusion pumps have been introduced to improve glycaemic control if repeated injections are inadequate in special situations, such as pregnancy (NCC, 2008a). These have proved popular with some women, as they allow a more flexible lifestyle (Gabbe et al., 2000). Most devices deliver a continuous infusion of soluble insulin into the subcutaneous tissues of the abdomen, and bolus doses are administered at mealtimes; this provides a more physiological replacement than repeated injections. The danger of nocturnal hypoglycaemia must be assessed, because some fatalities have occurred in the USA (Foster, 1991). If extra insulin is delivered, weight gain in pregnancy is more likely (Aronson, 2006). Technical problems can also occur, such as needle displacement, kinks in the tube, abscess formation and insulin reactions at the site. Exposing the pump to sunlight and heat can inactivate the stored insulin. Pump failure may be followed rapidly by ketoacidosis (Pryce, 2009).

Adverse effects of insulin

Hypoglycaemia

The most important adverse effect of insulin is hypoglycaemia. Hypoglycaemic attacks are dangerous, and if prolonged or repeated can lead to neurological damage to the woman or neonate. The onset of hypoglycaemia may be abrupt. Women and their families should be able to recognize the prodromal signs and symptoms of hypoglycaemia (Box 16.4). Hypoglycaemia causes a loss of consciousness, which may occur suddenly. It is therefore a particular hazard for drivers, who should check blood glucose concentrations before driving and every 2 hours, and have a supply of sugar available at all times (BNF, 2009).

Box 16.4 Signs and symptoms of hypoglycaemia

- Accidents – cuts, falls or road traffic accidents
- Mood changes, aggression, behaviour disturbance, anxiety, fatigue
- Sleep disturbances, nightmares
- Night sweats, morning headaches
- Nausea, sweating, numbness
- Hunger in the young

Practice points

■ If the patient is conscious, hypoglycaemia should be managed by oral administration of 10–20g of glucose as liquid or 2–4 teaspoons of sugar or 50–100 ml of Lucozade® or Glucogel®, repeated in 10 minutes if necessary, followed by milk and a snack. An unconscious patient should receive either glucagon (below) or intravenous glucose, for example 50 ml of 20% glucose (BNF, 2009) (Chapter 2, Buccal/sublingual administration).

■ Advise patients to record the time of day of all episodes in a diary, so that any relationship to time of injection may be ascertained. Mild hypoglycaemia should be reported, because it often precedes serious episodes (Aronson, 2006).

■ Advise 'medi-alert' identification.

■ In pregnancy, fluctuating glucose levels increase the risks of driving.

■ The fetus is more tolerant of hypoglycaemia than hyperglycaemia.

■ Overstimulation of the fetal pancreas may cause persistent hypoglycaemia in the neonate, lasting 24–48 hours after delivery. Early instigation of glucose feeds and blood glucose monitoring (hourly for the first 4 hours) can control the situation. Breastfeeding is ideal.

■ After delivery, the infant is usually monitored in special care baby units (Campbell and Lees, 2000).

Glucagon

The hormone glucagon is produced by the alpha cells of the islets of Langerhans of the pancreas and by the gastrointestinal tract. In health, glucagon is secreted between meals to mobilize carbohydrate stores from the liver, as blood glucose concentrations begin to fall. Glucagon is rapidly released in response to hypoglycaemia; however, this mechanism fails in diabetes. Glucagon is sometimes administered to manage hypoglycaemia. Glucagon is given by injection (by any route) in hypoglycaemic emergencies where intravenous glucose in impractical. However, it will be ineffective in chronic hypoglycaemia or starvation, as there will be no carbohydrate stores available to mobilize.

Weight gain is associated with insulin administration. This may worsen diabetes, increase the risk of cardiovascular disease and impact on compliance (DCCTRG, 2001).

Antibodies to insulin

The production of insulin antibodies is minimized (but not eliminated) by the use of human insulin. Antibodies delay and reduce the actions of insulin, necessitating higher doses. Insulin antibodies may cross the placenta and damage the fetal pancreas; therefore non-human insulin is rarely used in pregnancy.

Blurred vision

Changes in visual acuity may occur on initiation of insulin. It is usually transient.

Site reactions

Irritation at the injection site may be managed with antihistamine or hydrocortisone creams. Both lipoatrophy and lipohypertrophy cause irregular absorption of insulin. Lipohypertrophy is fat deposition and storage due to overexposure to insulin. Lipoatrophy is rarer, and is an immune response. Regular rotation of injection sites reduces these problems.

Postural hypotension, which may result from diabetic autonomic neuropathy, is exacerbated by insulin.

Practice point

■ Blood pressure should be monitored closely if drugs with potential to lower blood pressure are administered, for example opioids and local anaesthetics.

Drug interactions: insulin

Drug interactions may raise or lower blood glucose (Appendix 1). The following are possible:

- *Hyperglycaemia* is associated with: thiazides, thyroid hormones, amphetamines, cocaine, salbutamol, large quantities of caffeine, growth hormone, oestrogens, chlorpromazine, clozapine, olanzapine, lithium, corticosteroids, calcium channel antagonists, danazol, marijuana, nicotine, and medicines containing sugar.
- *Hypoglycaemia* is associated with: ACE inhibitors, salicylates (effects minimal), anabolic steroids, monoamine oxidise inhibitors, lithium, octreotide, disopyramide, cyclophosphamide, pentamidine, pyridoxine, and tetracyclines (rare).
- *Excess alcohol consumption* prolongs and/or delays hypoglycaemia. Any alcohol should be taken with food and limited to 2–3 drinks/day. Avoid driving (Baxter, 2006).
- *Beta blockers* and clonidine may: mask the warnings of hypoglycaemia, delay recovery from hypoglycaemia, and cause hypertension during hypoglycaemia.

- Diabetes complicates the management of *premature labour*. Beta$_2$ agonists (such as ritodrine) are contraindicated. The fetal lungs are particularly likely to be immature, but the administration of steroids dramatically increases the woman's requirements for insulin (Chapter 7).
- *Nicotine* reduces insulin absorption by causing vasoconstriction.

Labour and diabetes

In the past, the problems posed by placental insufficiency, macrosomia, shoulder dystocia and pre-eclampsia have discouraged obstetricians from advising vaginal delivery. The woman should be in a position to make a fully informed decision on mode of delivery (Boulvain et al., 2000).

Insulin needs fall rapidly with the onset of active labour and again on delivery of the placenta. Hence the demands for insulin and glucose change dramatically. If capillary blood glucose falls outside the range 4–7 mmol/l, insulin and dextrose will be infused (NCC, 2008a). This necessitates two separate intravenous infusion lines. (The infusions are incompatible.) Insulin is infused with sodium chloride or compound sodium lactate (BNF, 2009). Only soluble insulin is used in intravenous infusions. Insulin is not added directly to fluid bags (NICE, 2004a).

Practice points

- The tendency for insulin to adhere to plastic tubing means that infusion is unpredictable and must be titrated against the patient's response.
- Monitoring of capillary blood glucose should be undertaken hourly and maintained when insulin is discontinued.
- Blood glucose monitoring is needed to detect the fall in insulin requirements after delivery (NCC, 2008c).

Effective analgesia is important, and epidural infusions are recommended to reduce stress (NCC, 2008a). Continuous fetal heart rate monitoring is used routinely. Glucose infusion is continued until the next meal eaten without vomiting, as there is a danger of hypoglycaemia in the first 48–72 hours (Vaughan, 1995; Pangle, 2000).

Breastfeeding and diabetes

Breastfeeding reduces insulin requirements to below pre-pregnancy values and necessitates a high carbohydrate intake, for example snacks during feeding. Care should be taken to avoid hypoglycaemia when feeding at night. Although breastfeeding benefits the mother, careful glucose monitoring is required. The amount of insulin transferred to the neonate is considered too small to be harmful.

Metformin passes into breast milk. Manufacturers advise against breastfeeding, but the BNF (2009) does not contraindicate breastfeeding. Premature infants and those with poor renal function should not be breastfed by mothers taking metformin (Aronson, 2006).

Oral hypoglycaemics

Current guidelines sanction the administration of some oral antidiabetic agents, including metformin and glibenclamide (NCC, 2008a). Some of the other sulphonamides have been associated with congenital anomalies (Aronson, 2006). There is no evidence, to date, of **adverse events** associated with metformin in early pregnancy in women with polycystic ovary syndrome (Gilbert et al., 2006; Elizur and Tulandi, 2008) or type II diabetes (Ekpebegh et al., 2007). Animal studies have not demonstrated **teratogenicity** (Merck Serono, ABPI, 2009).

Actions and adverse effects: metformin

Metformin decreases glucose formation in the liver and enhances insulin's actions in fat and muscle. This reduces blood glucose concentrations without triggering weight gain.

Gastrointestinal disturbance

Most oral antidiabetic agents can cause gastrointestinal upset. A metallic taste may be experienced. Emesis or diarrhoea may make metformin intolerable.

Practice points

- Administration with meals may reduce nausea; when initiating therapy, increase dose gradually.
- Advise women that problems may ameliorate within a few weeks.

Long-term metformin may reduce absorption of vitamin B_{12} and folates. Monitoring and possible supplementation should be discussed with the prescriber (Davis, 2006).

Lactic acidosis

Metformin inhibits liver enzymes, including those that metabolize lactic acid, and can, rarely, allow this to accumulate, causing 'lactic acidosis'. Risks of lactic acidosis are increased if the patient becomes unwell or dehydrated, stops eating, intakes excess alcohol or develops renal impairment/pre-eclampsia.

Practice points

- If the patient develops fever, dehydration, sepsis, urinary tract infection or a cardiovascular event, seek urgent medical advice regarding administration.
- Women should be advised to avoid dieting or prolonged fasting.
- If diabetes is worsening, medication review should be sought.
- Check serum creatinine and creatinine clearance (Box 1.1): pre-therapy; during illness or suspected dehydration; if antihypertensives, diuretics or NSAIDs are co-prescribed; and regularly.
- Ensure the obstetric and anaesthetic team are aware of metformin administration, and medication for labour is planned. Medication may need review before labour.

Cautions and contraindications: metformin

- *Metformin is not prescribed* if the patient is dehydrated, prescribed diuretics, shocked or renal function tests indicate poor creatinine clearance or high serum creatinine (Box 1.1). It is not suitable for women who develop pre-eclampsia.
- *Liver impairment* and *heart failure* preclude administration of metformin.
- *Respiratory failure, anaemia or vascular disease* increase the risk of lactic acidosis.
- *Malnourished* patients require reduced doses. Metformin is less suitable for patients who fast for prolonged periods or adopt restrictive diets.
- *Hypothyroidism* or Addison's disease may increase the risk of hypoglycaemia.

V

Implications for practice: diabetes in pregnancy and childbirth

Potential problem	Management suggestions
Congenital anomalies and fetal loss	Maintain normoglycaemia from pre-conception
	Pre-conception folate supplements
	Ultrasound screening for congenital heart conditions
Hypoglycaemia	Rest and small meals. Minimize nausea
	Do not miss meals. Avoid alcohol
	Carry glucose and glucagon at all times. Instruct partner in administration
	Measure 3.00 a.m. blood glucose if nightmares or night sweats occur
	Evaluate risks of driving
Vomiting	Reduce nausea. Replace carbohydrate. Immediate referral on vomiting
Hyperglycaemia from 24 weeks	Monitor blood sugar. Be prepared to increase fast-acting or soluble insulin
	Aim for weight gain as in normal pregnancy
	Ensure client understands insulin regimen and injection administration techniques
Vascular disease	Antenatal examination for cardiovascular disease, which could compromise labour. Risk of thromboembolism (Chapter 8)
Ketoacidosis and fetal loss	Regular monitoring, regular diet, avoid alcohol
Diabetic retinopathy	Normoglycaemia, pre-conception and during pregnancy
	Retinal examinations and treatment by specialists
Diabetic nephropathy	Monitor urine for microalbuminuria and albumin loss Monitor serum creatinine
Increased risk of pre-eclampsia	Monitor BP very closely
Placental failure	Obstetricians may advise delivery at or before 39 weeks. Fetal monitoring
Macrosomia	Normoglycaemia during pregnancy. Establish definite date of conception
Shoulder dystocia	Prepare for Caesarean section
Fetal lung immaturity	Neonatal intensive care available
Neonatal hypoglycaemia	Immediate feeds, preferably breastfeeding, and at least every 2–3 hours
	Monitor blood glucose hourly for 4 hours, and 4-hourly for 48 hours
	Ensure tube feeds and intravenous dextrose available
Neonatal hypocalcaemia or hypomagnesaemia	Monitor if indicated. Calcium and magnesium injections available
Neonatal polycythaemia or hyperbilirubinaemia	Monitor if indicated. Exchange transfusion facilities available
Infections	Urine testing, skin inspection, prophylactic antibiotics, good breastfeeding technique essential to prevent abscesses
Poor control of diabetes	Monitor the cardiovascular system, kidneys, eyes, dental health, growth, thyroid function, celiac disease (NICE, 2004a)

Conclusion

Although considerable progress has been made in specialist centres, women who are diabetic run a high risk of obstetric and medical complications. Successful outcome of pregnancy requires meticulous attention to diet, monitoring and insulin regimens, which in turn demand commitment from both multidisciplinary teams and clients.

Further reading

- Jordan, S. (2008) *The Prescription Drug Guide for Nurses*. Open University Press/McGraw-Hill, Maidenhead; Chapter 16, insulin, Chapter 17, oral antidiabetic drugs.
- NCC (National Collaborating Centre for Women's and Children's Health) (2008) *Diabetes in Pregnancy: Clinical Guideline July 2008*. Commissioned by NICE. RCOG Press, London.

V

CHAPTER 17

Thyroid Disorders in Pregnancy

Sue Jordan

This chapter discusses thyroid imbalance and its recognition in pregnancy. Other endocrine disorders are mentioned briefly.

Chapter contents

- Thyroid hormones
- Thyroid function tests (TFTs) in pregnancy
- Hyperthyroidism
- Hypothyroidism
- Other endocrine disorders

Thyroid disease is the second commonest endocrine abnormality encountered in pregnancy; some 1–2% of pregnant women may be affected (Alexander et al., 2004; Cotzias et al., 2008). Like other endocrine disorders, thyroid imbalance may be a cause of infertility, but pregnancy can occur without correction of thyroid imbalance. Recognition of thyroid disorders in young women is not always easy, particularly when they arise *de novo* in pregnancy.

Thyroid hormones

The main function of the thyroid gland is to produce thyroid hormones – thyroxine (T_4) and tri-iodothyronine (T_3). In the tissues, T_4 is converted to T_3. Most of the actions of thyroid hormones are attributed to T_3. Thyroid disease disturbs the balance of thyroid hormone secretion, which upsets the regulation of:

- metabolic rate and heat production
- the central and peripheral nervous systems
- the sympathetic nervous system
- heart rate and cardiac contractility
- the absorption of glucose from the gastrointestinal tract
- reproduction and fertility
- the development of the central nervous system
- growth.

In health, the thyroid gland is controlled by thyroid-stimulating hormone (TSH) from the anterior pituitary gland, which, in turn, is controlled by thyrotropin-releasing hormone (TRH) from the hypothalamus. The release of TSH and TRH is regulated in a negative feedback mechanism by circulating thyroid hormones (T_4 and T_3). Raised TSH is associated with thyroid underactivity (hypothyroidism), while low or suppressed TSH indicates thyroid overactivity (hyperthyroidism).

Pregnancy and the associated increase in oestrogens almost immediately place additional demands on the thyroid gland. Normally, human chorionic gonadotropin from the placenta increases thyroxine secretion by 30–50% by weeks 16–20; however, women with underactive thyroids or subclinical thyroid disease are unable to meet the additional demands (Alexander et al., 2004).

The fetus is dependent on maternal thyroid hormones for the first 13 weeks. Therefore, the fetus is vulnerable to maternal thyroid disorder during the crucial stage of organogenesis when the woman may not realize she is pregnant.

Practice points

- Insufficient thyroxine in early pregnancy is associated with adverse outcomes (below).
- Women with thyroid disease or a history or family history of thyroid disease should contact their primary care team to organize thyroid function tests (TFTs) and optimize therapy before conception.
- Due to the high concentration of oestrogens associated with assisted reproduction, these women are more vulnerable to hypothyroidism (Alexander et al., 2004).

Fetal thyroid function becomes independent of the mother after 13 weeks' gestation. However, iodine and antithyroid drugs cross the placenta. Therefore:

- maternal iodine deficiency causes neonatal cretinism
- radioactive iodine (sometimes used to treat hyperthyroid conditions) destroys the fetal thyroid
- large doses of iodine cause fetal goitre.

Practice point

- Handling or application of iodine-containing preparations such as povidone iodine while pregnant or breastfeeding may allow sufficient iodine to enter the circulation to cause fetal goitre.

Several drugs interfere with the secretion, distribution and metabolism of thyroid hormones, and may affect thyroid status or TFTs. Examples include corticosteroids, heroin, methadone, lithium, amiodarone, iodine (including topical preparations), carbamazepine, NSAIDs, beta blockers, and interferons (British Thyroid Association, 2006).

Thyroid function tests (TFTs) in pregnancy

TFTs are undertaken on diagnosis of pregnancy when there is a current thyroid disorder, a personal or family history of thyroid disorder, type I diabetes, goitre, high cholesterol concentration or clinical suspicion of an abnormality. Ideally, such women should have their thyroid function tested when they plan to become pregnant. At present, it is not considered feasible to screen all pregnant women for thyroid disorders, but this is under discussion (British Thyroid Association, 2006).

Thyroid hormones exist in two forms: free and bound to plasma proteins (mainly thyroid-binding globulin). Only the free hormones are active (Chapter 1). When interpreting TFTs in pregnancy, it should be remembered that a goitre may be physiological and the concentrations of thyroid hormones are altered in normal pregnancy:

- the total quantity of thyroxine in the circulation is increased in the first trimester, but the concentration may be unchanged, due to the expanded plasma volume
- TSH is reduced between weeks 9–12
- in the last trimester, the concentrations of the free hormones are reduced (Girling, 1996).

Free thyroxine and tri-iodothyronine concentrations should be measured: raised and lowered concentrations are indicative of hyper- and hypothyroidism respectively. TFTs are interpreted in relation to the normal values for pregnancy, but there is no consensus as to treatment thresholds (Cotzias et al., 2008) (Table 17.1).

Practice points

When blood is taken from a pregnant woman for TFTs:
- free hormone concentrations must be requested
- thyroid antibody status should be included for women with type I diabetes
- it must be clearly stated on the form that the patient is pregnant
- dose and time of any thyroid-related medications must be noted
- all medications taken must be noted, as several interfere with TFTs.

Table 17.1 Diagnostic tests for thyroid function

Test	Normal values*	
	Non-pregnant	**Pregnant**
Free serum thyroxine (T_4)	9–25 pmol/l	10–16 pmol/l (first trimester)
		8–14.5 pmol/l (third trimester)
Total serum thyroxine (T_4)	60–160 nmol/l	64–142 nmol/l
Thyroid-stimulating hormone (TSH)**	0.4–4.5 mU/l**	0.4–2.0 mU/l (first and second trimesters)
		0.5–4.0 mU/l (third trimester)
Free serum tri-iodothyronine (T_3)	3.5–7.8 pmol/l	3–7 pmol/l (first trimester)
		2.5–5.5 pmol/l (third trimester)
Total serum tri-iodothyronine (T_3)	1.2–2.6 nmol/l	1.0–2.6 nmol/l
Thyroid peroxidise antibodies	Presence suggests Hashimoto's thyroiditis or Graves' disease or a high risk of these	
TSH receptor antibodies	Presence suggests Graves' disease	

Key: * Exact values depend on the laboratory undertaking the tests; ** some authors suggest that the upper limit of normal should be 2.5 mU/l.
Sources: British Thyroid Association (2006); Cotzias et al. (2008)

Hyperthyroidism

Hyperthyroidism affects individuals in a variety of ways. The insidious onset of the disease may allow it to go unrecognized for years. The classic symptoms of heat intolerance, sweating, increased appetite, nervousness, insomnia, irritability and short temper can also be features of normal pregnancy, also the hands usually feel warm and the pulse is rapid and bounding. A tremor may be seen if the fingers are outstretched. Other common, and easily overlooked, features of hyperthyroidism include: fatigue, muscle weakness or cramps, overactive reflexes, and increased frequency of bowel movements. Infrequent blinking and eyelid retraction give the classic 'staring' appearance of thyrotoxicosis. Inadequately treated hyperthyroidism is associated with miscarriage, low birth weight, pre-eclampsia, and fetal and neonatal hyperthyroidism.

In pregnancy, the thyroid gland may be palpably enlarged but the diagnosis of hyperthyroidism may be difficult, as a small goitre in pregnancy is normal, and does not usually indicate disease. Abnormal TFTs and hyperthyroidism before the 18th week of pregnancy are usually due to physiological changes of pregnancy, and may be associated with hyperemesis; there is no specific treatment. The commonest cause of hyperthyroidism in non-pregnant women is Graves' disease, which requires specialist management in pregnancy. It is distinguished from physiological hyperthyroidism by detection of thyroid receptor antibodies in venous blood samples (Muller et al., 2008).

Practice point

- Hyperthyroidism should always be considered if hyperemesis occurs, and TFTs undertaken (Abalovich et al., 2007). However, patients with hyperemesis gravidarum may have abnormal thyroid function test results without thyroid disease: therefore, it may be necessary to measure thyroid antibodies to assess the possibility of Graves' disease (Kametas and Nelson-Piercy, 2007).

If the mother has or has had Graves' disease, her autoantibodies cross the placenta. This may induce a goitre in the fetus and hyperthyroidism in the neonate. This is rare, but antibodies should be measured to assess this possibility. Fetal growth, goitre, cardiac function and heart rate are monitored regularly by ultrasound. Untreated neonatal hyperthyroidism carries a poor prognosis, and, in extreme cases, fetal goitre may obstruct the airway or impede delivery. Therefore these infants are carefully monitored.

Management of hyperthyroidism in pregnancy

Like other **autoimmune diseases**, hyperthyroidism may remit during pregnancy and rebound after delivery. Drug regimens must be monitored and adjusted accordingly. Subclinical hyperthyroidism is not treated in pregnancy (Abalovich et al., 2007). Hyperthyroidism is treated by antithyroid drugs alone, under specialist supervision. Antithyroid drugs cross the placenta, but thyroid hormones do not, therefore a blocking replacement regimen would render the fetus hypothyroid. Propylthiouracil is sometimes preferred to carbimazole because there is less placental transfer, and there may be fewer problems with breastfeeding (British Thyroid Association, 2006), and congenital anomalies (Aronson, 2006). The minimum effective dose is prescribed, often leaving a mild degree of maternal hyperthyroidism (Fitzgerald, 1995). Full TFTs should be taken prior to conception, on diagnosis, at booking, at least monthly, and after delivery (Hague, 1995; British Thyroid Association, 2006).

Antithyroid drugs may suppress fetal thyroid hormone production and stimulate TSH production, leading to fetal goitre and hypothyroidism. This is more likely with higher doses. In addition, there are reports of associations between carbimazole and methimazole and aplasia cutis and other congenital anomalies (Aronson, 2006).

Although carbimazole is generally well tolerated by the mother, it has the potential to cause **agranulocytosis**, and patients are advised to inform their doctors should they develop any signs of infection, particularly a sore throat. If agranulocytosis is suspected, a venous blood sample should be taken for a white cell count (BNF, 2009). Carbimazole may also cause nausea, rashes and hair loss.

If hyperthyroidism cannot be controlled by drugs, surgery is considered during the second trimester. However, ingestion of iodide in preparation for surgery may induce fetal goitre. Radio-iodine is **contraindicated** in pregnancy, breastfeeding and in children; 4 months should elapse between radioiodine treatment and pregnancy. Some endocrinologists prefer to avoid radioiodine in women under 40 (Conway and Betterbridge, 1996).

Uncontrolled or unrecognized hyperthyroidism may cause cardiac failure or even a thyroid storm. This emergency carries a high mortality rate and is managed in intensive care. High-risk situations include stress, labour, infection, trauma or operative delivery.

Note: a thyroid storm/crisis is a rare medical emergency, where very high concentrations of circulating thyroid hormones cause hyperpryrexia, delerium and extreme cardiovascular stress.

Breastfeeding

Both propylthiouracil and carbimazole appear in breast milk, and can cause thyroid enlargement and hypothyroidism in the infant. The transfer of propylthiouracil to breast milk is considered to be too low to damage the infant. Breastfeeding may be permissible with low-dose carbimazole. If possible, feeds should be given just before the mother takes the antithyroid drugs. The infant's development and thyroid function must be monitored (BNF, 2009), with the involvement of a paediatrician (Girling, 1996). Both iodine and technetium pass into breast milk and are concentrated in the thyroid gland of the infant; accordingly, women treated with radioactive isotopes of these elements are advised to discontinue breastfeeding.

Hypothyroidism

The thyroid gland may be unable to meet the extra demands of pregnancy. This may be recognized by increased TSH concentration in TFTs. Increased TSH production can lead to enlargement of the pituitary gland. Pregnancies in women with untreated hypothyroidism are at increased risk of hypertension or haemorrhage, miscarriage or premature birth, which may be due to the associated increased susceptibility to infection (Fitzgerald, 1995). In women with subclinical thyroid disease, prematurity and first trimester miscarriage can be substantially reduced by treatment with thyroid hormone replacement therapy (13/58 versus 4/57 and 8/58 versus 2/57) (Negro et al., 2006). Subnormal neonatal neurological, psychomotor and auditory development and low IQ are associated with untreated hypothyroidism in pregnancy (Hague, 1995; Glinoer and Abalovich, 2007).

Pregnancy-induced hypertension complicates 22–44% of pregnancies in hypothyroid women (Montoro, 1997). Some features of hypothyroidism, such as weight gain, tiredness, lethargy, constipation, goitre, fluid retention, memory loss, and joint pains, are easily confused with normal pregnancy; therefore TFTs are important in making a diagnosis. (In hypothyroidism, TSH is raised and free thyroid concentrations are reduced.)

Hypothyroidism is managed with thyroxine replacement therapy. If women are overtreated with thyroxine, the signs and symptoms of hyperthyroidism appear (see Implications for practice). Most authors emphasize the importance of regular monitoring of thyroid function (Montoro, 1997), and expect thyroxine requirements to rise by 30–50% in 85% of women with hypothyroidism during pregnancy. Some suggest that all women receiving thyroxine replacement therapy increase their dose by 30% as soon as pregnancy is confirmed (Alexander et al., 2004; Muller et al., 2008). Others suggest that overreplacement of thyroxine may be harmful and thyroxine doses should be adjusted according to the TSH concentration, rather than automatically increased (Girling and Nelson-Piercy, 2007). While some authorities consider TSH up to 4.0 mU/l as normal, others advocate therapy if TSH rises to 2.0 mU/l (British Thyroid Association, 2006; Glinoer and Abalovich, 2007), allowing a rise to 3.0 mU/l in the third trimester (Abalovich et al., 2007). Neonatal encephalopathy, with permanent sequelae, may occur more frequently in hypothyroid women who do not receive regular monitoring during pregnancy (Badawi et al., 2000).

Practice points

- As soon as women with hypothyroidism are confirmed pregnant, and again at booking, a blood sample should be taken for TFTs and a specialist referral arranged. A minimum of one full TFT each 4–6 weeks until the second trimester is suggested (British Thyroid Association, 2006; Glinoer and Abalovich, 2007).
- Women should be asked about any pre-pregnancy increases in thyroxine dose and noncompliance. These women are more likely to need an increase in thyroxine dose during pregnancy (Kothari and Girling, 2008).

Thryoxine requirements usually decline in the 2–6 weeks after birth, but may remain above pre-pregnancy levels during lactation. Breastfeeding is not contraindicated with replacement therapy.

Practice point

- Thyroid function should be monitored for 6 months after birth, with the first blood sample at 2–4 weeks.

Postpartum thyroiditis

Up to 5% of women are affected by this transient or permanent disorder in the first year after birth or pregnancy loss, although the diagnosis is often unrecognized, which causes much unnecessary distress. Postpartum thyroiditis is an autoimmune disorder, and many affected women develop thyroid disease later in life. Autoantibodies inflame and enlarge the thyroid gland, initially releasing thyroid hormones into the circulation and causing hyperthyroidism. This hyperthyroid phase is usually self-limiting and may not require treatment. Some 4–8 months later, the damaged thyroid is unable to maintain thyroxine output and hypothyroidism develops. This may be permanent and necessitate replacement therapy. Treatment of the hypothyroid phase may improve quality of life by relieving the symptoms of tiredness, lethargy and depression (Girling, 1996).

Practice point

- Women with signs and symptoms of thyroid disorder following delivery require long-term annual follow-up for hypothyroidism and specialist referral for subsequent pregnancies (British Thyroid Association, 2006; Muller et al., 2008).

Hypothyroidism may present with vague symptoms of tiredness or postpartum depression, and may arise any time within the first year of birth (Campbell and Lees, 2000).

Practice points

- TFTs may be indicated in women with postpartum depression, as hypothyroidism is readily treatable.
- Hypothyroidism may cause psychosis and hallucinations, which, without TFTs, can be mistaken for postpartum mental illness.

■ Untreated hypothyroidism causes failure of lactation. If this is suspected, TFTs are essential.

■ Women with thyroid antibodies or type I diabetes should be screened for postpartum thyroiditis at 3 and 6 months (Abalovich et al., 2007).

Neonates

Within a few days of postpartum life, TFTs assume adult values. All neonates have TSH measured at 2–7 days by a blood spot test. A positive screening result is rapidly followed by further blood tests in mother and infant. Treatment of neonatal hypothyroidism must be started within 18 days (British Thyroid Association, 2006).

Implications for practice: thyroxine sodium

Regular follow-up, assessment and blood tests are essential. When the patient is stabilized, annual appointments may be sufficient.

Potential problem	Management suggestions
Excessive doses	
Tachycardia	Instruct patients to check radial pulse weekly
	If resting pulse is above 85–100 bpm or irregular, withhold next dose and seek medical advice
Chest pain caused by myocardial ischaemia	ECG pre-therapy and follow-up
	Therapy is initiated cautiously, and evaluated regularly
	If patients report chest pain, withhold and inform prescriber. Dosage reduction may be necessary
	Ensure anaesthetic teams are informed of medication
	Advise 'medi-alert' identification
Cardiac dysrhythmia causing palpitations or syncope (fainting)	Monitor radial pulse and apex beat, simultaneously, to detect atrial fibrillation
	Arrange ECG if irregularities detected
Heart failure, poor exercise tolerance	Careful assessment and individualized dosage adjustments
Tremor	Ask patient to stretch out hands and fingers to assess any tremor. Inquire about difficulties with activities, such as writing
Restlessness, excitability, irritability, short temper, hypomania/mania Interpersonal skills and relationships may be affected	Advise patient to report these problems as they may indicate that dosage is excessive. Arrange TFTs
Insomnia	Administer thyroxine sodium first thing in the morning
Diarrhoea/nausea	Contact prescriber if bowel movements become more frequent than 3/day or if nausea develops
Increased absorption of glucose Hyperglycaemia within the first 2 hours after a meal	Check blood glucose on initiation of therapy and during medication review. Advise patients with diabetes to monitor glucose. Be prepared to increase insulin doses
Pyrexia, heat intolerance, sweating, flushing, muscle cramp or weakness	Arrange TFTs and report to prescriber
Weight loss despite increased appetite	Record weight weekly
Hair loss	Usually reverses as thyroid function normalizes

Increased risk of osteoporosis	No (or minimal) extra risk if thyroid status remains normal
Underdose of levothyroxine	
Tiredness, constipation, excessive menstrual loss, weight gain, depression, hair loss, dry skin	Assess patient. Monitor TFTs and serum cholesterol, which should be within normal range
	Emollients may help dry skin
	Dosage requirements increase during serious illness; arrange TFTs
On initiation of therapy	
Diabetes and adrenal disorders may be unmasked	Obtain venous blood samples to assess glucose and electrolytes
Diuresis for a few days	Warn patients. Ensure access to facilities
Therapeutic failure	
Slow initial response	Advise that it may take 4–6 weeks for benefits to be experienced. Arrange TFTs 4–6 weeks after each change of dose
The **half-life** of thyroxine is about 7 days, and full effects will not be achieved for 5 weeks. As metabolic rate increases, the rate of hormone clearance increases, and higher doses may be needed	Skin and hair texture may not return to a healthy 'normal' for 6 months
	Consider drug interactions (below)
Blood tests are within the normal range, but patient continues to feel unwell	Consider referral to specialist for consideration of regimen change, such as addition of liothyronine (Gitlin et al., 2004; Aronson, 2006)

Allergic reactions to levothyroxine are very rare.

Cautions and contraindications: thyroxine sodium

- If hypothyroidism has gone undiagnosed for a long time, adverse reactions are more likely; therefore, initial and incremental doses are lower.
- Disorders of the pituitary or adrenal complicate management. Seek specialist advice.
- Diabetes may be worsened.
- Missed doses – avoid administering 2 doses close together. If therapy is suspended for >7 days, symptoms of hypothyroidism are likely to appear.

Interactions: thyroxine sodium

Advise patients to inform all prescribers of thyroid hormone therapy and to seek advice from pharmacists before buying non-prescription products.

In health, opioids increase TSH production; however, opioids decrease TSH production in people suffering from stress or hypothyroidism (Ogrin and Schussler, 2005). Women with hypothyroidism may be extremely sensitive to sedatives and opioids; accordingly, some authorities advise avoiding preoperative sedation for elective surgery (Wall, 2002).

Practice point

■ Women with hypothyroidism may be unusually sensitive to opioids and may be severely sedated if administered an average dose of opioids, for example 50 mg pethidine for pain relief in labour (Malseed et al., 1995).

Other interactions include:

- Salbutamol, terbutaline, ketamine, dopamine, adrenaline/epinephrine, 'cold cures', amphetamines, and cocaine increase the risk of cardiac problems.
- Tricyclic antidepressants may increase the risk of cardiac dysrhythmias or alter thyroid function.
- Warfarin: anticoagulant dose may need reduction. Monitor blood clotting closely, particularly 4–6 weeks after changes in thyroid hormone dose.
- Oestrogens increase the dose requirements.
- Some antiepileptic drugs, rifampicin, some antimalarials and sertraline may reduce, and some antiviral drugs may increase, the effects of thyroxine. Thyroid function should be monitored carefully (McCowen et al., 1997).
- Digoxin and theophylline dose requirements vary according to thyroid status.
- Thyroid status may be altered by: lithium, quetiapine, amiodarone, interferons, steroids, and carbamazepine.
- Absorption of thyroxine is reduced by: preparations containing iron, aluminium or calcium, sucralfate, proton pump inhibitors, and soya protein. Administration should be separated by 4 hours.

Practice point

■ If iron or calcium supplements or antacid preparations are commenced, these should be at lunch time or later. Earlier administration may result in the woman becoming hypothyroid. Anaemia has many causes, including hypothyroidism.

Conclusion

If thyroid function is well controlled, the outcome of pregnancy is likely to be good. However, poorly controlled thyroid disease may result in intrauterine growth retardation, premature labour, increased perinatal mortality, or congenital abnormalities. It is important that healthcare professionals are aware of the protean and often confusing manifestations of thyroid disorders, and instigate the prompt measurement of thyroid function.

Other endocrine disorders

Pregnant women known to suffer from relatively rare conditions, such as adrenal or parathyroid disorders, will be referred to tertiary centres. Diagnostic difficulties can arise if endocrine disorders present for the first time in pregnancy. For example, raised blood pressure may be the only clue to an adrenal tumour. Disorders of the parathyroid glands and calcium metabolism are particularly threatening to the fetus (see de Swiet, 2002, Chs 13 and 14, for further information).

Further reading

■ British Thyroid Association (2006) *UK Guidelines for the Use of Thyroid Function Tests.* British Thyroid Association, www.british-thyroid-association.org.
■ Jordan, S. (2008) *The Prescription Drug Guide for Nurses.* Open University Press/McGraw-Hill, Maidenhead; Chapter 18.

Epilepsy in Pregnancy

Jennifer Sassarini, Nick Clerk and Sue Jordan

This chapter considers the difficult question of epilepsy in pregnancy. Many drugs prescribed for epilepsy are also prescribed in the management of mental illness. The reader will find that knowledge of the central nervous system and the normal physiological changes of pregnancy will facilitate understanding of this chapter.

Chapter contents

In 2001, a survey of the quality of information provision to women with epilepsy (n = 2,000) indicated that the most important issues for women aged 19–44 who were considering having children were:

- risk of epilepsy/medication affecting the unborn child (87%)
- effect of pregnancy on seizure control (49%)
- risk of the child developing epilepsy (42%) (NICE, 2004b).

V

Practice point

- All women should be counselled appropriately, in a timely manner, and helped to make informed choices about their treatment.

Epilepsy

Epilepsy is the commonest serious chronic neurological condition, occurring in 0.4–1% of the population (Hauser et al., 1996; Clinical Standards Advisory Group, 2000). Most of those affected, including women of child-bearing age, will require long-term treatment with antiepileptic drugs (AEDs) to prevent seizures. Three to four pregnancies in every 1,000 occur to women with active epilepsy (Dansky and Finnel, 1991; Olafsson et al., 1998), affecting 1,800–2,400 children each year in the UK.

Epilepsy is a long-term disorder characterized by recurrence of seizures that are often unprovoked and unpredictable (McNamara, 2006: 501). An epileptic seizure or fit is the result of a temporary physiologic dysfunction of the brain, caused by an abnormal electrical discharge of brain cells. There are different kinds of seizures. Each type is associated with a characteristic behavioural change and electrophysiological disturbance, usually detected by electroencephalography (EEG).

Note: a seizure is a transient alteration of behaviour due to disturbance of the firing of neurones in the brain, occurring in acute medical or neurologic illness.

Epilepsies can be classified as follows:

■ *Partial (focal) seizures:* These seizures originate from one part of the brain and may spread to become generalized seizures. These may or may not be associated with loss of consciousness.
■ *Generalized seizures:* These seizures involve the brain diffusely at onset. There is usually impaired consciousness and involuntary muscular activity.
■ *Unclassified seizures:* These do not fall into the first two groups and include neonatal seizures and febrile convulsions (Engel, 2001).

Practice point

■ When an epileptic fit occurs for the first time in the second half of pregnancy, eclampsia has to be excluded as a cause.

Untreated epilepsy may progress, therefore most specialists will prescribe an antiepileptic drug after 1 or 2 confirmed epileptic seizures, depending on the risk of recurrence (McNamara, 2006).

Pregnancy may influence the course of epilepsy by altering the seizure frequency. Epilepsy and its treatment with antiepileptic drugs (anticonvulsants) can also affect the course and outcome of pregnancy.

Effect of pregnancy on epilepsy

There is some evidence that the effect of pregnancy on seizure frequency can be predicted from the degree of pre-pregnancy control: women with long pre-pregnancy seizure-free periods are less likely to convulse in pregnancy (Donaldson, 1995).

In pregnancy, seizure frequency increases in some 35% of women due to hormonal changes, changes in the concentration of antiepileptic drugs in the circulation (Chapter 1; Morrell 2003), noncompliance, often due to fear of **teratogenesis**, sleep deprivation and alcohol consumption.

■ Changes in concentrations of oestrogens and progesterone can alter the threshold for seizures. Oestrogens are thought to decrease seizure threshold, whereas progesterone decreases neuronal excitability (Morrell, 1992).

▨ Changes in serum electrolytes (the decreased sodium and magnesium concentrations found in pregnancy) can predispose to seizures (Klingman, 1954).

▨ Concentrations of antiepileptics are reduced by:

  ▪ Expansion of the maternal extracellular fluid volume as well as development of an 'extra' fetal compartment.

  ▪ Reduced intestinal absorption, due to: reduced intestinal motility, and adsorption (binding) by medicines commonly used in pregnancy, such as antacids, notably gabapentin and phenytoin (BNF, 2009).

  ▪ Increased elimination of antiepileptics, which can result from a combination of decreased plasma protein binding and increased renal excretion (Chapter 1).

  ▪ Increased metabolism of drugs by maternal and fetal hepatic (liver) **enzymes** and the placenta (Lander et al., 1977).

Practice points

■ Relatives should know how to manage a fit, most particularly to place the patient in the recovery position once the fit is over. Pregnant women who are at risk of fits should be advised not to bathe alone. Ignoring such simple procedures may have contributed to maternal deaths (DH, 1998: 116).

■ Following a fit, the woman will be banned from driving for 1 year (BNF, 2009).

Physical and mental stress in labour can increase seizure frequency (Torbjörn and Vilho, 2007). Around 2–5% women with epilepsy experience seizures during labour or delivery (Tomson and Hillesmaa, 2007).

Effect of epilepsy on pregnancy

Although several obstetric complications have been reported to occur more frequently in women with epilepsy, there is little evidence to support these observations. Several authors have reported an increased rate of obstetric intervention during the delivery of women with epilepsy (Swartjes et al., 1998).

Generalized seizures are potentially dangerous for mother and fetus. Tonic-clonic seizures can cause fetal hypoxia and acidosis (Lipka and Burlow, 2003) and cardiotocographic changes have been described (Paul et al., 1978). Seizures in early pregnancy may cause hypoxic damage to the embryo and result in malformations. Cognitive defects in infants may be linked to the number of seizures in pregnancy (Byrne, 2001). Maternal experience of five or more tonic-clonic seizures in pregnancy is associated with an increased risk of developmental delay in exposed infants (Adab et al., 2004) and decreased verbal IQ (Harden, 2007).

Seizures are associated with risks of injury and, particularly if untreated, prolonged seizures can progress to **status epilepticus**, which carries an uncertain prognosis. The UK Confidential Enquiry into Maternal Deaths has identified women with epilepsy as at particular risk, reporting 11 deaths from 2003 to 2005. Six of these women met the criteria for sudden unexplained death in epilepsy (SUDEP), and a further two were reported as possibly due to SUDEP (DH, 2007).

Antiepileptic drugs (AEDs) and congenital anomalies

Up to 90% of infants born to women with epilepsy will be normal with appropriate management. When compared to the general population, women prescribed valproate or polytherapy have a two- to threefold increased risk of adverse outcomes, including: stillbirth, fetal loss prior to 20 weeks, congenital anomalies, and reduced birth weight, length and head circumference (Perucca, 2005).

Practice point

■ Women with epilepsy should be informed that although they are likely to have healthy pregnancies, their risk of certain complications during pregnancy and labour is higher than for women without epilepsy.

The potential for birth defects and delayed development due to AED exposure is recognized; however, there are still uncertainties about the precise risk (Winterbottom et al., 2007) especially for the newer AEDs (Adab et al., 2004). The UK Epilepsy and Pregnancy Register confirmed that the risk from major congenital malformation was significantly higher for infants exposed to multiple, rather than single, AED regimens. The crude rate for major congenital malformations with any polytherapy exposure was 6.0%, compared to 3.7% for pregnancies exposed to a single AED, with valproate posing the highest risk to the fetus, particularly at doses above 800–1,000 mg/day (Table 18.1) (Morrow et al., 2006).

Table 18.1 Risk of congenital anomalies

Valproate	6.2–13.3%
Carbamazepine	2.2–5.2%
Lamotrigine	1.4–4.4%
Phenobarbital	6.5%
Phenytoin	3.2–6.8%
Topiramate	0–7.1%

Sources: Data extracted from birth registries, with inconsistent definitions of anomalies; Tomson and Hillesmaa (2007); Walker et al. (2009)

The potential risks from AED treatment must be balanced against the potential risk from seizures in pregnancy.

Older antiepileptic drugs

The commonest major congenital malformations associated with established AEDs are:

■ neural tube defects (valproate 3%, usually severe open lumbosacral defect with hydrocephalus, carbamazepine 1%)
■ congenital heart anomalies
■ palatal and lip clefts
■ skeletal deformities and hypospadias (Rosa, 1991; Samrén et al., 1997).

The risk of minor malformations or anomalies including hypertelorism, epicanthic folds and digital hypoplasia is also increased (Holmes et al., 2001).

'Fetal anticonvulsant syndromes', comprising typical dysmorphic craniofacial appearances and a variety of musculoskeletal abnormalities, have been described. Features of fetal phenytoin syndrome include microcephaly and growth deficiency, with or without craniofacial and cardiac malformation (Clayton-Smith and Donnai, 1995; Moore et al., 2000). There is also a reported risk of malignant tumours in children with a history of intrauterine exposure (Singh et al., 2005).

For polytherapy combinations containing valproate, the major congenital malformation rates are between 2 and 3 times higher than combinations not containing valproate. Risks increase appreciably if the valproate dose exceeds 800–1,000 mg/day, with a rate of 9.1% at 1,000 mg (Morrow et al., 2006). These doses are not unusually high for treatment of either epilepsy or bipolar disorder. Effects on the fetus can be severe, and a 'fetal valproate syndrome' has been described, including: facial dysmorphic features, impaired psychomotor development, neural tube defects, digital defects, phocomelia, and urogenital malformations.

The impact of antiepileptics taken during pregnancy on the child's intellectual development is uncertain, but there are concerns over the effects of valproate on infant development, including autism (Duncan, 2007).

Some studies report no overall increased risk of congenital anomaly and developmental delay in association with carbamazepine monotherapy (Robert-Gnansia and Schaefer, 2007). However, effects on the fetus can be severe, and include: a 1% risk of neural tube defects, craniofacial defects, microcephaly, digital defects, cardiac malformations, hypospadias, and developmental delay.

Newer antiepileptic drugs (AEDs)

The safety of newer AEDs in pregnancy is yet to be established. Newer AEDs are no more effective, but are better tolerated than older drugs, and are indicated if seizure control has been difficult (Ben-Menachem, 2008). Lamotrigine has a spectrum of efficacy similar to valproate and is increasingly being prescribed as an alternative in epilepsy and mental illness. Infants exposed to lamotrigine alone are more likely to suffer major congenital malformations as the dose increases. However, at doses of 200 mg/day or less, lamotrigine has an overall lower risk of teratogenicity than valproate (Morrow et al., 2006). The major congenital malformations are similar to those associated with other AEDs; however, orofacial clefts, genitourinary abnormalities, for example hypospadias, and unusual gastrointestinal defects, such as duodenal and oesophageal atresia, appear to be more common. Pregnancy register data indicate an increased risk of orofacial clefts with lamotrigine compared to non-medicated controls – 5 cases occurred in 584 first trimester exposures (0.89%) (Shor et al., 2007).

Animal studies indicate that gabapentin, oxcarbazepine, tiagabine, topiramate and zonisamide may be teratogenic, and levetiracetam at high doses was associated with skeletal abnormalities and growth retardation, but no gross malformations. A report of 55 exposures to oxcarbazepine (20 polytherapy and 35 monotherapy) noted only one case of major congenital malformation (Morrow et al., 2006). Topiramate may only be prescribed if benefit outweighs risk (BNF, 2009).

Practice point

■ To reduce the risk of teratogenicity, in monotherapy, antiepileptic drugs are prescribed, where possible, as slow-release preparations or divided doses to avoid drug concentration peaks in maternal plasma.

Causes of malformations and anomalies

Although antiepileptics have been extensively studied, the mechanisms of teratogenesis are not clear (Lee and McManus, 1995). Genetic factors, both fetal and parental, probably play a part, as evidenced by the high rate of recurrence in sibships (Moore et al., 2000). Valproate may cause teratogenesis by altering gene expression during development.

One proposed mechanism of teratogenesis is folic acid deficiency (Pennell and Hovinga, 2008). Folic acid is a cofactor in the synthesis of DNA and cell division. Some antiepileptics decrease serum folate concentrations by decreasing absorption and accelerating hepatic metabolism. Low serum folate concentrations have been associated with increased rates of malformation, most specifically neural tube defects. Up to 90% of women receiving phenytoin, carbamazepine or barbiturates have reduced serum folate concentrations. Folate supplementation in these women can reduce the incidence of neural tube defects by up to 60% (Mulinare, 1988), but as few as 11% are taking folate supplementation appropriately (Fairgrieve et al., 2000) (Chapter 10).

V

Practice point

■ Women prescribed AEDs should consult specialists, as they may require folic acid supplementation at the higher dose, 5 mg (the usual dose is 400 micrograms), preferably pre-conception (BNF, 2009).

However, some authors question the role of folic acid deficiency in neural tube defects associated with antiepileptics (Byrne, 2001; Morrow et al., 2008). Another possible mechanism involves the formation of unstable oxides or **free radicals**, with known mutagenic properties, during the metabolism of antiepileptics. These oxides can be teratogenic and a genetic defect in the pathways responsible for their metabolism can contribute to fetal malformations. (The enzyme epoxide hydrolase is deficient.) The oxides can also be neutralized by antioxidants, including vitamin C. There is some evidence to suggest that low socioeconomic status in women with epilepsy increases the risk of teratogenesis, possibly *via* malnutrition (Malone and D'Alton, 1997; Blume, 1997).

Practice point

■ It would seem advisable to optimize the dietary intake of vitamin C by eating five portions of fresh fruit and vegetables each day. Dietary intake should be checked for consistency with health promotion guidelines.

Tests on fetal cells obtained by amniocentesis can determine the susceptibility of the fetus to toxic metabolites (Byrne, 2001).

Antiepileptic drugs (AEDs)

Therapy of epilepsy generally has three goals (Pedley et al., 1995):

1 To eliminate seizures or reduce their frequency to the maximum extent possible.
2 To avoid the **adverse effects** associated with long-term therapy.
3 To assist the woman to achieve normal psychosocial and vocational adjustment.

Drug therapy is the main treatment for epilepsy. Antiepileptic drugs should be prescribed when the risks of treatment outweigh the harms of uncontrolled seizures. The ideal antiepileptic would suppress seizures without causing any untoward effects to either woman or fetus. Drugs in current use eliminate or reduce seizures in about 75% of patients but frequently cause adverse effects. In the first year of therapy, 15% of patients prescribed an AED will experience an adverse reaction sufficiently severe to warrant changing therapy (McNamara, 2006). The degree of therapeutic success depends on several factors, such as seizure type, family history, neurological abnormalities, patient compliance and drug **pharmacokinetics**, which are notably altered in pregnancy (Breen and Davenport, 2006; Torbjörn and Vilho, 2007). There is often a very narrow therapeutic range between fits and sedation (Figure 1.1). For some people, even a delayed dose can allow seizure breakthrough.

Actions of antiepileptic drugs

AEDs reduce the activity of neurones (nerve cells) in the central nervous system. Each neurone's activity depends on the balance between positive and negative ions entering the cell. This balance may be disturbed in epilepsy and certain neurones repetitively generate action potentials; this is known as 'repetitive firing'. Drugs restore the balance or 'calm down' the neurones by decreasing the number of positive ions entering the cells or increasing the number of negative ions entering the cells. While this reduces the number of fits, it also suppresses the normal functions of the central nervous system. This may lead to sedation, incoordination or, in overdose, depression of vital signs.

There are four main mechanisms by which antiepileptics exert their effects:

1 Epilepsy and overactivity (or repetitive firing) of neurones are associated with excess sodium ion or calcium ion entry. Entry of these ions is blocked by some antiepileptics (carbamazepine, oxcarbazepine (very similar to carbamazepine), phenytoin, and lamotrigine). Since these ions are required by many cells, these drugs affect most body systems.
2 Enhancing the inhibitory **neurotransmitter**, gamma-aminobutyric acid (GABA). This increases the number of negative (chloride) ions entering the neurones. Some drugs (valproate, gabapentin and tiagabine) increase the amount of GABA in the **synapse**. Benzodiazepines and barbiturates increase the number of negative chloride ions entering the neurones, by acting on the GABA receptor.
3 Lamotrigine also acts by reducing the release of the excitatory neurotransmitter, glutamate.
4 Antiabsence antiepileptics (ethosuximide and valproate) act on calcium ion channels to inhibit neuronal transmission in the thalamus (the region of the brain just above the mid-brain), which plays an important role in the generation of electrical waves characteristic of absence seizures (McNamara, 2006).

AEDs depress neuronal activity throughout the brain, causing some degree of sedation and impaired coordination. Many newer AEDs, valproate and carbamazepine have been associated with an increased risk of suicidal ideation or behaviour, affecting 1 in 530 patients, particularly in the first weeks of therapy.

Practice point

■ Women prescribed AEDs for any reason should be monitored for excessive sedation or notable change in routine behaviour, particularly during vulnerable periods. Changes may include anxiety, aggression, and a preoccupation with dying (FDA, 2008).

AEDs interact with each other in a complex manner.

Two broad groups of antiepileptic drugs will be described: the older 'first-generation' drugs and the newer but less tried 'second-generation' drugs.

First-generation (older) antiepileptic drugs (AEDs)

With the exception of phenobarbitone, plasma concentrations are useful in monitoring therapy. These drugs are metabolized in the liver and excreted by the kidneys.

A detailed consideration of each of the commonly prescribed antiepileptics is outside the scope of this book, but relevant information, not all of which is readily available elsewhere, is summarized below.

Carbamazepine

Carbamazepine (Tegretol®) is commonly prescribed for partial seizures, secondary generalized seizures and trigeminal neuralgia. It is occasionally prescribed for management of bipolar affective disorders, but its efficacy has been questioned (Soares-Weiser et al., 2007).

Adverse effects of carbamazepine

Some of the unpleasant effects of carbamazepine may subside within the first few weeks of use. Acne and hirsuitism may affect the woman's body image, a problem that may be intensified in pregnancy and the puerperium. Other adverse effects include:

- *central nervous system:* dizziness, double vision, headaches, drowsiness, confusion or agitation. Some types of seizure may be worsened
- *eyes:* glaucoma
- *gastrointestinal tract:* nausea, dry mouth, decreased appetite, diarrhoea or constipation, cholestatic jaundice
- *skin:* rash, acne, hair loss or hirsuitism, hypersensitivity reactions
- *cardiovascular system:* **cardiac dysrhythmias**, thromboembolism, oedema
- *metabolic:* hypocalcaemia with rickets and osteomalacia, vitamin K and folic acid deficiency
- **hyponatraemia** (Chapter 6)
- *hypersensitivity responses:* these include bone marrow damage, enlarged lymph nodes, low white cell count (usually benign), **thrombocytopenia** (reduced platelet count), liver or kidney damage, and skin reactions (see lamotrigine, below).

Practice points

- Any signs of sore throat, fever, abnormal bruising or bleeding should be reported to the prescriber immediately. A full blood count should be arranged as an urgency.
- Weight gain in pregnancy must be monitored carefully if appetite is impaired.
- Supplements of folic acid, calcium, vitamin D and vitamin K may be advised. Transfer of vitamin K to the fetus/neonate is poor, and some authorities do not recommend maternal vitamin K supplementation. Intramuscular vitamin K should be administered at birth (Walker et al., 2009).

In overdose, carbamazepine also causes tremors, excitation, convulsions, BP changes and cardiac dysrhythmias.

Practice point

- Kidney and liver function should be monitored to ensure that the woman is able to eliminate carbamazepine (Robert-Gnansia and Schaefer, 2007).

Most drugs interact with carbamazepine. **Adverse effects** are enhanced by several drugs, including alcohol, antidepressants, erythromycin, cimetidine and grapefruit juice. The effectiveness of many drugs is reduced, including oral contraceptives (Chapter 1), nifedipine, corticosteroids, thyroid hormones, paracetamol, tramadol, and methadone (BNF, 2009).

There is no consensus on breastfeeding. The amount excreted in breast milk is probably too small to be harmful (BNF, 2009), but the neonate should be observed for tiredness, weakness or vomiting (Schaefer, 2007d).

Valproate

Valproate (Epilim® and Depakote®) (in various forms) is prescribed for generalized seizures, partial seizures and management of bipolar disorder. However, there is an increased risk of major congenital malformations (valproate 6.2% compared to lamotrigine 3.2% and carbamazepine 2.2% monotherapy) and developmental delay compared to other AEDs (Morrow et al., 2006).

Reviewers advise caution in the prescription of valproate to women planning to become pregnant, and suggest that other equally effective and safer AEDs should be considered (Aronson, 2006; Morrow et al., 2006), unless valproate is the only drug providing adequate seizure control (Tomson and Hillesmaa, 2007). Lamotrigine has a similar spectrum of efficacy, and has been suggested as an alternative in certain patient groups.

Adverse effects of valproate

Valproate is generally well tolerated; however, serious liver disorders or bleeding problems can arise:

- *central nervous system:* ataxia, tremors, sedation, hyperactivity and hallucinations
- *gastrointestinal tract:* increased appetite and weight gain, gastric irritation, liver dysfunction and pancreatitis
- *skin:* rash, acne, hirsuitism and transient hair loss
- *blood:* thrombocytopenia and inhibition of platelet aggregation, leucopenia and erythrocytopenia
- *cardiovascular system:* oedema
- *liver damage:* rare, but reported in neonates (Robert-Gnansia and Schaefer, 2007)
- *reproductive system:* high concentrations of androgens cause amenorrhoea, decreased libido, impaired fertility, and polycystic ovaries in susceptible women (more so than carbamazepine or gabapentin) (Morrell, 2003)
- *metabolism:* risk of fracture.

Neonatal respiratory distress and a withdrawal syndrome with severe hypoglycaemia have been reported.

Practice points

- In certain cases, with expert assessment, the dose of valproate can be lowered, or given in smaller doses more frequently, if the woman is seizure free and still in the first trimester.
- Weight should be monitored to pre-empt excessive weight gain.
- Any bruising and bleeding should be reported to the prescriber and a full blood count should be arranged urgently.
- Liver function tests are advisable, as pregnancy may compound any hepatic abnormalities.
- Oedema should be reported to prescribers: it should not be dismissed as a physiological response to pregnancy.
- Severe vomiting and abdominal pain should be reported to the prescriber, as it could represent pancreatitis or liver dysfunction. A venous blood sample for serum amylase and glucose estimations should be urgently arranged.
- Delivery should take place where paediatricians are available. Neonatal blood glucose should be monitored (Ebbesen et al., 2000).
- Dietary calcium and vitamin D should be optimized (Morrell, 2003).

In overdose, valproate causes sedation, loss of consciousness and respiratory depression, which may be fatal.

Drugs interacting with sodium valproate include: anticoagulant drugs, erythromycin, antipsychotics (including prochlorperazine), and antidepressants.

The literature offers no consensus on breastfeeding. The **half-life** of valproate is prolonged in breastfed infants, particularly in the first 10 days of life; therefore the drug may accumulate. A case is reported of a breastfed infant developing a low platelet count and anaemia, which resolved on the discontinuation of breastfeeding (Chaudron and Jefferson, 2000).

Phenytoin

Phenytoin (Epanutin®) is indicated for partial and generalized seizures, except absence seizures. It is occasionally used in the management of status epilepticus and cardiac dysrhythmias. Phenytoin is becoming less popular, due to its narrow therapeutic range, complicated pharmacokinetics, serious adverse effects and numerous drug interactions.

Adverse effects of phenytoin

Adverse effects of phenytoin include:

- *central nervous system:* **nystagmus**, slurred speech, ataxia, confusion, twitching, nervousness, insomnia and dystonic reactions
- *gastrointestinal tract:* nausea, vomiting and constipation
- *skin:* morbilliform rash with fever, bullous dermatitis, hirsuitism, **toxic epidermal necrolysis**
- *face:* gingival (gum) and lip hyperplasia and coarsening of facial features
- *blood:* megaloblastic anaemia responsive to folic acid, aplastic anaemia, lymphadenopathy thrombocytopenia, leucocytopenia, erythrocytopenia
- *metabolic:* hypocalcaemia with rickets and osteomalacia, vitamin K deficiency, folate deficiency
- *other:* systemic lupus erythromatosus, Dupuytren's contracture.

Practice points

- The physiological changes of pregnancy and the puerperium alter the plasma concentration of phenytoin. The woman should be carefully checked for signs of central nervous system toxicity, such as balance problems and confusion.
- Scrupulous attention to dental hygiene is required to minimize the risk of unsightly gum hyperplasia. (This problem occasionally arises with carbamazepine.)
- Vitamin supplements may be needed (see carbamazepine).

In overdose, phenytoin causes hyperglycaemia, nystagmus, ataxia, dysarthria, coma, cardiac dysrhythmias, hypotension and respiratory depression. The lethal dose is 2–5 g, which is 4–10 times the maximum recommended daily dose.

The literature offers no consensus on breastfeeding. While some authorities consider the amount of drug passed into breast milk too small to be harmful, manufacturers advise against breastfeeding (BNF, 2009).

Most drugs interact with phenytoin, including oral contraceptives, alcohol, antacids and other antiepileptics.

Benzodiazepines

Intravenous lorazepam and diazepam (Diazemuls® and Valium®), summarized in Table 18.2, are the benzodiazepines commonly used in the emergency treatment of epileptic seizures. Diazemuls® is diazepam formulated to reduce the risk of thrombophlebitis, associated with the intravenous administration of benzodiazepines. Benzodiazepines are also prescribed for short-term management of acute anxiety (Chapter 19).

Table 18.2 Diazepam and epilepsy: a summary

Indication	Treatment of epileptic fits. Not currently favoured for seizure prophylaxis
Preparations	Per rectum 0.5 mg/kg body weight, intravenous, 10–20 mg slowly
Contraindications	Previous drug sensitivity, respiratory depression, severe hepatic impairment
Adverse effects	Hypotension, respiratory depression
	Thrombophlebitis if administered into a vein (Chapter 2)
Overdose	CNS and severe respiratory depression, coma
Fetal effects	CNS and respiratory depression
	Neonatal withdrawal symptoms (long-term use)
	Hypotonia and hypothermia
Breastfeeding	Avoid if possible, too sedating (BNF, 2009)

Practice points

■ Diazemuls® or an alternative benzodiazepine should be available and protocols should be in place in the event of a seizure during or following labour.
■ Should intravenous benzodiazepines be administered in labour, fetal heart rate is likely to be abnormal for about 1 hour (Walker et al., 2009).
■ Facilities for resuscitation of mother and neonate must be in place.

Midazolam, as buccal liquid, is gaining popularity for management of seizures in some settings (Walker, 2005), following training (NICE, 2004b), but it remains unlicensed (BNF, 2009).

Barbiturates

Barbiturates, including primidone, are prescribed as drugs of 'last resort'. All barbiturates are sedating and interfere with learning. They also interact with several nutrients, resulting in a deficiency of vitamins D and K. Supplementation is necessary for both mother and neonate. Some authorities consider that barbiturates are less teratogenic than other antiepileptic drugs. However, the neonate may experience a severe withdrawal reaction. Breastfeeding is **contraindicated**.

Ethosuximide

Ethosuximide is prescribed for absence seizures. Since these often resolve in adulthood, and most prescribers review the need for medication as the woman approaches reproductive age, it is rarely encountered. Ethosuximide is associated with an increased risk of bleeding. It may be teratogenic. Breastfeeding is not advised by manufacturers (BNF, 2009).

Newer antiepileptic drugs (AEDs)

The newer or second-generation drugs include gabapentin, lamotrigine, oxcarbazepine, tiagabine, topiramate, levetiracetam and vigabatrin; these were appraised by NICE (2004b). Three further AEDs have been marketed in the UK since 2000, namely pregabalin, rufinamide and lacosamide (BNF, 2009). Animal studies on many of these AEDs are encouraging in comparison with the earlier drugs but human data are sparse (Morrow et al., 2006).

The International Lamotrigine Pregnancy Register's initial results are based on 334 pregnancies exposed to lamotrigine in the first trimester. They indicate that major congenital malformations occurred in 3/168 (1.8%) women receiving monotherapy and 10/166 (6.0%) women receiving polytherapy (Morrow et al., 2006).

Lamotrigine

Lamotrigine (Lamictal®) was first marketed in 1991 for patients with partial or generalized seizures. It blocks release of glutamate and modulates sodium ion channels. Concentration of lamotrigine may decrease by more than 50% during pregnancy, and return to pre-pregnancy values within 1–2 weeks of delivery (Tomson and Battino, 2007). Changes are lessened when carbamazepine is co-prescribed (Anderson, 2006). Regular (for example monthly) venous blood samples are needed in pregnancy and every few days postpartum; doses are adjusted accordingly (Brodtkorb and Reimers, 2008).

Adverse effects of lamotrigine

The adverse effects of lamotrigine include:

- *central nervous system:* dizziness, headache, ataxia, nystagmus, sleepiness or insomnia, confusion, tremor, nervousness, movement disorders, worsening seizures, tics
- *vision:* double or blurred vision, conjunctivitis
- *gastrointestinal tract:* nausea, vomiting and diarrhoea
- *hypersensitivity responses:* usually urticarial or maculopapular rash, occur in some 10% of patients, usually in the first 8 weeks of therapy (higher incidence in polytherapy). There are reports of **toxic epidermal necrolysis**, **Stevens Johnson syndrome**, and lymphadenopathy, which usually necessitate withdrawal (Aronson, 2006)
- *blood:* aplastic anaemia, thrombocytopenia, leucocytopenia, erythrocytopenia, disseminated intravascular coagulation are all rare
- *liver or pancreas damage:* see valproate
- *other:* systemic lupus erythromatosus, Dupuytren's contracture.

Practice point

- Patients who develop a rash should have their temperature taken and be seen by a doctor as soon as possible, always within 24 hours. Severe rash will necessitate hospital admission (Aronson, 2006).

Lamotrigine crosses the placenta and passes into breast milk. Concerns have been expressed regarding the possibility of infants developing rashes (Chaudron and Jefferson, 2000); however, breastfeeding is not contraindicated (BNF, 2009).

The concentration of lamotrigine is reduced by oestrogens and progestogens, whether from the placenta or the oral contraceptive pill. Lamotrigine also reduces the efficacy of the contraceptive pill (Schwenkhagen and Stodieck, 2008).

Levetiracetam

Levetiracetam (Keppra®) is prescribed for treatment of partial seizures, as adjunctive therapy for generalized seizures, and for refractory partial epilepsy. Its mode of action is currently thought to involve modulation of **neurotransmitter** release.

Like lamotrigine, the concentration in the serum decreases during pregnancy by up to 50%. Therapeutic drug monitoring and dosage adjustment may be required (Brodtkorb and Reimers, 2008). Levetiracetam crosses the placenta and passes into breast milk. It is generally well tolerated.

Adverse effects of levetiracetam

These include:

- *central nervous system:* emotional lability/irritability, behaviour disturbance, psychosis, dizziness, double vision, ataxia, tremor, headaches, drowsiness, fatigue or confusion, worsening seizures
- *gastrointestinal tract: nausea*, decreased appetite, diarrhoea, abdominal pain
- *skin:* rash, hair loss
- *blood:* very rarely, thrombocytopenia (reduced platelet count), leucocytopenia (reduced white cell counts), aplastic anaemia
- *immune system:* infections, colds, urinary tract infections.

Practice points

- The adverse effects of levetiracetam should not be mistaken for mental illness.
- Weight gain and food intake should be carefully monitored in pregnancy.

Withdrawal of antiepileptic drugs

Discontinuation of therapy may induce seizures, even status epilepticus, or behaviour disturbance.

Practice points

- If a dose has been omitted, a seizure may occur 2–3 days later.
- If no fits have occurred for 2–4 years, prescribers may gradually withdraw medication over 9–13 weeks or several months. Driving is not recommended during this time and for 6 months afterwards (BNF, 2009).
- Monitor patients for a recurrence of seizures during withdrawal and for 12 months.

Case report

Accurate appreciation of changing dose requirements facilitates care.

Following seizures at 27 weeks' gestation, a woman's dose of carbamazepine was increased from 600 to 800 mg/day. This was decreased immediately after delivery. Death occurred 17 days later. Carbamazepine was below the therapeutic range at postmortem.

This patient had followed advice, but the advice had been dangerously inaccurate and there was no evidence of therapeutic drug monitoring. Return to pre-pregnancy doses may be needed by end of the first week postpartum (Freyer, 2008) or not until 6–8 weeks after delivery (DH, 1998: 130).

Practice point

- Venous blood samples may be required every few days in the postnatal period if drug doses have been increased during pregnancy (Tomson and Battino, 2007).

V

Neonates of women taking antiepileptics frequently experience drug withdrawal reactions, which make breastfeeding difficult to establish (Schwartz, 1998). Breastfeeding may allow gradual withdrawal from *in utero* AEDs. However, infants are less efficient than adults at drug elimination and need to be carefully monitored.

Management of epilepsy in pregnancy

Management of epilepsy in pregnancy aims to reduce the risks of teratogenicity, while maintaining seizure control despite the physiological changes of pregnancy.

Pre-conception

Consideration should be given to:

- deferring pregnancy until seizure control is optimal
- re-evaluating the need for antiepileptic
- antiepileptic monotherapy, if possible
- obtaining venous blood samples to establish the concentration of antiepileptic at which therapy is optimized. This will serve as a baseline for comparison with samples in pregnancy
- folic acid supplementation (5 mg daily), under supervision
- lowest possible antiepileptic dose, in divided doses, if possible (Nulman et al., 1999)
- genetic counselling referral
- risks associated with medication and the methods of anomaly detection.

Pregnancy

Consideration should be given to:

- care by obstetrician and neurologist/epileptologist
- ultrasound screening for congenital abnormalities at 11–13 weeks and mid-trimester (Walker et al., 2009)
- continuing high-dose folic acid (5 mg) supplementation
- vitamin D and calcium supplements
- screening for congenital anomalies (ultrasound and blood tests) (Macara, 2008)
- monitoring antiepileptic concentrations in venous blood samples (most AEDs); dosage adjustment if clinically required, rather than routine increase of AED doses
- close obstetric monitoring for known complications, for example fetal growth restriction
- appropriate treatment of seizures
- oral vitamin K supplementation in the third trimester if certain AEDs are prescribed.

Labour and childbirth

Consideration should be given to:

- delivery in hospital with neonatal intensive care facilities
- one-to-one midwifery care during labour
- continuation of prescribed antiepileptics
- establishing intravenous access on admission to labour ward to facilitate management of any seizures
- avoiding factors predisposing to increased risk of seizures as much as possible – stress, exhaustion, pain, sleep deprivation, overbreathing and dehydration
- checking drugs administered in labour for drug interactions and seeking expert advice
- low threshold for epidural anaesthesia

- prompt treatment of seizures using parenteral administration of AEDs if necessary
- active management of third stage – risk of bleeding
- avoiding fetal scalp blood sampling if possible – risk of bleeding
- frequent tonic-clonic seizures are an indication for elective Caesarean delivery (Tomson and Hillesmaa, 2007)
- labouring in water is not recommended (Walker et al., 2009).

Postpartum

Consideration should be given to:

- all infants should receive vitamin K_1 1 mg intramuscular at birth (Chapter 8)
- examining neonate for congenital abnormalities and signs of central nervous system depression
- observation of neonate for antiepileptic withdrawal symptoms
- all mothers should be encouraged to breastfeed (NICE, 2004b), except in unusual circumstances. Discuss expressing breast milk to allow family members to give night-time feeds, thus minimizing sleep deprivation. Exercise caution with combination therapy, barbiturates, ethosuximide and benzodiazepines. There are few data for newer antiepileptics (Walker et al., 2009)
- offering extended hospital puerperium or discharge home to adequate domestic support
- offering practical advice on care to avoid trauma to mother and neonate, for example change nappies on the floor, avoid bathing infants alone, slings and stair climbing
- monitoring antiepileptic concentrations from venous blood samples. Dosage adjustment may be required
- contraceptive options. Some antiepileptics reduce the efficiency of all oral hormonal contraceptives as well as progesterone implants (Chapter 1)
- consultant follow-up for 3–6 months to: monitor seizure control and AED blood concentrations, and supervise dose titration towards pre-pregnancy dose requirements (Breen and Davenport, 2006; Torbjörn and Vilho, 2007; Battino and Tomson, 2007; Montouris, 2007; Walker et al., 2009).

Implications for practice: epilepsy in pregnancy

Potential problem	Management suggestions
Increased risks of seizures	Records of seizures should be maintained
	Discourage abrupt discontinuation of antiepileptics
	Ensure the family are able to manage seizures
	Minimize stress, allow plenty of rest and undisturbed sleep
	Avoid leaving the woman alone in a single room at night
	Some drugs, including some antidepressants, antipsychotics (prochlorperazine), metoclopramide, prostaglandins, quinolones, antimalarials, St John's wort, amphetamines, high doses of caffeine (used for management of postdural puncture headache (Chapter 2), increase the risks of seizures
Need to adjust medication	Advise that AED requirements are likely to increase during pregnancy and fall postnatally
	Ensure appropriate venous blood samples are taken, as directed
	Arrange help, if needed, for women to attend all appointments
	Advise regarding hazards of driving during periods of dose adjustment (increase and decrease)

Potential problem	Management suggestions
Appearance of adverse effects when doses are changed	Observe for adverse effects, particularly drowsiness/tiredness, constipation or nausea, which may be mistaken for signs and symptoms of pregnancy
	Women prescribed carbamazepine or phenytoin should be checked for nystagmus
Loss of oral medication during vomiting – oral medications are lost if vomiting occurs within 3 hours of administration	If vomiting occurs, ask the woman to note the time in relation to medication administration. Report problems to prescriber. If vomiting is severe, discuss alternative routes of administration, for example rectal carbamazepine for up to 7 days
Drug-induced nausea	Advise taking new tablets or increased doses with food to reduce the risk of nausea
Appetite changes	Monitor weight gain. Valproate may cause excessive weight gain, whereas carbamazepine may suppress appetite
Dietary deficiencies	An optimal diet, rich in vitamins B, C, D and K, calcium and folic acid is important. Consider referral to dietician
Emergency admission	Ensure patients wear identification with details of their medication
Teratogenesis	Help women to attend ultrasound screening (Macara, 2008). Ensure sonographer is informed of medication (name and dose)
	Encourage compliance with folic acid and other supplements, if prescribed
Contraception in the puerperium	Several anticonvulsants (phenytoin, carbamazepine, phenobarbitone and lamotrigine) interact with oral contraceptives. High doses are normally required, but this may be ill-advised during breastfeeding or prior to the establishment of regular menstrual cycles

Conclusion

All women should have the option of receiving combined care from an obstetrician and a neurologist. Where possible, antiepileptics should be reviewed prior to conception, with a view to gradual withdrawal and discontinuation if no fits have occurred for 4 years (Dichter, 1991) or even less (Bloomfield, 1996; SIGN, 2003). This will take several months. All patients should receive the minimum effective dose of AEDs. Monotherapy is associated with much lower risks for the fetus than polytherapy. Valproate appears to be the most teratogenic AED and should be avoided, if possible.

Women should realize that seizures pose greater risks than antiepileptic drugs. Sudden withdrawal of therapy may precipitate fits and, if untreated, epilepsy tends to worsen. Risks of congenital anomalies and adverse outcomes are higher in women with untreated epilepsy than in the general population. Risks may not be greatly increased by monotherapy, in association with careful monitoring.

Further reading

■ Jordan, S. (2008) *The Prescription Drug Guide for Nurses*. Open University Press/McGraw-Hill, Maidenhead; Chapter 14, Antiepileptics.
■ O'Donoghue, M.F. and Hayes, C.P. (2008) Managing epilepsy and anti-epileptic drugs during pregnancy, in Rubin, P. and Ramsay, M. (eds) *Prescribing in Pregnancy*, 4th edn. BMJ Group, London.
■ Walker, M. (2005) Status epilepticus: an evidence based guide. *BMJ*, 331: 673–7.

CHAPTER 19

Drugs and Mental Health

Sue Jordan and Billy Hardy

This chapter will discuss the drugs most commonly prescribed in the perinatal period for mental illness, the SSRI antidepressants, and briefly describe other drugs associated with the management of mental illness. Many of the adverse effects of antipsychotic medication are described with prochlorperazine (Chapter 5). (Other mood stabilizers, valproate and carbamazepine, are included in Chapter 18).

Chapter contents

- Childbirth and mental health problems/illness and pre-existing mental illness
- Drugs prescribed in the perinatal period
- Selective serotonin reuptake inhibitors (SSRIs)
- Tricyclic antidepressants (TCAs)
- Antipsychotics
- Anxiolytics
- Lithium therapy

Childbirth and mental health problems/mental illness

Definitions and diagnoses of mental illness remain symptom based, dependent, to some extent, on the clinical skills of practitioners (Bell, 1996). While aetiological debates persist (Brockington, 2004; Cox, 2004), authorities consider the putative neurobiological basis of mental illness justifies a pharmacotherapeutic approach (RCP, 2003; NICE, 2006).

Midwives encounter women with pre-existing mental health problems such as schizophrenia and bipolar disorder, sometimes known as serious mental illness, and women whose mental health problems emerge, and pose a risk, during the puerperium.

The puerperium is a crucial time for women's mental health. Across cultures, the incidence of mental health problems among women increases sharply in the puerperium (Oates, 2000; Wissart et al., 2005). Undiagnosed illness can, occasionally, progress to suicide and infanticide: one high-profile case concerned a psychiatrist whose bipolar disorder remained undertreated and who subsequently killed herself and her 3-month-old daughter (NHS, 2003; CEMACH, 2007; NICE, 2007).

Childbirth is associated with two distinct forms of mental health problems: puerperal psychosis and postnatal depression (Brockington, 2004; Nakku et al., 2006; NICE, 2007):

- *Puerperal psychosis* is potentially the most devastating mental illness associated with childbirth (NICE, 2007). Two in 1,000 women develop puerperal psychosis. Women with histories of psychosis or bipolar disorders, even if many years previously, have a 50% chance of developing serious mental illness in the first 3 months after birth. Onset of symptoms may be sudden and catastrophic (CEMACH, 2007). The mother's temporary loss of reality will, in many cases, require the intervention of psychiatric services offering complete intensive home support. The full range of treatment options will be considered in the most disturbed women, including prescriptions of antipsychotics and electroconvulsive therapy (Sharma et al., 2004).

Practice point

■ Routine questioning regarding previous mental health problems is recommended (CEMACH, 2007).

■ *Postnatal depression* must be distinguished from 'the blues', which are episodes of tearfulness and anxiety arising around postpartum day 5 and continuing episodically for several weeks, particularly when the mother is tired. Definitions of postnatal depression vary, but it is estimated that 10–13% women suffer depression in the year after birth, and a third to a half of these are seriously affected; a further 26% of women experience a self-limiting depressive episode (SIGN, 2002; Surkan et al., 2006; NICE, 2007). Prolonged postnatal depression is typically associated with adverse social circumstances; these women will benefit from postpartum screening, psychotherapeutic interventions and social support (Oates, 2000; Wisner et al., 2004; NICE, 2007). Although aetiological debates continue (Dennis and Stewart, 2004; Ward and Wisner, 2007), the most likely intervention remains the prescription of antidepressants.

Practice point

■ Severe depression requires immediate referral, whereas management of mild to moderate postnatal depression usually involves non-pharmacological treatments in the first instance (Musters and McDonald, 2008). Distinguishing between these conditions can be difficult, particularly during brief home visits.

In addition, women with *a pre-existing mental illness* will require extra help and support. The prevalence of depression and the relapse of a pre-existing depressive illness increases during pregnancy, particularly among women living in adverse circumstances or with poor social support. Some of this may be due to changes in the secretion of endogenous steroid hormones (O'Keane and Marsh, 2007). Mental health may be threatened not only by physiological changes, but also by sudden noncompliance with medication, often based on fears of **teratogenicity**. Therefore, pre-conception discussions between women and healthcare professionals are very important (CEMACH, 2007).

Community mental health teams or psychiatric services may offer specialist perinatal services for women with mental health problems, and they liaise closely with substance misuse teams, as needed (RCP, 1996; NICE, 2007). The midwife's knowledge and her relationship with her clients can be used effectively, in collaboration with primary healthcare teams or specialist services. Discontinuation of prescribed medications due to **adverse drug reactions** (both physical and psychological) is a key consideration (NICE, 2007; HCC, 2007a, 2007b; DH, 2008), and increasing women's understanding of pharmacological treatments may minimize any nonconcordance (Eberhard-Gran et al., 2006).

Case report

A young woman with a history of bipolar disorder, in stable circumstances, stopped her mood stabilizers before conception and remained well until after delivery. Nonspecific symptoms were followed by depression, which was not referred to the psychiatric services, and, later, suicide.

Because of her previous illness, this woman stood a 50% chance of relapse in the 3 months following childbirth. However, there was no attempt to refer her to mental health services with a view to restarting medication (CEMACH, 2007: 160).

Management of women with pre-existing mental illness presents difficult choices; the prescriber is often aware that attempts to prescribe 'the lowest possible dose' could result in relapse of major psychotic illness. Similarly, attempts to reduce doses 2–3 weeks before birth to minimize neonatal withdrawal symptoms may leave the woman vulnerable to a recurrence of mental illness post-partum, unless prompt action is taken to adjust medication on delivery.

Drugs prescribed for mental illness

The drugs used in mental illness are summarized in Table 19.1.

Table 19.1 Drugs prescribed for mental illness: summary and examples

Antidepressants	Selective serotonin reuptake inhibitors (SSRIs), for example fluoxetine, sertraline, paroxetine, and citalopram
	Inhibitors of both serotonin and noradrenaline reuptake, for example duloxetine and venlafaxine
	Tricyclic antidepressants (TCAs), for example imipramine, amitriptyline, dothiepin, and doxepin
	Monoamino-oxidase inhibitors (MAOIs), for example moclobemide and tranylcypromine (not recommended in pregnancy and breastfeeding)
	Others, such as tryptophan; see BNF for details
Antipsychotics	First-generation (typical) antipsychotics:
	• Oral medications, for example chlorpromazine, haloperidol, trifluoperazine, and prochlorperazine
	• Depot medications (intramuscular injections), for example fluphenzine, haloperidol (Haldol®), zuclopenthixol (Clopixol®), and flupenthixol (Depixol®)
	Second-generation (atypical) antipsychotics, for example risperidone, olanzapine, clozapine, quetiapine, aripiprazole, and amisulpride
Anxiolytics	Benzodiazepines, such as diazepam and temazepam
	Buspirone (manufacturers advise avoid in pregnancy and breastfeeding)
Antimanic agents	Lithium compounds
	Carbamazepine and sodium valproate (Chapter 18)

Selective serotonin reuptake inhibitors (SSRIs)

Evidence supports psychosocial interventions for depressive episodes following childbirth (Elliot et al., 1994, 2000; Hendrick, 2003; Dennis, 2004; Coyne and Mitchell, 2007). However, many women are prescribed antidepressants. While it can be argued that the quality and type of postnatal depression is different from other forms of clinical depression (Pitt, 1991), the antidepressants most likely to be prescribed during this period are those generally used in primary care, the selective serotonin reuptake inhibitors (SSRIs). These include fluoxetine (Prozac®), paroxetine (Seroxat®), sertraline (Lustral®), fluvoxamine, citalopram and related drugs, such as venlafaxine (Effexor®). SSRIs are also used in the treatment of obsessive compulsive disorders, anxiety, eating disorders and panic disorders.

Prescription of SSRIs has, in part, superseded both the older antidepressants (tricyclics) and the anxiolytics such as benzodiazepines (Medawar, 1997). Their introduction was facilitated by concerns over the dangers of overdose and the adverse drug reactions associated with older antidepressants (NICE, 2004c). Fatal overdoses of SSRIs have usually involved co-ingestion of alcohol or other drugs.

How the body handles SSRIs

Most SSRIs are available as tablets or capsules and liquids. Citalopram oral drops can be mixed with water or orange juice. Different brands and formulations may not be **bioequivalent**. Unlike the other SSRIs, fluoxetine and its main metabolite have unusually long **half-lives** of up to 10 days. While this is advantageous during withdrawal from fluoxetine, benefits may be delayed and fluoxetine will remain in the body several weeks after discontinuation. Thus there is potential for accumulation, and other SSRIs, such as sertraline, may be better choices when rapid symptom relief is needed, as in postpartum depression (Edwards and Anderson, 1999) or if a mother wishes to breastfeed. Sertraline is affected by these problems to a lesser degree; its active metabolites have half-lives of up to 3 days (Baldesssarini, 2006). SSRIs cross the placenta and enter breast milk.

Actions of SSRIs

Antidepressants may affect mood and behaviour by adjusting the operation of key **neurotransmitters**: serotonin (5HT, 5-hydroxytryptamine) and noradrenaline/norepinephrine. SSRIs increase the quantity of serotonin available in key **synapses** by blocking its reuptake into the neurones. Tricyclic antidepressants (TCAs) act similarly on noradrenaline. This alters the functioning of **receptors** and neurones, and tends to normalize circadian (24-hour) rhythms. Increase in serotonin availability is thought to be responsible for mood elevation, anxiety, anorexia, analgesia, and a change in libido. However, excess serotonin may disturb central nervous system functioning, and, rarely, extreme excess can produce hyperthermia and the 'serotonin syndrome' (below).

Adverse effects of SSRIs

Serotonin regulates the:

- gastrointestinal tract
- central nervous system
- cardiovascular system
- platelets.

Commonly reported adverse reactions are nausea, usually soon after starting treatment, feelings of nervousness, panic and insomnia. Serious adverse drug reactions occur in 1.5% of inpatients receiving SSRIs, mainly psychotic and neurological disturbances, which is slightly lower than the figure for TCAs (1.7%) (Grohmann et al., 1999). SSRIs are occasionally responsible for hypersensitivity reactions (below) and inappropriate secretion of ADH (SIADH). The **adverse effect** profile of SSRIs differs from TCAs, and, in general, they are better tolerated.

Gastrointestinal disturbances

Serotonin is important in controlling gastrointestinal motility and secretions. Some 18–26% of people taking SSRIs experience gastrointestinal disturbances, including anorexia, taste disturbance, nausea, diarrhoea, constipation, and indigestion.

Weight loss is usual, but this may be viewed positively by the woman. Maternal weight gain and mean birth weight may be reduced in women taking fluoxetine during the third trimester (Chambers et al., 1996); however, depressive illness can also be the cause of poor weight gain and premature birth (Wisner, 1999). In contrast, citalopram, like TCAs, can cause weight gain.

SSRIs increase both insulin sensitivity and, with regular use, the risk of hypoglycaemia in people with diabetes (Derijks et al., 2008).

Practice points

- Troublesome nocturnal gastrointestinal symptoms may cause noncompliance with medication.
- Regular recording of weight will facilitate assessment and reduce the risks of serious weight changes.
- Regular glucose monitoring should be undertaken by women with diabetes.

SSRIs may also cause hypersalivation or dry mouth, nasal congestion, cough, rhinitis, fever or flu-like symptoms.

Central nervous system

By blocking the reuptake of serotonin into presynaptic neurones, SSRIs increase the availability of bioamines in the synapses of the central nervous system. While this elevates mood, even to the extent of engendering hypomania, it is also responsible for insomnia, subjective feelings of agitation, anxiety, restlessness, inability to keep still, apprehension, helplessness, confusion, panic attacks, anger, aggression or violence, suicidal ideation and self-harm. There are anecdotal reports linking SSRIs to aggressive, violent behaviour and suicide (Boseley, 1999). Citalopram may cause somnolence.

Practice points

- Risk of suicide is increased during the first few weeks of therapy, and particular vigilance for ideation of violent behaviour or self-harm is required during this time (NICE, 2004c; Baldessarini, 2006).
- Refer to the prescriber *any clients who appear fidgety, are unable to sit still or complain of inner restlessness. Dose reduction may be needed.* Hallucinations may indicate that dose is excessive (Aronson, 2006).
- If insomnia emerges as a problem, medication can be administered in the morning.

In addition, increased concentrations of serotonin may antagonize dopamine. Neurotransmitter imbalance may also lead to amnesia, hallucinations, tremor, akathisia or, rarely, posture and movement disorders. Sensory disturbances are possible, including pins and needles, tinnitus, visual disturbances, taste disturbance and headache. Migraine may be worsened or occur for the first time. All antidepressants increase the likelihood of seizures in women with histories of convulsions.

Practice points

- SSRIs may worsen the symptoms of women who are already agitated.
- Antidepressants may impair driving skills, and women should be warned of this (BNF, 2009).

- If a tremor appears, consider excessive use of caffeine, bronchodilators or amphetamines.
- Neonates exposed to fluoxetine in the third trimester may experience poor neonatal adaption (Chambers et al., 1996), and extra help may be needed with breastfeeding.

With prolonged administration, SSRIs, particularly paroxetine, share the posture and movement adverse effects of antipsychotics and increase production of prolactin (below) (Aronson, 2006). Sudden onset of double vision has been associated with citalopram (Cowen, 2008). Dopamine inhibition may be the mechanism underlying sexual dysfunction and loss of libido, which are frequently reported adverse effects, particularly with paroxetine. Micturition may be increased.

Practice point

- When women are prescribed SSRIs, especially paroxetine, professionals should carefully observe for signs of tremor, restlessness, abnormal movements and stiffness.

Cardiovascular system

Although SSRIs are less cardiotoxic than other antidepressants, they may cause dysrhythmias, palpitations or alterations in heart rate. SSRIs antagonize the alpha receptors of the sympathetic nervous system, which are responsible for maintaining cardiac output and BP. This may result in postural hypotension or even heart failure, particularly with sertraline or paroxetine.

Case report

A woman with shortness of breath was prescribed citalopram and diazepam. Heart failure was only diagnosed at autopsy. The assessors considered that prescribed medication probably contributed to the outcome by blocking the stimulating effects of the sympathetic nervous system on the heart (CEMACH, 2007: 192).

Practice point

- Breathlessness is an important symptom of heart failure, which should be investigated.

Hypotension may compromise placental blood flow and intrauterine growth, without being detectable using standard measurement techniques.

Practice points

- Measuring BP in sitting and standing positions will assess the degree of postural hypotension.
- Regular monitoring of fetal growth is essential.

SSRIs may lead to increased sweating, acne, *Herpes simplex* reactivation and 'hot flushes'.

Bleeding and bruising

Serotonin is important in regulating the activity of platelets, and therefore blood clotting (Chapter 8). Bleeding, bruising or purpura may arise as a result of platelet dysfunction. This may present as haemoptysis, gastrointestinal bleeds or even a stroke (Taylor et al., 2007).

Hypersensitivity responses

Like all drugs, SSRIs can cause hypersensitivity responses in susceptible individuals. These are particularly common with fluoxetine. Rashes occur in 5–15% of clients. In a few cases, vasculitis and blood vessel necrosis have developed, jeopardizing the blood supply of the limb.

Practice point

■ Should pruritus (itching) develop, the woman should withhold further doses and seek immediate medical advice, as this may herald the onset of vasculitis (BNF, 2009).

Rare hypersensitivity responses include:

■ rashes, possibly associated with vasculitis (above)
■ alopecia (hair loss)
■ joint and muscle pains
■ angioedema
■ liver function disturbances
■ pancreatitis
■ bone marrow damage – aplastic anaemia or haemolytic anaemia
■ pulmonary fibrosis. *Dyspnoea is a warning sign*, which is easily overlooked.

Interactions: SSRIs

• SSRIs interact with many other medicines, particularly in those who are genetically susceptible. SSRIs inhibit key liver enzymes, reducing the elimination and causing the accumulation of several drugs, including phenothiazines (for example prochlorperazine – Stemetil®), carbamazepine, diazepam, lithium, phenytoin, procyclidine, tramadol, warfarin, ropivacaine, some antiarrhythmics, some antimalarials and antidepressants.

• The use of fluoxetine with diazepam should be treated with caution as it increases the half-life of diazepam, increasing sedation.

• Alcohol may intensify any sedation; experts advise all users to limit intake to 1 drink/day (Doran, 2003).

• Bleeding, without a change in prothrombin time, is more likely if NSAIDs, aspirin, clozapine, phenothiazines or anticoagulants are co-administered.

Practice point

■ SSRIs may intensify the hypotension and sedation associated with analgesics and antiemetics commonly used in labour.

Serotonin syndrome

The serotonin syndrome was first reported in the 1950s. It occurs in genetically susceptible people who combine SSRIs with other drugs that may increase serotonin availability in the central nervous system (for example MAOIs, tricyclic antidepressants, alcohol, diet pills, cold cures, amphetamines, such as methylphenidate or dexamfetamine prescribed for adult attention deficit disorder, cocaine, St John's wort, buspirone, sibutramine (for obesity), tramadol, tri-iodothyronine, triptans (for migraine), tryptophan, lithium or some antiviral drugs and possibly erythromycin and ergot derivatives) (Nolan and Scoggin, 1999). Reactions may occur several weeks after withdrawal of fluoxetine. The problem has also arisen in association with pethidine administration (Bowdle, 1998).

V

Serotonin syndrome results in uncontrollable hyperthermia (and occasionally death) associated with:

■ *mental state changes:* anxiety, hypomania, agitation
■ *cardiovascular problems:* tachycardia, blood pressure fluctuations
■ *gastrointestinal problems:* nausea, salivation
■ *motor abnormalities:* muscle rigidity, tremor, ataxia, shivering, **nystagmus**.

Practice point

■ Co-administration of recreational drugs may be dangerous: mania has been reported with co-administration of cannabis or amphetamines, and convulsions with LSD. Women should inform pharmacists of their medication and seek advice before using non-prescription remedies, particularly 'cold cures', 'stimulants', cimetidine and St John's wort.

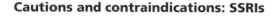

Cautions and contraindications: SSRIs

• Women with established history of mood disorder should be managed by specialists (O'Keane and March, 2007).

• SSRIs are not recommended for women with mania (or history of mania), agitation, need for sedation, suicidal ideation, previous panic attacks (may be worsened), epilepsy, parkinsonism, heart disease, hypertension, bleeding disorders, angle-closure glaucoma or previous hypersensitivity responses to SSRIs.

• Renal or hepatic impairment necessitate lower or less frequent doses.

• For people under 18, fluoxetine may be prescribed with careful monitoring. Most other SSRIs, mirtazepine and venlafaxine are not recommended for depression (CSM warning in BNF, 2009: 215).

SSRIs and pregnancy

The implications of investigations into exposure to SSRIs *in utero* or *via* breast milk are debated (Kallén, 2004b; Cowen, 2008). Manufacturers advise use in pregnancy only if potential benefits outweigh risks. Paroxetine and escitalopram demonstrated toxicity in animal studies (BNF, 2009), and authorities advise against paroxetine in pregnancy (Taylor et al., 2007). Meta-analysis of observation studies indicates an increased risk of low birth weight, prematurity and admission to special care facilities; however, these studies are unable to account for the effects of depression, social stress or smoking on birth weight. Some neurobehavioural effects of prenatal SSRIs have been demonstrated, but the evidence is not strong (Lattimore et al., 2005). A case control study (200 cases) suggested an increase in preterm birth, but no other adverse neonatal outcomes (Maschi et al., 2008). An older US case control study (n = 228) found that, in comparison with controls, women taking fluoxetine during the last trimester gained less weight and delivered smaller infants. There was also an increase in minor abnormalities (club feet, hydrocele, congenital hip dislocation and lacrimal stenosis) and evidence of poor neonatal adaptation, including jitteriness, respiratory disturbance and poor feeding (Chambers et al., 1996). Retrospective analyses suggest links with neonatal lung damage (Chambers et al., 2006) and, for paroxetine (Berard et al., 2007), sertraline, citalorpam (Pedersen et al., 2009) and possibly other SSRIs (Oberlander et al., 2008; Ververs et al., 2009), heart damage. Motor function difficulties, leading to increased referrals to physiotherapists, and constipation have been associated with

SSRI exposure *in utero* (Ververs et al., 2009). Risks are higher when benzodiazepines or several SSRIs are co-administered (Oberlander et al., 2008; Pedersen et al., 2009).

An older long-term study of preschool children exposed to antidepressants *in utero* found no performance deficits; this study included 55 children exposed to fluoxetine and 84 children exposed to a tricyclic antidepressant (Nulman et al., 1997).

Breastfeeding and SSRIs

SSRIs pass into breast milk and manufacturers advise against breastfeeding (BNF, 2009). Fluoxetine, escitalopram and citalopram may have a greater potential to accumulate than sertraline (Lattimore et al., 2005). Some authorities consider sertraline or paroxetine monotherapy to be more suitable (Schaefer, 2007e). In a comprehensive review, Yoshida et al. (1999) found few cases where neonates had suffered adverse effects due to SSRIs in breast milk; these included an infant with gastrointestinal problems and another with irritability. Preterm infants and those with a compromised hepatic or renal function are at increased risk. Chambers et al. (1999) found that infants (n = 26) breastfed by mothers taking fluoxetine gained significantly less weight than comparators (392 g over 6 months), although no infants showed signs of common adverse effects or malnutrition. Long-term studies to review behavioural development have not been located (Aronson, 2006).

Practice points

If a mother taking an SSRI decides to breastfeed (probably against medical advice):
- A blood sample should be obtained from the neonate to ensure that renal and hepatic function are normal before exposure (Yoshida et al., 1999).
- The neonate should be monitored closely for signs of colic, sedation, vomiting, crying, sleep disturbance and irritability, which may necessitate a change in feeding (Musters and McDonald, 2008).
- Weight gain, growth, feeding and ability to suck should be carefully monitored.
- Infants are most vulnerable in the first few days of life. Exposure to drugs *via* breast milk is less likely to be harmful when the infant is several months old (Kallén, 2007).
- Women should be informed that while there is little evidence of immediate serious harm to healthy term neonates (Hendrick et al., 2001), the effects on long-term development are uncertain (Cowen, 2008).

Implications for practice: SSRIs in pregnancy and the puerperium

Potential problem	Management suggestions
Hypomania/euphoria, agitation, anxiety, nervousness, amnesia, increased libido/promiscuity. Particular care on initiation or increase of therapy or for women with a history of bipolar disorder	Distinguish between adverse effects and 'normal' anxieties, behaviours and sleep loss. Consider alternative causes of overactivity: excess caffeine, non-prescribed stimulants, for example cold cures, recreational drugs, including cannabis, and amphetamines
	See women within days of initiation of therapy. Refer any problems to prescriber promptly
Headache within 1–2 hours of taking medication	Discuss with prescriber dividing the dose, administration at bedtime, and administration of paracetamol
Headache, migraine, tinnitus, paraesthesia	Seek medication review
Fever	Monitor vital signs pre-therapy and regularly. Report (see Serotonin syndrome, above)

V

Potential problem	Management suggestions
GI upsets	Administer with food to reduce nausea
	If faecal incontinence or sleep disturbance occur, seek alternative antidepressant
	Problems may subside after a few weeks
Dry mouth	Suggest regular water rinses
Weight changes	Record weight and dietary intake weekly
Cardiovascular changes	Check BP lying and standing
	Arrange ECG if pulse is abnormal or palpitations occur, and following overdose
Bleeding and bruising	Warn clients to inform doctor immediately if bleeding or bruising occur
	Advise against use of NSAIDs and analgesic doses of aspirin
Menstrual irregularities	Menstruation may be delayed, which could impact on estimation of delivery date
Increased frequency of micturition	Discuss any continence issues arising
Urine retention	Check urine sample for possible infection
Rash (often itching), which may indicate serious adverse reactions/vasculitis	Warn clients to inform doctor and withhold SSRIs or venlafaxine if a rash appears
Photosensitivity and sunburn (also with St John's wort)	Advise covering skin with clothing and high factor, high star sunscreen during exposure to direct sunlight
Rare adverse effects	Be prepared to take blood for liver function tests, amylase estimations and FBC if the patient develops abdominal pain and nausea or fever and sore throat

Tricyclic antidepressants (TCAs)

TCAs, such as amitriptyline, imipramine and dothiepin, are prescribed occasionally, because they may be more effective in severe depression (Barbui and Hotopf, 2001) and are not regarded as teratogenic. They are more dangerous than SSRIs in overdose, and were the immediate cause of death in two cases (DH, 1998).

Practice point

■ Families should be aware of the dangers of mental health medications (particularly TCAs, lithium and clozapine) in overdose, and ensure that tablets are stored securely away from young children.

For women stabilized on TCAs, the dose may need to be increased during pregnancy to maintain the clinical response; however, as mood often lifts in the third trimester, it may be possible to reduce the dose to minimize neonatal withdrawal reactions. Following delivery, the dose should be returned to pre-pregnancy values, and close observation maintained for emergent adverse effects (Wisner et al., 1999). The adverse effect profile of TCAs is similar in many ways to the phenothiazines. The **antimuscarinic** adverse effects are described in Table 5.2. Posture and movement disorders are associated with high doses. Tricyclics are also associated with agitation or even hypomania, particularly when treatment is initiated (see SSRIs, above).

Manufacturers advise avoiding tricyclics during breastfeeding (BNF, 2009), but, with the exception of doxepin, there is little evidence of harm (Yoshida et al., 1999).

Antidepressant withdrawal syndrome

If antidepressants, like phenothiazines, are abruptly discontinued, a withdrawal syndrome may be observed. Abrupt discontinuation often causes gastrointestinal upset, headache, flu-like symptoms, panic/anxiety, insomnia, hypomania, agitation, restlessness, confusion, dizziness, sensory disturbance, numbness, fatigue, tremor, depression, and (particularly fluoxetine) bleeding (Perahia et al., 2005). These problems can persist for several weeks.

Practice points

- These symptoms may be confused with the original problems.
- Antidepressants are discontinued gradually over several weeks or months (minimum 4 weeks), if possible. If symptoms occur, dose decrements are reduced. This is easier with liquid preparations.
- Withdrawal reactions may occur following missed doses if drugs with short half-lives are prescribed, for example paroxetine. Advise women not to miss or delay doses. There are fewer problems with fluoxetine, due to its very long half-life.

Neonates may experience withdrawal reactions or serotonin-related symptoms following use in late pregnancy. These include: jitteriness, excessive crying, sleep difficulties, feeding difficulties, hypoglycaemia, hypothermia, convulsions, gastrointestinal stasis, bladder retention, and respiratory distress (Aronson, 2006).

Practice point

- Neonates whose mothers have been prescribed antidepressants towards the end of pregnancy, particularly paroxetine, need careful surveillance for the emergence of these problems and to ensure adequate feeding. They are more likely to be admitted to a neonatal nursery (Aronson, 2006; O'Keane and Marsh, 2007). This will be facilitated if a full medication history is available.

Authorities suggest that partial breastfeeding will minimize withdrawal symptoms in neonates (Taylor et al., 2007).

Antipsychotics

Antipsychotics may be prescribed:

- for an acute episode of puerperal psychosis or mental illness
- as a component of the ongoing management of women with enduring mental illness, often as intramuscular 'depot' injections.

Perinatal mental health services may adopt specific care pathways and protocols, as discussed in SIGN (2002), NICE (2007) and CEMACH (2007).

Pregnancy and the puerperium are vulnerable periods for women and the potential for mental health problems, due to the physiological and psychosocial stresses associated with this highly scrutinized period of life (Oates, 2000). For women with pre-existing mental illness, it is possible that doses of medication will have been minimized during pregnancy, and this reduction of the 'pharmacological shield' will sometimes be insufficient to protect the mother in the puerperium (Dean et al., 1989).

Practice points

- Women with pre-existing mental illness should be reviewed by their mental health practitioners: throughout pregnancy; immediately after birth; and regularly during the puerperium. Psychiatrists frequently need to adjust medication upwards during this period.

- Women may be reassured to know that:
  - the risk of obstetric complications is not markedly increased in women with schizophrenia (Kendell et al., 2000)
  - observation studies conducted over several decades indicate that the traditional antipsychotics are unlikely to increase the risk of congenital anomalies substantially (Aronson, 2006).
- Antipsychotics cross the placenta and enter breast milk to varying degrees (Newport et al., 2007). Some women may become noncompliant with prescribed antipsychotic medication due to misplaced fears of damage to the fetus.

Practice points

- For women with pre-existing mental illness, noncompliance with prescribed antipsychotic medication carries a high risk of relapse, which poses more danger to mother and baby than the adverse effects of the drugs (Taylor et al., 2007; NICE, 2007).
- Early ultrasound scans will assist detection of congenital abnormalities.
- The effects of intramuscular 'depot' injections persist for up to 3 months after the last dose. If injections are discontinued, symptoms may re-emerge around this time.

Actions and adverse effects of antipsychotics

Many traditional antipsychotics are phenothiazines or related compounds, and therefore they have adverse effects similar to prochlorperazine (Stemetil®) (Chapter 5; Table 19.2). The hypotensive actions of these drugs may jeopardize the blood flow to the placenta (Pinkofsky, 1997).

The atypical antipsychotics (such as clozapine, olanzapine, risperidone, quetiapine and zotepine) are associated with weight gain, obesity, glucose intolerance and gestational diabetes (Taylor et al., 2007), which increase the risk of fetal macrosomia and adverse outcomes (Chapter 16). There are reports of an increased incidence of low birth weight and an increased risk of admission to neonatal intensive care with olanzapine (Newport et al., 2007).

Practice point

- For many reasons, regular antenatal checkups to monitor fetal growth are essential for women receiving antipsychotic medication.

Table 19.2 Summary of adverse effects of antipsychotics

Dopamine (D_2) antagonism	Posture and movement disorders
	Prolactin production
	Blunting of emotions
	Antiemetic
Antimuscarinic	Dry mouth, constipation (Table 5.2)
Antihistaminic	Sedation, rarely, impaired respiration
Antagonism of the alpha receptors	Hypotension
	Weight gain, glucose intolerance, diabetes
Increased excitability	Risk of **cardiac dysrhythmias** or seizures (people with epilepsy)
Hypersensitivity responses	**Agranulocytosis**

Practice points

■ Weight should be closely monitored.
■ Screening for gestational diabetes may be advisable.

Dopamine antagonism

Dopamine is an important neurotransmitter in the regulation of prolactin secretion, posture and movement, emotions, cognition, appetite, the gut, the eye, the cardiovascular system and the hypothalamus.

With long-term use, antipsychotics increase the production of prolactin. This may cause breast tenderness, galactorrhoea, hirsuitism and menstrual irregularities. Increased production of prolactin reduces, but does not abolish, fertility. Despite this, women with long-term use of antipsychotics should receive full contraceptive advice in the puerperium. Possible associations with breast tumours, some of which are prolactin dependent, require further investigation (Aronson, 2006).

Posture and movement disorders

When phenothiazines or other antipsychotics are used long term, for mental illness or hyper-emsis, the posture and movement adverse effects, attributed to blockade of the dopamine (D_2) receptors, are extremely important. Women are particularly vulnerable to these adverse effects postpartum, due to the rapid decline in oestrogen levels at this time. Although the long-acting intramuscular depot injections have the advantage of ensuring compliance in those with serious mental illness, they are associated with a high incidence of posture and movement adverse effects. These have also been reported in breastfed neonates (Loudon, 1995). There is a danger that some of these adverse effects, the tardive dyskinesias, associated with long-term use, *may be irreversible.*

Practice point

■ Women prescribed antipsychotic medications for more than a few days should be regularly assessed for stiffness and abnormal movements, which may herald the onset of pseudoparkinsonism and tardive dyskinesia. Scales, such as the AIMS (abnormal involuntary movement) scale, have been devised to assist professionals in this (DH/RCN, 1994; RCN, 1996; Jordan et al., 2004; NICE, 2007; DH, 2008). For further practice points, see Jordan (2008, Ch. 10).

With continuous use in the last 3 months of pregnancy, antipsychotics can cause prolonged movement disorders in neonates, lasting for up to 10 months (Cox and Nicholls, 1996).

The neuroleptic malignant syndrome is a rare complication of antipsychotic therapy, which can arise when medications are introduced or changed. It is characterized by fluctuating vital signs, autonomic instability, rigidity and muscle breakdown, leading to raised temperature and raised levels of creatine kinase in the plasma. Early recognition of the syndrome and withdrawal of D_2 antagonists is life-saving (Sharma et al., 1995; *Drug and Therapeutics Bulletin*, 1995).

Antipyschotics and the infant

Assessment of the effects of antipsychotic drugs is complicated by the higher rates of fetal loss, perinatal complications and congenital anomalies in drug-naive women with serious mental illness. Exposure to phenothiazines in weeks 4–10 may be linked with a small increase (0.4%) in birth defects (Austin and Mitchell, 1998).

There is little evidence that atypical antipsychotics (olanzapine, risperidone, quetiapine, and zotepine) are associated with congenital anomalies; however, due to the low numbers of pregnancies reported, manufacturers advise against their use in pregnancy and lactation unless potential benefits outweigh risks (BNF, 2009). Case study reviews found that 5 of 61 infants born to mothers taking clozapine had congenital anomalies, but many of the mothers were also taking other drugs (Dev and Krupp, 1995); reviewers indicate that there is no overall increase in congenital anomalies (Taylor et al., 2007).

Transfer across the placenta depends on the genetic makeup of the placenta and on the drug. Olanzapine is the most extensively transferred (Newport et al., 2007). The neonate is less able to eliminate these drugs than adults, so is at risk of developing movement disorders, hypotonia, sedation, jaundice, gastrointestinal obstruction, restlessness, poor suckling and bradykinesia, even if the mother is free of adverse effects (Aronson, 2006). Withdrawal symptoms, such as seizures, hyper-reflexia, tremor, and jitteriness, also require close observation.

Practice points

- These problems are likely to make effective latching to the nipple and breastfeeding difficult.
- Neonates should be closely observed for 2 days (Garbis and McElhatton, 2007).
- If the dose of antipsychotic has been reduced prior to delivery, in an attempt to ameliorate these problems, a return to pre-pregnancy dose should be planned immediately following delivery.

Breastfeeding and antipsychotics

Antipsychotics pass into breast milk, and during the puerperium high doses of drugs (>100 mg chlorpromazine/day) may be prescribed (Mortola, 1989). Animal studies and some reports have indicated that central nervous system development may be impaired, suggesting the need for formula feeding until further evidence is available (BNF, 2009). Dangers of developmental delay in the child's early years are increased if mothers are prescribed more than one drug (Yoshida et al., 1999; Taylor et al., 2007), if infants are small or premature, or if intramuscular medication is prescribed (Campbell and Lees, 2000). The infant may be sedated or have a poor suck reflex (Schaefer, 2007e), and failure to feed and gain weight are the most common problems (Suri et al., 1998).

Practice points

- When breastfeeding mothers are prescribed antipsychotics or benzodiazepines, careful records of infant weight gain and development must be kept. Review by paediatricians is advisable.
- Supplementary formula feeding should be considered.

Clozapine

Only four breastfed infants were identified, of whom one developed agranulocytosis and another became excessively sleepy; on the basis of these alarming reports, authorities recommend bottle feeding for infants of mothers taking clozapine (Dev and Krupp, 1995; Taylor et al., 2007).

Interactions: antipsychotics

A comprehensive list of interactions is beyond the scope of this book (see Baxter, 2006), but some of the drugs administered in labour can interact with antipsychotics, particularly chlorpromazine. For example, co-administration of opioids or prochlorperazine may induce problematic sedation, hypotension and respiratory depression. One fatal respiratory arrest, possibly associated with psychiatric medication, has been reported (CEMACH, 2005: 159).

The reactive metabolite of pethidine may cause problems, including central nervous system toxicity, hypotension and profound respiratory depression in susceptible individuals (Baldessarini, 2006). If local anaesthetics are used for pain relief, the risk of cardiac problems (heart block) is increased, necessitating careful monitoring of the mother in labour.

Anxiolytics

Prescription of benzodiazepines is declining, but non-prescription use may also need to be considered. In the management of anxiety, prescription is for a maximum of 4 weeks (BNF, 2009: 184). The longer acting benzodiazepines, such as diazepam (Valium®), are generally used to manage anxiety, and the shorter acting benzodiazpeines, such as temazepam, are used as hypnotics, but their actions are indistinguishable. Benzodiazepines pass into the lipid tissues of the body, where they are stored. Detection in urine is possible some 30 days after ingestion.

Use during pregnancy is complicated by reports of microcephaly, cleft palate, gastrointestinal malformations and vision defects (Laegreid, 1990; Medawar, 1992; Mulvihill et al., 2007; Wikner et al., 2007); most case reports of nervous system defects have been associated with non-prescription use. Analysis of the Swedish Medical Birth Register indicates an increased risk of preterm birth and low birth weight (Wikner et al., 2007). Benzodiazepenes reduce muscle tone, and, in the neonate, may cause the 'floppy baby syndrome', respiratory depression and hypothermia (Cox and Nicholls, 1996). Long-term use of benzodiazepines in the mother may cause a withdrawal syndrome in the neonate, therefore women may wish to discuss withdrawal of benzodiazepines. After long-term use, this is usually undertaken gradually by reducing the dose by 12.5% (range 10–25%) per fortnight. Abrupt withdrawal can cause insomnia, anxiety, anorexia, tremor, or even convulsions (BNF, 2009). Neonates are less able to eliminate benzodiazepines than adults; use during lactation may unduly sedate a breastfed infant.

Lithium therapy

Lithium is a mood stabilizer or antimanic agent with a very narrow therapeutic range. Lithium stabilizes intracellular enzymes and second messenger systems and enhances the uptake of noradrenaline/norepinephrine and serotonin. Lithium is only suitable for those who are able to comply closely with the prescribed regimen and attend for regular monitoring of venous blood samples.

V

Practice points

- Veins may become scarred and inaccessible from frequent access, for example in intravenous drug users or women who have received lithium or clozapine therapy.
- Withdrawal of lithium therapy, particularly if abrupt, is linked with a very high incidence of mania (Moncrieff, 1995; Silverstone and Romans, 1996).

Absorption of lithium is rapid and plasma concentrations peak 2–4 hours after ingestion. Absorption is optimized if lithium is taken with food (Genser, 2008). Lithium is distributed within the total body water, with slow passage across the **blood/brain barrier**. The concentration in the fetus and neonate equals that of maternal blood. As lithium is primarily excreted by the kidney, adequate salt and fluid intake is essential in order to avoid accumulation and possible intoxication. The half-life of lithium in adults is 12–24 hours but may be much longer in neonates, due to immaturity of the kidneys. Infants with higher serum concentrations are more likely to have low **Apgar scores**, neuromuscular complications and long hospital stays (El-Mallakh, 2008).

Adverse effects of lithium

Adverse effects include:

- *gastrointestinal:* nausea, vomiting, diarrhoea, dry mouth, weight gain or loss
- *neurological:* ataxia, tremor, weakness, muscle hyperirritability, facial muscle twitching, clonic movements, slurred speech, blurring of vision, headaches, seizures, psychomotor retardation, restlessness, stupor, coma, acute dystonia, EEG changes
- *cardiovascular:* hypotension, dysrhythmias, oedema, electrolyte imbalance
- *genitourinary:* glycosuria, polyuria, polydipsia, renal impairment
- *dermatological:* dryness and thinning of hair, skin rash, leg ulcers
- *haematological:* anaemia, leucocytosis
- *endocrine:* thyroid imbalance, weight gain and diabetes. Regular monitoring should be undertaken.

Most drugs interact with lithium, including those prescribed in mental illness. The concentration of lithium is increased by salt depletion, risking toxicity, and decreased by salt intake, risking mania. People prescribed lithium must therefore maintain regular fluid, salt and dietary intake, particularly during pregnancy.

The use of lithium in pregnancy, labour and the puerperium poses several problems:

- Lithium is teratogenic when administered during the first trimester, but the absolute risk is relatively low. Ultrasound scans and echocardiography (at 6 and 16–18 weeks) are needed to detect thyroid, renal and cardiac abnormalities, particularly defects in the tricuspid valve, which may be repaired *in utero* (Cox and Nicholls, 1996).
- The haemodilution of pregnancy increases the risk of mania, and close observation is needed, with blood tests monthly, then weekly in the last month and every 48 hours in the puerperium (Garbis and McElhatton, 2007).
- The rapid decrease in maternal circulatory volume following delivery may cause lithium toxicity, including damage to the kidneys and central nervous system.
- When lithium is discontinued during pregnancy, authorities recommend restarting before delivery or within 24 hours of delivery, to protect the mother during this vulnerable period (Silverstone and Romans, 1996; Viguera et al., 2008).
- The neonate is vulnerable to the adverse effects listed above. Neonates should be observed for hypoglycaemia and polyuria (Aronson, 2006). One infant exposed to lithium *via* breast milk was so hypoxic he became cyanosed (Suri et al., 1998). If fluid and electrolyte imbalance occur, lithium causes potentially irreversible neurotoxicity in the neonate, and breastfeeding is not advised by manufacturers (BNF, 2009).
- If a women wishes to breastfeed during lithium therapy, the neonate must be closely observed for dehydration, tremor, involuntary movements, cyanosis, muscle tone and other adverse effects. This involves measurement of lithium from neonatal blood samples. Supplementary formula feeds should be available if toxicity is suspected. There is no information on long-term effects (Aronson, 2006; Schaefer, 2007e).

Lithium may be considered in preference to the alternative drugs, valproate and carbamazepine, which may pose greater risks (Chapter 18) (Austin and Mitchell, 1998; Aronson, 2006).

Practice point

■ Women should be informed of the risks and need for any dietary supplementation before conception. A mental health services' case note review found no documentation of discussion of teratogenic risk and contraception for many women prescribed lithium, valproate, or carbamazepine (29/138 and 33/138 respectively), and that pre-conception folate is rarely discussed or prescribed (2/138) (James et al., 2007).

In women with bipolar disorder, the risks associated with a recurrence of mental illness are greater than those associated with teratogenicity or formula feeding, particularly if the woman has not been stable for at least 1 year before conception.

Case report

A woman of 35 had a 2-year history of bipolar disorder treated with lithium and citalopram. In a prenatal consultation, she made a decision to discontinue all medication during pregnancy and breastfeeding. She remained reasonably well during pregnancy and until the third postpartum night, when insomnia developed, and she became disorientated and paranoid. She was admitted to psychiatric services 5 days postpartum with agitation, confusion, delusions and auditory hallucinations. She refused all medications, and was restrained until her next of kin gave consent for administration of valproic acid, haloperidol and lorazepam. Sertaline was added 7 days later. She subsequently suffered a relapse and was hospitalized for electroconvulsive therapy. A decision was taken to restart lithium therapy and cease breastfeeding. Recovery took place over the next 3–4 weeks. A subsequent pregnancy was followed by a further episode of bipolar disorder, again with a full recovery.

This patient was highly educated and her symptoms fluctuated during her illness; at times she appeared well orientated, and at other times she did not recognize her baby and expressed a fear of harming him.

Practice point

■ Women with a history of bipolar illness should be intensively supervised, particularly during the post-partum period. While they may appear well during a short home visit, the risk of serious relapse of illness during this time may be as high as 90% (Viguera et al., 2008).

Conclusion

The guidelines by NICE (2004c, 2007), CEMACH (2007), SIGN (2002), DH (2002) and the NHS report on Emson (2003) all publicize the services available in the perinatal period. If mental health suddenly deteriorates, which is likely in the first 3 months after delivery, the risk of over-dose of prescribed and recreational drugs should be considered (Chapter 20) (CEMACH, 2007). Nine women died from overdose of psychiatric medication in 2002–4 (CEMACH, 2005).

Other issues are raised by women with less serious mental health problems, often in adverse social circumstances, where psychosocial interventions may be more appropriate. Such women would benefit from a thorough postpartum examination, including thyroid function tests, and a recognized screening instrument (Cox et al., 1987). For a discussion see Chetley (1995) and Medawar (1997).

Further research is needed to explore any connections between the medications administered in labour, such as ergometrine and corticosteroids, and postpartum illness.

Further reading

■ Doran, C. (2003) *Prescribing Mental Health Medication*. Routledge, London.
■ HCC (Healthcare Commission) (2007) *Talking about Medicines*. HCC, London.
■ Healy, D. (2009) *Psychiatric Drugs Explained*, 5th edn. Churchill Livingstone, London.
■ Jordan, S. (2008) *The Prescription Drug Guide for Nurses*. Open University Press/McGraw-Hill, Maidenhead; see Chapters 11 and 10 respectively for a full account of antidepressants and antipsychotics and implications for practice.
■ NICE (National Institute for Clinical Excellence) (2007) *Antenatal and Postnatal Mental Health*. NICE, London.
■ SIGN (Scottish Intercollegiate Guidelines Network) (2002) *Postnatal Depression and Puerperal Psychosis*. Royal College of Physicians, Edinburgh.
■ Taylor, D., Paton, C. and Kerwin, R. (2007) *The Maudsley Prescribing Guidelines*, 9th edn. Informa Healthcare, London.

CHAPTER 20

Recreational Drugs

Sue Jordan

This chapter considers the drugs commonly self-administered for non-medical purposes, together with some agents prescribed by substance misuse teams.

Chapter contents

- Alcohol/ethanol
- Caffeine
- Cigarettes
- Cannabis
- Recreational opioids
- Stimulants: amphetamines, cocaine, ketamine, khat

The history of the use of drugs for subjective purposes is inseparable from the history of medicine. Evidence for the use of **opioids** and alcohol has been found in human settlements dating back 4,000 years (Howe, 1972). Many drugs are used for subjective purposes, and not all users become addicted to or disabled by recreational drug use (Gossop, 2007). However, apart from any risk of addiction, overuse of these drugs often entails significant health hazards; therefore women should be followed up after childbirth, beyond the usual 6 weeks, even if the infant is transferred to other care (CEMACH, 2007).

Misuse of recreational drugs complicates pregnancy and increases risks of adverse outcomes: premature rupture of membranes, placental abruption, antepartum haemorrhage, stillbirth, premature birth, **Apgar score** at 5 minutes <7, low birth weight, admission to neonatal intensive care, and, in some cases, congenital anomalies. This suggests common biological mechanisms, such as disruption of the critical phases of neuronal migration or activation of stress hormones and **cytokines** (Huizink and Mulder, 2005). It is not always possible to identify a single causative agent as several recreational drugs are often used concurrently; infants exposed to both opioids and stimulants are particularly vulnerable (Burns et al., 2006; Bell and Harvey-Dodds, 2008).

Physical ill-health is relatively common in disadvantaged women, including those with mental health problems or misusing recreational drugs. Occasionally, symptoms of serious physical illness have been misdiagnosed; for example agitation associated with raised intracranial pressure or hypoxia has been attributed to mental health problems or substance misuse (CEMACH, 2005, 2007).

V

Practice points

■ The risk of pregnancy complications and/or neonatal withdrawal symptoms indicates that birth should take place where appropriate facilities are available.
■ Women with substance misuse problems should be managed by specialist teams, under supervision of an obstetrician (CEMACH, 2007).
■ Women known to misuse recreational drugs usually require more analgesia in labour; however, they are less likely to receive regional analgesia (Burns et al., 2006).

Testing of urine samples indicates that, in some communities, illicit drug use may occur in as many as 10% of pregnancies: 16/150 parous women who had previously denied drug use tested positive (in urine) for recreational drugs, mainly amphetamines (Sanaullah et al., 2006). Failure to report opiate and cocaine use is also likely, although injecting drug use complicates less than 1% of pregnancies (Burns et al., 2006; Wong et al., 2008).

Practice point

■ Routine questioning of all women regarding use of all recreational drugs, including tobacco and alcohol, is recommended (Chang, 2001; CEMACH, 2007).

Many women, but not their partners, reduce their use of tobacco, alcohol and cannabis during pregnancy, only to return to previous levels of consumption following delivery (Bailey et al., 2008). Women report that smoking is often the only available coping mechanism to relieve the stress induced by infants' crying for protracted periods (Gaffney et al., 2008).

Practice point

■ Strategies for support in the postpartum period should be explored to reduce the incidence of substance misuse.

Alcohol/ethanol

The alcohol most commonly consumed is ethanol or ethyl alcohol; other alcohols may be consumed in small quantities. Alcohol intake is often measured in units of 8–10 grams in the UK. A single drink (glass of wine, measure of shorts or half-pint of beer) contains 8–12 g or 150–270 mmol ethanol.

How the body handles ethanol

Ethanol is a small molecule that passes across biological membranes, including the placenta and blood/milk barrier, with ease. Some ethanol is absorbed through the stomach wall, but more is absorbed from the small intestine. Therefore, where transit into the small intestine is delayed, for example when a meal is eaten, absorption is slowed. Ethanol passes from the gut to the liver, where it is either metabolized or passed into the general circulation. Peak plasma concentrations are reached 30–90 minutes after ingestion on an empty stomach. Plasma and breast milk concentrations rapidly equalize (Lawrence and Schaefer, 2007).

Ethanol is metabolized to acetaldehyde and acetic acid, mainly in the liver, but also in the lining of the gut. It is suggested that the gut wall enzymes are less efficient in women than in men, possibly accounting for their increased susceptibility to **adverse effects** (Fleming et al., 2006). Acetic acid is metabolized to fatty acids, starch or proteins (Figure 20.1).

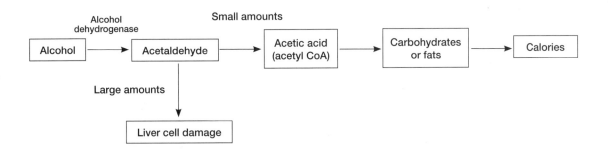

Practice point

■ If the liver is already stressed or damaged, it may lack the enzyme capacity to metabolize even moderate amounts of ethanol without sustaining cell damage. Therefore, women with, or at risk of, liver impairment, for example women with pregnancy-associated fatty liver or pre-eclampsia, are advised to abstain from ethanol.

Figure 20.1 Metabolism of ethanol

The most important enzyme group is alcohol dehydrogenase. The efficiency of these enzymes and the individual's capacity to metabolize ethanol depend on genetic makeup, gender and exposure to ethanol (see Chapter 1, Enzyme induction). If this capacity is exceeded, ethanol passes unchanged into the circulation. The plasma concentration (and central nervous system (CNS) effects) of a given quantity of ethanol will, therefore, depend on the rate at which the ethanol is drunk. On average, adults eliminate ethanol at a rate of 8–10 g (150–220 mmol or just over 1 unit)/hour. Consequently, if 10 pints of beer (or an equivalent 20 units) are consumed, high concentrations of ethanol may persist in the body the following day (Masters, 2001). If large quantities of ethanol are metabolized, energy substrates are expended, promoting accumulation of lactic acid and metabolic acidosis, which may be harmful. Infants metabolize alcohol more slowly, 4–5 g/hour, and heavy use of alcohol is considered incompatible with breastfeeding.

Practice points

■ An occasional single drink is generally regarded as safe when lactation is established. Following a single drink, women are advised against breastfeeding for 2 hours, which is sufficient time for elimination of 10g (1 unit) of alcohol.
■ Women are advised to consume a single drink over 30 minutes, to avoid any high concentrations in breast milk (Lawrence and Schaefer, 2007).
■ Women planning to drink may wish to express milk to cover a missed feed.

Small amounts of ethanol are metabolized by other, multifunctional enzymes. Regular intake of alcohol induces (speeds up) the action of these enzymes, increasing the rate of breakdown of other drugs, such as steroids and warfarin.

Actions and adverse effects of alcohol

Ethanol affects most body systems.

Central nervous system

The effects of ethanol on the cell membranes of nerve cells (neurones) depend on dose and previous exposure. The initial response is reduced excitability, brought about by inhibition of one type of glutamate receptor (the NMDA receptor) linked with learning and memory, which may explain why people often have no memory of events surrounding intoxication. With chronic ingestion, the number of NMDA receptors increases and **tolerance** develops, which may be associated with irritability and withdrawal symptoms. At higher doses, neurotransmitter release and nerve impulse transmission are depressed, particularly in the systems controlling balance. Ethanol is sedative and **anaesthetic**, imitating the actions of the brain's inhibitory transmitter (GABA), and, at very high doses, respiration is depressed. The blood ethanol concentration at which intoxication with psychomotor impairment appears varies with the individual and their habituated levels of consumption.

Practice point

■ Infants receiving breast milk following maternal drinking are too sedated to suckle or intake well. This is most important in the puerperium, before breastfeeding is established.

Long-term ethanol use can lead to cerebral atrophy, brain damage, and peripheral nerve damage, independent of vitamin deficiencies. This can be detected by computerized tomography (CT) or magnetic resonance imaging (MRI) while still at a reversible stage.

Practice point

■ Doctors may examine the nervous system and document any pre-existing nerve damage before administering regional anaesthesia to women known to be heavy drinkers (Kuczkowski, 2005).

Cardiovascular system

Low doses of ethanol alter the body's temperature regulation mechanisms in the hypothalamus, causing vasodilatation and sometimes sweating. In a cold environment, body temperature may fall. Epidemiological studies suggest that for adults over 55, 1–2 units of ethanol per day may reduce the risk of strokes (Reynolds et al., 2003) and coronary heart disease (Mukamal et al., 2003). This may be due to improvements in lipid profile. However, above this level, the risks of hypertension, stroke and other cardiovascular disease increase. Ethanol can cause cardiac arrhythmias and, rarely, cardiomyopathy.

Practice points

■ There are no physical health benefits associated with the consumption of alcohol in women of childbearing age.
■ Binge drinking is associated with stroke in young people.
■ Alcohol consumed within 24 hours increases BP. Women should therefore be asked about their alcohol intake in the previous 24 hours to assist in the interpretation of recordings (Fleming et al., 2006).

Endocrine system

Ethanol inhibits secretion of oxytocin and antidiuretic hormone, resulting in diuresis and dehydration; drinking alcohol is not advised during childbirth and until breastfeeding is established (Chapter

6). Ethanol decreases secretion of stress hormones and increases release of endorphins, the body's natural opioids, which may explain the potential for addiction. Immune function may be compromised, and white cell count reduced.

Gastrointestinal system and nutrition

Ethanol increases gastric acid secretion and gut motility; when taken with a meal, it aids digestion. However, particularly at higher concentrations, ethanol disrupts the lining of the gut, leading to alcoholic gastritis, blood loss, malabsorption, and diarrhoea.

Normally, the liver metabolizes ethanol into fatty acids and triglycerides (Figure 20.1). With heavy drinking, these can accumulate, causing 'fatty liver'. This stage of liver damage is potentially reversible, but with continued excessive intake, damage may progress. An inflammatory reaction ensues, causing formation of fibrous scar tissue (cirrhosis of the liver), which eventually blocks the venous drainage of the liver.

Practice point

- Blood clotting is impaired in women with liver dysfunction, increasing the risk of haemorrhage or haematoma. Coagulation tests will detect this.

Ethanol also damages the pancreas, causing recurrent pancreatitis, characterized by acute abdominal pain and nausea. Severe damage results in **shock** and organ failure.

People who use ethanol regularly may derive up to half their energy intake from drinking. Since alcoholic drinks contain few proteins and vitamins, this leads to nutritional deficiencies, particularly B vitamins, and anaemia. Ethanol inhibits the formation of new glucose in the liver (gluconeogenesis). If little food has been eaten and the liver's glycogen (starch) stores are low, the liver is unable to continue its normal outputting of glucose, resulting in hypoglycaemia. The brain and placenta depend on a steady supply of glucose from the liver, and hypoglycaemia may cause cerebral irritability and impair fetal metabolism (Chapter 16).

Effects on pregnancy

In pregnancy, ethanol intake above:

- 5 g/day (half a drink) adversely affects behaviour in 6–7-year-olds
- 10 g/day (1 drink) increases the risk of miscarriage and fetal death
- 17 g/day (2 drinks) increases the risk of preterm birth
- 12–30 g/day (2–3 drinks) suppresses fetal breathing movements
- 20 g/day (2–2.5 drinks) reduces fetal growth and birth weight
- 60 g/day (7+ drinks) increases the incidence of congenital anomalies
- 90 g/day (10+ drinks) may cause fetal alcohol syndrome (below).

There is less evidence of harm with lower intakes (Peters and Schaefer, 2007). However, absence of evidence cannot be taken as evidence of absence of effect. Whether intake below 10 g per day is associated with a slightly increased risk of miscarriage is unknown (NCC, 2008c); database analysis (n = 4,719) found no increased risk of preterm birth and intrauterine growth retardation at intakes below 60 g (6 drinks) per week if no single intake exceeded 2 drinks (20 g) (O'Leary et al., 2009). It is suggested that 2 drinks per day in the second trimester may be harmful (Fleming et al., 2006). A single 'binge' of more than 5 drinks (7.5 units, 60 g of ethanol), without regular drinking, may affect neurodevelopment and is particularly harmful in early pregnancy (Guerrini et al., 2009). Discontinuation of binge drinking before the second trimester does not reduce the risk of preterm birth (O'Leary et al., 2009).

Fetal alcohol syndrome

Alcohol (or acetaldehyde) causes the cells of the fetal brain to self-destruct (undergo apoptosis) (Farber and Olney, 2003). MRI studies indicate that key areas of the brain (cerebral hemispheres and centres for posture and movement) are reduced in volume (Fleming et al., 2006). Risk and severity of fetal alcohol syndrome increase with dose of ethanol and individual susceptibility.

Sustained heavy drinking during pregnancy is the cause of fetal alcohol syndrome, characterized by dysmorphic features, microcephaly, learning disabilities, low birth weight, stunted growth, neurodevelopmental delay, hearing, language and speech disorders, behavioural problems, hyperactivity, attention deficits, and, sometimes, cardiac, kidney or limb abnormalities. Infants with deficits, but without all the features of fetal alcohol syndrome, may be diagnosed with 'alcohol-related neurodevelopmental disorders' and 'fetal alcohol effects'. The mildest form of these is attention deficit (Fleming et al., 2006). Deficits may improve and growth at least partially catches up as the child grows, but much alcohol-related neurological damage is irreversible.

Practice points

■ A history of ethanol use should be obtained at the earliest opportunity. This should include direct inquiries regarding the number and nature of drinks for each day over the last 7–14 days (Dunkley-Brent, 2004).
■ Abstaining from alcohol during pregnancy is the most effective known public health strategy for prevention of birth defects (Peters and Schaefer, 2007).
■ Alcohol-based medicines, including some proprietary cough medicines, and chloral hydrate are best avoided.

Current guidelines on alcohol consumption in pregnancy recommend:

■ no alcohol during the first trimester, when risk of miscarriage is highest
■ binge drinking should be avoided
■ there is no evidence of harm associated with consumption of 1–2 units of alcohol once or twice a week in the second and third trimesters (NCC, 2008c).

Dependence and withdrawal

Habitual alcohol intake produces tolerance, both by enzyme induction and changes in the CNS **receptors**. The activity levels of the CNS receptors, including those associated with the sympathetic nervous system, increase to compensate for constant application of the sedative effects of alcohol. If alcohol is withdrawn, 6 hours to 10 days later, these increased activity levels are manifest as irritability, insomnia, tremor, muscle tension, overactive reflexes, sweating, nausea, thirst, cold skin and dehydration. Generalized seizures can occur in severe cases.

Practice points

■ Seizures or aggression may be due to hypoglycaemia, which can be corrected.
■ Abrupt cessation of alcohol intake is not usually advised for alcohol-dependent pregnant women (Guerrini et al., 2009).

A second stage of withdrawal can occur several days later in people with serious problems. This is known as 'delerium tremens' or 'DTs', characterized by fever, hallucinations, severe tachycardia, sweating, and profound vasodilation.

Practice point

■ If women are admitted to hospital, abstinence may be enforced. Therefore, women who use alcohol heavily should be closely observed for irritability, muscle tension, sweating, nausea, and thirst; medical input, including the testing of reflexes, should be sought if there are any concerns.

Delirium tremens is a serious condition, requiring specialist input. Specialists may prescribe benzodiazepines to prevent convulsions.

Caffeine

Caffeine and theobromine are among the active ingredients of tea, coffee, cocoa and chocolates, and may be included in some proprietary analgesics and cold cures.

Peak plasma concentrations occur 30–60 minutes after oral administration. Caffeine crosses the placenta and passes into breast milk, where it remains for 2 hours. Caffeine is metabolized more slowly in pregnancy (**half-life** increases from 3 to 7 or 11 hours), and women often voluntarily reduce their tea or coffee intake to compensate. Caffeine metabolism is slow in the fetus and neonate, prolonging and intensifying its effects. Half-life may be up to 80 hours in neonates, and approaches adult values by 6 months.

Practice points

■ Neonates may not be affected by maternal caffeine from breast milk until it has accumulated, which takes 3–5 half-lives (Chapter 1) or 7–10 days postpartum. All neonates should be observed for signs of irritability and frequent poor feeding at this age. If this reason for poor feeding is not recognized and actioned, breastfeeding may be abandoned unnecessarily.

■ Caffeine intake should be noted in all breastfeeding mothers to assist prompt recognition and prevention of poor feeding.

■ Women may be advised to restrict caffeine intake (to 300 mg/day maximum) during the first 3 months of feeding, by which time the infant's metabolism will be better able to cope (Lawrence and Schaefer, 2007).

The caffeine content of beverages varies considerably (Table 20.1). In general, beverages bought outside the home have higher caffeine content (Dixon, 2004). In addition, a 12 oz can of cola contains 30–65 mg caffeine and chocolate contains about 10 mg per ounce.

Table 20.1 Caffeine content for standard servings, mean 219 g

Beverage	Range (mg)	Mean (mg)
Coffee, ground	15–254	105
Coffee, instant	21–120	54
Tea	<1–90	40
Cocoa	10–15	
Decaffeinated tea and coffee	0.6–8	3

V

Actions of caffeine

Caffeine stimulates the central nervous system and the heart by:

- increasing the second messengers (Chapter 1, Pharmacodynamics) associated with central nervous system stimulation
- antagonizing the inhibitory transmitter adenosine.

Fatigue, concentration and learning are improved at low or normal doses, and driving is not adversely affected. Insomnia is commonly reported, and some people prefer to abstain from caffeine in the late evening. High doses may be associated with self-medication for fatigue or depression.

Practice points

- Direct inquiries about tea/coffee intake may offer clues as to general wellbeing postpartum.
- Evening caffeine intake may contribute to insomnia during pregnancy and the first weeks after birth, until the pre-pregnancy metabolic rate and half-life have returned.

Very high daily intakes (above 500 mg/day) can cause 'caffeinism', which presents as an anxiety disorder associated with agitation, dysphoria, insomnia, tachycardia, and gastrointestinal overactivity, and may possibly precipitate symptoms in people with schizophrenia or bipolar disorder. Withdrawal from caffeine doses above 250 mg/day may give fatigue, headaches, irritability, lethargy and nausea; however, caffeine is not considered addictive (O'Brien, 2006). Caffeine may affect the elimination of some antipsychotic medications; users are advised to maintain a constant intake of caffeine.

Caffeine causes tachycardia and maternal caffeine intake increases fetal heart rate (Peters and Schaefer, 2007). The well-known diuretic effects of caffeine are attributed to relaxation of renal arterioles.

Effects on pregnancy and the fetus

Minor developmental abnormalities were seen in animals whose caffeine intake was some 50 times normal human levels; this has not been supported by observation studies in humans (Peters and Schaefer, 2007). The mean caffeine intake of pregnant volunteers in the UK (n = 2,635) was 159 mg/day, mainly (62%) from tea. Intake fell during the early stages of pregnancy and increased in the third trimester. These data suggest that any level of caffeine consumption is associated with an increased risk of birth weight below the 10th centile, and caffeine consumption above 200 mg/day may decrease birth weight by 60–70g (CARE Study Group, 2008). Other studies have suggested increased risk of: fetal death at intakes above 300 mg/day; and intrauterine growth retardation and spontaneous abortion above 150 mg/day.

Practice point

- Some authorities suggest a 'safe' limit of caffeine consumption of 150 mg/day or 3 cups of tea or coffee (Peters and Schaefer, 2007), while others suggest 300 mg/day or 6 cups of tea or 4 cups of instant coffee (Dixon, 2004). However, not all the data support this (CARE Study Group, 2008). The wide variations in caffeine content (Table 20.1) complicate the imposition of 'safe limits'.

Cigarettes

In Europe, the problems associated with smoking tobacco have been discussed since the sixteenth century. Cigarettes deliver carcinogenic tars, carbon monoxide and nicotine – the last is the most addictive substance known. A cigarette contains just under a gram of tobacco and 6–11 mg of nicotine, 1–3 mg of which are absorbed. The amount absorbed is controlled by the smoker's technique and depth of inspiration.

How the body handles nicotine

Nicotine from tobacco, gum or patches is rapidly absorbed through the mucous membranes, lungs, skin, placenta and breast milk. Nicotine acts on the brain some 7 seconds after inhalation. It has a half-life of about 2 hours, which corresponds to a typical interval between cigarettes.

Practice point

■ Women, their family members and colleagues are likely to request a cigarette or smoking break every 2 hours.

Infants of mothers who smoke absorb nicotine by passive smoking and/or in breast milk, where concentrations reach 0.5 mg/l with 20 cigarettes per day. Nicotine is absorbed from the infant's gastrointestinal tract and may raise heart rate.

Practice point

■ To minimize the infant's intake of nicotine, women should be advised to allow as long as possible between smoking and feeding, providing this does not make them unduly anxious.

Nicotine is metabolized, mainly in the liver, to cotinine, which is excreted in the urine and breast milk. Excretion is reduced if the urine is alkaline (Taylor, 2006). The half-life of cotinine is 20 hours, making it a useful marker for the verification of self-reported smoking behaviour.

Actions and adverse effects of tobacco

The three main components of tobacco may be considered individually:

■ *Carbon monoxide* from the smoke of tobacco or cannabis cigarettes combines with heamoglobin, displacing oxygen and reducing the ability of red blood cells to deliver oxygen to the tissues. Most vulnerable to hypoxia are the heart, brain, placenta and fetus. Fetal haemoglobin has a higher affinity for carbon monoxide than adult haemoglobin, therefore proportionally less haemoglobin carries oxygen, and hypoxia and acidosis are more likely.
■ *Tar and irritants* damage cells and promote cancerous changes by altering the DNA-regulating oncogenes controlling cell division. Observation studies and databases indicate that the risk of lung cancer is proportionately related to tobacco use and exposure to tobacco smoke (Engeland et al., 1996). Childhood cancer may be more common following smoking in pregnancy, but the literature is inconclusive (Peters and Schaefer, 2007). It is unclear which component of tobacco smoke is responsible for the increase in cardiovascular mortality associated with smoking. Smoking irritates the mucous membranes of the respiratory tract and paralyses the respiratory cilia, increasing the risk of chest infections. Accordingly, general anaesthesia and intubation are avoided if at all possible in women who smoke (Kuczkowski, 2005). Traces of metals, such as cadmium and lead, are also present in tobacco.

V

■ *Nicotine* acts on receptors widely distributed throughout the central nervous system, causing both activation and relaxation. Smokers are able to induce muscle relaxation when they feel tense, and alertness when tired. Nicotine improves test performance and learning in rats and humans. Stimulation of the reward centres in the brain may explain its addictive potential. Nicotine stimulates release of the stress hormones: adrenaline/epinephrine, glucocorticoids, antidiuretic hormone, and endogenous opioids. Adrenaline release may be responsible for increased blood pressure and heart rate, vasoconstriction (including placenta), reduced gastrointestinal motility and appetite, and nausea in naive users. Nicotine crosses the placenta and can increase the heart rate of the fetus.

Practice point

■ Women unaccustomed to tobacco smoke may feel nauseous if exposed to cigarette smoke.

Prolactin secretion is diminished in smokers, but the wide variation in duration of breast-feeding among smokers suggests that psychological factors and feeding intentions are the main reasons why smokers abandon breastfeeding early (Amir and Donath, 2002).

Practice point

■ Women who smoke should receive the same encouragement to initiate and continue breastfeeding as non-smokers.

Thiocyanates in tobacco may adversely affect iodine status in infants at risk of deficiency. Thiocyanates inhibit iodine transport into the thyroid gland of the fetus, causing enlargement (Köksal et al., 2008), and breast milk, increasing the risk of iodine deficiency (Laurberg et al., 2004).

Effects on pregnancy and the fetus

The problems induced by tobacco smoke, including passive smoking, have been extensively reviewed, and include miscarriage, preterm birth, low birth weight, stillbirth, perinatal mortality, ectopic pregnancy, placental abruption, *placenta praevia*, premature rupture of membranes, cleft lip and cleft palate (NCC, 2008c). No associations were seen with other congenital anomalies (Morales-Suárez-Varela et al., 2006). Birth weight and prematurity are related to the number of cigarettes smoked daily. The incidence of either birth weight below 2,500 g or premature rupture of membranes before 33 weeks is doubled in women who smoke. Older women and nulliparae are most vulnerable (Peters and Schaefer, 2007).

Practice point

■ Smoking cessation during the early weeks of pregnancy is likely to normalize birth weight.

Nicotine replacement therapy may not be without risk. Examination of the Danish Birth Registry found that nicotine replacement therapy was associated with a higher risk of congenital anomalies (19/231), particularly musculoskeletal malformations, than either smoking or not smoking (Morales-Suárez-Varela et al., 2006), but not stillbirth (8/1,927) (Strandberg-Larsen et al., 2008).

Practice point

■ Nicotine patches are best use intermittently, and should be removed before retiring (NCC, 2008c).

The long-term harm associated with smoking is not easily separated from the effects of childhood exposure to tobacco or social and economic deprivation. Children exposed to tobacco smoke *in utero* have lower scores in some aspects of language development at age 6 (Lewis et al., 2007).

Dependence and withdrawal

The urge to smoke another cigarette is associated with falling or low nicotine concentrations. Many women find smoking cessation difficult. Symptoms of nicotine withdrawal are common, and include irritability, hostility, depression, concentration difficulties, bradycardia and weight gain (O'Brien, 2006). Therefore, the postnatal period may not be the easiest time for smoking cessation. Advice on smoking cessation should be tailored to the needs of individual clients and their attitudes to smoking (Dunkley-Brent, 2004: 362).

Nicotine patches deliver a constant concentration of nicotine, without the peaks experienced by smoking; however, they prevent withdrawal symptoms, and allow a gradual dose reduction. Long-term success is estimated to be 20% (O'Brien, 2006).

Cannabis

Cannabis is a general term for preparations of Indian hemp, which have been smoked for some 3,000 years. Of the 60 or so active cannabinoids in hemp, tetrahydrocannabinol (THC) and its metabolites are most important. The concentration of THC varies from 2 to 12%, depending on methods of production. Relatively few women report using cannabis without other recreational drugs, and separating the effects of cannabis from cigarette smoking is difficult in observation studies. Smoking cannabis raises carbon monoxide concentrations and exposes mother and infant to the same tars as tobacco smoke. Some cannabis plants may have been treated with herbicides, such as paraquat, which could be responsible for the associated lung damage (Gossop, 2007).

Cannabis passes rapidly into the brain, placenta, breast milk and the developing nervous system. Smoked cannabis becomes fully effective about an hour after inhalation and remains effective for 2–3 hours. It is highly lipid soluble, crosses all cell membranes, passes into adipose tissue and is excreted over 2–3 days. Metabolites can be detected in urine for at least 30 days after ingestion. The lethal dose is very high (40,000 times the effective dose) (Gossop, 2007).

Actions and adverse effects of cannabis

Tetrahydrocannabinol acts on the body's endogenous cannabinoid receptors, to produce relaxation, drowsiness, euphoria, increased appetite, heightened perception and pleasure, hallucinations and a feeling of 'reward'. The effects of cannabis are additive and prolonged. In some circumstances, cannabinoids are used medically to relieve pain, emesis, muscle spasm or appetite loss. In the UK, nabilone is available for treatment of emesis associated with cytotoxic therapy (BNF, 2009). The increase in appetite is useful in some clinical situations, but may promote unwanted weight gain. Cannabis has been used, successfully, for management of pregnancy-induced emesis (Westfall et al., 2006).

V

Practice point

■ In view of the uncertainties surrounding long-term effects of cannabis on brain development, it cannot be recommended in pregnancy without specialist input.

Central nervous system

Learning, memory, attention span, reaction time, psychomotor performance, coordination, balance, hand steadiness, muscle strength, perception, and information processing are adversely affected by cannabis, but self-confidence is not. These effects last 4–8 hours, longer than the subjective effects; the risk of road accidents is increased (Rang et al., 2007). Users recognize that this drug interferes with motivation and work (Gossop, 2007). Stroke, transient ischaemic attacks, and posture and movement disorders have been reported in young people (Wong et al., 2008).

Unpleasant reactions, including acute psychosis, are more likely with higher doses and oral ingestion, particularly in predisposed individuals. These include anxiety, hallucinations, delusions, paranoia, and depersonalization. First time use may induce panic. People with schizophrenia may suffer a relapse following cannabis use (O'Brien, 2006).

Cardiovascular system

High carbon monoxide concentrations and subsequent tissue hypoxia are responsible for an increased risk of cardiac and cerebrovascular disease. Cannabis raises heart rate and blood pressure, but at high doses reduces heart rate. Following maternal administration, fetal heart rate may decline (Peters and Schaefer, 2007). These effects can increase the oxygen needs of the heart and the risks of angina and **cardiac dysrhythmia**. Vasodilation causes the characteristic bloodshot eyes.

Case report

A 35-year-old woman with hypertension admitted the occasional use of cannabis. While in hospital, she smoked cannabis, and 30 minutes later developed palpitations, dyspnoea, hypertension and tachycardia. Her urine tested positive for cannabis. The hypertension resolved with medical treatment (Wong et al., 2008).

Respiratory system

Tetrahydrocannabinol is a bronchodilator. As with tobacco, the tar and carbon monoxide content of cigarettes may increase the risks of bronchitis, asthma and lung cancer. Smoking causes a dry mouth and oropharyngeal irritation.

Effects on pregnancy and the fetus

Pre-eclampsia, preterm delivery before 37 weeks, birth weight below 10th centile, Apgar score below 7 at 5 minutes, and admission to neonatal intensive care were all observed more frequently if the mother used cannabis, opioids or stimulants (n = 416,834) (Burns et al., 2006); however, it is uncertain if these effects are attributable to cannabinoids or hypoxia induced by carbon monoxide.

Chromosome damage has been seen in human white cells and in rodent fetuses, but no clinical consequences have been observed. THC acts on cannabinoid receptors in the fetal brain, particularly the prefrontal cortex. More hyperactivity and delinquent behaviour at 6 years, and impaired cognitive functioning at 9–12 years is observed in children of heavy cannabis users in pregnancy (Huizink and Mulder, 2006). Motor development of breastfed infants whose mothers use cannabis heavily is reported to be delayed (Lawrence and Schaefer, 2007).

Dependence and withdrawal

Tolerance to cannabis builds up in liver enzymes and other tissues, as with alcohol. Neither the withdrawal syndrome (restlessness, irritability, insomnia, nausea and cramps) nor addiction normally present clinical problems (O'Brien, 2006). The mental state of heavy users gradually normalizes during abstention.

Recreational opioids

Since the introduction of the hypodermic needle in the 1840s, recreational opioids have often been accompanied by the hazards of intravenous injections in non-sterile conditions. Opioids are taken to relieve depression and fatigue as well as for a 'kick' or 'rush', and tend to decrease pain, aggression and libido. Although opiate use is not incompatible with social stability, those addicted to intravenous use have a mortality rate several times that of age-matched controls (Gossop, 2007).

Opioids cross the placenta and enter breast milk. Heroin generates intense euphoria for some 45 minutes, followed by 3–5 hours of tranquility, so several doses may be needed each day. Higher plasma concentrations are achieved by intravenous injection than by smoking heroin; therefore, some clients ignore 'damage limitation' advice to revert to smoking heroin. Heroin is metabolized to 6-acetylmorphine and morphine, which disappears from urine 2 days after ingestion of high doses, and much sooner after low doses; therefore, unless amniotic fluid is sampled, midwives are reliant on women to self-report recreational use.

In addition to the adverse effects of opioids described in Chapter 4, which may complicate delivery, chronic ingestion of opioids is associated with:

- dysregulation of oestrogen and progestogen secretion
- impaired immunity
- transgenerational adverse effects
- dependence and withdrawal syndromes.

Reproductive system

Reduced secretion of gonadotrophic hormones (FSH and LH) from the anterior pituitary reduces secretion of oestrogen, which, together with increased secretion of prolactin, causes menstrual irregularities and amenorrhoea. Therefore, diagnosis of pregnancy may be delayed. Fertility is impaired by long-term use of many opioids, but not methadone (Schmittner et al., 2005).

Practice points

- Women who are switching from heroin to methadone or buprenorphine should receive adequate advice on their increased chances of conception and the need for effective contraception.
- Advice regarding contraception should be given before discharge from hospital. Long-acting reversible contraception may be most easily achieved by implants (CEMACH, 2005).

If amenorrhoea has lasted more than 1 year, this has an adverse effect on bone health. Stress fractures of the femoral neck have been reported in heroin users (Ghodse and Galea, 2008).

Impaired immunity

Opioids influence the cells of the immune system, including neutrophils, **lymphocytes**, natural killer cells, and **macrophages** (Chapter 14), *via* surface opioid receptors and second messenger systems (Chapter 1); mechanisms vary with different drugs. Endogenous opioids enhance the immune system, while long-term drug administration may be responsible for immunosuppression, an increased risk of bacterial infections, including TB, reactivation of *Herpes simplex* infections, and tumour spread (Gutstein and Akil, 2006; Roy et al., 2006). Depression of the cough reflex and respiratory cilia predispose to chest infections (Chapter 4). Lung damage, bronchoconstriction and immunosuppression increase the incidence of asthma. In addition, intravenous drug use is associated with serious infections, including endocarditis, hepatitis, HIV/AIDS, and pyelonephritis.

Practice point

■ The vulnerability of heroin users should promote prompt recognition and treatment of pneumonia, TB, streptococcal and other infections.

Both pain and opioids suppress the immune system. In acute situations, opioids boost the immune system by relieving acute pain, when present (Gutstein and Akil, 2006).

Transgenerational adverse effects

Effects on the fetus

Fetal bradycardia, reduced heart rate variability and reduced fetal movements are observed at peak methadone concentrations, despite no changes in maternal physiology (n = 42) (Jannson et al., 2005).

Intrauterine exposure to high concentrations of opioids may adversely affect the developing nervous system. Infants (n = 133) exposed *in utero* to prescribed methadone and, in some cases, other opioids are at increased risk of developmental delay, low IQ, attention deficits and behavioural problems; these problems may persist if the infants are adopted (Hunt et al., 2008). There are reports of permanent **nystagmus**, causing vision loss, in infants whose mothers used opioids, often with benzodiazepines; most affected infants also suffered developmental delay and microcephaly (n = 14) (Mulvihill et al., 2007).

Effects on pregnancy

Opioids are associated with premature rupture of membranes, placental abruption, antepartum haemorrhage, pre-eclampsia, stillbirth, premature delivery, low birth weight, anaemia, respiratory depression at birth, reduced head circumference, and neurodevelopmental delay. Birth weight is lower if heroin rather than methadone is used (Bell and Harvey-Dodds, 2008). Sudden opioid withdrawal during pregnancy can cause: fetal death; convulsions; premature rupture of membranes; uterine contractions; and premature labour (Peters and Schaefer, 2007).

Practice points

■ Women should be advised of the dangers of interruption of heroin supplies and the need to comply with substitution programmes.
■ Harm can be reduced by prompt recognition and treatment of infections, nutritional deficiencies, and use of other drugs, including alcohol.

Dependence and withdrawal

There may be no limit to opiate tolerance; injected doses above 1 g heroin/day have been reported (Gossop, 2007). Tolerance to opioid-induced euphoria may occur after 1 dose. However, not all the actions of opiates show tolerance; on long-term use, up to 50% of users experience excessive sweating, and 10–20% have chronic constipation, insomnia and loss of libido.

Opioid dependence is associated with an unpleasant physical withdrawal syndrome in adults and neonates. In adults, this comprises: lacrimation, runny nose, sweating and yawning starting 8–12 hours after last dose, followed by irritability, insomnia, weakness, anxiety, depression, anorexia, emesis, diarrhoea, dehydration, cramps, and fever peaking at 24–48 hours, lasting up to 7 days. Protracted withdrawal symptoms may persist for 6 months; as homeostatic mechanisms reset, the client experiences anxiety, insomnia, opiate craving, weight fluctuation, and altered breathing. Substitution therapy will need to be maintained during this time (Gutstein and Akil, 2006).

Practice points

■ Such symptoms are particularly distressing in the puerperium, and substance misuse specialists may increase the dose of heroin substitutes (methadone or buprenorthpine) at this time (CEMACH, 2005).
■ To minimize withdrawal symptoms, dose and preparation changes are undertaken gradually. If opioids are reduced, discontinued or modified, the woman should be observed for emergence of any rebound pain and other withdrawal symptoms. Dose reductions of 10–20% every other day may prevent withdrawal symptoms (Gutstein and Akil, 2006).
■ It may be difficult to achieve analgesia in labour.

Neonates born to mothers regularly using opioids, including methadone and buprenorphine, may display withdrawal symptoms 1–3 days after birth, but these may be delayed for 10–36 days, particularly if methadone has been ingested. Infants may be irritable and hyperactive, with abnormal reflexes and cry, rapid breathing, fever, tremor, diarrhoea, vomiting, convulsions and even coma (Bell and Harvey-Dodds, 2008). Oral morphine may be prescribed. Convulsions may not respond to standard therapy, and specialists may request administration of phenobarbitone (Peters and Schaefer, 2007; Dryden et al., 2009).

Practice points

■ Protocols for managing neonatal opioid withdrawal should be available in all units, as not all women disclose recreational drug use, and detection of opioids in urine samples is not always possible.
■ Close observation of neonates is needed for several weeks to detect delayed withdrawal (Peters and Schaefer, 2007).
■ Naloxone administration to these neonates should be avoided, as it may precipitate withdrawal symptoms and seizures (ILCR, 2006).

These symptoms may be alleviated by breastfeeding (Freyer, 2008), reducing the need for pharmacological interventions (Dryden et al., 2009), but, outside managed substitution programmes (Bell and Harvey-Dodds, 2008), this is not recommended by all authors (Peters and Schaefer, 2007).

Drugs prescribed as heroin substitutes

Either buprenorphine or methadone may be prescribed as heroin substitutes by substance misuse specialists, in conjunction with intensive support. Both regimens reduce the incidence of intrauterine growth retardation when compared with heroin (Binder and Vavrinková, 2008).

Buprenorphine

Buprenorphine has **agonist** and **antagonist** properties. It binds to opioid receptors but causes less respiratory depression than equivalent doses of morphine. However, because it blocks the actions of the body's own opioids, it can also cause opioid withdrawal symptoms, such as sweating, yawning or running eyes and nose. It may be superior to methadone for mood stabilization and constipation (Ghodse and Galea, 2008). It is sometimes preferred over methadone for pregnant women with opioid dependence, due to a lower incidence of preterm birth and neonatal with-

V

drawal symptoms (Kakko et al., 2008; Binder and Vavrinková, 2008). However, the short half-life (2–4 hours) necessitates more frequent dosing (Peters and Schaefer, 2007). Like other opioids, buprenorphine causes neonatal withdrawal symptoms, in proportion to dose administered, and is not recommended in pregnancy by manufacturers. Buprenorphine passes into breast milk, but in small quantities; its propensity to suppress lactation, explored in animal studies, requires further investigation (Schering-Plough, ABPI, 2009).

Practice point

■ Breastfeeding women prescribed buprenorphine and their infants are closely monitored to safeguard the infant's nutritional status.

Methadone

Methadone is a long-acting opioid (half-life 15–40 hours), and may be recommended for heroin substitution or chronic pain (Wolff et al., 2005; Peters and Schaefer, 2007). Methadone for oral administration is available in 4 concentrations (BNF, 2009). Following oral ingestion, peak effects are not experienced for 4 hours. Methadone binds to tissue proteins, which causes accumulation, slow release and a protracted withdrawal syndrome. Doses are usually administered once daily. The rate of elimination of methadone increases during pregnancy.

Practice point

■ Women prescribed methadone may find that, as pregnancy progresses, their previous dose becomes less effective at preventing withdrawal symptoms. Direct inquiries should be made, and any need for a shortening of dose interval or increased dose to cover the increased rate of metabolism should be discussed with prescribers. It is important that women do not resort to buying impure street drugs to compensate for this physiological change (Wolff et al., 2005).

Methadone's actions, tolerance and dependence are similar to morphine. Respiration is depressed for some 24 hours after ingestion. Sedation intensifies with repeated dosing, leaving some individuals markedly drowsy. **Cardiac dysrhythmias** similar to those associated with antipsychotic medication (long QTc interval) have been reported (Ghodse and Galea, 2008). Higher doses are associated with increased risk of neonatal withdrawal (Dryden et al., 2009). Methadone is not recommended for children (BNF, 2009).

Methadone concentrations in breast milk and breastfed infants are low (n = 8), and some authorities consider breastfeeding safe (Jannson et al., 2008; Dryden et al., 2009). However, abrupt weaning could induce withdrawal in infants, and co-administration of non-prescription opioids could introduce impurities or very high opioid concentrations. High doses of methadone may accumulate and induce drowsiness in the infant.

Practice point

■ Decisions to support women using methadone in breastfeeding their infants are taken on an individual basis by specialist teams. Intense supervision is needed to monitor infant sedation, nutrition and possible withdrawal symptoms over the first few months of life.

Pethidine

Pethidine (meperidine) is occasionally abused. It is an unusual opioid in that, in high doses, it causes dilated pupils (due to the anticholinergic actions of its metabolite, norpethidine), twitches, tremors, and seizures. On withdrawal, severe twitching is seen at 8–12 hours, earlier than other opioids. It is the only opioid that causes fits. However, some street drugs may contain barbiturates and quinine, which can cause fits on withdrawal.

Long-term use of opioids in association with chronic pain syndromes requires specialist advice.

Stimulants

The psychostimulants, amphetamines and cocaine, are **sympathomimetics**, that is, they potentiate the actions of the sympathetic nervous system by increasing the availability of catecholamine neurotransmitters: adrenaline/epinephrine, noradrenaline/norepinephrine and dopamine, and serotonin. These neurotransmitters are important not only for the 'fright, flight or fight' response, but also for constant control of the heart, blood pressure, gut, bladder and blood supply to vital organs. Consequently, stimulants may induce:

- central nervous system stimulation
- psychosis
- cardiovascular system stimulation, which may lead to heart attack or stroke
- dry mouth, dental caries
- gastrointestinal upset
- retention of urine, due to contraction of the internal urethral sphincter
- lung damage from inhalation
- pupil dilatation
- growth retardation
- organ damage
- adverse pregnancy outcome.

Release of dopamine in the forebrain is linked to addiction (Rang et al., 2007). The speed at which a drug enters the brain also determines its addictive potential. For example, cocaine has been progressively modified, from coca leaf, to hydrochlorride powder to freebase ('crack'), in order to achieve accelerated entry into neural tissue (Nutt, 1996). Intravenous methamphetamine is far more euphoriant and addictive than oral amphetamines. Similar differences exist between oral and intravenous benzodiazepines (Strang et al., 1994).

Pregnancy

Miscarriage, preterm birth, stillbirth, congenital anomalies, placental abruption, uterine rupture, cerebral infarction and maternal haemorrhage are all reported to be more common. Vasoconstriction of the placenta increases the likelihood of: intrauterine growth retardation, low birth weight and length, premature delivery, small head circumference, brain damage, and necrotizing enterocolitis (Peters and Schaefer, 2007). Anorexia is responsible for poor nutrition, vitamin deficiencies and dehydration, which adversely affect the infant. Reduced blood supply is likely to cause fetal acidosis, hypoxia and distress and low Apgar score.

V

Practice point

- Cocaine intake in the last trimester may cause fetal distress, necessitating emergency Caesarean delivery (Kuczkowski, 2004).

Cocaine-induced vasoconstriction in the fetus at varying stages of development may account for the variety of malformations reported in bones, limbs, eyes, heart or genitourinary tract (Peters and Schaefer, 2007).

Practice point

■ Detailed ultrasound investigations may be requested for investigation of possible congenital anomalies.

Long-term language development of children exposed to cocaine *in utero* is suboptimal and behavioural deficits persist at 6-year follow-up (Lewis et al., 2007; Wong et al., 2008).

The impact of stimulants on the developing fetus depends on the pattern of use. Some authorities suggest that occasional or sporadic use in early pregnancy in comfortable social circumstances without co-administration of other drugs may not be harmful to the fetus (Peters and Schaefer, 2007).

Overdose

Overdose of cocaine or amphetamines may present as overactivity, aggression, stereotypical behaviour, paranoia, hallucinations or an acute psychotic episode followed by exhaustion, hyperthermia, dehydration, and convulsions. BP may be dangerously elevated. Coma, respiratory arrest, cardiovascular collapse and rhabdomyolysis (muscle breakdown) may follow. The breakdown products of muscle may damage the kidneys or liver or cause disseminated intravascular coagulation. Hospital admission is essential for sedation, airway maintenance and control of cardiac arrhythmias. Management centres on control of individual symptoms, and usually involves benzodiazepine administration (BNF, 2009). There are individual differences in sensitivity, and acute intoxication may occur with first use.

Dependence and withdrawal

Stimulant use is characterized by tolerance and withdrawal symptoms. Tolerance to CNS effects may result in regular users requiring increased doses to obtain either the same sensation of euphoria or relief of opioid-induced sedation. A pattern of 'bingeing' and prolonged intoxication with a risk of overdose may emerge (Rang et al., 2007).

Practice point

■ Sudden discontinuation of stimulants, for example during hospital admission, may induce depression and craving.

Withdrawal from amphetamines or cocaine is followed by a craving for the drug, depression, anxiety, general fatigue and sleep – a 'crash'. On awakening, appetite is increased. Somnolence, fatigue, depression and anhedonia persist for days or weeks, with fluctuating craving and sometimes suicidal ideation. These symptoms are attributed to abrupt cessation of dopamine release, so that the levels of this neurotransmitter in the forebrain fall below normal (Nutt, 1996). After amphetamine discontinuation, sleep patterns take 2 months to normalize.

Neonates suffering withdrawal from stimulants feed and sleep poorly, and may develop tremors. Neonates are more likely to experience toxicity and fetal distress than withdrawal. Small frequent feeds are advised (Peters and Schaefer, 2007).

Amphetamines

Amphetamines were introduced in the 1930s, as the benzedrine inhaler for asthma; their use soon spread to include the treatment of alcoholism, epilepsy and migraine. Amphetamines were used in the 1939–45 war, and by US forces in the 1960s, to improve performance and delay fatigue (Gossop, 2007); they are used illegally in sports to improve sprint performance (Rang et al., 2007). Although mainly encountered as drugs of abuse, amphetamines and related drugs are prescribed for narcolepsy and as part of 'comprehensive programmes' for attention-deficit hyperactivity disorder, but are either **contraindicated** or not advised in pregnancy (BNF, 2009). They are no longer prescribed for the management of obesity.

Amphetamines, including metamphetamine, may be administered orally, intravenously or by smoking. They cross all biological membranes, including the **blood/brain barrier**, placenta and blood/milk barrier. Half-life ranges from 5 to 30 hours, longer if the urine is alkaline; effects can be prolonged by the ingestion of antacids. They can be detected in urine for 1–2 days after ingestion.

Actions of amphetamines

Central nervous system

Release of catecholamines increases alertness, excitement, self-confidence, libido, motor activity, energy, attention and concentration and elevates mood; fatigue and boredom may be overcome, so that performance remains high, particularly in subjects deprived of sleep. However, complex tasks, such as driving, are increasingly subject to errors. Although short-term learning is initially improved with methylphenidate (Ritalin®), the long-term value of these drugs has been questioned (Chetley, 1995). Insomnia, headache, anxiety, tension, hostility, irrational fears, anorexia, confusion and irritability are common effects of amphetamine use. Stereotypical behaviours occur at higher doses. Euphoric or dysphoric moods may be induced. Intravenous injection produces the sensation of a 'high' or a 'rush'.

Prolonged use of amphetamines in high dose causes neuronal damage, cognitive impairment, anxiety, depression or psychotic symptoms (Rang et al., 2007). Amphetamine-induced psychosis resembles paranoid schizophrenia, with intense fear, persecutory symptoms, visual and tactile hallucinations and delirium; it usually disappears with a week of abstinence. Intoxication with any CNS stimulant, hallucinogen or cannabis may mimic the symptoms of mania or schizophrenia. These symptoms may be exacerbated by either the use of or the withdrawal from alcohol (Milton and Jann, 1995). Drug-induced psychosis is an increasingly common reason for acute psychiatric admission; a history of repeated admissions, with rapid recovery and relapse on discharge, should trigger suspicion of drug abuse (Cohen, 1995).

Cardiovascular system

Amphetamines mimic the actions of the sympathetic nervous system, raising blood pressure, altering heart rate, and inducing flushing and sweating. The increased activity of the heart, coupled with coronary vasoconstriction, may cause angina, cardiac arrhythmias, myocardial infarction, or pulmonary hypertension, pulmonary oedema, and heart failure due to an excessively high cardiac output (high output cardiac failure). Prolonged amphetamine use may lead to cardiomyopathy. Stroke or transient cerebral ischaemia may arise from cerebrovascular spasm or intracerebral haemorrhage.

Practice point

■ Women using amphetamines may be at increased risk of hypertensive complications of pregnancy.

V

The gut may be stimulated or inhibited by amphetamines and the patient may contact the emergency services complaining of severe, acute abdominal pain accompanied by diarrhoea and vomiting.

Ecstasy

Ecstasy (MDMA or 3,4-methylenedioxymethamphetamine) is an amphetamine with some hallucinogenic properties. It is becoming less widely used (Wong et al., 2008). It has also been used for the promotion of communication and counselling in the care of the dying.

Release of the neurotransmitter serotonin is responsible for the characteristic euphoria, lasting some 4 hours. Tolerance develops rapidly, which may account for both chronic bingeing and sparing use patterns (Wong et al., 2008). MDMA actions on the cardiovascular and central nervous systems resemble other stimulants, and include bruxism, paranoid delusions, anxiety, angina, fits, hyperthermia and organ failure; these problems are often compounded by dehydration. Occasionally, release of antidiuretic hormone is increased, causing fluid retention (Chapter 6). MDMA has the potential to produce lasting changes in human brain function and structure analogous to the damage seen in monkeys (Kalant, 2007b).

Cocaine

The leaves of the coca plant (*Erythroxylon coca*) have been used by the Andean Indians for 4,000 years to increase endurance, strength and work capacity, enabling them to work at high altitude. Cocaine entered Western medicine in the last century, superseding opium as a popular prescribed drug (Medawar, 1992; Gossop, 2007). Until the 1970s, cocaine was mainly used intranasally as cocaine hydrochloride, and not regarded as dangerous. This changed with the development of almost 100% pure forms of cocaine base, 'crack' cocaine, which can be smoked. Cocaine combines local anaesthesia with intense vasoconstriction of mucous membranes; however, since it is more toxic than alternative local anaesthetics, it is rarely prescribed.

Cocaine rapidly crosses all mucous membranes, the blood/brain barrier, placenta and blood/milk barrier. Smoking or intravenous injection both afford very rapid actions. The duration of action of cocaine is 30 minutes. (Half-life is 30–90 minutes in adults and 30–40 minutes in neonates.) Cocaine appears in breast milk some 15 minutes after maternal intake and persists for 24 hours. Cocaine's metabolites can be detected in adult urine for 2–3 days after ingestion and in neonates' urine for 3–4 days. Cocaine can be detected in meconium or the hair of users and neonates (Rang et al., 2007).

Practice point

■ Breastfeeding is not advised for 24 hours after cocaine ingestion.

Actions of cocaine

Cocaine increases the concentration of dopamine (and noradrenaline/norepinephrine) in the brain by blocking reuptake into neurones. The euphoriant and unwanted effects of cocaine are similar to those of amphetamine, but paranoia, hallucinations and stereotypical behaviour are less common and shorter in duration.

Central nervous system

Cocaine is a stimulant, causing euphoria, excitement, talkativeness, increased libido, impaired judgement, emotional instability, grandiose delusions, increase in energy and alertness, assertiveness, anorexia, nausea, headache, overactive reflexes and at high dose, tremors, anxiety, confusion, depression, seizures, dilated pupils, hyperthermia, bronchospasm and respiratory arrest.

Practice points

- These effects may be intensified by administration of other local anaesthetics (such as lidocaine/lignocaine or bupivacaine), and there are reports of aggressive behaviour, therefore close observation is required (Kuczkowski, 2004).
- Pain perception may be heightened, and women may be dissatisfied with prescribed regional analgesia despite sensory blockade (Chapter 4).

The high doses of cocaine absorbed by inhalation by 'freebasing' give the sought-after rush without intravenous injection. Prolonged use leads to insomnia, inability to concentrate, irritability, depression, sexual dysfunction, hypervigilance, loss of insight and a paranoid psychotic state. Compulsive behaviour may lead to bingeing to exhaustion as doses are administered every 15 minutes.

Neonates exposed to cocaine *in utero* show signs of central nervous system stimulation (irritability, tremors, poor sleep, high pitched cries, vomiting, fever, sneezing, and rapid breathing) and feed poorly until are able to clear the drug from their bodies. These symptoms may also appear in breastfed infants, and women using cocaine regularly may be advised against breastfeeding (Peters and Schaefer, 2007).

Cardiovascular system

Blood pressure, heart rate and respiratory rate are increased in both user and fetus, as with amphetamines. Vasoconstriction may injure the endothelial lining of blood vessels, and activate platelets. This may lead to subarachnoid haemorrhage, aortic dissection, or premature atherosclerosis. Thrombus may form at any time, causing stroke, heart attack or heart failure in user or neonate. Cocaine-induced vasoconstriction may also jeopardize the gut. Cardiovascular sensitivity to cocaine, and other local anaesthetics (Chapter 4), is increased during pregnancy and serious cardiovascular events can follow small doses of cocaine in healthy women up to 24 hours after ingestion (Kuczkowski, 2004).

Practice points

- Cocaine use may cause seizures, hypertension, oedema and proteinuria. If renal and hepatic function tests are not done, this could be confused with eclampsia.
- Low platelet counts may complicate misuse of cocaine or opioids, increasing the risk of haemorrhage (Kuczkowski, 2004).

Cocaine constricts both diseased and non-diseased coronary arteries, and this is exacerbated by tobacco. Recognition of the role of stimulants in patients presenting with chest pain or a possible myocardial infarction is essential, as both the interpretation of diagnostic tests and treatment will depend on the history of cocaine consumption. Use of beta blockers in cocaine-induced myocardial ischaemia is likely to induce seizures, intensified coronary vasoconstriction, or a catastrophic rise in BP (Hollander, 1995). Rather, management centres on benzodiazepines, aspirin and nitrates.

V

Case report

An obese woman with a history of non-prescription use of heroin, cocaine and amphetamines was prescribed labetolol (a beta blocker) for pre-eclampsia. A few weeks after birth, her blood pressure rose and she had a seizure. Cerebral and subarachnoid haemorrhages were found on CT scan.

It is possible that cocaine and amphetamine use contributed to the hypertension and subsequent cerebral haemorrhages. Whether prescription of a beta blocker compounded the problems remains unknown (CEMACH, 2007: 194).

Organ damage

Smoking or nasal administration frequently traumatizes the epithelia lining the respiratory passages, causing ulceration and bleeding. Inhalation of cocaine can cause acute lung injury, either pneumothorax, or acute respiratory failure, with widespread alveolar damage, alveolar haemorrhage, pulmonary oedema, and infiltration (Restrepo et al., 2007). Long-term use of cocaine may cause kidney or liver damage.

Ketamine

Ketamine is a liquid or powder that can be injected, ingested or smoked with other materials. Mind-altering effects last about 1 hour, which can lead to repetitive dosing. It is occasionally prescribed as an anaesthetic, and, in low doses, for some chronic pain conditions, and in veterinary medicine. Manu-facturers do not recommend use in pregnancy and breastfeeding, outside delivery (Pfizer, ABPI, 2009).

Ketamine acts on glutamate receptors, responsible for central nervous system stimulation, and dopamine receptors, responsible for memory. Recreational use is associated with impaired memory and cognition, agitation and paranoid psychosis. Like other stimulants, ketamine increases heart rate, BP and body temperature. Seizures have been reported (Welters and Leuwer, 2008). Ketamine may cause cell death in the developing brain, by the same mechanisms as alcohol (Farber and Olney, 2003).

Khat

The leaves of the plant *Catha edulis* may be chewed, brewed or smoked. Stimulant compounds (cathinone), similar to amphetamines, increase the availability of the neurotransmitter dopamine. The effects on the cardiovascular system are similar to those of other stimulants. Khat also causes constipation and may be linked to mental health problems. Reduced birth weight and lactation have been reported in khat users (Wong et al., 2008).

Conclusion

The 'wonder drugs' of their day, most recreational drugs now have few uses in clinical practice, and considerable potential for abuse. Although many people use drugs for recreation without requiring medical help, their widespread use means that professionals should be aware of the link between these drugs and a wide variety of presentations, such as accidents, hypertension, prema-ture labour, seizures, stroke, chest pain, and violent behaviour. Just as no patient history is complete without a detailed drug history, so no drug history is complete without a record of recreational drug use. By virtue of their close relationships with patients, the time they spend at the bedside and their communication skills, midwives are well placed to uncover vital informa-tion that will allow clinically appropriate referral and treatment.

Further reading

■ Chang, G. (2001) Alcohol screening instruments for pregnant women. *Alcohol Research and Health*, 25: 204–9, http://pubs.ni.nih.gov/publications/arh25-3/204-209.htm.
■ Peters, P.W. and Schaefer, C. (2007) Recreational drugs, in Schaefer, C., Peters, P.W. and Miller, R.K. (eds) *Drugs during Pregnancy and Lactation: Treatment Options and Risk Assessment*, 2nd edn. Elsevier, Oxford.

Quick Reference for Major Drug Groups/Drugs

The most important drugs in midwifery are summarized under the headings: uses, adverse effects; cautions and contraindications; and interactions. The drugs are listed alphabetically. The lists are not exclusive.

Contents

- Beta$_2$ adrenoreceptor agonists
- Corticosteroids
- D$_2$ antagonist antiemetics
- Heparin
- Histamine, receptor antagonists (antiemetics)
- Insulin
- Iron (oral preparations)
- Laxatives
- Local anaesthetics
- Magnesium
- Nifedipine
- Nitrous oxide
- Opioids
- Oxytocin
- Prostaglandins
- SSRIs (selective serotonin reuptake inhibitors)

BETA$_2$ ADRENOCEPTOR AGONISTS

Uses

Premature labour

Rescue medication for asthma

Adverse effects

Cardiovascular system

Bleeding tendency

Cardiac dysrhythmias

Chest pain

Flushing

Lowered diastolic BP

Overactive thyroid worsened

Peripheral vasodilation

Postural hypotension

Pulmonary oedema

Raised systolic BP

Sweating, erythema

Tachycardia

Transient hypoxia

Central nervous system

Anxiety/agitation

Behaviour disturbances

Confusion

Dizziness

Hallucinations

Headache

Insomnia

Irritability

Paranoia/fear

Restlessness

Tension

Tremor

Smooth muscle inhibition

Constipation

Glaucoma

Heartburn

Ileus

Nausea/anorexia

Urine retention/dysuria

Vomiting

Metabolic

Anorexia

Drying of mucous secretions

Hyperglycaemia – rarely
  ketoacidosis

Hypokalaemia/cramps, weakness,
  cardiac dysrhythmias

Increased lactate and free
  fatty acids

Lactic acidosis and
  hyperventilation

Neonatal hypoglycaemia

Hypersensitivity responses

Anaphylaxis

Bronchospasm/wheezing

LFT changes

Rash/itching

Cautions and contraindications

Acute angle glaucoma

Cardiac disease (high risk of
  myocardial infarction)

Cardiac dysrhythmias

Diabetes

Haemorrhage

Hypertension (any cause)

Hyperthyroidism

Hypokalaemia

Intrauterine infection

Liver or kidney impairment

Phaeochromocytoma

Severe, worsening asthma

Interactions

Amphetamines (including
  those prescribed for
  attention deficit disorder)

Beta blockers

Caffeine

Cocaine

Methyldopa (those prescribed)

Muscle relaxants (some)

Oxytocin

continued on next page

Anaesthetic gases (some)	'Cold cures'	Salbutamol
Antidepressants (MAOIs)	Digoxin	Steroids
Antipsychotics (possible)	Diuretics	Theophylline
Atropine	Glycopyrronium	

CORTICOSTEROIDS

Uses

Arthritis	Immunosuppression	Prematurity
Asthma	Inflammatory bowel disease	Replacement therapy for
Dermatology	Neoplastic disease	Addison's disease
Emesis	Nephrotic syndrome	

Adverse effects

Anti-inflammatory

Acne	Impaired healing	Infections

Metabolic

Appetite increased	Hypokalaemia/cramps	Telangiectasia
Avascular necrosis of bone	Muscle wasting/weakness	Tendon rupture
Body fat redistribution	Oesophageal ulceration	Thin skin
Fluid retention	Osteoporosis/fractures	Waist expansion
Growth impairment	Pancreatitis	Weakness
Hyperglycaemia	Peptic ulceration	Weight gain
Hypertension	Raised intracranial pressure	Worsened lipid profile
Hypocalcaemia	Striae	

Endocrine

Adrenal suppression	Hirsuitism/acne	Oligomenorrhoea

Eyes

Cataracts	Glaucoma
Infections	Papilloedema

Central nervous system

Emotional lability/depression	Insomnia	Seizures
Fatigue	Malaise	Steroid abuse/dependence
Hallucinations	Nausea	
Hiccups	Psychoses	

Cardiovascular system

Bleeding/bruising	Hypertension	Low platelets
Fluid retention/heart failure	Increase in red cells	Thromboembolism

Hypersensitivity responses

Anaphylaxis	Contact allergy/rash

continued on next page

Cautions and contraindications

Diabetes

Diverticulitis, colitis

Epilepsy

Glaucoma

Heart failure/attack

HIV/AIDS

Hypertension

Hypothyroidism

Infections

Live vaccines

Liver failure

Mental illness

Migraine

Myasthenia gravis

Osteoporosis

Peptic ulceration

Renal insufficiency

TB

Thrombophilia

Interactions

Alcohol

Aloe

Antacids

Anticoagulants

Antidiabetics

Antiepileptics

Antihypertensives

Antivirals and antifungals (some)

Asian herbal mixtures (some)

Beta$_2$ adrenoceptor agonists

Ciclosporin

Digoxin

Diuretics

Erythromycin (related drugs)

Hypoglycaemia agents

Liquorice

NSAIDs

Oestrogens

Salt (in food or intravenous infusion)

Sympathomimetics

Vaccines

D$_2$ ANTAGONIST ANTIEMETICS (e.g. prochlorperazine, but see also histamine antagonists)

Uses
Emesis in labour or due to: migraine, ergot alkaloids, opioids or anaesthetics
Hyperemesis gravidarum

Adverse effects

Alterations in BP	Dizziness	Neuroleptic malignant
Anxiety	Drying of secretions	syndrome (rare)
Blood glucose changes	Headache	SIADH (rare)
Blurred vision	Hypersensitivity responses	Urine retention
Breast tenderness	Impaired fertility	Weight gain (long term)
Cardiac dysrhythmias	Insomnia or sedation	
Diarrhoea or constipation	Metallic taste	

Depression of:

Alertness	Mood	Thermoregulation
Cough	Respiration	

Posture and movement disorders

Abnormal movements/	Acute dystonia (rare)	Tremors
parkinsonism (long term)	Restlessness	

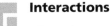

Cautions and contraindications

Atopy (metoclopramide)	For 3–4 days after	Phaeochromocytoma
Blood dyscrasias	gastrointestinal surgery	Porphyria
Breastfeeding	G6PD deficiency	Respiratory disorders
Cardiovascular disease	Glaucoma	Serious CNS conditions
Diabetes	Hepatic or renal impairment	Young people (metoclopramide)
Epilepsy	Masking serious pathology	

Interactions

All CNS depressants	Antipsychotics	Insulin
Anticoagulants	Ciclosporin	Lithium
Antidepressants	Corticosteroids	Suxamethonium
Antiepileptics	Desferoxamine	(metoclopramide)
Antihistamines	Diuretics	Tetrabenazine
Antihypertensives	Drugs for parkinsonism	

HEPARIN

Uses
Prevention and management of thromboembolic disorders

Adverse effects

Bleeding	Thrombocytopenia
Diuresis @ 36–48 hrs	(delayed – severe, early – mild)
Hyperkalaemia	Vasospastic reaction (rare)

Hypersensitivity responses

Anaphylaxis	Lacrimation	Rash/itching/urticaria
Bronchospasm	Nasal congestion	Site reactions
Chills/fever/headache	Necrosis of skin	

Long-term use only

Hair loss	Osteoporosis
Heparin resistance	Raised liver enzymes

Cautions and contraindications

Aortic aneurysm	Hypertension	Severe diabetes
Bleeding tendencies	Lesions in GI, GU or	Threatened abortion
Cerebral aneurysm	respiratory tracts	Thrombocytopenia
Cerebrovascular haemorrhage	Liver disease/alcoholism	Thrombophilias
Deficiency of vitamin K or C	Pericarditis/endocarditis	Trauma/surgery
Drainage tubes *in situ*	Prematurity	Tuberculosis
Epidural or spinal puncture	Renal impairment	
Haemophilias	Retinopathy	

Interactions

ACE inhibitors (related drugs)	Dipyridamole	Oral hypoglycaemics (some, rare)
Acid-citrate-dextrose	Drotrecogin alfa	Quinine
Alcohol	Guar gum	Salicylates
Antibiotics (some)	Iloprost	SSRIs
Clopidogrel	Ketorolac	Thrombolytic therapy
Corticosteroids	Nitrates	Tobacco
Dextrans	NSAIDs	Valproate
Digoxin	Oral anticoagulants	

HISTAMINE$_1$ RECEPTOR ANTAGONISTS (antiemetics)

Uses

Allergic disorders	Sedation
Antiemetics	Vertigo

Adverse effects

Central nervous system

Confusion	Incoordination	Sedation
Depression	Insomnia	Seizures (rare)
Hallucinations	Irritability	Tinnitus
Headache	Movement disorders (rare)	

Drying of secretions

Dry eyes	Inability to sweat	Xerostomia (dry mouth)
Dry skin	Risk of chest infection	
Ear infections	Sore mouth	

Cardiovascular system

Hypotension	Tachycardia

Gastrointestinal system

Anorexia	Gastric upset
Constipation	Ileus

Renal system

Urine retention

Eyes

Blurred vision	Glaucoma	Photophobia

Hypersensitivity responses (rare)

Angioedema/anaphylaxis	Bronchospasm	Rash
Blood dyscrasia	Photosensitivity	

Cautions

Asthma	GI obstruction	Porphyria
Breastfeeding	Glaucoma	Renal impairment
Cardiovascular disease	History of seizures	Retention of urine
Diabetes	Liver disease	

Interactions

Anaesthetics	Antivirals (some)	Sedatives, for example alcohol,
Antiarrhythmics	Drugs for parkinsonism	opioids, tricyclic
Antifungals (some)	Erythromycin (related drugs)	antidepressants,
		antipsychotics

INSULIN

Uses

Ketoacidosis

Maintenance of normoglycaemia in diabetes

Adverse effects

Antibody formation

Hypoglycaemia

Hypokalaemia (infusions)

Insulin resistance

Loss of hypoglycaemic awareness

Oedema

Postural hypotension

Vision impairment

Weight gain

Injection site problems

Bruising

Itching

Lipoatrophy

Lipohypertrophy

Cautions and contraindications

Hypersensitivity

Hypoglycaemia

Interactions

Drugs causing hyperglycaemia

Amphetamines, cocaine

Antipsychotics

Caffeine (large doses)

Calcium antagonists

Diuretics

Glucosamine

Marijuana

Nicotine

Phenytoin

Pyridoxine

Steroids (oestrogens,
    progesterone,
    glucocorticoids)

Sympathomimetics

Thyroxine

Drugs causing hypoglycaemia

ACEIs

Alcohol

Anabolic steroids

Fibrates

Lanreotide

MAOIs

Salicylates

Some NSAIDs

Tetracyclines

Loss of hypoglycaemic awareness

Beta blockers

IRON (oral preparations)

Uses
Iron deficiency anaemia

Adverse effects
Gastrointestinal system

Anorexia	Nausea	Stool and urine discolouration
Constipation	Painful swallowing	Teeth staining
Diarrhoea	Stomach cramps	Vomiting
Indigestion		

Impaired absorption
Phosphate deficiency (rare)   Zinc or calcium deficiency

Haematological

Folic acid deficiency	Headache	Iron overload

Cautions and contraindications

Haemolytic anaemia	Liver disease	Sensitivity to iron
Haemosiderosis	Peptic ulcer	Ulcerative colitis

Interactions

Alcohol	Cholestyramine	Quinolones
Antacids	Cimetidine	Tea (tannins)
Bisphophonates	Ciprofloxacin	Tetracyclines (including doxycycline)
Caffeine	Histamine$_2$ antagonists	Vitamin C
Calcium supplements	Methyldopa	Vitamin E
Cereals (phytates)	Milk, eggs	

LAXATIVES

Uses

Bowel disease and investigations	Conditions exacerbated by straining at stool	Opioid administration (several days)

Adverse effects

Abdominal cramps	Flatulence	Nausea/anorexia
Dehydration	Hypokalaemia	Throat irritation
Diarrhoea	Intestinal obstruction	

Prolonged use

Absorption of the laxative	Loss of protein, calcium and other minerals	Rectal irritation/worsening of haemorrhoids
Colonic atony		
Dependence		
Fluid retention due to sodium content		

Cautions and contraindications

Atonic colon	Dehydration	Hypersensitivity responses
Colostomy/ileostomy	Diabetes (some products)	Intestinal obstruction
Debility	Eating disorders	Swallowing difficulties

Interactions

Administer at least 2 hours apart from other drugs and food	Corticosteroids	Loss of other drugs or minerals due to diarrhoea
Beta$_2$ agonists	Digoxin	
	Diuretics	

LOCAL ANAESTHETICS

Uses

Epidural/regional
  anaesthesia/analgesia
Nerve block

Suturing and minor procedures
Topical, e.g. intravenous access

Adverse effects: maternal
Cardiovascular

Cardiovascular collapse/dysrhythmia   Hypertension   Hypotension

Central nervous system

Anxiety	Fever	Shivering
Confusion	Nausea	Thermoregulation failure
Convulsions	Paraesthesia/paralysis	Tremor
Dyspnoea	Restlessness	

Smooth muscle relaxation

Incontinence of urine or faeces   Prolongation of labour   Retention of urine

Hypersensitivity reactions

Problems associated with dural puncture such as headache

Adverse effects: fetal/neonatal

Depression of CNS	Neonatal hypothermia	Respiratory depression
Fetal bradycardia	Pyrexia	

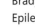

Cautions

Bradycardia, heart block	Malignant hyperthermia	Previous hypersensitivity
Epilepsy	Methaemoglobinaemia	Porphyria
Hypovolaemia	Myasthenia gravis	
Liver, kidney, respiratory or thyroid disease		

Interactions

5HT3 antagonists	Benzodiazeipines	Diuretics
Antiarrhythmics	Beta antagonists (blockers)	Muscle relaxants
Antipsychotics	Calcium antagonists	Sedatives (alcohol,
Antivirals (some)	Cimetidine, possibly ranitidine	prochlorperazine)

MAGNESIUM

Uses (parenteral)

Acute severe asthma

Anticonvulsant prophylaxis in
  eclampsia

Cardiac dysrhythmias

Hypomagnesemia

Uses (oral)

Laxative

Adverse effects: maternal

Nervous system

Dizziness

Double vision

Drowsiness/sedation

Flaccid paralysis

Headache

Loss of deep tendon reflexes

Reduced muscle tone

Respiratory paralysis

Slurred speech

Tetany

Weakness, lethargy, depression

Cardiovascular system

Asystole

Chest pain

Complete heart block

Flushing

Hypotension

Hypothermia

Hypoxia

Impaired coagulation

Palpitations

Pulmonary oedema

Sweating

Smooth muscle relaxation

Abdominal cramps

Diarrhoea

Ileus

Nausea

Tocolysis

Vomiting

Renal system

Osmotic diuresis

Protein loss

Other

Decreased bone density with
  long-term use

Dry mouth/thirst

Urticaria with intravenous use

Adverse effects: neonatal/fetal

Blunting of reflexes

Congenital rickets (long-term use)

Convulsions

Decreased HR variability

Drowsiness

Hypothermia

Meconium ileus

Neonatal convulsions

Poor muscle tone

Respiratory depression/apnoea

Cautions and contraindications

Cardiac disease

Heart block

Hepatic impairment

Gastrointestinal conditions (serious)

Myasthenia gravis

Renal impairment

Respiratory impairment

---

continued on next page

Interactions

Aminoglycosides	Calcium antagonists	Opioids
Benzodiazepines	General anaesthetics	Phenothiazines
Beta$_2$ adrenoreceptor agonists (salbutamol)	Local anaesthetics	
	Muscle relaxants	

NIFEDIPINE

Uses

Angina	Raynaud's phenomenon
Hypertension	Tocolysis

Adverse effects: maternal

Angina	Dizziness	Oedema
Blurred vision	Eye pain/vision disturbance	Palpitations
Breast tenderness	Flushing	Polyuria/dysuria
Breathlessness	Heart rate changes	Prolonged labour
Bruising/bleeding	Hypotension	Pulmonary oedema
Cough	Hypothermia	Sweating
Chills	Joint pain	Tinnitus
Cramps/stiffness		

Gastrointestinal

Constipation	Gastric upset	Heartburn
Dry mouth	Gum overgrowth	Nausea

Central nervous system

Fatigue	Insomnia	Posture and movement disorders
Headache/migraine	Nervousness	Tremor

Hypersensitivity

Bronchospasm	Photosensitivity
Hepatotoxicity	Rashes/itching

Adverse effects: neonatal/fetal

Possibly IUGR	Possibly prematurity

Cautions and contraindications

Abrupt withdrawal	Heart failure	Liver or kidney impairment
Breastfeeding	Hypotension	Porphyria
Diabetes	Ischaemic heart disease	Unstable angina/recent MI

continued on next page

Interactions

Alcohol
Anaesthetics
Antiarrhythmics
Antidepressants (some)
Antiepileptics
Antifungals (some)
Antihypertensives (all)
Beta blockers
Ciclosporin
Cimetidine, ranitidine

Digoxin
Grapefruit juice
Ionic X-ray contrast media
Khat
Magnesium
Muscle relaxants (non-depolarizing)
NSAIDs
Rifampicin
Ritonavir

Some antiemetics
   (prochlorperazine)
Steroids
Sympathomimetics (including
   OTC cold cures)
Theophylline
Tobacco
Vancomycin
Vasodilators

NITROUS OXIDE

Uses

Anaesthesia when combined with
   other agents

Dressing changes
Inhalation analgesia

Trauma

Adverse effects: maternal

Alkalosis
Dizziness
Hallucinations

Hypoxia
Light-headedness
Nausea

Sedation
Vomiting

Adverse effects: neonatal

Hypoxia

Sedation

Adverse effects: healthcare workers

Impaired fertility

Leucopenia

Vitamin B_{12} deficiency

Cautions

Air embolism
Bowel distension
Family history of malignant
   hyperthermia

First 16 weeks of pregnancy
Intoxication
Occluded middle ear
Pneumothorax

Prolonged exposure
   (>24 hours)
Respiratory impairment
Storage precautions

Interactions

Antihypertensives
Methotrexate
Opioids

Other anaesthetics (such as
   halothane)

Sedatives
Vitamin B_{12}

OPIOIDS

Uses
Acute pulmonary oedema/MI
Analgesia
Anxioloysis
Cough (not recommended)
Sedation
Ventilator management

Adverse effects
Depression of:
Blood pressure
Breastfeeding
Central nervous system/sedation
Cough/chest infections
Fertility (long-term use)
Gag reflex
GI tract motility – delayed gastric
  emptying, ileus, constipation,
  biliary colic
Heart rate
Immune system (long-term use)
Respiration
Thermoregulation
Uterine contractility

Other
Bronchospasm
Confusion and hallucinations
Convulsions
Cramps
Dry mouth
Miosis (except pethidine)
Mood changes
Myoclonus
Nausea/vomiting
Pruritus
Retention of urine
SIADH
Tinnitus
Vision disturbance (temporary)

Cautions and contraindications
Addison's disease
Alcohol intoxication
Asthma attack
Biliary colic
Convulsions (particularly
  pethidine)
Decreased respiratory reserve
Dependence
Head injury/raised intracranial
  pressure
Hypotension
Hypothyroidism/thyroid disease
Known allergy to opioids
Liver failure
Myasthenia gravis
Pancreatitis
Paralytic ileus
Phaeochromocytoma
Renal impairment

Interactions
All central nervous system
  depressants (including
  alcohol, antipsychotics)
Antiarrhythmics
Antidepressants
Antiepileptics
Antifungals
Antihistamines
Antimalarials
Antiparkinsonism drugs
  (Selegiline)
Antivirals
Benzodiazeipines
Carbamazepine
Cimetidine
Cyclizine
Erythromycin
Ketoconazole
MAOIs (pethidine)
Metoclopramide
Midazolam (with fentanyl)
Nitrous oxide
Phenothiazines
Promethazine
Rifampicin
Ritonavir (other antivirals)
Sedatives
Sodium oxybate
Tobacco

OXYTOCIN

Uses

Augmentation of labour

Induction of labour

Missed or incomplete abortion

Postpartum haemorrhage

Adverse effects: maternal
Overstimulation of the uterus

Abruptio placenta

Amniotic fluid embolus

Painful contractions

Pelvic haematoma

Postpartum haemorrhage

Trauma

Uterine rupture

Cardiovascular system

Cardiac arrhythmia

Cardiovascular collapse

Cerebrovascular accident

DIVC

Fluid retention

Headache

Hypersensitivity responses

Hypertension

Hypotension

Nausea and vomiting

Water intoxication

Adverse effects: fetal/neonatal

Acidosis

Asphyxia

Birth trauma

Cardiac dysrhythmias

Hypoxia

Neonatal jaundice

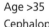

Cautions and contraindications

Age >35

Cephalopelvic disproportion

Difficult delivery (prolapsed cord, *placenta praevia*)

DIVC risk

Eclampsia/pre-eclampsia

Fetal distress

Fetal malposition

Grand multiparae

Heart disease

History of uterine sepsis

Hypersensitivity

Hypertension (pregnancy induced)

Hypertonic uterus

Obstetric emergencies

Overdistension of uterus

Placental abruption

Premature labour

Previous sections

Undilated cervix

Uterine or cervical surgery

Uterine inertia

Interactions

Adrenaline

Anaesthetics

Carbamazepine

Cyclophosphamide

Ephedrine

Opioids

Prostaglandins

Sympathomimetics

PROSTAGLANDINS

Uses in childbirth

Evacuation of the uterus	Induction of labour	Postpartum haemorrhage

Adverse effects

Gastrointestinal

Abdominal pain	Hiccups
Diarrhoea	Nausea, vomiting

Uterine hyperstimulation (as for oxytocin)

Fetal compromise	Pain	Rupture of uterus

Cardiovascular

BP alterations	Flushing	Raised white cell count
Cardiac dysrhythmias	Hypoxia	Sweating
Diuresis	Pulmonary oedema	Tachycardia
DIVC	Pyrexia/chills	

Respiratory system

Bronchospasm	Choking	Wheezing

Nervous system

Back pain	Seizures
Increase in intraocular pressure (glaucoma)	Tremor

Vaginal irritation

Adverse effects: fetal/neonatal

Acidosis	Birth trauma	Hypoxia
Asphyxia	Cardiac dysrhythmias	

Cautions and contraindications

Asthma	Grand multiparas	Pelvic infection
BP abnormalities	High risk of uterine rupture	Previous section/uterine surgery
Cardiac disease	Hypersensitivity	Pulmonary disease
Epilepsy	Hypertension/hypotension	Risk of DIVC
Fetal compromise/disproportion	Kidney disease	Ruptured membranes
Glaucoma/raised intraocular pressure	Liver disease	Unexplained vaginal bleeding

---

Interactions

Alcohol	Aspirin/NSAIDs
Antihypertensives	Oxytocin

SSRIs (selective serotonin reuptake inhibitors, e.g. fluoxetine/ Prozac®)

Uses

Bulimia nervosa
Depression

Obsessive/compulsive disorders
Panic disorder

Social phobia

Adverse effects
Central nervous system

Aggression
Agitation
Amnesia
Anxiety
Blurred vision
Convulsions
Dizziness
Fever
Hallucinations

Headache
Hypomania/maina
Insomnia
Loss of libido
Migraine
Neuroleptic malignant syndrome
Panic attacks
Pins and needles
Posture and movement disorders

Restlessness/behaviour
  disturbance
Sedation (some SSRIs,
  e.g. citalopram)
Tinnitus
Tremor
Vision disturbance
Weakness

Cardiovascular system

Bleeding/bruising
Flushes

Palpitations/dysrhythmias
Postural hypotension

SIADH
Sweating

Gastrointestinal system

Anorexia
Diarrhoea or constipation
Dry mouth

Glucose changes
Hypersalivation/nasal congestion
Indigestion

Nausea/vomiting
Taste disturbance
Weight changes

Other

Breast tenderness
Frequent micturition

Glaucoma
Menstrual irregularities

Serotonin syndrome
Skin infections

Hypersensitivity responses

Angioedema
Arthralgia
Bone marrow damage
Hair loss

Liver damage
Lung damage
Myalgia
Pancreatitis

Photosensitivity
Rash/itching
Vasculitis

Cautions and contraindications

Abrupt withdrawal
Agitation
Bleeding disorders
Breastfeeding
Cardiac disease
Diabetes

ECT
Glaucoma
Hepatic impairment
History of mania
Parkinsonism

Pregnancy
Renal impairment
Risk of convulsions
Suicidal ideation
Young people <18

continued on next page

Interactions

Alcohol

Amphetamines, cocaine

Antiarrhythmics

Anticoagulants

Antiepileptics

Antihistamines

Antiparkinsonian drugs

Antipsychotics

Antivirals

Benzodiazepines/buspirone

Bupropion

Calcium blockers

Cannabis

Carbamazepine

Cimetidine

Cold cures

Digoxin

Erythromycin

Lithium

LSD

NSAIDs

Other antidepressants

Pentazocine

Prochlorperazine

Ropivacaine

Sedatives

St John's wort

Theophylline

Tramadol

Triptans

Warfarin

APPENDIX II

Glossary

These words are highlighted in **bold** *within the text.*

achlorhydria Deficiency in hydrochloric acid production by the stomach.

acidosis A pathological condition resulting from accumulation of acid or loss of base, and characterized by increase in hydrogen ion concentration (and decrease in pH). The usual cause is poor oxygenation of tissues.

adsorption The formation of a layer of a substance on the surface of a solid by chemical attraction.

adverse drug reaction Any untoward and unintended response in a patient or investigational subject to a medicinal product, which is related to any dose administered (ICH, 1996).

adverse effect The impact on the patient of an adverse reaction (Edwards and Aronson, 2000).

adverse event Any untoward medical occurrence in a patient or participant in a drug trial to whom a medicinal product has been administered, including occurrences that are not necessarily caused by or related to that product (ICH, 1996).

agonist A substance having a specific cellular affinity that produces a predictable response; also, a chemical capable of stimulating a cell receptor.

agranulocytosis A marked reduction in the number of circulating granular leukocytes, particularly neutrophils. This renders the patient very liable to serious infections. Unrecognized and untreated, these overwhelming infections can be fatal.

AIDS Acquired immune deficiency syndrome, a disease associated with the HIV virus.

alkalosis A pathological condition resulting from accumulation of base or loss of acid, and characterized by decrease in hydrogen ion concentration (and increase in pH).

alpha (α) agonist A drug that stimulates the alpha receptors.

alpha$_1$ receptors These receptors normally respond to noradrenaline/norepinephrine and adrenaline/epinephrine. They form an important component of the sympathetic nervous system. One of their important functions is the control of blood pressure.

anaesthetic An agent causing reversible loss of sensation.

anaphylaxis A severe hypersensitivity response (allergic reaction) to a chemical introduced into the body. The response is characterized by histamine release in the tissues, causing bronchospasm, swelling and severe hypotension. Immediate treatment is needed to avert fatality.

antagonist A chemical that can occupy a cell receptor without stimulating it and thereby block the action of agonists for that receptor.

antibacterial A substance that inhibits the growth of, or kills, a bacterium.

antibiotic A natural substance that inhibits the growth of, or kills, a bacterium. Sometimes widened to substances that inhibit all microorganisms.

antigen Any molecule, usually a protein or polysaccharide, that interacts with an antibody. The term antigen is usually used in immunology to describe foreign material, although antigens can be generated within the body, for example A and B antigens on the surface of erythrocytes.

antibodies Immunoglobulin proteins secreted by B lymphocytes. Antibody synthesis is induced by specific antigens, and they combine with these specific antigens usually to initiate pathogen destruction.

antifungal A substance that inhibits the growth of, or kills, a fungus.

antimicrobial A substance that inhibits the growth of, or kills, a microorganism.

antimuscarinic A substance that blocks the actions of the parasympathetic nervous system by acting on the postganglionic muscarinic receptors.

antiviral A substance that inhibits the replication of, or destroys, a virus.

Apgar score This system was named after Virginia Apgar, an anaesthetist. It was introduced to standardize the observation of all neonates. It combines measures of heart rate and respiratory effort with observations of muscle tone, skin colour and reflex irritability. A score of 9 or 10 indicates a healthy baby. A score of 4–6 indicates mild or moderate neonatal depression. A non-responsive baby will score 4 or less. Assessments are made 1, 5 and 10 minutes after delivery.

aPTT   Activated partial thromboplastin time. A coagulation test of the entire coagulation mechanism that detects deficiencies in the formation of thromboplastin (factor Xa). Normal range 30–40 seconds.

atelectasis   In adults, collapse of the lungs, usually the lower lobes. At birth, incomplete expansion of the lungs.

atopy/atopic   A condition characterized by hypersensitivity responses, including asthma, eczema, hay fever.

autoimmune diseases   Disorders of the body's defence system in which components of the immune system attack the body's own tissues. Rheumatoid arthritis and systemic lupus erythematosis are examples.

bacteraemia   The presence of bacteria in the blood.

beta (β) lactamase   A penicillin-degrading enzyme produced by some bacteria.

beta (β) agonist   A drug that stimulates the beta receptors. These receptors normally respond to adrenaline/epinephrine and noradrenaline/norepinephrine. Their important functions include the control of the heart, bronchioles and blood vessels. There are several subtypes of beta receptors. The best studied are the β_1 (mainly in the heart) and β_2 receptors, which are associated with the fright and flight response.

bioavailability   A measure of absorption or the fractional extent to which the drug dose reaches its site of action.

bioequivalence   Two forms of a drug are said to be bioequivalent if their rates and extent of absorption of their active ingredients are the same under test conditions.

blood/brain barrier   The structure separating the blood from the brain tissue and the cerebrospinal fluid. It is composed of the capillary endothelium and the astrocyte end-feet. In adults, it protects the brain tissue from fluctuations in the plasma. It is not fully developed in neonates.

BMI (body mass index)   This represents weight in kilograms divided by height in metres squared. It takes no account of the composition of tissue. A convenient calculator can be found on the BNF website (bnf.org).

broad-spectrum antibiotic   An antibiotic that is active against many types of Gram-positive and Gram-negative bacteria.

capsule   A gelatine case surrounding an oral preparation.

cardiac dysrhythmias   Disordered rhythms of the heart, usually due to disturbance of the conducting system.

They range in severity from benign to lethal. They may be symptomless, or give rise to vague symptoms such as breathlessness or palpitations.

cardiac output   Cardiac output is the volume of blood pumped into the dorsal aorta each minute by the left ventricle of the heart. This is the quantity of blood flowing through the circulation each minute, transporting substances (including oxygen and carbon dioxide) to and from the tissues.

chemotherapeutic agent   An antimicrobial that is used to treat infections inside the human body.

common law   This refers to legal principles derived from cases decided in the higher courts, which are then binding on lower courts through a system of precedence. This allows for a degree of certainty in the law to be maintained.

confidence intervals (CI)   The range of values around the mean or the effect, within which the true mean or effect is located. Often interpreted as: authors are 95% confident that the true effect (or mean) lies within the range stated as the 95% confidence interval.

conjugation   The joining of two compounds to produce another compound. The compound produced is usually less toxic than the original. This occurs in the liver, where glucuronic acid is added to drug molecules to make them water soluble, so that they can be eliminated by the kidneys.

contraindicated   Not recommended for clinical use.

cytokines   Any soluble factor secreted by cells of the lymphoid system that signals to other lymphoid cells.

dystocia   Abnormal labour or childbirth.

dystocia, shoulder   Due to failure of rotation, after delivery of the baby's head, the shoulders impact on the pelvic brim, with the anterior shoulder trapped under the pubis. Without very prompt action to deliver the baby, intrapartum death will occur.

endothelial cells/endothelium   The layer of epithelial cells lining the heart, blood vessels, lymph vessels and serous cavities of the body.

enteric coating   A layer of material on the outer surface of a tablet or capsule that prevents dissolution in the stomach, and thereby both delays absorption and protects the lining of the stomach.

enterohepatic recycling   Several substances, including steroids and bile salts, are excreted in the bile and reabsorbed into the liver lower down the intestine via the hepatic protal vein. This recycling and reusing reduces the loss in the faeces.

enzymes   Enzymes are proteins that act as catalysts in biochemical reactions. Each enzyme is specific to one reaction or a group of similar reactions. Catalysts are substances that increase the rate of chemical reactions without undergoing any permanent change.

free radical   A free radical is an atom or a group of

atoms with an unpaired valence electron. Because of the unpaired electron, free radicals are extremely reactive, and can easily damage cell membranes.

G6PD (glucose-6-phosphate dehydrogenase) deficiency   Hereditary deficiency of a key enzyme in one of the metabolic pathways breaking down glucose in red blood cells. This causes haemolysis (bursting of red cells) and jaundice. Problems often arise for the first time on exposure to certain drugs, such as dapsone, nitrofurantion, and some quinolones. It is possible for haemolysis to occur in the neonates of unaffected mothers.

general anaesthetic   An anaesthetic causing loss of consciousness in addition to loss of sensation.

glomerular filtration rate (GFR)   The volume of fluid passing into the Bowman's capsules each minute in all nephrons in both kidneys is the glomerular filtration rate. The normal value is about 125 ml/minute or 180 litres/day. Normally, 99% of this is reabsorbed by the renal tubules. GFR is measured by inulin or creatinine clearance. Serum creatinine values give an approximation of GFR.

Gram-negative   A major class of bacteria that have a thin cell wall and an outer membrane on their surface.

Gram-positive   A major class of bacteria that have a thick cell wall and no outer membrane on their surface.

ground substance   The intercellular matrix of connective tissue in which cells and fibres are embedded. It is composed of mucopolysaccharides/ proteoglycans, such as chondroitin-4- sulphate, chondroitin-6-sulphate and hyaluronic acid.

haemolysis   Destruction of the red blood cells, liberating haemoglobin into the surrounding fluid.

half-life   The time it takes for one-half of an observed change to occur. In pharmacology, the half-life usually referred to is the 'elimination half-life'. Elimination half-life is the time taken for the concentration of the drug in blood or plasma to fall to half its maximum value. For some drugs, elimination half-life has three distinct phases (is triphasic). 1. Distribution phase, where the drug enters the tissues. 2. A phase where the drug is moving from the tissues into the circulation and simultaneously being excreted. 3. Excretion phase, where the drug is removed from the body.

heterozygous   Describing an organism with two different alleles (genes) at a given locus on a pair of homologous chromosomes.

homozygous   Describing an organism with two identical alleles (genes) at a given locus on a pair of homologous chromosomes.

hyperkalaemia   Serum potassium ion concentration above normal values. This may lead to dangerous cardiac dysrhythmias (ventricular tachycardia and ventricular fibrillation), with characteristic ECG changes and cardiac arrest. The initial effects are a twitchiness and paraesthesia, followed by cramps, weakness, paralysis and paralytic ileus.

hypersensitivity   A response quantitatively greater than is usual for a given dose.

hypertonic   A hypertonic solution has a higher osmotic pressure than normal plasma.

hypokalaemia   Serum potassium concentration below normal values. These are 3.5–5.1 mmol/l. Hypokaleamia may cause a range of problems from vague symptoms of weakness, constipation, depression to sudden cardiac events.

hyponatraemia   Serum sodium ion concentration below normal values. In the third trimester, these are 133–143 mmol/l. Serious symptoms develop if serum sodium concentration falls below 120 mmol/l.

hypotonic   A hypotonic solution has a lower osmotic pressure than normal plasma.

international normalized ratio (INR)   The ratio of the prothrombin time of the patient's blood sample to the prothrombin time of a standard blood sample. The prothrombin time is a measure of the time taken for clot formation when a tissue thromboplastin reagent is added. It effectively measures the activity of prothrombin, fibrinogen, and factors V, VII and X.

intrathecal administration   The introduction of a drug or other substance into the cerebrospinal fluid.

ionized   Containing ions. An ion is an atom or group of atoms that carries either a positive or a negative charge as a result of either losing or gaining an electron.

isotonic   An isotonic solution has the same osmotic pressure as normal plasma.

kernicterus   High plasma concentrations of bilirubin in the neonate, leading to neurological damage.

leucocytosis   An increased concentration of white blood cells in the circulation. Normal value 4,000–11,000 cells/microlitre.

ligand   Any substance that binds to a particular type of receptor.

lipophilic   Having an affinity for lipids (fats). A lipid is a substance insoluble in water, but soluble in ether; examples include fats, fatty acids, steroids, phospholipids, oils.

lymphocytes   White blood cells, which occur as two major populations. B lymphocytes mature in the bone marrow and can transform into antibody-secreting plasma cells when exposed to antigen. T lymphocytes mature in the thymus gland and regulate the activities of B cells and participate in cell-mediated immunity.

macrocytosis   Circulating red blood cells are larger than normal. Normal red cell volume is 78–95 femto-litres. The commonest causes of macrocytosis are folate or vitamin B_{12} deficiency.

macrophages   These develop from monocytes, a group of white blood cells. They follow neutrophils into infected or damaged tissues and phagocytose (ingest and destroy) bacteria, dead neutrophils, tumour cells and other foreign material, acting as a second line of defence and a 'rubbish collection system'. Unlike neutrophils, they can survive this process, and live for months.

methaemoglobinaemia Methaemoglobin is formed, in genetically susceptible individuals, when the iron atoms in haemoglobin are oxidized, usually as a result of ingesting oxidizing drugs. Methaemoglobin cannot transport oxygen around the body. Therefore, if it builds up in the circulation (methaemoglobinaemia), the patient will develop a life-threatening cyanotic condition. Severe methaemoglobinaemia is incompatible with life. Management involves intravenous injection of methylthioninium chloride (methylene blue) (BNF, 2009).

microflora The community of microorganisms in a micro-environment such as the gut.

microorganism An organism that can only be seen with the aid of a microscope.

mOsm/kg (milliosmoles/kilogram) Unit of measurement for osmotic pressure. In health, human plasma has an osmotic pressure 280–296 mOsm/kg.

MRSA Methicillin-resistant staphylococcus aureus.

myoclonus Myoclonus is repetitive involuntary muscle contraction, jerking, or shaking due to imbalance in the normal controls of skeletal muscle tension. It may be distressing to both patients and carers.

narrow-spectrum antibiotic An antibiotic that is active against a narrow range of bacteria.

neurotransmitter A chemical messenger passing from one neurone to the next, across the synaptic cleft; for example acetylcholine, dopamine, and noradrenaline/ norepineprhine. Some neurotransmitters are also hormones; for example noradrenaline/norepineprhine and antidiuretic hormone.

nocebo Harmful effects brought on by administration of a placebo treatment (see below). Usually common ailments such as headache, nausea.

nystagmus Involuntary rapid movements of the eyeballs. Movements may be horizontal, vertical or rotatory.

obtunding Rendering dull or reducing sensitivity, for example to pain.

odds ratio (OR) An estimate of an effect. The odds of an event occurring in one group compared to another. If the odds ratio is one, the odds are equal in the two groups, and there is no difference.

opioids This term describes any preparation acting on the body's opioid receptors, for example morphine, diamorphine, codeine, and naloxone.

opportunistic pathogen A normally harmless microorganism that can cause disease when the body is weakened.

osmosis The movement of water across a differentially permeable membrane separating two solutions of unequal concentration of solutes or osmotic pressure.

osmotic pressure or osmolality of a solution The force or pressure required to prevent the movement of pure water into that solution. This depends on the number of osmotically active particles in the solution, or its effective concentration.

over the counter (OTC) drug A medicine sold directly to the public, without a prescription.

oxytocic An agent that hastens the evacuation of the uterus by increasing contraction of the myometrium.

partial pressure of a gas This refers to mixtures of gases. It is the pressure that gas would exert, if it were present alone, occupying the same volume. The 'partial pressure' is effectively the concentration of the gas.

pathogen A microorganism that causes disease.

peptidoglycan The polymer that makes up most bacterial cell walls.

pH The pH scale is a logarithmic scale of hydrogen ion concentration expressing the acidity or alkalinity of a solution. A neutral solution at 25°C has a pH of 7. An acid solution has a pH below 7. An alkaline solution has a pH above 7. The pH of normal adult arterial blood is 7.35–7.45. Venous blood has a lower pH.

pharmacodynamics The science and study of the actions and effects of chemicals on living material.

pharmacokinetics The science and study of the factors that determine the amount of a drug present at biologically effective sites at various times after its introduction to a biological system.

placebo An inactive preparation administered in the guise of a therapeutic agent, originally as a placating measure.

polymer A substance made up of large molecules, which consist of repeating units of identical chemical composition (the monomers). Examples include polysaccharides and plastics.

porphyria The porphyrias are a group of rare inherited conditions, in which enzymes needed to make haemoglobin are deficient or absent. Therefore, intermediate compounds accumulate, and can cause neurological disturbance, psychosis, abdominal pain, skin changes, or urine pigmentation. In susceptible, but asymptomatic, people, this condition can be triggered by administration of certain medications.

receptor A specialized configuration of molecules on the cell membrane or within the cell that responds to neurotransmitters, hormones, paracrines or drugs with similar structures.

relative risk (or risk ratio) (RR) An estimate of an effect. The risk or chance of an event occurring in one group compared to another. If the relative risk is one, the risks are equal in the two groups, and there is no difference.

renin-angiotensin-aldosterone axis Renin is secreted by the juxtaglomerular apparatus of the kidneys, in response to changes in blood pressure, salt and water balance and the sympathetic nervous system. Renin triggers the release of several other hormones that regulate blood pressure and salt and water balance. See Chapter 7, beta$_2$ adrenoreceptor agonists.

reticuloendothelial system   A network of macrophages (or similar cells) associated with lymphocytes, dispersed throughout the organs of the body and the lymph nodes. It is important in initiation of the immune response.

serum   Plasma with the clotting factors removed.

shock   Inadequate delivery of oxygen to the tissues, due to acute failure of the peripheral circulation. Causes include: excessive fluid loss such as haemorrhage; acute cardiac failure; sepsis; and adrenal failure.

SIADH (syndrome inappropriate ADH – antidiuretic hormone)   Production of ADH in excess of the body's requirements, leading to water retention, hyponatraemia and eventually water intoxication. This is an occasional complication of therapy with several drugs, including SSRIs and opioids. Similar effects are seen with overuse of oxytocin.

side effect   A physiological effect other than that for which a given drug is administered.

status epilepticus   A state of repeated epileptic fits with no period of consciousness between them. About 30% of survivors have permanent brain damage.

Stevens Johnson syndrome   A hypersensitivity response involving the deposition of immune complexes and haemorrhagic ulceration in skin and mucous membranes, including the conjunctiva, oral cavity, respiratory tract, and other epithelial surfaces. Rash and multi-organ involvement may be preceded by fever. Early recognition and intervention are essential to prevent loss of sight.

sympathomimetic   A drug whose actions resemble those of the stimulant neurotransmitters of the sympathetic nervous system.

synapse/synaptic junction   The contact between two neurones, where action potentials are transmitted from one neurone to the next.

synaptic inhibition   Inhibiting the transmission of excitatory signals between neurones at the synapse.

tablet   A preparation of powdered drug compressed or moulded into discs. In addition to the active drug, a tablet usually contains excipients, such as binders or lubricants.

teratogen   A chemical that causes malformation of a fetus.

teratogenesis   The impaired development of fetal organs, leading to structural or functional abnormalities.

T helper lymphocytes   These cells enhance the effects of other cells of the immune system.

thrombocytopenia   A concentration of platelets in the circulation below the normal limits (150,000–400,000/microlitre). If the concentration falls below 50,000/microlitre, severe bleeding disorders will ensue.

thrombosis   Blood vessel occlusion by a platelet aggregate and/or a fibrin clot.

thromboxanes   Derivatives of the phospholipids of plasma membranes, which promote platelet aggregation and vasoconstriction.

tocolytic   An agent that delays evacuation of the uterus by inhibiting contraction of the uterine muscle.

tolerance   Decreased responsiveness acquired after exposure to a drug.

tort   A civil wrong for which one may seek compensation in a court of law.

toxic epidermal necrolysis   A life-threatening reaction to drugs, chemicals or microorganisms resulting in destruction of the whole epidermal layer, blisters and loss of skin. As skin peels away, fluid balance, thermoregulation and barrier defences to infection are jeopardized. If the causative agent can be identified and removed, the epidermal layer can recover. Early recognition and treatment are vital.

underpowered   This is a term used in statistics. It refers to studies with too few subjects to be able to determine whether there or not there are statistically significant differences between the study groups in the variable under consideration. Studies examining the occurrence of rare events, such as eclamptic fits or certain congenital malformations, must recruit large numbers of women to avoid being underpowered.

uterotonics   Agents that increase the tone or tension of the uterine muscle.

vaccine   A suspension of inactivated or dead microorganisms that stimulates the body to develop immunity to a disease.

venous return   This is the quantity of blood flowing into the right atrium each minute. Generally, this is equal to the cardiac output.

ventilation   The ventilation rate is the volume of air breathed in per minute, that is, the volume of air inspired times the number of breaths per minute.

References

AAGBI (Association of Anaesthetists of Great Britain and Ireland) (1996) *A Report Received by Council of the Association of Anaesthetists on Blood Borne Viruses and Anaesthesia*, www.aagbi.org/publications/guidelines/archive/docs/hivinsert96.pdf.

Abalos, E., Duley, L., Steyn, D.W. and Henderson-Smart, D.J. (2007) Antihypertensive drug therapy for mild to moderate hypertension during pregnancy. *Cochrane Database of Systematic Reviews*, Issue 1. Art. No.: CD002252. DOI: 10.1002/14651858.CD002252.pub2.

Abalovich, M., Amino, N. and Barbour, L.A. (2007) Management of thyroid dysfunction during pregnancy and postpartum: an Endocrine Society Clinical Practice Guideline. *J Clin Endocrinol Metab*, 92(8S): 1–47.

Abbas, A.K. and Lichtman, A.H. (2004) *Basic Immunology: Functions and Disorders of the Immune System*, 2nd edn. W.B. Saunders, Philadelphia.

ABPI (Association of the British Pharmaceutical Industry) (2008) *Compendium of Data Sheets and Summaries of Product Characteristics* (updated yearly). Datapharm Publications, London, http://emc.medicines.org.uk/.

ABPI (Association of the British Pharmaceutical Industry) (2009) *Compendium of Data Sheets and Summaries of Product Characteristics* (updated yearly). Datapharm Publications, London (Pharmacy Dept), http://emc.medicines.org.uk/.

Abramsky, L., Botting, B., Chapple, J. and Stone, D. (1999) Has advice on periconceptual folate supplementation reduced neural tube defect? Research letter. *Lancet*, 354: 998.

Adab, N., Tudur Smith, C., Vinten, J. et al. (2004) Common antiepileptic drugs in pregnancy in women with epilepsy. *Cochrane Database of Syst Rev*, Issue 3: CD004848.

Ahn, E., Pairaudeau, N., Pairaudeau, N. Jr et al. (2006) A randomized cross over trial of tolerability and compliance of a micronutrient supplement with low iron separated from calcium vs high iron combined with calcium in pregnant women. *BMC Pregnancy Childbirth*, 6: 6–10.

Aldrich, C.J., D'Antona, D., Spencer, J. et al. (1995) The effect of maternal posture on fetal cerebral oxygenation during labour. *British Journal of Obstetrics and Gynaecology*, 102: 14–19.

Alef, K. (1999) Clostridium difficile-associated disease. *Journal of Nurse Midwifery*, 44: 19–29.

Alexander, E., Marqusee, E., Lawrence, J. et al. (2004) Timing and magnitude of increases in levothyroxine requirements during pregnancy in women with hypothroidism. *New England Journal of Medicine*, 351: 241–9.

Alexander, J.M., Sharma, S.K., McIntire, D.D. and Leveno K.J. (2002) Epidural analgesia lengthens the Friedman active phase of labor. *Obstetrics and Gynecology*, 100(1): 46–50.

Allman, A.C., Genevier, E.S., Johnson, M.R. and Steer, P.J. (1996) Head-to-cervix force: an important physiological variable in labour. *British Journal of Obstetrics and Gynaecology*, 103: 763–8.

Al-Mufti, R., Morey, R., Shennan, A. and Morgan, B. (1997) Blood pressure and fetal heart rate changes with patient-controlled combined spinal epidural analgesia while ambulating in labour. *British Journal of Obstetrics and Gynaecology*, 104(5): 554–8.

Amant, F., Spitz, B., Timmerman, D. et al. (1999) Misoprostol compared with methylergometrine for the prevention of postpartum haemorrhage. *British Journal of Obstetrics and Gynaecology*, 106: 1066–70.

Amedee-Manesme, O., Lambert, W.E., Alagille, D. and de Leenheer, A.P. (1992) Pharmacokinetics and safety of a new solution of vitamin K1(20) in children with cholestasis. *Journal of Paediatric Gastroenterology and Nutrition*, 14: 160–5.

Amir, L.H. and Donath, S.M. (2002) Does maternal smoking have a negative physiological effect on breastfeeding? The epidemiological evidence. *Birth*, 29(2): 112–23.

Anderson, G.D. (2006) Using pharmacokinetics to predict the effects of pregnancy and maternal-infant transfer of drugs during lactation. *Expert Opin Drug Metabolism and Toxicology*, 2(6): 947–60.

Anim-Somuah, M., Smyth, R. and Howell, C. (2005) Epidural versus non-epidural or no analgesia in labour. *Cochrane Database of Systematic Reviews*, Issue 4. Art. No.: CD000331. DOI: 10.1002/14651858.CD000331.pub2.

Ansell, P., Bull, D. and Roman, E. (1996) Childhood leukaemia and intramuscular vitamin K: findings from a case control study. *BMJ*, 313: 204–5.

Arfeen, Z., Armstron, P.J. and Whitfield, A. (1994) The effects of Entonox and epidural analgesia on arterial oxygen saturation of women in labour. *Anaesthesia*, 49(1): 32–4.

Arkoosh, V. (1991) Guidelines for regional anesthesia in obstetrics: viewpoint of an anesthesiologist in a tertiary care center. Cleveland Clinic Foundation, sector for anaesthesia for obstetrics, www.anes.ccf.org:8080/soap/guideline.htm.

Arkoosh, V., Palmer, C., Yun, E. et al. (2008) A randomized, double-masked, multicenter comparison of the safety of continuous intrathecal labor analgesia using a 28-gauge catheter versus continuous epidural labor analgesia. *Anesthesiology*, 108(2): 286–98.

Armand, S., Jasson, J., Talafre, M. and Tison, C. (1993) The effects of regional analgesia on the newborn, in Reynolds, F. (ed.) *Effects on the Baby of Maternal Analgesia and Anaesthesia*. Saunders, London.

Arner, S. and Meyerson, B. (1988) Lack of analgesic effect of opioids on neuropathic and idiopathic forms of pain. *Pain*, 33: 11–23.

Aronin, S.I., Peduzzi, P. and Quagliarello, V.J. (1998) Community-acquired bacterial meningitis: risk stratification for adverse clinical outcome and effect of antibiotic timing. *Annals Intern Medicine*, 129: 862–9.

Aronson, J.K. (ed.) (2006) *Meyler's Side Effects of Drugs: The International Encyclopedia of Adverse Drug Reactions and Interactions*. Elsevier, New York. Shortcut URL to www.sciencedirect.com/science/referenceworks/0444510052 requires subscription.

Askie, L.M., Duley, L., Henderson-Smart, D.J., Stewart L.A., PARIS Collaborative Group (2007) Antiplatelet agents for prevention of pre-eclampsia: a meta-analysis of individual patient data. *Lancet*, 369(9575): 1791–8.

Assaley, J., Baron, J. and Cibils, L. (1998) Effects of magnesium sulphate infusion upon clotting parameters in patients with pre-eclampsia. *Journal of Perinatal Medicine*, 26(2): 115–19.

Association of Anaesthetists of Great Britain and Northern Ireland (2007) *Guidelines for the Management of Severe Local Anaesthetic Toxicity*, www.aagbi.org/publications/guidelines/docs/latoxicity07.pdf.

Atienzar, M. Palanca, J., Torres, F. et al. (2008) A randomized comparison of levobupivacaine, bupivacaine and ropivacaine with fentanyl, for labor analgesia. *Int J Obstetrics Anesth*, 17(2): 106–11.

Austin, J., Kaur, B., Anderson, H.R. et al. (1999) Hay fever, eczema, and wheeze: a nationwide UK study (ISAAC, international study of asthma and allergies in childhood). *Archives of Disease in Childhood*, 81: 225–30.

Austin, M. and Mitchell, P. (1998) Psychotropic medications in pregnant women: treatment dilemmas. *Medical Journal of Australia*, 169(8): 428–31.

Badawi, N., Kurinczuk, J., Mackenzie, C. et al. (2000) Maternal thyroid disease: a risk factor for newborn encephalopathy in term infants. *British Journal of Obstetrics and Gynaecology*, 107: 798–801.

Bader, A., Fragneto, R., Terui, K. et al. (1995) Maternal and neonatal fentanyl and bupivacaine concentrations after epidural infusion during labor. *Anesthetic Analgesia*, 81: 829–32.

Badr, K. and Brenner, B. (1991) Vascular injury to the kidney, in Wilson, J., Braunwald, E., Isselbacher, K. et al. (eds) *Harrison's Principles of Internal Medicine*, 12th edn, McGraw-Hill, New York.

Bahl, R., Frost, C., Kirkwood, B.R. et al. (2005) Infant feeding patterns and risks of death and hospitalization in the first half of infancy: multicentre cohort study. *Bull World Health Organ*, 83(6): 418–26.

Bailey, J.A., Hill, K.G., Hawkins, J.D. et al. (2008) Men's and women's patterns of substance use around pregnancy. *Birth*, 35(1): 50–9.

Bais, J.M., Eskes, M., Pel, M. et al. (2004) Postpartum haemorrhage in nulliparous women: incidence and risk factors in low and high risk women. A Dutch population-based cohort study on standard (> or = 500 ml) and severe (> or = 1000 ml) postpartum haemorrhage. *European J Obstetrics Gynecology and Reproductive Biology*, 15: 166–72.

Bajekal, R., Turner, R. and Yentis, S. (2000) Anti-infective measures and Entonox equipment: a survey. *Anaesthesia*, 55: 153–4.

Baker, K. (2006) *Obstetrics by Ten Teachers*, 18th edn. Hodder Arnold, London.

Bakhireva, L.N., Jones, K.L., Schatz, M. et al., Organization of Teratology Information Specialists Collaborative Research Group (2007) Safety of leukotriene receptor antagonists in pregnancy. *J Allergy Clin Immunol*, 119(3): 618–25.

Baldessarini, R. (2006) Drug therapy of depression and anxiety disorders, in Brunton L., Lazo, J. and Parker, K. (eds) *Goodman & Gilman's: The Pharmacological Basis of Therapeutics*, 11th edn. McGraw-Hill, New York.

Baldessarini, R. and Tarazi, F. (2006) Pharmacotherapy of psychosis and mania, in Brunton, L., Lazo, J. and Parker, K. (eds) *Goodman & Gilman's: The Pharmacological Basis of Therapeutics*, 11th edn. McGraw-Hill, New York.

Bancroft, K., Tuffnell, D., Mason, G. et al. (2000) A randomised controlled pilot study of the management of gestational impaired glucose tolerance. *British Journal of Obstetrics and Gynaecology*, 107: 959–63.

Bangh, S.A., Hughes, K.A., Roberts, D.J. and Kovarik, S.M. (2005) Neonatal ergot poisoning: a persistent iatrogenic illness. *American Journal of Perinatology*, 22(5): 239–43.

Banks, B.A., Macones, G., Cnaan, A. et al. (2002) Multiple courses of antenatal corticosteroids are associated with early severe lung disease in preterm neonates. *J Perinatol*, 22(2): 101–7.

Baraz, R. and Collis, R.E. (2005) The management of accidental dural puncture during labour epidural analgesia: a survey of UK practice. *Anaesthesia*, 60(7): 673–9.

Barbour, L., Kick, S., Steiner, J. et al. (1994) A prospective study of heparin-induced osteoporosis in pregnancy using bone densitometry. *American Journal of Obstetrics and Gynaecology*, 170: 862–9.

Barbui, C. and Hotopf, M. (2001) Amitriptyline v. the rest: still the leading antidepressant after 40 years of randomised controlled trials. *British Journal of Psychiatry*, 178: 129–44.

Barker, D., Bull, A., Osmond, C. and Simmonds, S. (1990) Fetal and placental size and risk of hypertension in adult life, *BMJ*, 301: 259–62.

Baron, T., Ramirez, B. and Richter, J.E. (1993) Gastrointestinal motility disorders during pregnancy. *Annals of Internal Medicine*, 118(5): 366–75.

Barrett, J., Whittaker, P., Williams, J. and Lind, T. (1994) Absorption of non-haem iron from food during normal pregnancy. *BMJ*, 309: 79–82.

Bartfai, Z., Kocsis, J., Puho, E. and Czeizel, A. (2007) A population-based case-control teratologic study of promethazine use during pregnancy. *Science Direct: Reproductive Toxicology*, 25: 276–85.

Barzo, B., Moretti, M., Mareels, G. et al. (1999) Reporting bias in retrospective ascertainment of drug-induced embryopathy. *Lancet*, 354: 1700–1.

Bates, S.M., Greer, I.A., Hirsh, J. and Ginsberg, J.S. (2004) Use of antithrombotic agents during pregnancy: the Seventh ACCP Conference on Antithrombotic and Thrombolytic Therapy. *Chest*, 126(3 Suppl): 627–44.

Battino, D. and Tomson, T. (2007) Management of epilepsy during pregnancy. *Drugs*, 67(18): 2727–46.

Baxi, L.V., Petrie, R.H. and James, L.H. (1988) Human fetal oxygenation, heart rate variability and uterine activity following maternal administration of meperidine. *Journal of Perinatal Medicine*, 16: 23–30.

Baxter, K. (2006) *Stockley's Drug Interactions*, 7th edn. Blackwell Science, Oxford.

Begley, C. (1990a) A comparison of 'active' and 'physiological' management of the third stage of labour. *Midwifery*, 6: 3–17.

Begley, C. (1990b) The effect of Ergometrine on breast feeding. *Midwifery*, 6: 60–72.

Begley, C. (1990c) The effect of Ergometrine on breast feeding (reply to letter). *Midwifery*, 6: 232–3.

Beilin, Y., Bodian, C., Weiser, J. et al. (2005) Effect of labor analgesia with and without fentanyl on infant breast-feeding: a prospective, randomized double-blind study. *Anesthesiology*, 103: 1211–17.

Beischer, N., Mackay, E. and Colditz, P. (1997) *Obstetrics and the Newborn*, 3rd edn. London, Saunders.

Bell, G. (1996) Psychological medicine, in Axford, J. (ed.) *Medicine*. Blackwell, Oxford.

Bell, J. and Harvey-Dodds, L. (2008) Pregnancy and injecting drug use. *BMJ*, 336(7656): 1303–5.

Bem, M., Roddam, P. and Wheatley, R. (1996) Patient controlled analgesia in critically ill patients. *Care of the Critically Ill*, 12(1): 10–14.

Ben-Arush, M. and Berant, M. (1996) Retention of drugs in venous access port chamber: a note of caution. *BMJ*, 312: 496–7.

Benet, L. (1996) General principles, in Hardman, J., Limbard, L., Molinoff, P. et al. (eds) *Goodman and Gilman's: The Pharmacological Basis of Therapeutics*, 9th edn. McGraw-Hill, New York.

Ben-Menachem, E. (2008) Strategy for utilization of new antiepileptics. *Curr Opin Neurol*, 21: 167–72.

Bennett, V.R. and Brown, L.K. (1993) *Myles Textbook for Midwives*, 12th edn. Churchill Livingstone, Edinburgh.

Berman, A., Snyder, S., Kozier, B. and Erb, G. (2008) *Kozier & Erb's Fundamentals of Nursing*, 8th edn. Pearson, Upper Saddle River, NJ.

Bieber, T. (2008) Atopic dermatitis. *New England of Medicine*, 358(14): 1483–94.

Binder, T. and Vavrinková, B. (2008) Prospective randomised comparative study of the effect of buprenorphine, methadone and heroin on the course of pregnancy, birthweight of newborns, early postpartum adaptation and course of the neonatal abstinence syndrome (NAS) in women followed up in the outpatient department. *Neuro Endocrinol Lett*, 29(1): 80–6.

Blair, D.T. and Dauner, A. (1992) Extrapyramidal symptoms are serious side-effects of antipsychotics and other drugs. *Nurse Practitioner*, 17(11): 56–67.

Blair, F., Tassone, S., Pearman, C. et al. (1998) Inducing labor with a sustained-release PGE2 vaginal insert. *Journal of Reproductive Medicine*, 43(5): 408–12.

Blanch, G., Lavender, T., Walkinshaw, S. and Alfirevic, Z. (1998) Dysfunctional labour: a randomised trial. *British Journal of Obstetrics and Gynaecology*, 105: 117–20.

Bloomfield, T. (1996) Principles of prescribing in pregnancy. *Prescriber*, 7(1): 66–70.

Blossom, D.B., Kallen, A.J., Patel, P.R. et al. (2008) Outbreak of adverse reactions associated with contaminated heparin. *New England Journal of Medicine*, 359(25): 2674–84.

Blume, W.T. (1997) Epilepsy: advances in management. *European Neurology*, 38: 198–208.

BNF (2009) *British National Formulary*, no.57. London, British Medical Association/ Pharmaceutical Society of Great Britain.

BOC (2004) Medical Entonox Data sheet, www.bocsds.com/uk/sds/medical%5Centonox.pdf.

Bootman, L. and Milne, R. (1996) Costs, innovation and efficiency in anti-infective therapy. *Pharmacoeconomics*, 9(S1): 31–9.

Boseley, S. (1999) Prozac: can it make you kill? *Guardian Weekend*, 30 October: 13–16.

Boulvain, M., Kelly, A.J. and Irion, O. (2008) Intracervical prostaglandins for induction of labour. *Cochrane Database of Systematic Reviews*, Issue 1. Art. No.: CD006971. DOI: 10.1002/14651858.CD006971.

Boulvain, M., Stan, C. and Irion, O. (2000) Elective delivery in diabetic pregnant women. *Cochrane Database Systematic Review* (issue 2). Update Software, Oxford.

Bowdle, T. (1998) Adverse effects of opioid agonists and agonist-antagonists in anaesthesia. *Drug Safety*, 19(3): 173–89.

Bradley, C.S., Kennedy, C.M., Turcea, A.M. et al. (2007) Constipation in pregnancy: prevalence, symptoms and risk factors. *Obstetrics & Gynecology*, 110(6): 1351–7.

Bramadat, I.J. (1994) Induction of labor: an integrated review. *Health Care for Women International*, 15(2): 135–48.

Brancazio, L., Laifer, S. and Schwartz, T. (1997) Peak expiratory flow in normal pregnancy. *Obstetrics and Gynecology*, 89: 383–6.

Bray, J., Clarke, C., Brennan, G. and Muncey, T. (2008) Should we be 'pushing meds'? The implications of pharmacogenomics. *Journal of Psychiatric and Mental Health Nursing*, 15(5): 357–64.

Breen, D.P. and Davenport, R.J. (2006) Teratogenicity of antiepileptic drugs. *BMJ*, 333: 615–16.

British Thyroid Association (2006) *UK Guidelines for the Use of Thyroid Function Tests*. British Thyroid Association/ British Thyroid Foundation, www.british-thyroid-association.org.

Brockington, I. (2004) Diagnosis and management of post-partum disorders: a review. *World Psychiatry*, 3(2): 89–95.

Brocklehurst, P., Gates, S., McHarg, K.M. et al. (1999) Are we prescribing multiple courses of antenatal corticosteroids? A survey of practice in the UK. *British Journal of Obstetrics and Gynaecology*, 106: 977–9.

Brodtkorb, E. and Reimers, A. (2008) Seizure control and pharmacokinetics of antiepileptic drugs in pregnant women with epilepsy. *Seizure*, 17(2): 160–5.

Broussard, C. and Richter, J. (1998) Treating gastro-oesophageal reflux disease during pregnancy and lactation: what are the safest therapy options? *Drug Safety*, 19(4): 325–37.

Brown, H.C., Paranjothy, S., Dowswell, T. and Thomas, J. (2008) Package of care for active management in labour for reducing caesarean section rates in low-risk women. *Cochrane Database of Systematic Reviews*, Issue 4. Art. No.: CD004907. DOI: 10.1002/14651858.CD004907.pub2.

Brown, M. (1997) Pre-eclampsia: a case of nerves? *Lancet*, 349: 297–8.

Brown, M. and Buddle, M. (1996) Hypertension in pregnancy. *Med. J. Australia*, 165(7): 360–5.

Brownfoot, F.C., Crowther, C.A. and Middleton, P. (2008) Different corticosteroids and regimens for accelerating fetal lung maturation for women at risk of preterm birth. *Cochrane Database of Systematic Reviews*, Issue 4. Art. No.: CD006764. DOI: 10.1002/14651858.CD006764.pub2.

Brownridge, P. (1991) Treatment options for the relief of pain during childbirth. *Drugs*, 41(1): 69–80.

Brucker, M. and Faucher, M. (1997) Pharmacologic management of common gastrointestinal health problems in women. *Journal of Nurse Midwifery*, 42(3): 145–62.

Brunton, L. (1996) Agents affecting gastrointestinal water flux and motility: emesis and antiemetics: bile acids and pancreatic enzymes, in Hardman, J., Limbard, L., Molinoff, P. et al. (eds) *Goodman & Gilman's: The Pharmacological Basis of Therapeutics*, 9th edn. McGraw-Hill, New York.

Brunton, L., Lazo, J. and Parker, K. (eds) (2006) *Goodman & Gilman's: The Pharmacological Basis of Therapeutics*, 11th edn. McGraw-Hill, New York.

Bryant, H. and Yerby, M. (2004) Pain relief during labour, in Henderson, C. and MacDonald, S. (eds) *Mayes' Midwifery: A Textbook for Midwives*, 13th edn. Baillière Tindall, Edinburgh.

Bsat, F.A., Hoffman, D.E. and Seubert, D.E. (2003) Comparison of three outpatient regimens in the management of nausea and vomiting in pregnancy. *Journal of Perinatology*, 23(7): 531–5.

BTS (British Thoracic Society) (2008) *British Guideline on the Management of Asthma*. BTS, Scottish Intercollegiate Guideline Network, London/Edinburgh, www.brit-thoracic.org.uk/Portals/0/Clinical%20Information/Asthma/Guidelines/qrg101%20revised%202009.pdf.

Buchan, P.C. (1979) Pathogenesis of neonatal hyperbilirubinaemia after induction of labour with oxytocin. *BMJ*, 2: 1255–7.

Buckley, K. (1990) Abnormalities of the postpartum period, in Buckley, K. and Kulb, N. (eds) *High Risk Maternity Nursing Manual*. Williams & Wilkins, Baltimore.

Burm, A.G. (2003) Occupational hazards of inhalational anaesthetics. *Best Practice and Research in Clinical Anaesthesiology*, 17(1): 147–61.

Burns, L., Mattick, R.P. and Cooke, M. (2006) The use of record linkage to examine illicit drug use in pregnancy. *Addiction*, 101(6): 873–82.

Burr, M.L., Wat, D., Evans, C. et al. (2006) Asthma prevalence in 1973, 1988 and 2003. *Thorax*, 61(4): 296–9.

Bushnell, T. and Justins, D. (1993) Choosing the right analgesic. *Drugs*, 46: 394–408.

Busowski, J.D. and Parsons, M.T. (1995) Amniotomy to induce labor. *Clinical Obstetrics and Gynecology*, 38(2): 232–45.

Butler, R. and Fuller, J. (1998) Back pain following epidural anaesthesia in labour. *Can J Anaesth*, 45(8): 724–8.

Buxton, I. (2006) Pharmacokinetics and pharmacodynamics, in Brunton L., Lazo, J. and Parker, K. (eds) *Goodman & Gilman's: The Pharmacological Basis of Therapeutics*, 11th edn. McGraw-Hill, New York.

Bygdeman, M. (2003) Pharmacokinetics of prostaglandins. *Best Practice and Research in Clinical Obstetrics and Gynaecology*, 17(5): 707–16.

Byrne, B. (2001) Management of epilepsy in pregnancy, in Bonnar, J. (ed.) *Recent Advances in Obstetrics and Gynaecology 21*. Churchill Livingstone, Edinburgh.

Byrne, C., Saxton, D., Pelikan, P. and Nugent, P. (1986) *Laboratory Tests: Implications for Nursing Care*. Addison-Wesley, Menlo Park.

Byron, M. (1995) Treatment of rheumatic diseases, in Rubin, P. (ed.) *Prescribing in Pregnancy*. BMJ Group, London.

Caminiti, F., de Murtas, M., Parodo, G. et al. (1980) Decrease in human plasma prolactin levels by oral prostaglandin E2 in early puerperium. *Journal of Endocrinology*, 87: 333–7.

Cammu, H. and Eeckhout, E.V. (1996) A randomised controlled trial of early versus delayed use of amniotomy and oxytocin infusion in nulliparous labour. *British Journal of Obstetrics and Gynaecology*, 103: 313–18.

Campbell, S. and Lees, C. (eds) (2000) *Obstetrics by Ten Teachers*, 17th edn. Arnold, London.

Campbell, W. and Halushka, P. (1996) Lipid-derived autacoids, in Hardman, J., Limbard, L., Molinoff, P. et al. (eds) *Goodman & Gilman's: The Pharmacological Basis of Therapeutics*, 9th edn. McGraw-Hill, New York.

Canales, E., Garrido, J., Zarate, A. et al. (1976) Effect of ergonovine on prolactin secretion and milk letdown. *Obstetrics and Gynecology*, 48: 228–9.

Cao, Z., Bideau, R., Valdes, R. and Elin, R. (1999) Acute hypermagnesemia and respiratory arrest following infusion of MgSO4 for tocolysis. *Clinica Chimica Acta*, 285: 191–3.

Capogna, G. and Celleno, D. (1993) The effects of anaesthetic agents on the newborn, in Reynolds, F. (ed.) *Effects on the Baby of Maternal Analgesia and Anaesthesia*. Saunders, London.

Capogna, G., Celleno, D., Lyons, G. et al. (1998) Minimum local analgesic concentration of extradural bupivacaine increase with progression in labour. *British Journal of Anaesthesia*, 80(1): 11–13.

Cappell, M. and Garcia, A. (1998) Gastric and duodenal ulcers during pregnancy. *Gastroenterological Clinics of North America*, 27(1): 169–95.

Cararach, V., Palacio, M., Martínez, S. et al. (2006) Comparison of their efficacy and secondary effects. *European J Obstetrics Gynecol Reprod Biol*, 127(2): 204–8.

CARE Study Group (2008) Maternal caffeine intake during pregnancy and risk of fetal growth restriction: a large prospective observational study. *BMJ*, 337: a2332; doi: 10.1136/bmj.a2332.

CARIS (Congenital Anomaly Register and Information Service) (2008) *CARIS Review: 10 Years of Reporting*. CARIS, Singleton Hospital, Swansea, www.wales.nhs.uk/sites3/Documents/416/Caris%20Ann%20rep%20%28Eng%29%20final.pdf.

Carli, F., Creagh-Barry, P., Gordan, H. et al. (1993) Does epidural analgesia influence the mode of delivery in primiparae managed actively? *International Journal of Obstetric Anesthesia*, 2: 15–20.

Carlson, J. and Byington, K. (1998) Fundamental principles of pharmacology, in Williams, B. and Baer, C. (eds) *Essentials of Clinical Pharmacology in Nursing*, 3rd edn. Springhouse, Springhouse, PA.

Carmichael, F., Haas, D. and Chan, V. (2007) General anaesthetics, in Kalant, H., Grant, D. and Mitchell, J. (eds) *Principles of Medical Pharmacology*, 7th edn. Saunders, Toronto.

Carmichael, S.L., Shaw, G.M., Schaffer, D.M. et al. (2003) Dieting behaviors and risk of neural tube defects. *American J Epidemiol*, 158(12): 1127–31.

Carson, R. (1996) The administration of analgesics. *Modern Midwife*, November: 12–16.

Carstoniu, J., Levytam, S. and Norman, P. (1994) Nitrous oxide in early labour: safety and analgesic efficacy assessed by a double-blind, placebo-controlled study. *Anesthesiology*, 80(1): 30–35.

Carter, C.S. (2003) Developmental consequences of oxytocin. *Physiol Behav*, 79(3): 383–97.

Casson, I., Clarke, C., Howard, C. et al. (1997) Outcomes of pregnancy in insulin dependent diabetic women: results of a five year population cohort study. *BMJ*, 315: 275–8.

Cassoni, P., Marrocco, T., Sapino, A. et al. (2006) Oxytocin synthesis within the normal and neoplastic breast: first evidence of a local peptide source. *International Journal of Oncology*, 28(5): 1263–8.

Catling, S. (2008) Major obstetric haemorrhage, in Clyburn, P., Collis, R., Harries, S. and Davies, S. (eds) *Obstetric Anaesthesia*. Oxford University Press, Oxford.

Catterall, W. and Mackie, K. (2006) Local anaesthetics, in Brunton L., Lazo J. and Parker, K. (eds) *Goodman & Gilman's: The Pharmacological Basis of Therapeutics*, 11th edn. McGraw-Hill, New York.

Cederholm, I. (1997) Preliminary risk–benefit analysis of ropivacaine in labour and following surgery. *Drug Safety*, 16(6): 391–402.

CEMACH (Confidential Enquiries into Maternal and Child Health) (2005) *Why Mothers Die 2000–2002: The Sixth Report of the Confidential Enquiries into Maternal Deaths in the United Kingdom*. CEMACH, London.

CEMACH (Confidential Enquiries into Maternal and Child Health) (2007) *Saving Mothers' Lives: Reviewing Maternal Deaths to Make Motherhood Safer – 2003–2005: The Seventh Report of the Confidential Enquiries into Maternal Deaths in the United Kingdom*. CEMACH, London.

Chadwick, C. and Forbes, A. (1996) Pharmaceutical problems for the nutrition team pharmacist. *The Hospital Pharmacist*, 3(6): 139–43.

Chaim, W., Bashiri, A., Bar-David, J. et al. (2000) Prevalence and clinical significance of postpartum endometritis and wound infection. *Infectious Disease in Obstetrics and Gynecology*, 8(2): 77–82.

Chaiyakunapruk, N., Kitikannakorn, N., Nathisuwan, S. et al. (2006) The efficacy of ginger for the prevention of postoperative nausea and vomiting: a meta-analysis. *American J Obstetrics Gynecol*, 194(1): 95–9.

Chamberlain, G. (1975) *Lecture Notes on Obstetrics*, 3rd edn. Blackwell Scientific, Oxford.

Chamberlain, G. and Zander, L. (1999) Induction. *BMJ*, 318: 995–8.

Chambers, C., Anderson, P., Thomas, R. et al. (1999) Weight gain in infants breastfed by mothers who take fluoxetine. *Pediatrics*, 104(5): 1010–15.

Chambers, C., Johnson, K., Dick, L. et al. (1996) Birth outcomes in pregnancy women taking fluoxetine. *New England Journal of Medicine*, 335: 1010–15.

Chambers, C.D., Hernandez-Diaz, S., Van Marter, L.J. et al. (2006) Selective serotonin-reuptake inhibitors and risk of persistent pulmonary hypertension of the newborn. *New England Journal of Medicine*, 354(6): 579–87.

Chambers, H. (2006) General principles of antimicrobial therapy, in Brunton, L., Lazo, J. and Parker, K. (eds) *Goodman & Gilman's: The Pharmacological Basis of Therapeutics*, 11th edn. McGraw-Hill, New York.

Chambers, H. and Sande, M. (1996) Antimicrobial agents: general considerations, in Hardman, J., Limbard, L., Molinoff, P. et al. (eds) *Goodman & Gilman's: The Pharmacological Basis of Therapeutics*, 9th edn. McGraw-Hill, New York.

Chang, G. (2001) Alcohol screening instruments for pregnant women. *Alcohol Research and Health*, 25: 204–9, http://pubs.niaaa.nih.gov/publications/arh25-3/204-209.htm.

Chapel, H., Haeney, H., Misbah, S. and Snowden, N. (2006) *Essentials of Clinical Immunology*, 5th edn. Blackwell, Malden, MA.

Chappell, L., Poulton, L., Halligan, A. and Shennan, A. (1999) Lack of consistency in research papers over the definition of pre-eclampsia. *British Journal of Obstetrics and Gynaecology*, 106: 983–5.

Chappell, L.C. and Shennan, A.H. (2008) Assessment of proteinuria in pregnancy. *BMJ*, 336(7651): 968–9.

Chaudron, L. and Jefferson, J. (2000) Mood stabilisers during breastfeeding. *Journal of Clinical Psychiatry*, 61: 79–90.

Chen, F.P., Chang, S.D. and Chuu, K.K. (1995) Expectant management in severe pre-eclampsia: does magnesium sulfate prevent the development of eclampsia? *Acta Obstetricia et Gynecologica Scandinavia*, 74: 181–5.

Cherny, N. (1996) Opioid analgesics. *Drugs*, 51: 713–37.

Chetley, A. (1995) *Problem Drugs*. Zed Books, London.

Chien, P., Khan, K. and Arnott, N. (1996) Magnesium sulphate in the treatment of eclampsia and pre-eclampsia: an overview of the evidence from randomised trials. *British Journal of Obstetrics and Gynaecology*, 103: 1085–91.

Chilvers, R. and Weisz, M. (2000) Entonox equipment as a potential source of cross-infection. *Anaesthesia*, 55(2): 176–9.

Chittumma, P., Kaewkiattikun, K. and Wiriyasiriwach, B. (2007) Comparison of the effectiveness of ginger and vitamin B6 for treatment of nausea and vomiting in early pregnancy: a randomized double-blind controlled trial. *J Ed Assoc Thai*, 90(1): 15–20.

Choy, J. (2000) Mortality from peripartum meningitis. *Anaesthesia and Intensive Care*, 28: 328–30.

Chrubasik, J., Chrubasik, S. and Martin, E. (1992) Patient-controlled spinal opiate analgesia in terminal cancer. *Drugs*, 43: 799–804.

Churchill, D., Beevers, G.D., Meher, S. and Rhodes, C. (2007) Diuretics for preventing pre-eclampsia. *Cochrane Database of Systematic Reviews*, Issue 1. Art. No.: CD004451. DOI: 10.1002/14651858.CD004451.pub2.

Clark, A.J. (1933) *The Mode of Action of Drugs on Cells*. Edward Arnold, London.

Clark, D. and Lipworth, B. (1997) Dose-response of inhaled drugs in asthma. *Clinical Pharmacokinetics*, 32(1): 58–74.

CLASP Collaborative Group (1994) A randomised trial of low-dose aspirin for the prevention and treatment of pre-eclampsia among 9364 pregnant women. *Lancet*, 343: 619–29.

Clayton, B. and Stock, Y. (1993) *Basic Pharmacology for Nurses*, 10th edn. Mosby, London.

Clayton-Smith, J. and Donnai, D. (1995) Fetal valproate syndrome. *J Med Genet*, 32: 724–7.

Clayworth, S. (2000) The nurse's role during oxytocin administration. *MCN: American Journal of Maternal and Child Nursing*, 25(2): 80–5.

Clinical Standards Advisory Group (2000) *Services for Patients with Epilepsy*. DH, London.

Clyburn, P. and Rosen, M. (1993) The effects of opioid and inhalational analgesia on the newborn, in Reynolds, F. (ed.) *Effects on the Baby of Maternal Analgesia and Anaesthesia*. Saunders, London.

Clyburn, P., Adekanye, K. and Gupta, S. (2008a) Maternal physiology, in Clyburn, P., Collis, R., Harries, S. and Davies, S. (eds) *Obstetric Anaesthesia*. Oxford University Press, Oxford.

Clyburn, P., Adekanye, K. and Gupta, S. (2008b) Maternal pathophysiology, in Clyburn, P., Collis, R., Harries S. and Davies, S. (eds) *Obstetric Anaesthesia*. Oxford University Press, Oxford.

Cochrane, G. and Rees, P. (1989) *A Colour Atlas of Asthma*. Wolfe Medical, London.

Cockshott, W.P., Thompson, G.T., Howlett, L. and Seeley, E. (1982) Intramuscular or intralipomatous injections? *New England Journal of Medicine*, 307(6): 356–8.

Coetzee, E., Dommisse, J. and Anthony, J. (1998) A randomised controlled trial of intravenous magnesium sulphate versus placebo in the management of women with severe pre-eclampsia. *British Journal of Obstetrics and Gynaecology*, 105: 300–3.

Cohen, S. (1995) Overdiagnosis of schizophrenia: role of alcohol and drug misuse. *Lancet*, 346: 1541–2.

Cole, P.V. (1975) Entonox at St Bartholomew's Hospital, proceedings of symposium on Entonox held at St Bartholomew's Hospital, London, in *Entonox Digest*. Medishield, London.

Collaris, R. and Tan, P.C. (2009) Oral nifepidine versus subcutaneous terbutaline tocolysis for external cephalic version: a double-blind randomised trial. *BJOG*, 116(1): 74–80.

Collis, R. and Harries, S. (2005) A subdural abscess and infected blood patch complicating regional analgesia for labour. *International Journal of Obstetric Anesthesia*, 14: 246–51.

Collis, R., Harries, S., Lewis, E. and Hussain, S. (2008) Regional analgesia for labour, in Clyburn, P., Collis, R., Harries, S. and Davies, S. (eds) *Obstetric Anaesthesia*. Oxford University Press.

COMET (Comparative Obstetric Mobile Epidural Trial) Study Group UK (2001) Effect of low-dose mobile versus traditional epidural techniques on mode of delivery: a randomised controlled trial. *Lancet*, 358(9275): 19–23.

Connor, C. (2008) Effects of analgesia and anaesthesia on the fetus, in Clyburn, P., Collis, R., Harries, S. and Davies, S. (eds) *Obstetric Anaesthesia*. Oxford University Press.

Conway, G. and Betteridge, D. (1996) Endocrine disease, in Axfor, J. (ed.) *1996 Medicine*. Blackwell Science, Oxford.

Cook, C., Spurrett, B. and Murray, H. (1999) A randomized clinical trial comparing oral misoprostol with synthetic oxytocin or syntometrine in the third stage of labour. *Australian and New Zealand Journal of Obstetrics and Gynecology*, 39(4): 414–19.

Cooper, P.R. and Panettieri, R.A. Jr (2008) Steroids completely reverse albuterol-induced beta(2)-adrenergic receptor tolerance in human small airways. *Journal of Allergy and Clinical Immunology*, 122(4): 734–40.

Cornelissen, M., von Kries, R, Loughnan, P. and Schubiger, G. (1997) Prevention of vitamin K deficiency bleeding: efficacy of different multiple oral dose schedules of vitamin K. *European Journal of Paediatrics*, 156(2): 414–19.

Cotter, A., Ness, A. and Tolosa, J. (2001) Prophylactic oxytocin for the third stage of labour. *Cochrane Database of Systematic Reviews*, Issue 4. Art. No.: CD001808.DOI: 10.1002/14651858.CD001808.

Cotzias, C., Wong, S.J., Taylor, E. et al. (2008) A study to establish gestation-specific reference intervals for thyroid function tests in normal singleton pregnancy. *European J Obstetrics Gynecol Reprod Biol*, 137(1): 61–9.

Cousins, D.H. (1994) Stop these parenteral blunders. *Hospital Pharmacy Practice*, 4(10): 387–9.

Cousins, D.H. (1995) A patient dies after receiving vancomycin. *Hospital Pharmacy Practice*, 5(5): 227–8.

Coutts, A. (2000) Nutrition and the life cycle: maternal nutrition and pregnancy. *British Journal of Nursing*, 9: 1133–8.

Cowan, L.D., Leviton, A. and Dammann, O. (2000) New research directions in neuroepidemiology. *Epidemiology Review*, 22(1): 18–23.

Cowen, P.J. (2008) Antidepressant drugs, in Aronson J.K. (ed.) *Side Effects of Drug Annual* 30. Elsevier, Amsterdam.

Cox, J. (2004) Postnatal mental disorder: towards ICD-11. *World Psychiatry*, 3(2): 96–7.

Cox, J. and Nicholls, K. (1996) Prescribing psychotropic drugs for pregnant patients. *Prescribers' Journal*, 36(4): 192–7.

Cox, J., Holden, J. and Sagovsky, R. (1987) Detection of postnatal depression: development of the 10-item Edinburgh Postnatal Depression Scale. *British Journal of Psychiatry*, 150: 782–6.

Cox, S. (2007) Taking medicine during pregnancy. *Journal of Midwifery & Women's Health*, 52(5): 519–20.

Coyne, J.C. and Mitchell, A.J. (2007) Postpartum depression: NICE may be discouraging detection of postpartum depression. *BMJ*, 334(7593): 550.

Craig, J., Haynes, A., McClelland, D. and Ludlam, C. (2002) Blood disorders, in Haslett, C., Chilvers, E., Boon, N. and Colledge, N. (eds) *Davidson's Principles and Practice of Medicine*. Churchill Livingstone, Edinburgh.

Crowell, M.K., Hill, P. and Humenick, S. (1994) Relationship between obstetric analgesia and time of effective breast feeding. *Journal of Nurse-Midwifery*, 39(3): 150–6.

Crowley, P. (1999) Corticosteroids prior to preterm delivery. *Cochrane Database of Systematic Reviews*, Issue 3. Oxford, Update Software.

Crowther, C. (1990) Magnesium sulphate versus diazepam in the management of eclampsia: a randomised controlled trial. *British Journal of Obstetrics and Gynaecology*, 97: 110–17.

Crowther, C. and Middleton, P. (1997) Anti-D administration after childbirth for preventing Rhesus alloimmunisation. *Cochrane Database Syst Rev*, (2): CD000021. DOI: 10.1002/14651858.CD000021.

Crowther, C. and Middleton, P. (1999) Anti-D administration in pregnancy for preventing rhesus alloimmunisation. *Cochrane Database Syst Rev*, (2): CD000020. DOI: 10.1002/14651858.CD000020.

Crowther, C., Hiller, J., Moss, J. et al. (2005) Effect of treatment of gestational diabetes mellitus on pregnancy outcomes. *New England Journal of Medicine*, 352(24): 2477–86.

Crowther, C.A. and Harding, J.E. (2007) Repeat doses of prenatal corticosteroids for women at risk of preterm birth for preventing neonatal respiratory disease. *Cochrane Database of Systematic Reviews*, Issue 3. Art. No.: CD003935. DOI: 10.1002/14651858.CD003935.pub2.

Crowther, C.A, Haslam, R.R., Hiller, J.E. et al.; ACTORDS Study Group (2006) Neonatal respiratory distress syndrome after repeat exposure to antenatal corticosteroids: a randomised controlled trial. *Lancet*, 367(9526): 1913–19.

Crowther, C.A., Doyle, L.W., Haslam, R.R. et al.; ACTORDS Study Group (2007) Outcomes at 2 years of age after repeat doses of antenatal corticosteroids. *New England Journal of Medicine*, 357(12): 1179–89.

Crowther, C.A., Hiller, J.E. and Doyle, L.W. (2002) Magnesium sulphate for preventing preterm birth in threatened preterm labour. *Cochrane Database of Systematic Reviews*, Issue 4. Art. No.: CD001060. DOI: 10.1002/14651858. CD001060.

Cullen, G. and O'Donoghue, D. (2007) Constipation and pregnancy. *Best Practice & Research Clinical Gastroenterology*, 21(5): 807–18.

Cummings, K. and Dolak, J. (2006) Obstetrical and pediatric anesthesia, case report: epidural abscess in a parturient with pruritic urticarial papules and plaques of pregnancy (PUPPP). *Canadian Journal of Anesthesia*, 53(10): 1010–14.

Currier, G. and Simpson, G. (2001) Risperidone liquid concentrate and oral lorazepam versus intramuscular haloperidol and intramuscular lorazepam for treatment of psychotic patients. *Journal of Clinical Psychiatry*, 62(3): 153–7.

Cuskelly, G., McNulty, H. and Scott, J. (1996) Effect of increasing dietary folate on red-cell folate: implications for prevention of neural tube defects. *Lancet*, 347: 657–9.

Czeizel, A. and Dudas, I. (1992) Prevention of the first occurrence of neural-tube defects by periconceptual vitamin supplementation. *New England Journal of Medicine*, 327: 1832–5.

Dahlman, T.C. (1993) Osteoporotic fractures and the recurrence of thromboembolism during pregnancy and the puerperium in 184 women undergoing thromboprophylaxis with heparin. *American Journal of Obstetrics and Gynecology*, 168: 1265–70.

Dahlman, T.C., Sjoberg, H. and Ringertz, H. (1994) Bone mineral density during long-term prophylaxis with heparin in pregnancy. *American Journal of Obstetrics and Gynecology*, 170: 1315–20.

Daly, S., Mills, J., Molloy, A. et al. (1997) Minimum effective dose of folic acid for food fortification to prevent neural tube defects. *Lancet*, 350: 1666–9.

Daniel-Spiegel, E., Weiner, Z., Ben-Shlomo, I. and Shalve, E. (2004) For how long should oxytocin be continued during induction of labour? *BJOG*, 111: 331–4.

Dansky, L.V. and Finnell, R.H. (1991) Parental epilepsy, anticonvulsant drugs, and reproductive outcome: epidemiological and experimental findings spanning 3 decades. *Reproductive Toxicology*, 5: 301–35.

Darroca, R., Buttino, L., Miller, J. and Khamis, H. (1996) Prostaglandin E2 gel for cervical ripening in patients with an indication for delivery. *Obstetrics and Gynecology*, 87: 228–30.

Darwish, M., Kirby, M., Robertson, P. Jr. et al. (2006) Comparison of equivalent doses of fentanyl buccal tablets and arteriovenous differences in fentanyl pharmacokinetics. *Clinical Pharmacokinetics*, 45(8): 843–50.

Davis, N.M. (1992) Local and topical anaesthetic agents, in Baer, C. and Williams, B. (eds) *Clinical Pharmacology and Nursing*, 2nd edn. Springhouse, Springhouse, PA.

Davis, S. (2006) Insulin, oral hypoglycaemic agents, and the pharmacology of the endocrine pancreas, in Brunton, L., Lazo, J. and Parker, K. (eds) *Goodman and Gilman's: The Pharmacological Basis of Therapeutics*, 11th edn. McGraw-Hill, New York.

Davis, W., Wells, S., Kuller, J. and Thorp, J. (1997) Analysis of the risks associated with calcium channel blockade: implications for the obstetrician-gynecologist. *Obstetric and Gynecological Survey*, 52: 198–201.

Dawood, M.Y. (1995) Pharmacologic stimulation of uterine contraction. *Seminars in Perinatology*, 19:1: 73–83.

DCCTRG (Diabetes Control and Complications Trial Research Group) (2001) Influence of intensive diabetes treatment on body weight and composition of adults with type 1 diabetes in the Diabetes Control and Complications Trial. *Diabetes Care*, 24(10): 1711–21.

De Abajo, F.J., Meseguer, C.M. and Antiñolo, G. (2004) Labor induction with dinoprostone or oxytocine and postpartum disseminated intravascular coagulation: a hospital-based case-control study. *American Journal of Obstetrics and Gynecology*, 191(5): 1637–43.

De Arcos, F., Gratacos, E., Palacio, M. and Cararach, V. (1996) Toxic hepatitis: a rare complication associated with the use of ritodrine during pregnancy. *Acta Obstetricia et Gynecologica Scandinavica*, 75(4): 340–2.

De Groot, A., van Dongen, P., Vree, T. et al. (1998) Ergot alkaloids. *Drugs*, 56: 523–35.

De Jong, P., Johanson, R., Baxen, P. et al. (1997) Randomised trial comparing the upright and supine positions for the second stage of labour. *British Journal of Obstetrics and Gynaecology*, 104: 567–71.

De Swiet, M. (1995) Anticoagulants, in Rubin, P. (ed.) *Prescribing in Pregnancy*, 2nd edn. BMJ Group, London.

De Swiet, M. (2000) Maternal blood pressure and birthweight. *Lancet*, 355: 81–2.

De Swiet, M. (2002) *Medical Disorders in Obstetric Practice*, 4th edn. Blackwell, Oxford.

De Vries, E.N., Ramrattan, M.A., Smorenburg, S.M. et al. (2008) The incidence and nature of in-hospital adverse events: a systematic review. *Quality and Safety in Health Care*, 17(3): 216–23.

Dean, B. (1996) Are incompatibilities a problem? *Pharmacy in Practice*, November: 371–2.

Dean, C., Williams, R.J. and Brockington, I.F (1989) Is puerperal psychosis the same as bipolar manic depressive disorder? A family study. *Psychological Medicine*, 19: 637–47.

Dennesen, P., Bonten, M. and Weinstein, R. (1998) Multiresistant bacteria as a hospital epidemic problem. *Annals of Medicine*, 30(2): 176–85.

Dennis, C.L. (2004) Treatment of postpartum depression, part 2: a critical review of non biological interventions. *Journal of Clinical Psychiatry*, 65: 1252–65.

Dennis, C.L. and Stewart, D.E. (2004) Treatment of postpartum depression, part 1: a critical review of biological interventions. *Journal of Clinical Psychiatry*, 65: 1242–51.

Derbyshire, E. (2007) The importance of adequate fluid and fibre intake during pregnancy. *Nursing Standard*, 21(24): 40–3.

Derbyshire, E., Davies, J. and Dettmar, P. (2007) Changes in bowel function: pregnancy and the puerperium. *Dig Dis Sci*, 52: 324–8.

Derbyshire, E., Davies, J., Costarelli, V. and Dettmar, P. (2006) Diet, physical inactivity and the prevalence of constipation throughout and after pregnancy. *Maternal and Child Nutrition*, 2: 127–34.

Derijks, H.J., Heerdink, E.R., de Koning, F.H. et al. (2008) The association between antidepressant use and hypoglycaemia in diabetic patients: a nested case control study. *Pharmacoepidemiol Drug Safety*, 17(4): 336–44.

Desprats, R., Dumas, J.C., Giroux, M. et al. (1991) Maternal and umbilical cord concentrations of fentanyl after epidural analgesia for caesarean section. *European Journal of Obstetrics & Gynaecology & Reproductive Biology*, 42: 89–94.

Dev, V. and Krupp, P. (1995) Adverse event profile and safety of clozapine. *Review of Contemporary Pharmacotherapeutics*, 6: 197–208.

Dever, L., China, C., Eng, R. et al. (1998) Vancomycin-resistant *Enterococcus faecium* in a Veterans' Affairs Medical Center: association with antibiotic usage. *American Journal of Infection Control*, 26(1): 40–6.

Dewan, D. and Cohen, S. (1994) Epidural analgesia and the incidence of Caesarean section. *Anesthesiology*, 80(6): 1189–92.

Dewey, K. (2001) Maternal and fetal stress are associated with impaired lactogenesis in humans. *Journal of Nutrition*, 131(S): 3012–15.

Dewey, K.G., Nommsen-Rivers, L.A., Heinig, M.J. and Cohen R.J. (2003) Risk factors for suboptimal infant breastfeeding behavior, delayed onset of lactation, and excess neonatal weight loss. *Pediatrics*, 112(3 Pt 1): 607–19.

DH (Department of Health) (1991) *Report on Confidential Enquiries into Maternal Deaths in the United Kingdom 1985–7*. HMSO, London.

DH (Department of Health) (1994) *Report on Confidential Enquiries into Maternal Deaths in the United Kingdom 1988–90*. HMSO, London.

DH (Department of Health) (1996) *Report on Confidential Enquiries into Maternal Deaths in the United Kingdom 1991–3*. HMSO, London.

DH (Department of Health) (1998) *Why Mothers Die. Report on Confidential Enquiries into Maternal Deaths in the United Kingdom 1994–6*. HMSO, London.

DH (Department of Health) (2002) *Women's Mental Health: Into the Mainstream – Strategic Development of Mental Health Care for Women*. DH, London.

DH (Department of Health) (2003) *An Organisation with a Memory*. TSO, London.

DH (Department of Health) (2006) *Immunisation Against Infectious Disease: The Green Book*, updated 2008. TSO, Norwich, www.dh.gov.uk/en/Publichealth/Healthprotection/Immunisation/Greenbook/DH_4097254.

DH (Department of Health) (2007) *Why Mothers Die: Report on Confidential Enquiries into Maternal Deaths 2003–2005*. TSO, London.

DH (Department of Health) (2008) *Medicines Management: Everybody's Business*. TSO, London.

DH/RCN (Department of Health/Royal College of Nursing) (1994) *Good Practice in the Administration of Depot Neuroleptics: A Guidance Document for Mental Health and Practice Nurses*. HMSO, London.

Diav-Citrin, O., Shechtman, S., Aharonovich, A. et al. (2003) Pregnancy outcome after gestational exposure to loratadine or antihistamines: a prospective controlled cohort study. *J Allergy Clin Immunol*, 111: 1239–43.

Dichter, M. (1991) The epilepsies and convulsive disorders, in Wilson, J., Braunwald, E., Isselbacher, K. et al. (eds) *Harrison's Principles of Internal Medicine*, 12th edn, McGraw-Hill, New York.

Dickersin, K. (1989) Pharmacological control of pain during labour, in Chalmers, I., Enkin, M. and Kierse, M.J. (eds) *Effective Care in Pregnancy and Childbirth*. Oxford Medical, Oxford.

Dixon, W. (2004) *Survey of Caffeine Levels in Hot Beverages*, 53/04. Food Standards Agency, London, www.food.gov.uk/multimedia/pdfs/fsis5304.pdf.

Doan, T., Melvold, R. and Waltenbaugh, C. (2005) *Concise Medical Immunology*. Lippincott Williams & Wilkins, Springhouse, PA.

Dodd, J.M., Crowther, C.A., Dare, M.R. and Middleton P. (2006) Oral betamimetics for maintenance therapy after threatened preterm labour. *Cochrane Database of Systematic Reviews*, Issue 1. Art. No.: CD003927. DOI:10.1002/14651858.CD003927.pub2.

Doepp, F., Schreiber, S., Munster, T. et al. (2004) How does the blood leave the brain? A systematic ultrasound analysis of cerebral venous drainage patterns. *Neuroradiology*, 46: 565–70.

Donaldson, J.O. (1995) Neurologic disorders, in de Swiet, M. (ed.) *Medical Disorders in Obstetric Practice*, 3rd edn. Blackwell Science, Oxford.

Donders, G. (2000) Treatment of sexually transmitted bacterial diseases in pregnant women. *Drugs*, 59: 477–85.

Doran, C. (2003) *Prescribing Mental Health Medication*. Routledge, London.

Doran, M., Rassam, S., Jones, L. and Underhill, S. (2004) Lesson of the week: toxicity after intermittent inhalation of nitrous oxide for analgesia. *BMJ*, 328: 1364–5.

Dornhorst, A. and Frost, G. (2000) Jelly-beans, only a colourful distraction from gestational glucose-challenge tests. *Lancet*, 355: 674.

Dounas, M., O'Kelly, B., Jamali, S. et al. (1996) Maternal and fetal effects of adrenaline with bupivacaine (0.25%) for epidural analgesia during labour. *European Journal of Anaesthesiology*, 13(6): 594–8.

Downing, J. and Ramasubramanian, R. (1993) Effects of analgesia and anaesthesia on fetal acid-base balance and respiratory gas exchange, in Reynolds, F. (ed.) *Effects on the Baby of Maternal Analgesia and Anaesthesia*. Saunders, London.

Dresser, G., Bailey, D., Leake, B.F. et al. (2002) Fruit juices inhibit organic anion transporting polypeptide-mediated drug uptake to decrease the oral availability of fexofenadine. *Clinical Pharmacology and Therapeutics*, 71(1): 11–20.

Dresser, G., Spence, J. and Bailey, D. (2000) Pharmacokinetic-pharmacodynamic consequences and clinical relevance of cytochrome P450 3A4 inhibition. *Clinical Pharmacokinetics*, 38: 41–57.

Drife, J.O. (1996) Choice and instrumental delivery. *British Journal of Obstetrics and Gynaecology*, 103(7): 608–11.

Drug and Therapeutics Bulletin (1995) The drug treatment of patients with schizophrenia. *Drug and Therapeutics Bulletin*, 33(11): 81–6.

Drug and Therapeutics Bulletin (2007) Understanding monoclonal antibodies. *Drug and Therapeutics Bulletin*, 45(7): 55–6.

Drugs and Therapy Perspectives (1993) Antiemetic selection depends on cause of emesis. *Drugs and Therapy Perspectives*, 1(8): 9–11.

Drugs and Therapy Perspectives (1996) Plenty of scope for individualised pain control during labour and delivery. *Drugs and Therapy Perspectives*, 7(4): 7–10.

Dryden, C., Young, D., Hepburn, M. and Mactier, H. (2009) Maternal methadone use in pregnancy: factors associated with the development of neonatal abstinence syndrome and implications for healthcare resources. *BJOG*, 116(5): 665–71.

Dubus, J., Marguet, C., Le Roux, P. et al. (2001) Local side-effects of inhaled corticosteroids in asthmatic children. *Allergy*, 56(10): 944–9.

Duley, L. (1996) Magnesium sulphate regimens for women with eclampsia: messages from the Collaborative Eclampsia Trial. *British Journal of Obstetrics and Gynaecology*, 103: 103–5.

Duley, L. (1999) Aspirin for preventing and treating pre-eclampsia. *BMJ*, 318: 751–2.

Duley, L. and Neilson, J. (1999) Magnesium sulphate and pre-eclampsia. *BMJ*, 319: 3–4.

Duley, L., Gulmezoglu, A. and Henderson-Smart, D. (2000) Anticonvulsants for women with pre-eclampsia. *Cochrane Pregnancy and Childbirth Database* (issue 2). Oxford, Update Software.

Duley, L., Gülmezoglu, A.M. and Henderson-Smart, D.J. (2003) Magnesium sulphate and other anticonvulsants for women with pre-eclampsia. *Cochrane Database of Systematic Reviews*, Issue 2. Art. No.: CD000025. DOI: 10.1002/14651858.CD000025.

Duley, L., Henderson-Smart, D.J. and Meher, S. (2006) Drugs for treatment of very high blood pressure during pregnancy. *Cochrane Database of Systematic Reviews*, Issue 3. Art. No.: CD001449. DOI: 10.1002/14651858.CD001449.pub2.

Duley, L., Henderson-Smart, D.J., Meher, S. and King, J.F. (2007) Antiplatelet agents for preventing pre-eclampsia and its complications. *Cochrane Database of Systematic Reviews*, Issue 2. Art. No.: CD004659. DOI: 10.1002/14651858.CD004659.pub2.

Duncan, S. (2007) Teratogenesis of sodium valproate. *Current Opinion in Neurology*, 20(2): 175–80.

Dunkley-Brent, J. (2004) Health promotion in midwifery, in Henderson, C. and MacDonald, S. (eds) *Mayes' Midwifery: A Textbook for Midwives*, 13th edn. Baillière Tindall, Edinburgh.

Ebbesen, F., Joergensen, A., Hoseth, E. et al. (2000) Neonatal hypoglycaemia and withdrawal symptoms after exposure in utero to valproate. *Archives of Disease in Childhood: Fetal and Neonatal Edition*, 83(2): F124–9.

Ebden, P. and Evans, E. (1996) Management of asthmatic conditions in pregnancy. *Prescriber*, 7(3): 21–5.

Eberhard-Gran, M., Esklid, A. and Opjordsmoen, S. (2006) Use of psychotropic medication in treating mood disorders during lactation: practical recommendations. *CNS Drugs*, 20: 187–98.

Eberle, R. and Norris, M. (1996) Labour analgesia: a risk–benefit analysis. *Drug Safety*, 14(4): 239–51.

EBM (Evidence-Based Medicine) Working Group (1992) Evidence-based medicine: a new approach to teaching the practice of medicine. *JAMA*, 268: 2420–5.

Eclampsia Trial Collaborative Group (1995) Which anticonvulsant for women with eclampsia? Evidence from the Collaborative Eclampsia Trial. *Lancet*, 345: 1455–63.

Edwards, G. and Anderson, I. (1999) Systematic review and guide to selection of selective serotonin reuptake inhibitors. *Drugs*, 57: 507–33.

Edwards, I.R. and Aronson, J.K. (2000) Adverse drug reactions: definitions, diagnosis, and management. *Lancet*, 356: 1255–9.

Egerman, R., Mercer, B., Doss, J. and Sibai, B. (1998) A randomized controlled trial of oral and intramuscular dexamethasone in the prevention of neonatal respiratory distress syndrome. *American Journal of Obstetrics and Gynecology*, 179: 1120–3.

Eggers, K., Chawathe, M., Benjamin, F. et al. (2008) Anaesthesia for Caesarean section, in Clyburn, P., Collis, R., Harries, S. and Davies, S. (eds) *Obstetric Anaesthesia*. Oxford University Press, Oxford.

Einarson, A., Ho, E. and Koren, G. (2000) Can we use metronidazole during pregnancy and breastfeeding? *Canadian Family Physician*, 46: 1053–4.

Ekpebegh, C.O., Coetzee, E.J., van der Merwe, L. and Levitt, N.S. (2007) A 10-year retrospective analysis of pregnancy outcome in pregestational Type 2 diabetes: comparison of insulin and oral glucose-lowering agents. *Diabet Medicine*, 24(3): 253–8.

Elbourne, D. and Wiseman, R. (2000) Types of intramuscular opioids for maternal pain relief. *Cochrane Database Systematic Review* (issue 2). Update Software, Oxford.

Elimian, A., Garry, D., Figueroa, R. et al. (2007) Antenatal betamethasone compared with dexamethasone (betacode trial): a randomized controlled trial. *Obstetrics Gynecol*, 110(1): 26–30.

Elizur, S.E. and Tulandi, T. (2008) Drugs in infertility and fetal safety. *Fertil Steril*, 89(6): 1595–602.

Elliot, S., Gerrard, J. and Holden, J. (1994) *The Management of Postnatal Depression in Primary Care*. Sainsbury Centre for Mental Health, London.

Elliott, S.A., Leverton, T.J., Sanjack, M. et al. (2000) Promoting mental health after childbirth: a controlled trial of primary prevention of postnatal depression. *British Journal of Clinical Psychology*, 39: 223–41.

Ellis, M., Manandhar, N., Manandhar, D. and Costello, A. (2000) Risk factors for neonatal encephalopathy in Kathmandu, Nepal, a developing country. *BMJ*, 320: 1229–36.

Ellison, J., Walker, I. and Greer, I. (2000) Antenatal use of enoxaparin for prevention and treatment of thromboembolism in pregnancy. *British Journal of Obstetrics and Gynaecology*, 107: 1116–21.

El-Mallakh, R. (2008) Lithium, in Aronson, J.K. (ed.) *Side Effects of Drug Annual* 30. Elsevier, Amsterdam.

El-Refaey, H., Nooh, R., O'Brien, P. et al. (2000) The misoprostol third stage of labour: a randomised controlled comparison between orally administered misoprostol and standard management. *British Journal of Obstetrics and Gynaecology*, 107: 1104–10.

ElSedeek, M.S., Awad, E.E. and ElSebaey, S.M. (2009) Evaluation of post-partum blood loss after misoprostol induced labour. *BJOG*, 116(3): 431–5.

Eltzschig, H., Lieberman, E., Camann, P. and Camann, W. (2003) Regional anesthesia and analgesia for labor and delivery. *New England Journal of Medicine*, 348(4): 319–32.

Empson, M.B., Lassere, M., Craig, J.C. and Scott, J.R. (2005) Prevention of recurrent miscarriage for women with antiphospholipid antibody or lupus anticoagulant. *Cochrane Database of Systematic Reviews*, Issue 2. Art. No.: CD002859. DOI: 10.1002/14651858.CD002859.pub2.

Endrenyi, L. (2007) Pharmacokinetics: principles and clinical applications, in Kalant, H., Grant, D. and Mitchell, J. (eds) *Principles of Medical Pharmacology*, 7th edn. Saunders, Elsevier, Toronto.

Engel, J. (2001) ILAE Commission Report: a proposed diagnostic scheme for people with epileptic seizures and with epilepsy: Report of the ILAE Task Force on Classification and Terminology. *Epilepsia*, 42(6): 796–803.

Engeland, A., Haldorsen, T., Andersen, A. and Tretli, S. (1996) The impact of smoking habits on lung cancer risk: 28 years' observation of 26,000 Norwegian man and women. *Cancer Causes & Control*, 7: 366–76.

England, M.J., Tjallinks, A., Hofmeyr, J. and Harber, J. (1988) Suppression of lactation: a comparison of bromocriptine and prostaglandin E2. *Journal of Reproductive Medicine*, 33: 630–2.

Engstrom, J. and Sittler, C. (1994) Nurse-midwifery management of iron-deficiency anaemia during pregnancy. *Journal of Nurse Midwifery*, 39(2S): 20–43.

Euphrates Group (2005) *European Consensus on Prevention and Management of Post Partum Haemorrhage*, www.euphrates.inserm.fr/inserm/euphrates.nsf/ViewAllDocumentsByUNID/95A14F46F31A5246C125707400485AED/$File/EuphratesConsensus.pdf?OpenElement.

Evans, P. and Misra, U. (2003) Poor outcome following epidural abscess complicating epidural analgesia for labour. *European Journal of Obstetrics & Gynecology and Reproductive Biology*, 109: 102–5.

Evers, A., Crowder, M. and Balser, J. (2006) General anesthetics, in Brunton, L., Lazo, J. and Parker, K. (eds) *Goodman & Gilman's: The Pharmacological Basis of Therapeutics*, 11th edn. McGraw-Hill, New York.

Facchinetti, F., Venturini, P., Blasi, I. and Giannella, L. (2005) Changes in the cervical competence in preterm labour. *BJOG*, 112(S1): 23–7.

Fairgrieve, S., Jackson, M., Jonas, P. et al. (2000) Population based, prospective study of the care of women with epilepsy in pregnancy. *BMJ*, 321: 674–5.

Fairlie, F., Walker, J., Marchall, L. and Elbourne, D. (1999) Intramuscular opioids for maternal pain relief in labour: a randomised controlled trial comparing pethidine with diamorphine. *British Journal of Obstetrics and Gynaecology*, 106: 1181–7.

Farber, N.B. and Olney, J.W. (2003) Drugs of abuse that cause developing neurons to commit suicide. *Brain Res Dev Brain Res*, 147(1/2): 37–45.

FDA (US Food and Drugs Administration) (2008) *Suicidal Behaviour and Ideation and Antiepileptic Drugs*. Centre for Drug Evaluation and Research, Silver Spring, MD, www.fda.gov/Cder/drug/InfoSheets/HCP/antiepileptics200812.htm.

Feldman, R., Weller, A., Zagoory-Sharon, O. and Levine, A. (2007) Evidence for a neuroendocrinological foundation of human affiliation: plasma oxytocin levels across pregnancy and the postpartum period predict mother-infant bonding. *Psychological Science*, 18(11): 965–70.

Fernandez, S. (2000) Hamochromatosis mutations. Unpublished research project. Cardiff, University of Wales.

Fernando, R., Bonello, E., Gill, P. et al. (1997) Neonatal welfare and placental transfer of fentanyl and bupivacaine during ambulatory combined spinal epidural analgesia for labour. *Anaesthesia*, 52: 517–24.

Fewtrell, M., Loh, K., Blake, A. et al. (2006) Randomised, double blind trial of oxytocin nasal spray in mothers expressing breast milk for preterm infants. *Archives of Disease in Childhood, Fetal and Neonatal Edition*, 91: F169–74.

Findley, I. and Chamberlain, G. (1999) Relief of pain. *BMJ*, 318: 927–30.

Finning, K., Martin, P., Summers, J. et al. (2008) Effect of high throughput RHD typing of fetal DNA in maternal plasma on use of anti-RhD immunoglobulin in RhD negative pregnant women: prospective feasibility study. *BMJ*, 336(7648): 816–18.

Fischer, C., Blank, P., Jaouen, E. et al. (2000) Ropivacaine, 0.1%, plus sufentanil. *Anesthesiology*, 92(6): 1588–93.

Fitzgerald, P. (1995) Endocrine disorders, in Tierney, L., McPhee, S. and Papadakis, M. (eds) *Current Medical Diagnosis and Treatment*. Appleton & Lange, Norwalk, CT.

Fleming, M., Mihic, S.J. and Harris, A. (2006) Ethanol, in Brunton, L., Lazo, J. and Parker, K. (eds) *Goodman & Gilman's: The Pharmacological Basis of Therapeutics*, 11th edn. McGraw-Hill, New York.

Foix-L'Helias, L., Marret, S., Ancel, P.-Y. et al. (2008) Impact of the use of antenatal corticosteroids on mortality, cerebral lesions and 5-year neurodevelopmental outcomes of very preterm infants: the EPIPAGE cohort study. *BJOG*, 115: 275–82.

Forster, M., Nimmo, G. and Brown, A. (1996) Prolapsed intervertebral disc after epidural analgesia in labour. *Anaesthesia*, 51(8): 773–5.

Foster, D. (1991) Diabetes Mellitus, in Wilson, J., Braunwald, E., Isselbacher, K. et al. (eds) *Harrison's Principles of Internal Medicine*, 12th edn. McGraw-Hill, New York.

Foster, P.R., McIntosh, R.V. and Welch, A.G. (1995) Hepatitis C infection from anti-D immunoglobulin. *Lancet*, 345: 372.

Fox, R. and Draycott, T. (1996) Diazepam is more useful than magnesium for immediate control of eclampsia (letter). *BMJ*, 312: 1668–9.

Fraser, C. and Arieff, A. (1990) Water metabolism and its disorders, in Cohen, R., Lewis, B., Alberti, K. and Denman, A. (eds) *The Metabolic and Molecular Basis of Acquired Disease*. Baillière Tindall, London.

Fraser, W., Vendittelli, F., Krauss, I. and Breart, G. (1998) Effects of early augmentation of labour with amniotomy and oxytocin in nulliparous women: a meta-analysis. *British Journal of Obstetrics and Gynaecology*, 105: 189–94.

French, N.P., Hagan, R., Evans, S. et al. (1999) Repeated antenatal corticosteroids: size at birth and subsequent development. *American Journal of Obstetrics and Gynecology*, 180: 114–21.

Freyer, A. (2008) Drug-prescribing challenges during pregnancy. *Obstetrics, Gynaecology and Reproductive Medicine*, 18(7): 180–6.

Friedman, L. and Isselbacher, K. (1991) Anorexia, nausea, vomiting and indigestion, in Wilson, J., Braunwald, E., Isselbacher, K. et al. (eds) *Harrison's Principles of Internal Medicine*, 12th edn. McGraw-Hill, New York.

Friedman, L., Lewis, P.J., Clifton, P. and Bulpitt, C.J. (1978) Factors influencing the incidence of neonatal jaundice. *BMJ*, 1: 1235–7.

Frigoletto, F., Lieberman, E., Lang, J. et al. (1995) A clinical trial of active management of labor. *New England Journal of Medicine*, 333: 745–50.

Fujii, Y., Tanaka, H. and Toyooka, H. (1998) Prevention of nausea and vomiting with granisetron, droperidol and metoclopramide during and after spinal anaesthesia for caesarean section. *Acta Anaesthesiologica Scandinavia*, 42(8): 921–5.

Fung, B. (2000) Continuous epidural analgesia for painless labor does not increase the incidence of cesarean delivery. *Acta Anaesthesiologia Sinica*, 38: 79–84.

Gabbe, S., Holing, E., Temple, P. and Brown, Z. (2000) Benefits, risks, costs, and patient satisfaction associated with insulin pump therapy for the pregnancy complicated by type 1 diabetes mellitus. *American Journal of Obstetrics and Gynecology*, 182: 1283–91.

Gaffney, K.F., Beckwitt, A.E. and Friesen, M.A. (2008) Mothers' reflections about infant irritability and postpartum tobacco use. *Birth*, 35(1): 66–72.

Gaiser, R., Cheek, T. and Gutsche, B. (1998) Comparison of three different doses of intrathecal fentanyl and sufentanil for labor analgesia. *Journal of Clinical Anesthetics*, 10: 488–93.

Galbraith, A., Bullock, S., Manias, E. et al. (2007) *Fundamentals of Pharmacology*, 2nd edn. Addison Wesley, Harlow.

Gallery, E. (1995) Hypertension in pregnancy. *Drugs*, 49: 555–62.

Ganong, W.F. (1999) *Review of Medical Physiology*, 19th edn. Appleton & Lange, Norwalk, CT.

Ganong, W.F. (2005) *Review of Medical Physiology*, 22nd edn. McGraw Hill, New York.

Garbis, H. (2007) Antiasthmatic and cough medication, in Schaefer, C., Peters, P.W. and Miller, R.K. (eds) *Drugs during Pregnancy and Lactation: Treatment Options and Risk Assessment*, 2nd edn. Elsevier, Oxford.

Garbis, H. and McElhatton, P. (2007) Psychotropic drugs, in Schaefer C., Peters P.W. and Miller, R.K. (eds) *Drugs during Pregnancy and Lactation: Treatment Options and Risk Assessment*, 2nd edn. Elsevier, Oxford.

Garbis, H., van Tonningen, M.R. and Reuvers, M. (2007) Anti-infective agents, in Schaefer, C., Peters, P.W. and Miller, R.K. (eds) *Drugs during Pregnancy and Lactation: Treatment Options and Risk Assessment*, 2nd edn. Elsevier, Oxford.

Gardiner, H. and Fouron, J. (2009) Folic acid fortification and congenital heart disease. *BMJ*, 338: 1221–2.

Garland, H.O. (1985) Maternal adjustments to pregnancy, in Case, R.M. (ed.) *Variations in Human Physiology*. Manchester University Press, Manchester.

Garret, A. and Fitzgerald, M. (2004) Coxibs and cardiovascular disease. *New England Journal of Medicine*, 351: 1709–11.

Gautier, P., Derby, F., Fanard, L. et al. (1997) Ambulatory CSE analgesia for labor. *Regional Anesthesia*, 22: 143–9.

Geerts, W., Jay, R., Code, K. et al. (1996) A comparison of low-dose heparin with low-molecular weight heparin as prophylaxis against venous thromboembolism after major trauma. *New England Journal of Medicine*, 335: 701–7.

Geha, R.S. and Rosen, F.S. (2008) *Case Studies in Immunology: A Clinical Companion*, 5th edn. Garland Science, New York.

Genser, D. (2008) Food and drug interaction: consequences for the nutrition/health status. *Annals Nutr Metab*, 52(S1): 29–32.

Ghodse, A.H. and Galea, S. (2008) Opioid analgesics, in Aronson, J.K. (ed.) *Side Effects of Drug Annual* 30. Elsevier, Amsterdam.

Gibb, D. and Arulkumaran, S. (1997) *Fetal Monitoring in Practice*, 2nd edn. Butterworth-Heinemann, Oxford.

Gilbert, C., Valois, M. and Koren, G. (2006) Pregnancy outcome after first-trimester exposure to metformin: a meta-analysis. *Fertil Steril*, 86(3): 658–63.

Gilbert, L., Porter, W. and Brown, V.A. (1987) Postpartum haemorrhage: a continuing problem. *British Journal of Obstetrics Gynaecology*, 94(1): 67–71.

Gill, A.W. and Colvin, J. (2007) Use of naloxone during neonatal resuscitation in Australia: compliance with published guidelines. *J Paediatr Child Health*, 43(12): 795–8.

Gillmer, M. (1996) Management of pre-existing disorders in pregnancy: diabetes mellitus. *Prescribers' Journal*, 36: 159–64.

Giménez-Arnau, A.M., Toll, A. and Pujol, R.M. (2005) Immediate cutaneous hypersensitivity response to phytomenadione induced by vitamin K in skin diagnostic procedure. *Contact Dermatitis*, 52(5): 284–5.

Gimpl, G. and Fahrenholz, F. (2001) The oxytocin receptor system: structure, function, and regulation. *Physiology Review*, 81(2): 629–83.

Ginsberg, J. (1996) Management of venous thromboembolism. *New England Journal of Medicine*, 335: 1816–28.

Girling, J. (1996) Thyroid disease in pregnancy. *British Journal of Hospital Medicine*, 56: 316–20.

Girling, J. and de Swiet, M. (1996) Pre-eclampsia. *Update*, 16(10): 338–42.

Girling, J. and Nelson-Piercy, C. (2007) Hypothyroidism in pregnancy: three unresolved issues. *BMJ*, 335(7616): 362.

Gitlin, M., Altshuler, L.L., Frye, M.A. et al. (2004) Peripheral thyroid hormones and response to selective serotonin reuptake inhibitors. *J Psychiatry Neurosci*, 29(5): 383–6.

Glinoer, D. and Abalovich, M. (2007) Unresolved questions in managing hypothyroidism during pregnancy. *BMJ*, 335: 300–2.

Goadsby, P., Goldberg, J. and Silberstein, S. (2008) Migraine in pregnancy. *BMJ*, 336(7659): 1502–4.

Golding, J., Greenwood, R., Birmingham, K. and Mott, M. (1992) Childhood cancer, intramuscular vitamin K, and pethidine given during labour. *BMJ*, 305: 341–6.

Golding, J., Paterson, M. and Kinlen, L.J. (1990) Factors associated with childhood cancer in a national cohort study. *British Journal of Cancer*, 62: 304–8.

Goldstein, L. and Berkovitch, M. (2007) Antiemetics, in Schaefer, C., Peters, P.W. and Miller, R.K. (eds) *Drugs during Pregnancy and Lactation: Treatment Options and Risk Assessment*, 2nd edn. Elsevier, Oxford.

Goma, H.M., Said, R.N. and El-Ela, A.M. (2008) Study of the newborn feeding behaviors and fentanyl concentration in colostrum after an analgesic dose of epidural and intravenous fentanyl in cesarean section. *Saudi Medicine J*, 29(5): 678–82.

Gonser, M. (1995) Labor induction and augmentation with oxytocin: pharmacokinetic considerations. *Archives of Gynecology and Obstetrics*, 256: 63–6.

Gooch, K., Culleton, B.F., Manns, B.J. et al. (2007) NSAID use and progression of chronic kidney disease. *American Journal of Medicine*, 120(3): 280, e1–7.

Gossop, M. (2007) *Living with Drugs*, 6th edn. Ashgate, Aldershot.

Graham, K. (1998) Magnesium sulphate in eclampsia. *Lancet*, 351: 1061.

Grahame-Smith, P. and Aronson, J.K. (1985) *The Oxford Textbook of Clinical Pharmacology and Drug Therapy*. Oxford University Press, Oxford.

Graves, C. (1996) Agents that cause contraction or relaxation of the uterus, in Hardman, J., Limbard, L., Molinoff, P. et al. (eds) *Goodman & Gilman's: The Pharmacological Basis of Therapeutics*, 9th edn. McGraw-Hill, New York.

Gray, G. and Saloojee, H. (2008) Breast-feeding, antiretroviral prophylaxis, and HIV. *New England Journal of Medicine*, 359: 2.

Greaves, M. (1999) Antiphospholipid antibodies and thrombosis. *Lancet*, 353: 1348–53.

Greene, M. and Solomon, C. (2005) Gestational diabetes mellitus: time to treat. *New England Journal of Medicine*, 352(24): 2544–6.

Greer, F., Marchall, S., Severson, R. et al. (1998) A new mixed micellar preparation for oral vitamin K prophylaxis. *Archives of Disease in Childhood*, 79(4): 300–5.

Greer, I. (1999) Thrombosis in pregnancy: maternal and fetal issues. *Lancet*, 353: 1258–65.

Griffith, D., Betteridge, D. and Axford, J. (1996) Diabetes mellitus, lipoprotein disorders and other metabolic diseases, in Axford, J. (ed.) *Medicine*. Blackwell, Oxford.

Griffith, R. (2005) Managing difficulties in swallowing solid medication: the need for caution. *Nurse Prescriber*, 3: 201–3.

Griffith, R., Griffiths, H. and Jordan, S. (2003) Continuing professional development: administration of medicines, part 1: the law. *Nursing Standard*, 18(2): 47–54.

Grohmann, R., Ruther, E., Engel, R. and Hippius, R. (1999) Assessment of adverse drug reactions in psychiatric inpatients. *Pharmacopsychiatry*, 32(1): 21–8.

Grossman, E., Messerli, F., Grodzicki, T. and Kowey, P. (1996) Should a moratorium be placed on sublingual nifedipine capsules given for hypertensive emergencies and pseudoemergencies? *JAMA*, 276: 1328–31.

Guerrini, I., Jackson, S. and Keaney, F. (2009) Pregnancy and alcohol misuse. *BMJ*, 338: b845, doi: 10.1136/bmj.b845.

Guidolin, L., Vignoli, A. and Ganger, R. (1998) Worsening in seizure frequency and severity in relation to folic acid administration. *European Journal of Neurology*, 5: 301–3.

Gulmezoglu, A. (2000) Prostaglandins for prevention of postpartum harmorrhage. *Cochrane Database Systematic Review* (issue 2). Update Software, Oxford.

Gulmezoglu, A.M., Forna, F., Villar, J. and Hofmeyr, G.J. (2007) Prostaglandins for preventing postpartum haemorrhage. *Cochrane Database of Systematic Reviews*, Issue 3. Art. No.: CD000494. DOI: 10.1002/14651858.CD000494.pub3.

Gutstein, H. and Akil, H. (2006) Opioid analgesics, in Brunton, L., Lazo, J. and Parker, K. (eds) *Goodman & Gilman's: The Pharmacological Basis of Therapeutics*, 11th edn. McGraw-Hill, New York.

Guyton, A. (1996) *Textbook of Medical Physiology*, 9th edn. Saunders, Philadelphia.

Gyetvai, K., Hannah, M., Hodnett, E. and Ohlsson, A. (1999) Tocolytics for preterm labor: a systematic review. *Obstetrics and Gynecology*, 94: 869–77 .

Hague, W. (1995) Treatment of endocrine diseases, in Rubin, P. (ed.) *Prescribing in Pregnancy*, 2nd edn. BMJ Group, London.

Haider, B.A. and Bhutta, Z.A. (2005) Effects of interventions for helminthic infections in pregnancy (Protocol). *Cochrane Database of Systematic Reviews*, Issue 4. Art. No.: CD005547. DOI: 10.1002/14651858.CD005547.

Halken, S. (2004) Prevention of allergic disease in childhood: clinical and epidemiological aspects of primary and secondary allergy prevention. *Pediatric Allergy and Immunology*, Suppl, 16(4/5): 9–32.

Hall, D., Odendaal, H. and Smith, M. (2000) Is the prophylactic administration of magnesium sulphate in women with pre-eclampsia indicated prior to labour? *British Journal of Obstetrics and Gynaecology*, 107: 903–8.

Hall, J., Pauli, R. and Wilson, K.M. (1980) Maternal and fetal sequelae of anti-coagulation during pregnancy. *American Journal of Medicine*, 68: 122–40.

Hall, R. (1996) Intrathecal opioids for labor analgesia in a community hospital. Cleveland Clinic Foundation, sector for anaesthesia for obstetrics, www.anes.ccf.org:8080/soap/itnarc.htm.

Halligan, A., Bell, S. and Taylor, D. (1999) Dipstick proteinuris: caveat emptor. *British Journal of Obstetrics and Gynaecology*, 106: 1113–15.

Halpern, S., Leighton, B., Ohlsson, A. et al. (1998) Effect of epidural vs. parenteral opioid analgesia on the progress of labour: a meta-analysis. *JAMA*, 280(24): 2105–10.

Halpern, S., Levine, T., Wilson, D. et al. (1999) Effect of labor analgesia on breastfeeding success. *Birth*, 26(2): 83–8.

Hannah, M., Ohlsson, A., Farine, D. et al. (1996) Induction of labor compared with expectant management for prelabor rupture of the membranes at term. *New England Journal of Medicine*, 334: 1005–10.

Hansen, D., Lou, H. and Olsen, J. (2000) Serious life events and congential malformations: a national study with complete follow-up. *Lancet*, 356: 875–80.

Haram, K., Hervig, T., Thordarson, H. and Aksnes, L. (1993) Osteopenia caused by heparin treatment in pregnancy. *Acta Obstetrica et Gynecologica Scandanavia*, 72(8): 674–5.

Harden, C.L. (2007) Pregnancy and epilepsy. *Seminars in Neurology*, 27(5): 453–9.

Harms, C., Sigemund, M., Marsch, S. et al. (1999) Initiating extradural analgesia during labour: comparison of three different bupivacaine concentrations used as the loading dose. *Fetal Diagnostics and Therapeutics*, 14: 368–74.

Harries, S. and Turner, M. (2008) Non-regional labour analgesia, in Clyburn, P., Collis, R., Harries, S. and Davies, S. (eds) *Obstetric Anaesthesia*. Oxford University Press, Oxford.

Harries, S., Garry, M. and Ratnalikar, V. (2008) Anaesthesia for Caesarean section, in Clyburn, P., Collis, R., Harries, S. and Davies, S. (eds) *Obstetric Anaesthesia*. Oxford University Press, Oxford.

Harris, T. (2004) Care in the third stage of labour, in Henderson, C. and MacDonald, S. (eds) *Mayes' Midwifery: A Textbook for Midwives*, 13th edn. Baillière Tindall, Edinburgh.

Harris, T., Cameron, P.A. and Ugoni, A. (2001) The use of pre-cannulation local anaesthetic and factors affecting pain perception in the emergency department setting. *Emerg Med Journal*, 18: 175–7.

Harsten, A., Gillberg, L., Hakansson, L. and Olsson, M. (1997) Intrathecal sufentanil compared with epidural bupivacaine analgesia in labour. *European Journal of Anaesthesiology*, 14: 642–5.

Hassain, A. and Ahsan, F. (2005) The vagina as a route for systemic drug delivery. *Journal of Controlled Release*, 103: 301–13.

Haste, F., Brooke, O., Anderson, H. and Bland, J. (1991) The effect of nutritional intake on outcome of pregnancy in smokers and non-smokers. *British Journal of Nutrition*, 65(3): 347–54.

Hauser, W.A., Annegers, J.F. and Rocca, W.A. (1996) Descriptive epidemiology of epilepsy: contributions of population-based studies from Rochester, Minnesota. *Mayo Clinic Proc*, 71: 5776–86.

Hawthorne, G., Robson, S., Ryall, E. et al. (1997) Prospective population based survey of outcome of pregnancy in diabetic women: results of the Northern Diabetic Pregnancy Audit (1994). *BMJ*, 315: 279–81.

Hayashi, R. (1990) The role of prostaglandin in the treatment of postpartum haemorrhage. *Journal of Obstetrics and Gynaecology*, 10(S2): 521–4.

Hayes, D., Hendler, C.B., Tscheschlog, B. et al. (eds) (2003) *Medication Administration Made Incredibly Easy*. Lippincott, Williams & Wilkins, Springhouse, PA.

HCC (Healthcare Commission) (2007a) *Talking about Medicines*. HCC, London.

HCC (Healthcare Commission) (2007b) *Improvements in Medicines Management*. HCC, London.

Heaton, D. and Pearce, M. (1995) Low molecular weight versus unfractionated heparin. *Pharmacoeconomics*, 8(2): 91–9.

Helbo-Hansen, H. (1995) Neonatal effects of maternally administered fentanyl, alfentanil and sufentanil, in Bogod, D. (ed.) *Baillière's Clinical Anaesthesiology: Obstetric Anaesthesia*. Baillière Tindall, London.

Helewa, M., Burrows, R, Smith, J. et al. (1997) Report of the Canadian Hypertension Society Consensus Conference, 1. Definitions, evaluation and classification of hypertensive disorders in pregnancy. *Canadian Medical Association Journal*, 157(6): 715–25.

Henderson, J.J., Dickinson, J.E., Evans, S.F. et al. (2003) Impact of intrapartum epidural analgesia on breast-feeding duration. *Aust N Z J Obstetrics Gynaecol*, 43: 372–7.

Hendrick, V. (2003) Treatment of postnatal depression: effective interventions are available, but the condition remains under diagnosed. *BMJ*, 327(7422): 1003–4.

Hendrick, V., Fukuchi, A., Altshuler, L. et al. (2001) Use of sertraline, paroxetine and fluvoxamine by nursing women. *British Journal of Psychiatry*, 179: 163–6.

Hengge, U.R., Ruzicka, T., Schwartz, R.A. and Cork, M.J. (2006) Adverse effects of topical glucocorticosteroids. *J American Acad Dermatol*, 54(1): 1–15.

Herman, N., Choi, K., Affleck, P. et al. (1999) Analgesia, pruritus, and ventilation exhibit a dose-response relationship in parturients receiving intrathecal fentanyl during labor. *Anesthesia and Analgesia*, 89: 378–83.

Herpolsheimer, A. and Schretenthaler, J. (1994) The use of intrapartum intrathecal narcotic analgesia in a community-based hospital. *Obstetrics and Gynaecology*, 84(6): 931–6.

Hess, P., Pratt, S., Soni, A. et al. (2000) An association between severe labor pain and cesarean delivery. *Anesthetic Analgesia*, 90: 881–6.

Hess, P.E., Pratt, S.D. and Oriol, N.E. (2006) An analysis of the need for anesthetic interventions with differing concentrations of labor epidural bupivacaine: an observational study. *International Journal of Obstetric Anesthesiology*, 15(3): 195–200.

Hibbard, B.M. (1988) *Principles of Obstetrics*. Butterworth, London.

Hibbard, E. and Smithells, R. (1965) Folic acid metabolism and human embryopathy. *Lancet*, 1: 1254–6.

Hijazi, R., Taylor, D. and Richardson, J. (2009) Effect of topical alkane vapocoolant spray on pain with intravenous cannulation in patients in emergency departments: randomised double blind placebo controlled trial. *BMJ*, 338: 457–60, b215. doi: 10.1136/bmj.b215.

Hildebrandt, H. (1999) Maternal perception of lactogenesis time: a clinical report. *Journal of Human Lactation*, 15(4): 317–23.

Hill, W.C. (1995) Risks and complications of tocolysis. *Clinical Obstetrics and Gynecology*, 38(4): 725–45.

Hillman, R. (1996) Hematopoietic agents, in Hardman, J., Limbard, L., Molinoff, P. et al. (eds) *Goodman & Gilman's: The Pharmacological Basis of Therapeutics*, 9th edn. McGraw-Hill, New York.

Hindmarsh, P., Geary, M., Rodeck, C. et al. (2000) Effect of early maternal iron stores on placental weight and structure. *Lancet*, 356: 719–23.

Hinshaw, K., Simpson, S., Cummings, S. et al. (2008) A randomised controlled trial of early versus delayed oxytocin augmentation to treat primary dysfunctional labour in nulliparous women. *BJOG*, 115(10): 1289–95.

Hirsch, I. (2005) Insulin analogues. *New England Journal of Medicine*, 352(2): 174–83.

Hirst, J., Chibbar, R and Mitchell, B. (1993) Role of oxytocin in the regulation of uterine activity during pregnancy and in the initiation of labor. *Seminars in Reproductive Endocrinology*, 11: 219–23.

Hoffman, B.B. (2006) Therapy of hypertension, in Brunton, L., Lazo, J. and Parker, K. (eds) *Goodman & Gilman's: The Pharmacological Basis of Therapeutics*, 11th edn. McGraw-Hill, New York.

Hofmeyr, G. (1995) Prophylactic intravenous preloading before epidural anaesthesia in labour. *Cochrane Pregnancy and Childbirth Database*, Issue 2. Update Software, Oxford.

Hofmeyr, G. and Gulmezoglu, A. (2000) Vaginal misoprostol for cervical ripening and labour induction in late pregnancy. *Cochrane Pregnancy and Childbirth Database*, Issue 2. Update Software, Oxford.

Hofmeyr, G., Gulmezoglu, A. and Alfirevic, Z. (2000) Misoprostol for induction of labour at term (letter). *British Journal of Obstetrics and Gynaecology*, 107: 576.

Holford, N. (2001) Pharmacokinetics and pharmacodynamics, in Katzung, B. (ed.) *Basic and Clinical Pharmacology*, 8th edn. McGraw-Hill, New York.

Holgate, S. (1997) The cellular and mediator basis of asthma in relation to natural history. *Lancet*, 350(s2): 5–9.

Hollander, J. (1995) The management of cocaine-associated myocardial ischaemia. *New England Journal of Medicine*, 333(19): 1267–72.

Holleboom, C., Merkus, J., van Elfereen, L. and Keirse, M. (1996) Randomised comparison between a loading and incremental dose model for ritodrine administration in preterm labour. *British Journal of Obstetrics and Gynaecology*, 103: 695–701.

Hollmen, A. (1993) The effects of regional anaesthesia on utero and fetoplacental blood flow, in Reynolds, F. (ed.) *Effects on the Baby of Maternal Analgesia and Anaesthesia*. Saunders, London.

Holmér Pettersson, P., Jakobsson, J. and Owall A. (2006) Plasma concentrations following repeated rectal or intravenous administration of paracetamol after heart surgery. *Acta Anaesthesiol Scand*, 50(6): 673–7.

Holmes, L.B., Harvey, E.A., Coull, B.A. et al. (2001) The teratogenicity of anticonvulsant drugs. *N Engl J Med*, 344: 1132–8.

Hoogerwerf, W. and Pasricha, S. (2006) Pharmacotherapy of gastric acidity, in Brunton L., Lazo, J. and Parke, K. (eds) *Goodman & Gilman's: The Pharmacological Basis of Therapeutics*, 11th edn. McGraw-Hill, New York.

Hopkinson, H. (1995) Treatment of cardiovascular diseases, in Rubin, P. (ed.) *Prescribing in Pregnancy*, 2nd edn. BMJ Group, London.

Howden, C. (1995) Treatment of common minor ailments, in Rubin, P. (ed.) *Prescribing in Pregnancy*, 2nd edn. BMJ Group, London.

Howe, G.M. (1972) *Man, Environment and Disease in Britain*. Penguin, Harmondsworth.

Howell, C. and Chalmers, I. (1992) A review of prospectively controlled comparisons of epidural with non-epidural forms of pain relief during labour. *International Journal of Obstetric Anesthesia*, 1: 93–110.

Howell, C.J. (1994) Systemic narcotics for analgesia in labour *Cochrane Database of Systemic Reviews*, 03398. Update Software, Oxford.

Howell, C.J. (1995a) Epidural top-ups on maternal request vs scheduled top-ups. *Cochrane Pregnancy and Childbirth Database*, Issue 2. Update Software, Oxford.

Howell, C.J. (1995b) Prophylactic blood patch for dural puncture. *Cochrane Pregnancy and Childbirth Database*, Issue 2. Update Software, Oxford.

Howell, C.J. (1995c) Epidural vs non-epidural analgesia in labour. *Cochrane Pregnancy and Childbirth Database*, Issue 2. Update Software, Oxford.

Howell, C.J., Dean, T., Lucking, L. et al. (2002) Randomised study of long-term outcome after epidural versus non-epidural analgesia during labour. *BMJ*, 325(7360): 357.

Howell, C.J., Kidd, C., Roberts, W. et al. (2001) A randomised controlled trial of epidural compared with non-epidural analgesia in labour. *BJOG*, 108(1): 27–33.

Hughes, S. (1992) Analgesia methods during labour and delivery. *Canadian Journal of Anaesthesia*, 39(5): R18–23.

Huizink, A.C. and Mulder, E.J. (2006) Maternal smoking, drinking or cannabis use during pregnancy and neurobehavioral and cognitive functioning in human offspring. *Neurosci Biobehav Rev*, 30(1): 24–41.

Hunt, R.W., Tzioumi, D., Collins, E. and Jeffery, H.E. (2008) Adverse neurodevelopmental outcome of infants exposed to opiate in-utero. *Early Hum Dev*, 84(1): 29–35.

IASP Subcommittee on Taxonomy (1986) Classification of chronic pain. *Pain Supplement*, 3: 216–21.

ICH (International Conference on Harmonisation) (1996) *ICH Harmonised Tripartite Guideline for Good Clinical Practice*. Institute of Clinical Research, Marlow.

Idama, T. and Lindow, S. (1998) Magnesium sulphate: a review of clinical pharmacology applied to obstetrics. *British Journal of Obstetrics and Gynaecology*, 105: 260–8.

ILCOR (International Liaison Committee on Resuscitation) (2006) Consensus on science with treatment recommendations for pediatric and neonatal patients: pediatric basic and advanced life support. *Pediatrics*, 117(5): e955–77.

ILCR (International Liaison Committee on Resuscitation) (2006) Consensus on science with treatment recommendations for pediatric and neonatal patients: neonatal resuscitation. *Pediatrics*, 117(5): e978–88.

Irestedt, L., Ekblom, A., Olofsson, C. et al. (1998) Pharmacokinetics and clinical effect during continuous epidural infusion with ropivacaine 2.5 mg/ml or bupivacaine 2.5 mg/ml for labour pain relief. *Acta Anaesthesiologica Scandinavia*, 42(8): 890–6.

Isarangkura, P., Shearer, M.J., Pindit, P. et al. (1994) Vitamin K (Konakion MM) by oral route in the prevention of the haemorrhagic disease of the newborn and idiopathic vitamin K deficiency in infants. International Symposium Vitamin K in Infancy, 7–8 October, Basel, Switzerland.

Jadad, A., Sigouin, C., Mohide, P. et al. (2000) Risk of congenital malformations associated with treatment of asthma during early pregnancy. *Lancet*, 355: 119.

James, L., Barnes, T.R., Lelliott P. et al. (2007) Informing patients of the teratogenic potential of mood stabilizing drugs: a case note review of the practice of psychiatrists. *J Psychopharmacol*, 21(8): 815–19.

Jansson, L.M., Choo, R. and Velez, M.L. et al. (2008) Methadone maintenance and breastfeeding in the neonatal period. *Pediatrics*, 121(1): 106–14.

Jansson, L.M., Dipietro, J. and Elko, A. (2005) Fetal response to maternal methadone administration. *American J Obstetrics Gynecol*, 193(3 Pt 1): 611–17.

Jarrett, R. (1997) Should we screen for gestational diabetes? *BMJ*, 315: 736–7.

Jenkins, C., Costello, J. and Hodge, L. (2004) Systematic review of prevalence of aspirin induced asthma and its implications for clinical practice. *BMJ*, 328(7437): 434.

Jevon, P. and Ewens, B. (2002) *Monitoring the Critically Ill Patient*. Blackwell Science, Oxford.

Jewell, D. and Young, G. (2000) Interventions for nausea and vomiting in early pregnancy. *Cochrane Database Systematic Review* (issue 2). Update Software, Oxford.

Jonas, W., Nissen, E., Ransjö-Arvidson, A.B. et al. (2008) Influence of oxytocin or epidural analgesia on personality profile in breastfeeding women: a comparative study. *Arch Womens Ment Health*, 11(5/6): 334–45.

Jones, M.L., Wray, J. and Wight, J. (2004) A review of the clinical effectiveness of routine antenatal anti-D prophylaxis for rhesus-negative women who are pregnant. *BJOG*, 111(9): 892–902.

Jordan, S. (1998) From classroom theory to clinical practice: evaluating the impact of a post-registration course. *Nurse Education Today*, 18: 293–302.

Jordan, S. (2002) Managing adverse drug reactions: an orphan task. Developing nurse-administered evaluation checklists. *Journal of Advanced Nursing*, 38(5): 437–48.

Jordan, S. (2006) Infant feeding and analgesia in labour: the evidence is accumulating. *International Breastfeeding Journal Research*, 1: 25; doi: 10.1186/1746-4358-1-25.

Jordan, S. (2007) Adverse drug reactions: reducing the burden of treatment. *Nursing Standard*, 21(34): 35–41.

Jordan, S. (2008) *The Prescription Drug Guide for Nurses*. Open University Press/McGraw-Hill, Maidenhead.

Jordan, S. (2009) Medication errors in an intensive care unit: systems, pressures and prioritising. *Journal of Advanced Nursing*, 16(10): 2258–9.

Jordan, S. and Segrott, J. (2008) Evidence based practice: the debate (editorial). *Journal of Nursing Management*, 16(4): 385–7.

Jordan, S. and Tait, M. (1999) Antibiotic therapy. *Nursing Standard*, 13(45): 49–54.

Jordan, S. and Torrance, C. (1995) Bionursing: explaining falls in elderly people. *Nursing Standard*, 9(50): 30–2.

Jordan, S. and White, J. (2001) Bronchodilators: implications for nursing practice. *Nursing Standard*, 15: 45–52.

Jordan, S., Emery, S., Bradshaw, C. et al. (2005) The impact of intrapartum analgesia on infant feeding. *BJOG*, 112: 927–34.

Jordan, S., Jones, R. and Sargeant, M. (2009a) Adverse drug reactions: managing the risk. *Journal of Nursing Management*, 17: 175–84.

Jordan, S., Emery, S., Watkins, A. et al. (2009b) Associations of drugs routinely given in labour with breastfeeding at 48 hours: analysis of the Cardiff Births Survey. *BJOG*, 116(12): 1622–9.

Jordan, S., Knight, J. and Pointon, D. (2004) Monitoring adverse drug reactions: scales, profiles and checklists. *International Nursing Review*, 51: 208–21.

Jordan, S., Storey, M. and Morgan, G. (2008) Antibiotics and allergic disorders in childhood. *Open Nursing Journal*, 2: 48–57.

Jordan, S., Tunnicliffe C. and Sykes, A. (2002) Minimising side effects: the clinical impact of nurse-administered 'side effect' checklists. *Journal of Advanced Nursing*, 37(2): 155–65.

Jorgensen, J., Romsing, J., Rasmussen, M. et al. (1996) Pain assessment of subcutaneous injections. *Annals of Pharmacotherapy*, 30: 729–32.

JSC (Joint Specialty Committee on Renal Medicine of the Royal College of Physicians of London and the Renal Association) (2006) *Chronic Kidney Disease in Adults: UK Guidelines for Identification, Management and Referral*. Royal College of Physicians, London.

Kakko, J., Heilig, M. and Sarman, I. (2008) Buprenorphine and methadone treatment of opiate dependence during pregnancy: comparison of fetal growth and neonatal outcomes in two consecutive case series. *Drug Alcohol Depend*, 96(1/2): 69–78.

Kalant, H. (2007a) Opioid analgesics and antagonists, in Kalant, H., Grant, D. and Mitchell, J. (eds) *Principles of Medical Pharmacology*, 7th edn. Saunders, Toronto.

Kalant, H. (2007b) Hallucinogens and psychomimetics, in Kalant, H., Grant, D. and Mitchell, J. (eds) *Principles of Medical Pharmacology*, 7th edn. Saunders, Toronto.

Källén, B. (2004a) Use of folic acid supplementation and risk for dizygotic twinning. *Early Human Development*, 80(2): 143–51. Erratum in: *Early Hum Dev*, 2005, 81(5): 471.

Källén, B. (2004b) Neonate characteristics after maternal use of antidepressants in late pregnancy. *Archives of Pediatric and Adolescent Medicine*, 158: 312–16.

Källén, B. (2007) The safety of anti-depressant drugs during pregnancy. *Expert Opinion on Drug Safety*, 6(4): 357–70.

Källén, B. and Mottet, I. (2003) Delivery outcome after the use of meclozine in early pregnancy. *European Journal Epidemiol*, 18(7): 665–9.

Kametas, N. and Nelson-Piercy, C. (2007) Hyperemesis gravidarum, gastrointestinal and liver disease in pregnancy. *Obstetrics, Gynecology and Reproductive Medicine*, 18(3): 69–75.

Kan, R. and Hughes, S. (1995) Recent developments in analgesia during labour. *Drugs*, 50: 417–22.

Karemaker, R., Kavelaars, A., ter Wolbeek M. et al. (2008) Neonatal dexamethasone treatment for chronic lung disease of prematurity alters the hypothalamus-pituitary-adrenal axis and immune system activity at school age. *Pediatrics*, 121(4): e870–8.

Katz, P. and Castell, D. (1998) Gastroesophageal reflux disease during pregnancy. *Gastroenterology Clinics of North America*, 27(1): 153–67.

Katz, V., Farmer, R. and Kuller, J. (2000) Pre-eclampsia into eclampsia: toward a new paradigm. *American Journal of Obstetrics*, 182: 1389–96.

Kawabata, K.M. (1996) Two cases of asthmatic attack caused by spinal anaesthesia. *Masui*, 45(1): 102–6.

Kelly, A.J., Kavanagh, J. and Thomas, J. (2003) Vaginal prostaglandin (PGE2 and PGF2a) for induction of labour at term. *Cochrane Database of Systematic Reviews*, Issue 4. Art. No.: CD003101. DOI: 10.1002/14651858.CD003101.

Kelsey, J. and Prevost, R. (1994) Drug therapy during labour and delivery. *American Journal of Hospital Pharmacy*, 51: 2394–402.

Kendell, R., McInneny, K., Juszczak, E. and Bain, M. (2000) Obstetric complications and schizophrenia. *British Journal of Psychiatry*, 176: 516–22.

Kennedy, S. and Longnecker, D. (1996) History and principles of anaesthesiology, in Hardman, J., Limbird, L., Molinoff, P. et al. (eds) *The Pharmacological Basis of Therapeutics*, 9th edn. McGraw Hill, New York.

Kenyon, S., Boulvain, M. and Neilson, J.P. (2003) Antibiotics for preterm rupture of membranes. *Cochrane Database of Systematic Reviews*, Issue 2. Art. No.: CD001058. DOI: 10.1002/14651858.CD001058.

Khan, G., John, I., Chan, T. et al. (1995) Abu Dhabi third stage trial. *European Journal of Obstetrics and Gynecology*, 58: 147–51.

Khan, K. and Chien, P. (1997) Seizure prophylaxis in hypertensive pregnancies: a framework for making clinical decisions. *British Journal of Obstetrics and Gynaecology*, 104: 1173–9.

King, J., Flenady, V., Cole, S. and Thornton, S. (2005) Cyclo-oxygenase (COX) inhibitors for treating preterm labour. *Cochrane Database of Systematic Reviews*, Issue 2. Art. No.: CD001992. DOI: 10.1002/14651858.CD001992.pub2.

King, J., Flenady, V.J., Papatsonis, D.N. et al. (2003) Calcium channel blockers for inhibiting preterm labour. *Cochrane Database of Systematic Reviews*, Issue 1. Art. No.: CD002255. DOI: 10.1002/14651858.CD002255.

Kinsley, B. (2007) Achieving better outcomes in pregnancies complicated by type 1 and type 2 diabetes mellitus. *Clinical Therapeutics*, 29(Suppl D): S153–60.

Klein, M.C. (2006) Does epidural analgesia increase rate of Cesarean section? *Canadian Family Physician*, 52(4): 419–21, 426–8.

Klinger, G. and Koren, G. (2000) Controversies in antenatal corticosteroid treatment. *Canadian Family Physician*, 46: 1571–3.

Klingman, W.O. (1954) The effect of ion exchange resins in the paroxysmal disorders of the nervous system. *American Journal of Psychiatry*, 111: 184–95.

Knight, M. on behalf of UKOSS (2008) Antenatal pulmonary embolism: risk factors, management and outcomes. *BJOG*, 115: 453–61.

Knight, M., Duley, L., Henderson-Smart, D. and King, J. (2000) Antiplatelet agents for preventing and treating pre-eclampsia. *Cochrane Pregnancy and Childbirth Database*, Issue 2. Update Software, Oxford.

Knox, T. and Olans, L. (1996) Liver disease in pregnancy. *New England Journal of Medicine*, 335(8): 569–76.

Koehntop, D., Rodman, J., Brundage, D. et al. (1986) Pharmacokinetics of fentanyl in neonates. *Anesthetic Analgesia*, 65: 227–32.

Koelewijn, J.M., de Haas, M., Vrijkotte, T.G. et al. (2009) Risk factors for RhD immunisation despite antenatal and postnatal anti-D prophylaxis. *BJOG*, Jun 17. Epub ahead of print, PMID: 19538414.

Köksal, N., Aktürk, B., Saglam, H. et al. (2008) Reference values for neonatal thyroid volumes in a moderately iodine-deficient area. *J Endocrinol Invest*, 31(7): 642–6.

Koopmans, C.M., Bijlenga, D., Groen, H. et al. for the HYPITAT study group (2009) Induction of labour versus expectant monitoring for gestational hypertension or mild pre-eclampsia after 36 weeks' gestation (HYPITAT): a multicentre, open-label randomised controlled trial. *Lancet*, DOI:10.1016/S0140-6736(09)60736-4.

Korytkowski, M., Bell. D., Jacobsen, C., Suwannasari, R. for the FlexPen Study Team (2003) A multicenter, randomized open-label, comparative, two-period crossover trial of preference, efficacy and safety profile of a prefilled disposable pen and conventional vial/syringe for insulin injections in patients with type 1 or 2 diabetes mellitus. *Clinical Therapeutics*, 25: 2836–48.

Koscielniak-Nielsen, Z., Hesselbjerg, L., Brushoj, J. et al. (1998) Use of EMLA cream for topical analgesia prior to spinal puncture. *Anaesthesia*, 53: 1218–22.

Kotaska, A., Klein, M. and Liston, R. (2006) Epidural analgesia associated with low-dose oxytocin augmentation increases cesarean births: a critical look at the external validity of randomized trials. *American Journal of Obstetrics & Gyncology*, 194: 809–14.

Kothari, A. and Girling, J. (2008) Hypothyroidism in pregnancy: pre-pregnancy thyroid status influences gestational thyroxine requirements. *BJOG*, 115(13): 1704–8.

Kramer, M., Coates, A., Michoud, M. et al. (1995) Maternal asthma and idiopathic preterm labor. *American Journal of Epidemiology*, 142(10): 1078–88.

Kuczkowski, K.M. (2004) The cocaine abusing parturient: a review of anesthetic considerations. *Can J Anaesth*, 51(2): 145–54.

Kuczkowski, K.M. (2005) Labor analgesia for the tobacco and ethanol abusing pregnant patient: a routine management? *Arch Gynecol Obstetrics*, 271(1): 6–10.

Kuhnert, B. (1993) Human perinatal pharmacology: recent controversies, in Reynolds, F. (ed.) *Effects on the Baby of Maternal Analgesia and Anaesthesia*. Saunders, London.

Kulb, N. (1990) Oxytocin induction/augmentation of labor, in Buckley, K. and Kulb, N. (eds) *High Risk Maternity Nursing Manual*. Williams & Wilkins, Baltimore.

Kumar, S. and Regan, F. (2005) Management of pregnancies with RhD alloimmunisation. *BMJ*, 330(7502): 1255–8.

Kuoppala, T. (1988) Alterations in vitamin D metabolites and minerals in diabetic pregnancy. *Gynecologic and Obstetric Investigation*, 25: 99–105.

Kyle, P., Fielder, J., Pullar, B. et al. (2008) Comparison of methods to identify significant proteinuria in pregnancy in the outpatient setting. *BJOG*, 115: 523–7.

Lack, G. (2008a) Food allergy. *New England Journal of Medicine*, 359(12): 1252–60.

Lack, G. (2008b) Epidemiologic risks for food allergy. *Journal of Allergy and Clinical Immunology*, 121: 1331–6.

Laegreid, L. (1990) Clinical observations in children after prenatal benzodiazepine exposure. *Dev Pharmacol Ther*, 15(3/4): 186–8.

Lake, R. and Jordan, S. (2005) Prescription drugs: uses and effects: anticoagulants. *Nursing Standard*, 19(19): S1–2.

Lalloo, D.G., Shingadia, D., Pasvol, G. et al. (2007) UK malaria treatment guidelines. *Journal of Infection*, 54: 111–21.

Lamont, R. (2000) The pathophysiology of pulmonary oedema with the use of beta-agonists. *British Journal of Obstetrics and Gynaecology*, 107: 439–44.

Lamont, R., Mason, R. and Adinkra, P. (2001) Advances in the use of antibiotics in the prevention of preterm birth, in Bonnar, J. (ed.) *Recent Advances in Obstetrics and Gynaecology 21*. Churchill Livingstone, Edinburgh.

Lander, C.M., Edwards, V.E., Eadie, M.J. and Tyrer, J.H. (1977) Plasma anticonvulsant concentrations during pregnancy. *Neurology*, 27: 128–31.

Lane, P.A. and Hathaway, W.E. (1985) Vitamin K in infancy. *J Pediatr*, 106(3): 351–9.

Larimore, W. and Cline, M. (2000) Keeping normal labor normal. *Primary Care*, 27: 221–36.

Laskin, C., Bombardier, C., Hannah, M. et al. (1997) Prednisone and aspirin in women with autoantibodies and unexplained recurrent fetal loss. *New England Journal of Medicine*, 337: 148–53.

Lattimore, K., Donn, S., Kaciroti, N. et al. (2005) Selective serotonin reuptake inhibitor (SSRI) use during pregnancy and effects on the fetus and neonate. *Journal of Perinatology*, 25: 595–604.

Laurberg, P., Nøhr, S.B., Pedersen, K.M. and Fuglsang, E. (2004) Iodine nutrition in breast-fed infants is impaired by maternal smoking. *J Clin Endocrinol Metab*, 89(1): 181–7.

Laurence, KM., James, N., Miller, M. et al. (1981) Double-blind randomised controlled trial of folate treatment before conception to prevent recurrence of neural-tube defects. *BMJ*, 282: 1509–11.

Lauszus, F., Klebe, J. and Bek, T. (2000) Diabetic retinopathy in pregnancy during tight metabolic control. *Acta Obstetrica Gynecologica*, 79: 367–70.

Lawrence, R. and Schaefer, C. (2007) General commentary on drug therapy and drug risk during lactation, in Schaefer, C., Peters, P.W. and Miller, R.K. (eds) *Drugs during Pregnancy and Lactation: Treatment Options and Risk Assessment*, 2nd edn. Elsevier, Oxford.

Le Coq, G., Ducot, B. and Benhamou, D. (1998) Risk factors of inadequate pain relief during epidural analgesia for labour and delivery. *Canadian Journal of Anaesthesia*, 45(8): 719–23.

Lee, A. and McManus, P. (1995) Psychiatric and neurological disorders: part 2. *The Pharmaceutical Journal*, 254: 118–21.

Lee, M.-J., Davies, J., Guinn, D. et al. (2004) Single versus weekly courses of antenatal corticosteroids in preterm premature rupture of membranes. *American College of Obstetricians and Gynecologists*, 103(2): 274–81.

Leighton, B. and Halpern, S. (2002) Epidural analgesia: effects on labor progress and maternal and neonatal outcomes. *Seminars in Perinatology*, 26(2): 122–35.

Leng, G., Caquineau, C. and Sabatier, N. (2005) Regulation of oxytocin secretion. *Vitam Horm*, 71: 27–58.

Leng, G., Meddle, S.L. and Douglas, A.J. (2008) Oxytocin and the maternal brain. *Current Opinion in Pharmacology*, 8(6): 731–4.

Lensing, A., Prandoni, P., Prins, M. and Buller, H. (1999) Deep-vein thrombosis. *Lancet*, 353: 479–85.

Letsky, E.A. and Warwick, R. (1994) Haematological problems, in James, D.K., Steer, PT, Weiner, C.P. and Gonik, B. (eds) *High Risk Pregnancy: Management Options*. W.B. Saunders, Philadelphia.

Leung, G., Lam, T. and Ho, L. (2002) Breast-feeding and its relation to smoking and mode of delivery. *Obstetrics and Gynecology*, 99: 785–94.

Levey, A., Bosch, J., Lewis, J. et al. (1999) A more accurate method to estimate glomerular filtration rate from serum creatinine: a new prediction equation. *Annals of Internal Medicine*, 130: 461–70.

Levine, R., Hauth, J. Curet, L. et al. (1997) Trial of calcium to prevent pre-eclampsia. *New England Journal of Medicine*, 337: 69–76.

Levy, J., Montes, F., Szalam, F. and Hillyer, C. (2000) The in vitro effects of antithrombin III on the activated coagulation time in patients on heparin therapy. *Anesthetic Analgesia*, 90(5): 1076–9.

Lewis, B.A., Kirchner, H.L., Short, E.J. et al. (2007) Prenatal cocaine and tobacco effects on children's language trajectories. *Pediatrics*, 120(1): e78–85.

Li, Z., Gindler, J., Wang, H. et al. (2003) Folic acid supplements during early pregnancy and likelihood of multiple births: a population-based cohort study. *Lancet*, 361: 380–4.

Lieberman, E. and O'Donoghue, C. (2002) Unintended effects of epidural analgesia during labor: a systematic review. *American J Obstetrics Gynecol*, 186: S31–68.

Lieberman, E., Lang, J., Richardson, D. et al. (2000) Intrapartum maternal fever and neonatal outcomes. *Pediatrics*, 105(1): 8–13.

Liljestrand, J. (1999) Reducing perinatal and maternal mortality in the world: the major challenges. *British Journal of Obstetrics and Gynaecology*, 106: 877–80.

Lilley, L.L., Aucker, A.S. and Albanese, J.A. (1996) *Pharmacology and the Nursing Process*. Mosby, St Louis, MO.

Lima, F., Khamashta, M., Buchanan, N. et al. (1996) A study of sixty pregnancies in patients with the anti-phospholipid syndrome. *Clinical and Experimental Rheumatology*, 14(2): 131–6.

Lindhoff-Last, E., Willeke, A., Thalhammer, C. et al. (2000) Hirudin treatment in a breastfeeding woman. *Lancet*, 355: 467–8.

Lindow, S., Dhillon, A., Husaini, S. and Russell, I. (2004) A randomised double-blind comparison of epidural fentanyl versus fentanyl and bupivicaine for pain relief in the second stage of labour. *BJOG*, 111: 1075–80.

Lindow, S., Hendricks, M., Nugest, F. et al. (1999) Morphine suppresses the oxytocin response in breastfeeding women. *Gynecol Obstetrics Invest*, 48(1): 33–7.

Lipka, K. and Burlow, H. (2003) Lactic acidosis following convulsions. *Acta Anaesthesiol Scand*, 47: 616–18.

Lipkin, G. (1993) Drug therapy in maternal care, in Spencer, R.T., Nicolls, L., Lipkin, G. et al. (eds) *Clinical Pharmacology and Nursing Management*, 4th edn. Lippincott, Philadelphia.

Lister, S. (2004) Drug administration: general principles, in Dougherty, L. and Lister, S. (eds) *The Royal Marsden Hospital Manual of Clinical Nursing Procedures*, 6th edn. Blackwell Science, Oxford.

Little, R., Kirkman, E., Driscoll, P. et al. (1995) Preventable deaths after injury: why are the traditional 'vital' signs poor indicators of blood loss? *Journal of Accident and Emergency Medicine*, 12: 1–14.

Lockwood, C.J. (1997) Calcium-channel blockers in the management of preterm labour. *Lancet*, 350: 1339–40.

Loeb, S., Holmes, N.H., Charnow, J. et al. (1993) *Clinical Skill-builders: Medication Administration and IV Therapy Manual*, 2nd edn. Springhouse, Springhouse, PA.

Loeser, J. and Melzack, R. (1999) Pain: an overview. *Lancet*, 353: 1607–9.

Loftus, J., Hill, H. and Cohen, S. (1995) Placental transfer and neonatal effects of epidural sufentanil and fentanyl administered with bupivacaine during labour. *Anaesthesiology*, 83: 300–8.

Long, P. (1995) Rethinking iron supplementation during pregnancy. *Journal of Nurse-Midwifery*, 40(1): 36–40.

Loose, D. and Stancel, G. (2006) Estrogens and progestins, in Brunton, L., Lazo J. and Parker, K. (eds) *Goodman & Gilman's: The Pharmacological Basis of Therapeutics*, 11th edn. McGraw-Hill, New York.

Loudon, J. (1995) Psychotropic drugs, in Rubin, P. (ed.) *Prescribing in Pregnancy.* BMJ Publishing, London.

Lu, J. and Nightingale, C. (2000) Magnesium sulfate in eclampsia and pre-eclampsia: pharmacokinetic principles. *Clinical Pharmacokinetics*, 38: 305–15.

Lumbiganon, P. and Laopaiboon, M. (2008) Monitoring in pre-eclampsia, in Glasziou, P., Irwig, L. and Aronson, J.K. (eds) *Evidence-based Medical Monitoring*. Blackwell Publishing/BMJ Books, Oxford.

Lumbiganon, P., Hofmeyr, J., Gulmezoglu, A. et al. (1999) Misoprostol dose-related shivering and pyrexia in the third stage of labour. *British Journal of Obstetrics and Gynaecology*, 106: 304–8.

Lumbiganon, P., Villar, J., Piaggio, G. et al. (2002) Side effects of oral misoprostol during the first 24 hours after administration in the third stage of labour. *BJOG*, 109: 1222–6.

Luppi, P. (2003) How immune mechanisms are affected by pregnancy. *Vaccine*, 21(24): 3352–7.

Lutomski, D., Bottorff, M. and Sangha, K. (1995) Pharmacokinetic optimisation of the treatment of embolic disorders. *Clinical Pharmacokinetics*, 28(1): 67–92.

Lyons, G., Columb, M., Hawthorne, L. and Dresner, M. (1997) Extradural pain relief in labour: bupivacaine sparing by extradural fentanyl is dose dependent. *British Journal of Anaesthesia*, 78: 493–7.

Macara, L.M. (2008) Identifying fetal abnormalities, in Rubin, P. and Ramsay, M. (eds) *Prescribing in Pregnancy*, 4th edn. BMJ Group, London.

MacArthur, C., Lewis, M., Knox, E.G. and Crawford, J.S. (1990) Epidural analgesia and long term backache after childbirth. *BMJ*, 301: 9–12.

McAtamney, D., O'Hare, R., Hughes, D. et al. (1998) Evaluation of remifentanil for control of haemodynamic response to tracheal intubation. *Anaesthesia*, 53(12): 1223–7.

McBride, W.G. (1969) An aetiological study of drug ingestion by women who gave birth to babies with cleft palate. *Austalian and New Zealand Journal of Obstetrics and Gynaecology*, 9(2): 103–4.

McCartney, D. (1995) Constipation. *Update*, May 5: 597–8.

McCowan, L., Buist, R., North, R. and Gamble, G. (1996) Perinatal morbidity in chronic hypertension. *British Journal of Obstetrics and Gynaecology*, 103: 123–9.

McCrae, A.F., Jozwiak, H. and McClure, J.H. (1995) Comparison of ropivacaine and bupivacaine in extradural analgesia for the relief of pain in labour. *British Journal of Anaesthesia*, 74(3): 261–5.

McDonagh, M.S., Osterweil, P. and Guise, J.M. (2005) The benefits and risks of inducing labour in patients with prior caesarean delivery: a systematic review. *BJOG*, 112(8): 1007–15.

McDonald, H.M., Brocklehurst, P. and Gordon, A. (2007) Antibiotics for treating bacterial vaginosis in pregnancy. *Cochrane Database of Systematic Reviews*, Issue 1. Art. No.: CD000262. DOI: 10.1002/14651858.CD000262.pub3.

McDonald, S., Prendiville, W. and Blair, E. (1993) Randomised trial of oxytocin alone versus oxytocin and ergometrine in active management of third stage of labour. *BMJ*, 307: 1167–71.

McDonald, S.J., Abbott, J.M. and Higgins, S.P. (2004) Prophylactic ergometrine-oxytocin versus oxytocin for the third stage of labour. *Cochrane Database of Systematic Reviews*, Issue 1. Art. No.: CD000201. DOI: 10.1002/14651858. CD000201.pub2.

McEwan, A. (2007) Induction of labour. *Obstetrics, Gynaecology and Reproductive Medicine*, 18(1): 1–6.

McFadden, E.R. (1991) Asthma, in Wilson, J., Braunwald, E., Isselbacher, K. et al. *Harrison's Principles of Internal Medicine*, 12th edn. McGraw-Hill, New York.

Macfarlane, A., Gissler, M., Bolumnar, F. and Rasmussen, S. (2003) The availability of perinatal health indicators in Europe. *European Journal of Obstetrics and Gynecology and Reproductive Biology*, 111: S15–32.

MacKay, H.T. and Evans, A. (1995) Gynecology and obstetrics, in Tierney, L., McPhee, S. and Papadakis, M. (eds) *Current Medical Diagnosis and Treatment*. Appleton & Lange, Norwalk, CT.

McKenry, L. and Salerno, E. (1995) *Pharmacology in Nursing*, 19th edn. Mosby, St Louis, MO.

McKenry, L. and Salerno, E. (2003) *Pharmacology in Nursing*, 21st edn. Elsevier, Mosby, St Louis, MO.

McKenry, L., Tessier, E. and Hogan, M. (2006) *Mosby's Pharmacology in Nursing*, 22nd edn. Elsevier Mosby, St Louis, MO.

McLaughlin, J. and Thompson, D. (1995) Drugs for the treatment of nausea and vertigo. *Prescriber*, 6(9): 31–8.

McNamara, J.O. (2006) Pharmacotherapy of the epilepsies, in Brunton, L., Lazo, J. and Parker, K. (eds) *Goodman & Gilman's: The Pharmacological Basis of Therapeutics*, 11th edn. McGraw-Hill, New York.

McNinch, A. and Tripp, J. (1991) Haemorrhagic disease of the newborn in the British Isles; two year prospective study. *BMJ*, 303: 1105–9.

McNinch, A., Upton, C., Samuels, M. et al. (1985) Plasma concentrations after oral and intramuscular vitamin K1 in neonates. *Archives of Disease in Childhood*, 60: 814–18.

McQuaid, K. (1995) Alimentary tract, in Tierney, L., McPhee, S. and Papadakis, M. (eds) *Current Medical Diagnosis and Treatment*. Appleton & Lange, Norwalk, CT.

McRae-Bergeron, C., Andrews, C. and Lupe, P. (1998) The effect of epidural analgesia on the second stage of labor. *American Association of Nurse Anaesthetists Journal*, 66(2): 177–82.

Magann, E.F., Evans, S., Hutchinson, M. et al. (2005) Postpartum hemorrhage after vaginal birth: an analysis of risk factors. *Southern Medical Journal*, 98(4): 419–22.

Magee, L. and Koren, G. (2007) Perinatal Pharmacology, in Kalant, H., Grant, D. and Mitchell, J. (eds) *Principles of Medical Pharmacology*, 7th edn. Elsevier, Toronto.

Magee, L., Ornstein, M. and Dadelszen, P. (1999) Management of hypertension in pregnancy. *BMJ*, 318: 1332–6.

Maggioni, A., Franzosi, M. and Latini, R. (2008) Beta-adrenoceptor antagonists and antianginal drugs, in Aronson JK (ed.) *Side Effects of Drug Annual* 30. Elsevier, Amsterdam.

Magpie Trial Collaborative Group (2002) Do women with pre-eclampsia, and their babies, benefit from magnesium sulphate? The Magpie Trial: a randomised placebo-controlled trial. *Lancet*, 359: 1877–90.

Magpie Trial Follow-Up Study Collaborative Group (2007a) The Magpie Trial: a randomised trial comparing magnesium sulphate with placebo for pre-eclampsia: outcome for children at 18 months. *BJOG*, 114(3): 289–99.

Magpie Trial Follow-Up Study Collaborative Group (2007b) The Magpie Trial: a randomised trial comparing magnesium sulphate with placebo for pre-eclampsia: outcome for women at 2 years. *BJOG*, 114(3): 300–9.

Mahadevan, U. (2007) Gastrointestinal medications in pregnancy. *Best Practice & Research Clinical Gastroenterology*, 21(5): 849–77.

Mahadevan, U. and Kane, S. (2006) Use of gastrointestinal medications in pregnancy. *Gastroenterology*, 131(1): 278–82.

Mahmood, K. (2000) Zinc supplementation in pregnancy. *Cochrane Pregnancy and Childbirth Database*, Issue 2. Update Software, Oxford.

Mahmood, T., Rayner, A., Smith, N. and Beat, I. (1995) A randomized prospective trial comparing single dose prostaglandin E2 vaginal gel with forewater amniotomy for induction of labour. *European Journal of Obstetrics and Gynecology and Reproductive Biology*, 58: 111–17.

Majerus, P. and Tollefsen, D. (2006) Blood coagulation and anticoagulant, thrombolytic and anti-platelet drugs, in Brunton, L., Lazo, J. and Parker, K. (eds) *Goodman & Gilman's: The Pharmacological Basis of Therapeutics*, 11th edn, McGraw-Hill, New York.

Majkowska-Wojciechowska, B., Pelka, J., Korzon, L. et al. (2007) Prevalence of allergy, patterns of allergic sensitization and allergy risk factors in rural and urban children. *Allergy*, 62(9): 1044–50.

Makrides, M. and Crowther, C. (2000) Magnesium supplementation in pregnancy. *Cochrane Pregnancy and Childbirth Database* (issue 2). Update Software, Oxford.

Malone, F.D. and D'Alton, M.E. (1997) Drugs in pregnancy: antiepileptics. *Seminars in Perinatology*, 21(2): 114–25.

Malseed, R.T., Goldstein, F.J. and Balkon, N. (1995) *Pharmacology: Drug Therapy and Nursing Considerations*, 4th edn. Lippincott, Philadelphia.

Mander, R. (1994) Epidural analgesia 2: research basis. *British Journal of Midwifery*, 2(1): 12–16.

Marcus, R. and Coulston, A. (1996) Fat-soluble vitamins, in Hardman, J., Limbard, L., Molinoff, P. et al. (eds) *Goodman & Gilman's: The Pharmacological Basis of Therapeutics*, 9th edn. McGraw-Hill, New York.

Marik, P. and Plante, L. (2008) Venous thromboembolic disease and pregnancy. *New England Journal of Medicine*, 359: 2025–33.

Martinsen, T.C., Bergh, K. and Waldum, H.L. (2005) Gastric juice: a barrier against infectious diseases. *Basic and Clinical Pharmacology and Toxicology*, 96(2): 94–102.

Maschi, S., Clavenna, A., Campi, R. et al. (2008) Neonatal outcome following pregnancy exposure to antidepressants: a prospective controled cohort study. *BJOG*, 115: 283–9.

Masters, S. (2001) The alcohols, in Katzung, B. (ed.) *Basic and Clinical Pharmacology*, 8th edn. McGraw-Hill, New York.

Mathews, F., Yudkin, P. and Neil, A. (1998) Folates in the periconceptual period: are women getting enough? *British Journal of Obstetrics and Gynaecology*, 105: 954–9.

Mathiesen, E.R., Kinsley, B., Amiel, S.A. et al. on behalf of Insulin Aspart Pregnancy Study Group (2007) Maternal glycemic control and hypoglycemia in type 1 diabetic pregnancy: a randomized trial of insulin aspart versus human insulin in 322 pregnant women. *Diabetes Care*, 30(4): 771–6.

Matz, H., Orion, E. and Wolf, R. (2006) Pruritic urticarial paules and plaques of pregnancy: polymorphic eruption of pregnancy (PUPP). *Clinics in Dermatology*, 24: 105–8.

Mayberry, L.J., Clemmens, D. and De, A. (2002) Epidural analgesia side effects, co-interventions, and care of women during childbirth: a systematic review. *American J Obstetrics Gynecol*, 186(5 Suppl Nature): S81–93.

Mazzotta, P. and Magee, L. (2000) A risk–benefit assessment of pharmacological and nonpharmacological treatments for nausea and vomiting of pregnancy. *Drugs*, 59: 781–800.

MCHRC (Maternal and Child Health Research Consortium) (1997) *Confidential Enquiry into Stillbirths and Deaths in Infancy. 4th Annual Report.* MCHRC, London.

MCHRC (Maternal and Child Health Research Consortium) (2000) *Confidential Enquiry into Stillbirths and Deaths in Infancy. 7th Annual Report.* MCHRC, London.

Medawar, C. (1992) *Power and Dependence: Social Audit on the Safety of Medicines.* Social Audit, London.

Medawar, C. (1997) The antidepressant web: marketing depression and making medicines work. *International Journal of Risk and Safety in Medicine*, 10(2): 75–126.

Mehta, K., Kalkwarf, H., Mimouni, F. et al. (1998) Randomized trial of magnesium administration to prevent hypocalcemia in infants of diabetic mothers. *Journal of Perinatalogy*, 18: 352–6.

Melzack, R. and Wall, P. (1996) *The Challenge of Pain.* Penguin, London.

Mentes, A. (2001) pH changes in dental plaque after using sugar-free paediatric medicine. *Journal of Clinical Paediatric Dentistry*, 25(4): 307–12.

MHRA (Medicines and Healthcare products Regulatory Agency) (2003) *Supplementary Prescribing.* MHRA, London.

MHRA (Medicines and Healthcare products Regulatory Agency) (2007) Codeine: very rare risk of side-effects in breast-fed babies. *Drug Safety Update*, 1(4): 6.

MHRA (Medicines and Healthcare products Regulatory Agency) (2008) *Drug Analysis Prints*, www.mhra.gov.uk/Safetyinformation/Howwemonitorthesafetyofproducts/Medicines/TheYellowCardScheme/YellowCarddata/Druganalysisprints/index.htm?indexChar=A.

Michel, T. (2006) Treatment of myocardial ischaemia, in Brunton, L., Lazo, J., Parker, K. (eds) *Goodman & Gilman's: The Pharmacological Basis of Therapeutics*, 11th edn. McGraw-Hill, New York.

Midtvedt, T. (2008) Penicillins, cephalosporins, other beta lactam antibiotics and tetracyclines, in Aronson, J.K. (ed.) *Side Effects of Drug Annual* 30. Elsevier, Amsterdam.

Miller, N.M., Fisk, N.M., Modi, N. and Glover, V. (2005) Stress responses at birth: determinants of cord arterial cortisol and links with cortisol response in infancy. *BJOG*, 112(7): 921–6.

Miller, R.K., Peters, P.W. and Schaefer, C. (2007) Genereal commentary on drug therapy and risks in pregnancy, in Schaefer, C., Peters, P.W. and Miller, R.K. (eds) *Drugs during Pregnancy and Lactation: Treatment Options and Risk Assessment*, 2nd edn. Elsevier, Oxford.

Milman, N. (2008) Prepartum anaemia: prevention and treatment. *Annals Hematol*, 87(12): 949–59.

Milman, N., Bergholt, T., Byg, K. et al. (1999) Iron status and iron balance during pregnancy: a critical reappraisal of iron supplementation. *Acta Obstetrica Gynecoligica Scandinavia*, 78(9): 749–57.

Milman, N., Byg, K.E., Bergholt, T. and Eriksen, L. (2006) Side effects of oral iron prophylaxis in pregnancy: myth or reality? *Acta Haematol*, 115(1/2): 53–7.

Milton, G. and Jann, M. (1995) Emergency treatment of psychotic symptoms. *Clinical Pharmacokinetics*, 28(6): 494–504.

Mitchelson, F. (1992a) Pharmacological agents affecting emesis: a review (Part I). *Drugs*, 43: 295–315.

Mitchelson, F. (1992b) Pharmacological agents affecting emesis: a review (Part II). *Drugs*, 43: 443–63.

Moen, V., Brudin, L., Rundgren, M. and Irestedt, L. (2009) Hyponatraemia complicating labour – rare or recognised? A prospective observational study. *BJOG*, 116(4): 552–61.

Moise, K. (2002) Management of rhesus allommunisation in pregnancy. *Obstetrics and Gynecology*, 100: 600–11.

Moldin, P.G. and Sundell, G. (1996) Induction of labour: a randomised clinical trial of amniotomy versus amniotomy with oxytocin infusion. *British Journal of Obstetrics and Gynaecology*, 103: 306–12.

Moncrieff, J. (1995) Lithium revisited. *British Journal of Psychiatry*, 167: 569–74.

Montan, S. and Arulkumaran, S. (2006) Neonatal respiratory distress syndrome. *Lancet*, 367: 1878–9.

Montoro, M. (1997) Management of hypothyroidism during pregnancy. *Clinical Obstetrics and Gynecology*, 40(1): 65–80.

Montouris, G. (2007) Importance of monotherapy in women across the reproductive cycle. *Neurology*, 69(24 Suppl 3): S10–16.

Moore, S., Turnpenny, P., Quinn, A. et al. (2000) A clinical study of 57 children with fetal anticonvulsant syndromes. *Journal of Medical Genetics*, 37: 489–97.

Morales-Suárez-Varela, M.M., Bille, C., Christensen, K. and Olsen, J. (2006) Smoking habits, nicotine use, and congenital malformations. *Obstetrics Gynecol*, 107(1): 51–7.

Morisaki, H., Yamamoto, S., Morita, Y. et al. (2000) Hypermagnesemia-induced cardiopulmonary arrest. *Journal of Clinical Anesthesia*, 12: 224–6.

Morrell, M.J. (1992) Hormones and epilepsy through the lifetime. *Epilepsia*, 33: S49–561.

Morrell, M.J. (2003) Reproductive and metabolic disorders in women with epilepsy. *Epilepsia*, 44(Suppl 4): 11–20.

Morrow, J.I., Hunt, S.J., Russell, A.J. et al. (2008) Folic acid use and major congenital malformations in offspring of women with epilepsy: a prospective study from the UK Epilepsy and Pregnancy Register. *Journal of Neurology and Neurosurgical Psychiatry*, 77: 193–8.

Morrow, J.I., Russell, A., Guthrie, E. et al. (2006) Malformation risks of anti-epileptic drugs in pregnancy: a prospective study fro the UK Epilepsy and Pregnancy Register. *J Neurol Neurosurg Psychiatry*, 77(1): 101–3.

Mortola, J.F. (1989) The use of psychotropic agents in pregnancy and lactation. *Psychiatric Clinics of North America*, 12: 53–68.

Mousa, H., McKinley, C. and Thong, J. (2000) Acute postpartum myocardial infarction after ergometrine administration in a woman with familial hypacholsterolaemia. *British Journal of Obstetrics and Gynaecology*, 107: 939–40.

Mousa, H.A. and Alfirevic, Z. (2007) Treatment for primary postpartum haemorrhage. *Cochrane Database of Systematic Reviews*, Issue 1. Art. No.: CD003249. DOI: 10.1002/14651858.CD003249.pub2.

Moutquin, J.M., Sherman, D., Cohen, H. et al. (2000) Double-blind, randomized, controlled trial of atosiban and ritodrine in the treatment of preterm labor: a multicenter effectiveness and safety study. *Am J Obstet Gynecol*, 182(5): 1191–9.

MRC Vitamin Study Research Group (1991) Prevention of neural tube defects: results of the MRC vitamin study. *Lancet*, 338: 132–7.

Muir, H., Writer, D., Douglas, J. et al. (1997) Double-blind comparison of epidural ropivacaine 0.25% and bupivacaine 0.25% for the relief of childbirth pain. *Canadian Journal of Anaesthesia*, 44: 599–604.

Mukamal, K., Conigrave, K., Mittleman, M. et al. (2003) Roles of drinking pattern and type of alcohol consumed in coronary heart disease in men. *New England Journal of Medicine*, 348(2): 109–18.

Mulder, E., Derks, J. and Visser, G. (1997) Antenatal corticosteroids therapy and fetal behaviour: a randomised study of the effects of betamethasone and dexamethasone. *British Journal of Obstetrics and Gynaecology*, 104: 1239–47.

Mulinare, J., Cordero, J.F., Erickson, J.D. and Berry, R.J. (1988) Periconceptual use of multivitamins and the occurrence of neural tube defects. *Journal of the American Medical Association*, 260: 3141–5.

Muller, A.F., Berghout, A., Wiersinga, W.M. et al., Working Group Thyroid Function Disorders of the Netherlands Association of Internal Medicine (2008) Thyroid function disorders: guidelines of the Netherlands Association of Internal Medicine. *Neth J Medicine*, 66(3): 134–42.

Mulvihill, A.O., Cackett, P.D., George, N.D. and Fleck, B.W. (2007) Nystagmus secondary to drug exposure in utero. *British Journal J Ophthalmol*, 91(5): 613–5.

Munn, M., Groome, L., Atterbury, J. et al. (1999) Pneumonia as a complication of pregnancy. *Journal of Maternal and Fetal Medicine*, 8: 151–4.

Murphy, V.E., Clifton, V.L. and Gibson, P.G. (2006) Asthma exacerbations during pregnancy: incidence and association with adverse pregnancy outcomes. *Thorax*, 61(2): 169–76.

Murphy, V.E., Gibson, P., Talbot, P.I. and Clifton, V.L. (2005) Severe asthma exacerbations during pregnancy. *Obstetrics Gynecol*, 106(5 Pt 1): 1046–54.

Musters, C. and McDonald, E. (2008) Management of postnatal depression. *BMJ*, 337: 399–403.

Nagelhout, J. (1992) General anaesthetic agents, in Baer, C. and Williams, B. (eds) *Clinical Pharmacology and Nursing*, 2nd edn. Springhouse, Springhouse, PA.

Naidu, S., Payne, A.J., Moodley, J. et al. (1996) Randomised study assessing the effect of phenytoin and magnesium sulphate on maternal cerebral circulation in eclampsia using transcranial Doppler ultrasound. *British Journal of Obstetrics and Gynaecology*, 103: 111–16.

Nakku, J., Nakasi, G. and Mirembe, F. (2006) Postpartum major depression at six weeks in primary health care: prevalence and associated factors. *African Health Sciences*, 6(4): 207–14.

NCC (National Collaborating Centre for Women's and Children's Health) (2004) *Caesarean Section: Clinical Guideline*. Commissioned by NICE. RCOG Press, London.

NCC (National Collaborating Centre for Women's and Children's Health) (2007) *Intrapartum Care: Care of Healthy Women and their Babies during Childbirth: Clinical Guideline*. Commissioned by NICE. RCOG Press, London.

NCC (National Collaborating Centre for Women's and Children's Health) (2008a) *Diabetes in Pregnancy: Clinical Guideline*. Commissioned by NICE. RCOG Press, London.

NCC (National Collaborating Centre for Women's and Children's Health) (2008b) *Induction of Labour: Clinical Guideline*. Commissioned by NICE. RCOG Press, London.

NCC (National Collaborating Centre for Women's and Children's Health) (2008c) *Antenatal Care: Clinical Guideline*. Commissioned by NICE. RCOG Press, London.

NCC MERP (National Coordinating Council for Medication Error Reporting and Prevention) (2005) *NCC MERP: The First Ten Years: 'Defining the Problem and Developing Solutions'*. United States Pharmacopia, Rockville, MA, www.nccmerp.org/pdf/reportFinal2005-11-29.pdf.

NCCMH (National Collaborating Centre for Mental Health) (2004) *Depression: Management of Depression in Primary and Secondary Care*. British Psychological Society/Royal College of Psychiatrists, London/Leicester.

Neale, R. (1996) Intrapartum stillbirths and deaths in infancy: the first CESDI report, in Studd, J. (ed.) *Progress in Obstetrics and Gynaecology*, vol. 12. Churchill Livingstone, Edinburgh.

Negro, R., Formoso, G., Mangieri, T. et al. (2006) Levothyroxine treatment in euthyroid pregnant women with autoimmune thyroid disease: effects on obstetrical complications. *J Clin Endocrinol Metab*, 91(7): 2587–91.

Nelson-Piercy, C. (1996) Decisions in prescribing for hypertension in pregnancy. *Prescriber*, 7(2): 29–36.

Nelson-Piercy, C. (1997) Hazards of heparin: allergy, heparin-induced thrombocytopenia and osteoporosis. *Ballière's Clinical Obstetrics and Gynaecology*, 11(3): 489–509.

Nelson-Piercy, C. and Moore-Gillon, J. (1995) Treatment of asthma, in Rubin, P. (ed.) *Prescribing in Pregnancy*, 2nd edn. BMJ Group, London.

Nelson-Piercy, C., Letsky, E. and de Swiet, M. (1997) Low-molecular-weight heparin for obstetric thromboprophylaxis. *American Journal of Obstetrics and Gynecology*, 176: 1062–8.

Neri, I., Blasi, I., Castro, P. et al. (2004) Polyethylene glycol electrolyte solution (isocolan) for constipation during pregnancy: an observational open-label study. *J Midwifery Womens Health*, 49: 355–8.

Newcomer, J.W., Selke, G., Melson, A.K. et al. (1999) Decreased memory performance in healthy humans induced by stress-level cortisol treatment. *Arch Gen Psychiatry*, 56(6): 527–33.

Newport, D.J., Calamaras, M.R., DeVane, C.L. et al. (2007) Atypical antipsychotic administration during late pregnancy: placental passage and obstetrical outcomes. *American Journal Psychiatry*, 164(8): 1214–20.

Ngai, S., Chan, Y., Lam, S. and Lao, T. (2000) Labour characteristics and uterine activity. *British Journal of Obstetrics and Gynaecology*, 107: 222–7.

NHS (National Health Service) (2003) *Inquiry into the Care and Treatment of Daksha Emson*. North East London Strategic Health Authority, London.

NICE (National Institute for Health and Clinical Excellence) (2002) *Guidance on the Use of Routine Antenatal Anti-D Prophylaxis for Women who are Rhesus D (RhD) Negative*. Technology Appraisal Guidance 41. NICE, London.

NICE (National Institute for Health and Clinical Excellence) (2004a) *Type 1 Diabetes: Diagnosis and Management of Type 1 Diabetes in Children, Young People And Adults*. Clinical Guideline 15. NICE, London.

NICE (National Institute for Health and Clinical Excellence) (2004b) Stokes T, Shaw EJ, Juarez-Garcia A, Camosso-Stefinovic J, Baker R (eds) *Clinical Guidelines and Evidence Review for the Epilepsies: Diagnosis and Management in Adults and Children in Primary and Secondary Care*. Royal College of General Practitioners, London.

NICE (National Institute for Health and Clinical Excellence) (2006) *Bipolar Disorder: Management of Bipolar Disorder in Adults, Children and Adolescents in Primary and Secondary Care*. Clinical Guideline 38. NICE, London.

NICE (National Institute for Health and Clinical Excellence) (2007) *Antenatal and Postnatal Mental Health*. NICE, London.

NICE (National Institute for Health and Clinical Excellence) (2008) *Routine Antenatal Anti-D Prophylaxis for Women who are Rhesus D (RhD) Negative*. Review of NICE Technology Appraisal Guidance 41. NICE, London.

Nichols, L. (1993) Drug reactions and interactions, in Spencer, R.T., Nichols, L., Lipkin, G. et al. (eds) *Clinical Pharmacology and Nursing Management*. Lippincott, Philadelphia.

NIH Consensus Development Panel on the Effect of Corticosteroids for Fetal Maturation on Perinatal Outcomes (1995) Effect of corticosteroids for fetal maturation on perinatal outcomes. *JAMA*, 273: 413–18.

Nisbet, A. (2006) Intramuscular gluteal injections in the increasingly obese population. *BMJ*, 332: 637–8.

Nisell, H., Lintu, H., Lunen, N. et al. (1995) Blood pressure and renal function seven years after pregnancy complicated by hypertension. *British Journal of Obstetrics and Gynaecology*, 102: 876–81.

Nishiguchi, T., Saga, K., Sumimoto, K. et al. (1996) Vitamin K prophylaxis to prevent neonatal vitamin K deficient intercranial haemorrage in Shizuka prefecture. *British Journal of Obstetrics and Gynaecology*: 103(11): 1078–84.

Nissen, E., Gustavsson, P., Widstrom, A.M. and Uvnas-Moberg, K. (1998) Oxytocin, prolactin, milk production and their relationship with personality traits in women after vaginal delivery or Cesarean section. *Journal of Psychosomatic Obstetrics and Gynaecology*, 19: 49–58.

Nissen, E., Lilja, G., Matthiesen, A. et al. (1995) Effects of maternal pethidine on infants' developing breast feeding. *Acta Paediatrica*, 84(2): 140–5.

Nissen, E., Uvnas-Moberg, K., Svensson, K. et al. (1996) Different patterns of oxytocin, prolactin but not cortisol release during breastfeeding in women delivered by caesarean section or by the vaginal route. *Early Human Development*, 45(1/2): 103–18.

Nissen, E., Widstrom, A., Lilja, G. et al. (1997) Effects of routinely given pethidine during labour on infants' developing breastfeeding behaviour. *Acta Paediatrica*, 86(2): 201–8.

Niven, C. (1992) *Psychological Care for Families: Before, During and After Birth*. Butterworth Heinemann, Oxford.

Nkata, M. (1996) Rupture of uterus: a review of 32 cases in a general hospital in Zambia. *BMJ*, 312: 1204–5.

NMC (Nursing and Midwifery Council) (2003) Nurse cautioned about prescribing without qualification. NMC press release 390. NMC, London.

NMC (Nursing and Midwifery Council) (2004) *Midwives Rules and Standards*. NMC, London.

NMC (Nursing and Midwifery Council) (2006) *Standards of Proficiency for Nurse and Midwife Prescribers*. NMC, London.

NMC (Nursing and Midwifery Council) (2007) *Standards for Medicines Management*. NMC, London, www.nmc-uk.org/aDisplayDocument.aspx?DocumentID=6228.

NMC (Nursing and Midwifery Council) (2008a) *The Code: Standards of Conduct, Performance and Ethics for Nurses and Midwives*. NMC, London.

NMC (Nursing and Midwifery Council) (2008b) *Fitness to Practise: Annual Report 2007–08*. NMC, London.

Nolan, S. and Scoggin, J.A. (1999) Serotonin syndrome: recognition and management. www.uspharmacist.com.

Nordstrom, L., Fogeistam, K., Fridman, G. et al. (1997) Routine oxytocin in the third stage of labour: a placebo controlled randomised trial. *British Journal of Obstetrics and Gynaecology*, 104: 781–6.

Norris, M., Grieco, W., Borkowski, M. et al. (1994) Complications of labor analgesia: epidural versus combined spinal epidural techniques. *Anesthesia and Analgesia*, 79: 529–37.

NPC (National Prescribing Centre) (2004) *Patient Group Directions: A Practical Guide and Framework of Competencies for all Professionals Using Patient Group Directions*. NPC, London.

NPSA (National Patient Safety Agency) (2009) Safety in doses. National Reporting and Learning Service, NPSA, London, www.nrls.npsa.nhs.uk/resources/?entryid45=61625.

Nulman, I., Laslo, D. and Koren, G. (1999) Treatment of epilepsy in pregnancy. *Drugs*, 57: 535–44.

Nulman, I., Rovet, J., Stewart, D. et al. (1997) Neurodevelopment of children exposed in utero to antidepressant drugs. *New England Journal of Medicine*, 336: 258–62.

Nutt, D. (1996) Addiction: brain mechanims and their treatment implications. *Lancet*, 347(8993): 31–6.

Nuutila, M. and Kajanoja, P. (1996) Local administration of prostaglandin E2 for cervical ripening and labor induction: the appropriate route and dose. *Acta Ostetrica et Gynecologica Scandinavica*, 75(2): 135–8.

Oates, J. (1996) Antihypertensive agents and the drug therapy of hypertension, in Hardman, J., Limbard, L., Molinoff, P. et al. (eds) *Goodman & Gilman's: The Pharmacological Basis of Therapeutics*, 9th edn. McGraw-Hill, New York.

Oates, M. (2000) *Perinatal Maternal Mental Health Services*. Council Report CR88. Royal College of Psychiatrists, London.

Oberlander, T.F., Warburton, W., Misri, S. et al. (2008) Major congenital malformations following prenatal exposure to serotonin reuptake inhibitors and benzodiazepines using population-based health data. *Birth Defects Research*, 83(1): 68–76.

O'Brien, C. (2006) Drug addiction and drug abuse, in Brunton, L., Lazo, J. and Parker, K. (eds) *Goodman & Gilman's: The Pharmacological Basis of Therapeutics*, 11th edn. McGraw-Hill, New York.

O'Connor, R.A. (1995) Induction of labour: not how but why? *British Journal of Hospital Medicine*, 52(11): 559–63.

Ofori, B., Oraichi, D., Blais, L. et al. (2006) Risk of congenital anomalies in pregnant users of non-steroidal anti-inflammatory drugs: a nested case-control study. *Birth Defects Research. Part B, Developmental and Reproductive Toxicology*, 77(4): 268–79.

Ogrin, C. and Schussler, G.C. (2005) Suppression of thyrotropin by morphine in a severely stressed patient. *Endocrinology Journal*, 52(2): 265–9.

O'Keane, V. and Marsh, M. (2007) Depression during pregnancy. *BMJ*, 334: 1003–5.

Okojie, P. and Cook, P. (1999) Update on some aspects of the use of epidural analgesia in labour. *International Journal of Clinical Practice*, 53(6): 418–20.

Olafsson, E., Hallgrimsson, J.T., Hauser, W.A. et al. (1998) Pregnancies of women with epilepsy: a population-based study in Iceland. *Epilepsia*, 39: 887–92.

Olah, K. and Gee, H. (1996) The active mismanagement of labour. *British Journal of Obstetrics and Gynaecology*, 103(8): 729–31.

O'Leary, C.M., Nassar, N., Kurinczuk, J.J. and Bower, C. (2009) The effect of maternal alcohol consumption on fetal growth and preterm birth. *BJOG*, 116(3): 390–400.

Olfert, S.M. (2006) Reproductive outcomes among dental personnel: a review of selected exposures. *Journal of the Canadian Dental Association*, 72(9): 821–5.

Olofsson, C. and Irestedt, L. (1998) Traditional analgesic agents: are parenteral narcotics passé and do inhalational agents still have a place in labour? *Ballière's Clinical Obstetrics and Gynaecology*, 12(3): 409–21.

Olofsson, C., Ekblom, A., Ekman-Ordeberg, G. and Irestedt, L. (1998) Obstetric outcome following epidural analgesia with bupivacaine-adrenaline 0.25% or bupivacaine 0.125% with sufentanil. *Acta Anaesthesiologica Scandinavia*, 42: 284–92.

Olofsson, C., Ekblom, A., Ekman-Ordeberg, G. et al. (1996) Lack of analgesic effect of systemically administered morphine or pethidine on labour pain. *British Journal of Obstetrics and Gynaecology*, 103: 968–72.

Olsen, K. and D'Oria, L. (1992) Uterine motility agents, in Baer, C. and Williams, B. (eds) *Clinical Pharmacology and Nursing*. Springhouse, Springhouse, PA.

Olsen, S., Secher, N., Tabor, A. et al. (2000) Randomised clinical trials of fish oil supplementation in high risk pregnancies. *British Journal of Obstetrics and Gynaecology*, 107: 382–95.

Orioli, I. and Castilla, E. (2000) Epidemiological assessment of misoprostol teratogenicity. *British Journal of Obstetrics and Gynaecology*, 107: 519–23.

Orlikowski, C., Dickinson, J., Paech, M. et al. (2006) Intrapartum analgesia and its association with post-partum back pain and headache in nulliparous women. *Australian and New Zealand Journal of Obstetrics and Gynaecology*, 46: 395–401.

Osler, M. (1987) A double blind study comparing meptazinol and pethidine for pain relief in labour. *European Journal of Obstetrics, Gynecology and Reproductive Biology*, 26(1): 15–18.

Ostrow, C.L. and McCoy, C.A. (1998) Hematinic agents, in Williams, B. and Baer, C. (eds) *Essentials of Clinical Pharmacology in Nursing*. Springhouse, Springhouse, PA.

Ounsted, M.K., Hendrick, M., Mutch, L.M. et al. (1978) Induction of labour by different methods in primiparous women. 1: Some perinatal and postnatal problems. *Early Hum Dev*, 2: 227–39.

Out, J.J., Vierhout, M.E. and Wallenburg, H.C. (1988) Breast-feeding following spontaneous and induced labour. *Eur J Obstet Gynecol Reprod Biol*, 29: 275–9.

Pacheco, L.D., Ghulmiyyah, L.M., Snodgrass, W.R. and Hankins, G.D. (2007) Pharmacokinetics of corticosteroids during pregnancy. *American Journal of Perinatology*, 24(2): 79–82.

Paech, M. (1998) New epidural techniques for labour analgesia: patient-controlled epidural analgesia and combined spinal-epidural analgesia. *Baillière's Clin Obstet Gynaecol*, 12(3): 377–95.

Palmer, A., Waugaman, W., Conklin, K. and Kotelko, D. (1991) Does the administration of oral Bicitra before elective cesarean section affect the incidence of nausea and vomiting in the parturient? *Nurse Anesthetist*, 2(3): 126–33.

Palmon, S.C., Lloyd, A.T. and Kirsch, J.R. (1998) The effect of needle gauge and lidocaine pH on pain during intradermal injection. *Anesth Analg*, 86(2): 379–81.

Pandey, M.K., Rani, R. and Agrawal, S. (2005) An update in recurrent spontaneous abortion. *Archives of Gynecology and Obstetrics*, 272(2): 95–108.

Pang, D. and O'Sullivan, G. (2008) Analgesia and anaesthesia in labour. *Obstetrics, Gynecology and Reproductive Medicine*, 18(4): 87–92.

Pangle, B. (2000) Drugs in pregnancy and lactation, in Herfindal, E. and Gourley, D. (eds) *Textbook of Therapeutics: Drug and Disease Management*, 7th edn. Lippincott, Williams &Wilkins, Philadelphia.

Papatsonis, D., Flenady, V., Cole, S. and Liley, H. (2005) Oxytocin receptor antagonists for inhibiting preterm labour. *Cochrane Database of Systematic Reviews*, Issue 3. Art. No.: CD004452. DOI: 10.1002/14651858.CD004452.pub2.

Pare, P., Ferrazzi, S., Thompson, W.G. et al. (2001) Epidemiological survey of constipation in Canada: rates, demographics, and predictors of health. *American J Gastroenterol*, 96: 3130–7.

Parker, K. and Schimmer, B. (2006) Pituitary hormones and their hypothalamic releasing hormones, in Brunton, L., Lazo, J. and Parker, K. (eds) *Goodman & Gilman's: The Pharmacological Basis of Therapeutics*, 11th edn. McGraw-Hill, New York.

Parker, L., Cole, M., Craft, A. and Hey, E. (1998) Neonatal vitamin K administration and childhood cancer in the north of England: retrospective case-control study. *BMJ*, 316: 189–93.

Pasricha, P. (2006) Treatment of disorders of bowel motility and water flux, in Brunton, L., Lazo, J. and Parker, K. (eds) *Goodman & Gilman's: The Pharmacological Basis of Therapeutics*, 11th edn. McGraw-Hill, New York.

Passmore, S., Draper, G., Brownhill, P. and Kroll, M. (1998a) Case-control studies of relation between childhood cancer and neonatal vitamin K administration. *BMJ*, 316: 178–84.

Passmore, S., Draper, G., Brownhill, P. and Kroll, M. (1998b) Ecological studies of relation between hospital policies on vitamin K administration and subsequent occurrence of childhood cancer. *BMJ*, 316: 184–9.

Pattee, C., Ballantyne, M. and Milne, B. (1997) Epidural analgesia for labour and delivery: informed consent issues. *Canadian Journal of Anaesthesia*, 44: 918–23.

Paul, R.H., Koh, K.S. and Berstein, S.G. (1978) Changes in fetal heart rate-uterine contraction patterns associated with eclampsia. *American Journal of Obstetrics and Gynecology*, 130: 165–9.

Pedersen, L.H., Henriksen, T.B., Vestergaard, M. et al. (2009) Selective serotonin reuptake inhibitors in pregnancy and congenital malformations: population based cohort study. *BMJ*, 23(339): b3569, doi: 10.1136/bmj.b3569.

Pediani, R. (2003) Patient-administered inhalation of nitrous oxide and oxygen gas for procedural pain relief. World Wide Wounds, www.worldwidewounds.com/2003/october/Pediani/Entonox-Pain-Relief.html.

Pedley, T.A., Scheuer, M.L. and Walczak, T.S. (1995) Epilepsy, in Rowlands, L.P. (ed.) *Merritt's Textbook of Neurology*, 9th edn. Williams & Wilkins, New York.

Pennell, P.B. and Hovinga, C.A. (2008) Antiepileptic drug therapy in pregnancy 1: gestational-induced effects on AED pharmokinetics. *Int Rev Neurobiol*, 83: 227–40.

Perahia, D.G., Kajdasz, D.K., Desaiah, D. and Haddad, P.M. (2005) Symptoms following abrupt discontinuation of duloxetine treatment in patients with major depressive disorder. *Journal of Affective Disorders*, 89(1/3): 207–12.

Perrone, R.D., Madias, N.E. and Levey, A.S. (1992) Serum creatinine as an index of renal function: new insights into old concepts. *Clin Chem*, 38(10): 1933–53.

Perry, K., Morrison, J., Rust, O. et al. (1995) Incidence of adverse cardiopulmonary effects with low-dose continuous terbutaline infusion. *American Journal of Obstetrics and Gynecology*, 173: 1273–7.

Perucca, E. (2005) Birth defects after prenatal exposure to antiepileptic drugs. *Lancet Neurol*, 4: 781–6.

Perucchini, D., Fischer, U., Spinas, G. et al. (1999) Using fasting plasma glucose concentrations to screen for gestational diabetes mellitus: prospective population based study. *BMJ*, 319: 812–15.

Peschman, P. (1992) Vitamin, mineral and other nutritional agents, in Baer, C. and Williams, B. (eds) *Clinical Pharmacology and Nursing*, 2nd edn. Springhouse, Springhouse, PA.

Peters, P. and Schaefer, C. (2007) Recreational drugs, in Schaefer, C., Peters, P.W. and Miller, R.K. (eds) *Drugs during Pregnancy and Lactation: Treatment Options and Risk Assessment*, 2nd edn. Elsevier, Oxford.

Pfaffenrath, V. and Rehm, M. (1998) Migraine in pregnancy: what are the safest treatment options. *Drug Safety*, 19: 383–8.

Philipson, E.H., Kalhan, S.C., Riha, M.M. and Pimentel, R. (1987) Effects of maternal glucose infusion on fetal acid-base status in human pregnancy. *American J Obstetrics Gynecol*, 157(4 Pt 1): 866–73.

Pignotti, M.S., Indolfi, G., Ciuti, R. and Donzelli, G. (2005) Perinatal asphyxia and inadvertent neonatal intoxication from local anaesthetics given to the mother during labour. *BMJ*, 330(7481): 34–5.

Pinkofsky, H. (1997) Psychosis during pregnancy: treatment considerations. *Annals of Clinical Psychiatry*, 9(3): 175–9.

Pipkin, F.B., de Swiet, M., Duley, L. et al. (1996) Where next for prophylaxis against pre-eclampsia? *British Journal of Obstetrics and Gynaecology*, 103: 603–7.

Pitt, B. (1991) Postnatal depression. *Hospital Update*, 17(2): 133–40.

Plested, C.P. and Bernal, A.L. (2001) Desensitisation of the oxytocin receptor and other G-protein coupled receptors in the human myometrium. *Experimental Physiology*, 86(2): 303–12.

Plouin, P., Breart, G., Llado, J. et al. (1990) A randomized comparison of early with conservative use of antihypertensive drugs in the management of pregnancy-induced hypertension. *British Journal of Obstetrics and Gynaecology*, 97: 134–41.

Po, A.L. and Po, G.L. (1992) *OTC Medications*. Blackwell Scientific, Oxford.

Poirier, M., Olivero, O., Walker, D. and Walker, V. (2004) Perinatal genotoxicity and carcinogenicity of anti-retroviral nucleoside analog drugs. *Toxicology and Applied Pharmacology*, 199: 151–61.

Ponce, J., Martínez, B., Fernández, A. et al. (2008) Constipation during pregnancy: a longitudinal survey based on self-reported symptoms and the Rome II criteria. *European Journal of Gastroenterology and Hepatology*, 20(1): 56–61.

Porter, J., Bonello, E. and Reynolds, F. (1998) Effect of epidural fentanyl on neonatal respiration. *Anaesthesiology*, 89: 79–85.

Posfay-Barbe, K.M., Zerr, D.M. and Pittet, D. (2008) Infection control in paediatrics. *Lancet Infectious Diseases*, 8(1): 19–31.

Potts, J. (1991) Diseases of the parathyroid gland and other hyper- and hypo-calcaemic disorders, in Wilson, J., Braunwald, E., Isselbacher, K. et al. (eds) *Harrison's Principles of Internal Medicine*, 12th edn. McGraw-Hill, New York.

Prather, C.M. (2004) Pregnancy related constipation. *Current Gastroenterology Reports*, 6(5): 402–4.

Pratt, R.J., Pellowe, C.M., Wilson, J.A. et al. (2007) National evidence-based guidelines for preventing healthcare-associated infections in NHS hospitals in England: epic2. *Journal of Hospital Infection*, 65(Suppl 1): S1–64.

Prendiville, W., Elbourne, D. and McDonald, S. (2000) Active versus expectant management in the third stage of labour. *Cochrane Database Systematic Review* (issue 2). Update Software, Oxford.

Prescott, S.L., Macaubas, C., Smallacombe, T. et al. (1999) Development of allergen-specific T-cell memory in atopic and normal children. *Lancet*, 353(9148): 196–200.

Pritchard, J., Cunningham, F. and Pritchard, S. (1984) The Parkland Memorial Hospital protocol for treatment of eclampsia: evaluation of 245 cases. *American Journal of Obstetrics and Gynecology*, 148: 951–63.

Pryce, R. (2009) Diabetic ketoacidosis caused by exposure of insulin pump to heat and sunlight. *BMJ*, 338: a2218.

Qarmalawi, A., Morsy, A., Fadly, A. et al. (1995) Labetolol vs. methyldopa in the treatment of pregnancy-induced hypertension. *Int. J Gynaecol. Obstet.*, 49(2): 125–30.

Quigley, M.A., Kelly, Y.J. and Sacker, A. (2007) Breastfeeding and hospitalization for diarrheal and respiratory infection in the United Kingdom Millennium Cohort Study. *Pediatrics*, 119(4): e837–42.

Quintiliani, R. Sr and Quintiliani, R. Jr. (2008) Pharmacokinetics/pharmacodynamics for critical care clinicians. *Crit Care Clin*, 24(2): 335–48.

Rabl, M., Joura, E.A., Yücel, Y. and Egarter, C. (2002) A randomized trial of vaginal prostaglandin E2 for induction of labor: insert vs. tablet. *Journal of Reproductive Medicine*, 47(2): 115–19.

Rahm, V.A., Hallgren, A., Högberg, H. et al. (2002) Plasma oxytocin levels in women during labor with or without epidural analgesia: a prospective study. *Acta Obstetrics Gynecol Scand*, 81(11): 1033–9.

Rai, R., Cohen, H., Dave, M. and Regan, L. (1997) Randomised controlled trial of aspirin and aspirin plus heparin in pregnant women with recurrent miscarriage associated with phosphorlipid antibodies. *BMJ*, 314: 253–7.

Rajan, L. (1993) Perceptions of pain and pain relief in labour: the gulf between theory and observation. *Midwifery*, 9(3): 136–45.

Rajan, L. (1994) The impact of obstetric procedures and analgesia/anaesthesia during labour and delivery on breast feeding. *Midwifery*, 10(2): 87–103.

Rang, H., Dale, M., Ritter, J. and Flower, R. (2007) *Pharmacology*, 6th edn. Elsevier, Churchill Livingstone, Edinburgh.

Ranta, P., Spalding, M., Kangas-Saarela, T. et al. (1995) Maternal expectations and experiences of labour pain. *Acta Anaesthesiologica Scandinavia*, 31(1): 60–6.

Rascol, O., Hain, T.C., Brefel, C. et al. (1995) Antivertigo medications and drug-induced vertigo. *Drugs*, 50: 777–91.

Rayburn, W.F. and Conover, E.A. (1993) Non-prescription drugs and pregnancy, in Studd, J. (ed.) *Progress in Obstetrics and Gynaecology*, vol. 10. Churchill Livingstone, Edinburgh.

RCN (Royal College of Nursing) (1996) *Nurses' Involvement in the Use of Neuroleptic Drugs*. Record no. 000 562. RCN, London.

RCOG (Royal College of Obstetricians and Gynaecologists) (1999) *Use of Anti-D Immunoglobulins for Rh Prophylaxis*. Revised 2002. RCOG Press, London.

RCOG (Royal College of Obstetricians and Gynaecologists) (2002) *Tocolytic Drugs for Women in Preterm Labour*. RCOG Press, London.

RCOG (Royal College of Obstetricians and Gynaecologists) (2007) *Thrombombolic Disease in Pregnancy and the Puerperium: Acute Management*. Green top guideline no. 28. RCOG Press, London.

RCP (Royal College of Psychiatrists) (1996) *A Handbook on Perinatal Maternal Mental Health Services*. RCP, London.

RCP/BHS (Royal College of Psychiatrists/British Hypertension Society) (2006) *Management of Hypertension in Adults in Primary Care*. RCP, London.

RCP/BPS (Royal College of Psychiatrists/British Psychological Society) (2003) *Schizophrenia: Full National Clinical Guideline on Core Interventions in Primary and Secondary Care*. RCP/BPS, London.

Redline, R.W. (2004) Placental inflammation. *Seminars in Neonatology*, 9(4): 265–74.

Redman, C. and Jefferies, M. (1988) Revised definition of pre-eclampsia. *Lancet*, 8589: 809–12.

Renfrew, M., Lang, S. and Woolridge, M. (2000) Oxytocin for promoting successful lactation. *Cochrane Pregnancy and Childbirth Database* (issue 2). Update Software, Oxford.

Restrepo, C.S., Carrillo, J.A., Martínez, S. et al. (2007) Pulmonary complications from cocaine and cocaine-based substances: imaging manifestations. *Radiographics*, 27(4): 941–56.

Reuvers, M. (2007) Anticoagulant and fibrinolytic drugs, in Schaefer, C., Peters, PW. and Miller, RK. (eds) *Drugs during Pregnancy and Lactation: Treatment Options and Risk Assessment*, 2nd edn. Elsevier, Oxford.

Reveiz, L., Gaitán, H.G. and Cuervo, L.G. (2007b) Enemas during labour. *Cochrane Database of Systematic Reviews*, Issue 4. Art. No.: CD000330. DOI: 10.1002/14651858.CD000330.pub2.

Reveiz, L., Gyte, G.M. and Cuervo, L.G. (2007a) Treatments for iron-deficiency anaemia in pregnancy. *Cochrane Database of Systematic Reviews*, Issue 2. Art. No.: CD003094. DOI: 10.1002/14651858.CD003094.pub2.

Rey, E. and Boulet, L.P. (2007) Asthma in pregnancy. *BMJ*, 334(7593): 582–5.

Reynolds, F. (1993a) Principles of placental drug transfer, in Reynolds, F. (ed.) *Effects on the Baby of Maternal Analgesia and Anaesthesia*. Saunders, London.

Reynolds, F. (1993b) Pain relief in labour. *British Journal of Obstetrics and Gynaecology*, 100: 979–83.

Reynolds, F. and Crowhurst, J. (1997) Opioids in labour: no analgesic effect. *Lancet*, 349: 4–5.

Reynolds, F., Sharma, S.K. and Seed, P.T. (2002) Analgesia in labour and fetal acid-base balance: a meta-analysis comparing epidural with systemic opioid analgesia. *BJOG*, 109(12): 1344–53.

Reynolds, K., Lewis, L., Nolen, J. et al. (2003) Alcohol consumption and risk of stroke: a meta-analysis. *JAMA*, 289(5): 579–88.

Riaz, M., Porat, R., Brodsky, N. and Hurt, H. (1998) The effects of magnesium sulfate treatment on newborns: a prospective controlled study. *Journal of Perinatology*, 18: 449–54.

Rice, I., Wee, M. and Thomson, K. (2004) Obstetrics epidurals and chronic adhesive arachnoiditis. *British Journal of Anaesthesia*, 92(1): 109–20.

Richardson, M. (2000) Regional anesthesia for obstetrics. *Anesthesiology Clinics of North America*, 18: 383–406.

Richter, J.E. (2005) Review article: the management of heartburn in pregnancy. *Aliment Pharmacol Ther*, 22(9): 749–57.

Rix, P., Ladehoff, P., Moller, A.M. et al. (1996) Cervical ripening and induction of delivery by local administration of prostaglandin E2 gel or vaginal tablets is equally effective. *Acta Ostetrica et Gynecologica Scandinavica*, 75(1): 45–7.

Robert-Gnansia, E. and Schaefer, C. (2007) Antiepileptics, in Schaefer, C., Peters, P.W. and Miller, R.K. (eds) *Drugs during Pregnancy and Lactation: Treatment Options and Risk Assessment*, 2nd edn. Elsevier, Oxford.

Roberts, A., Leveno, K., Sidawi, E. et al. (1995) Fetal acidaemia associated with regional anesthesia for elective Caesarean delivery. *Obstetrics and Gynecology*, 85(1): 79–83.

Roberts, C.L., Torvaldsen, S., Cameron, C.A. and Olive, E. (2004) Delayed versus early pushing in women with epidural analgesia: a systematic review and meta-analysis. *BJOG*, 111(12): 1333–40.

Roberts, D. and Dalziel, S. (2006) Antenatal corticosteroids for accelerating fetal lung maturation for women at risk of preterm birth. *Cochrane Database Syst Rev*, Jul 19;3:CD004454.

Roberts, J. and Hubel, C. (1999) Is oxidative stress the link in the two-stage model of pre-eclampsia? *Lancet*, 354(9181): 788–9.

Robertson, R. and Robertson, D. (1996) Drugs used for the treatment of myocardial ischaemia, in Hardman, J., Limbard, L., Molinoff, P. et al. (eds) *Goodman & Gilman's: The Pharmacological Basis of Therapeutics*, 9th edn. McGraw-Hill, New York.

Robinson, C., Schumann, R., Zhang, P. and Young, R.C. (2003) Oxytocin-induced desensitization of the oxytocin receptor. *American Journal of Obstetrics and Gynecology*, 188(2): 497–502.

Robson, S.C. (1996) Magnesium sulphate: the time of reckoning. *British Journal of Obstetrics and Gynaecology*, 103: 99–102.

Rodger, M. and King, L. (2000) Drawing up and administering intramuscular injections: a review of the literature. *Journal of Advanced Nursing*, 31(3): 574–82.

Rogers, C. (1995) *The Women's Guide to Herbal Medicine*. BCA, London.

Rogers, J., Wood, J., McCandish, R. et al. (1998) Active versus expectant management of third stage of labour. *Lancet*, 351: 693–9.

Rosa, F.W. (1991) Spina bifida in infants of women treated with carbamazepine during pregnancy. *N Engl J Med*, 324: 674–7.

Rosenberg, G.A. (2002) Matrix metalloproteinases in neuroinflammation. *Glia*, 39(3): 279–91.

Ross, S. and Soltes, D. (1995) Heparin and haematoma: does ice make a difference? *Journal of Advanced Nursing*, 21: 434–9.

Rossoni, E., Feng, J., Tirozzi, B. et al. (2008) Emergent synchronous bursting of oxytocin neuronal network. *PLoS Comput Biol*, 4(7): e1000123.

Rotchell, Y., Cruickshank, J., Gay, M.P. et al. (1998) Barbados low dose aspirin study in pregnancy: a randomised trial for the prevention of pre-eclampsia and its complications. *British Journal of Obstetrics and Gynaecology*, 105: 286–92.

Rothman, K., Moore, L., Singer, M. et al. (1995) Teratogenicity of high vitamin A intake. *New England Journal of Medicine*, 333: 1369–73.

Rotmensch, S., Liberati, M., Celentano, C. et al. (1999) The effect of betamethasone on fetal biophysical activities and Doppler velocimetry of umbilical and middle cerebral arteries. *Acta Obstetrics Gynecol Scand*, 78(9): 768–73.

Rouse, D.J., Hirtz, D.G., Thom, E. et al. (2008) A randomized, controlled trial of magnesium sulfate for the prevention of cerebral palsy. *New England Journal of Medicine*, 359(9): 895–905.

Routeledge, P. (2004) Adverse drug reactions and interactions, in Talbot, J. and Walker, P. (eds) *Stephens' Detection of New Adverse Drug Reactions*. Wiley, Chichester.

Roy, S., Wang, J., Kelschenbach, J. et al. (2006) Modulation of immune function by morphine: implications for susceptibility to infection. *J Neuroimmune Pharmacol*, 1(1): 77–89.

Rubin, P.C., Butters, L., Clark, D.M. et al. (1983) Placebo-controlled trial of atenolol in treatment of pregnancy-associated hypertension. *Lancet*, 1(8322): 431–4.

Rude, R. and Oldham, S. (1990) Disorders of magnesium metabolism, in Cohen, R., Lewis, B., Alberti, K. and Denman, A. (eds) *The Metabolic and Molecular Basis of Acquired Disease*. Baillière Tindall, London.

Ruggiero, R. (2006) Visible embryo pharmaceutical guide to drugs in pregnancy, www.visembryo.com/baby/pharmaceuticals.html.

Ruigomez, A., Rodriguez, G.L., Cattatuzzi, C. and Troncon, M. (1999) Use of cimetidine, omeprazole and ranitidine in pregnant women and pregnancy outcomes. *American Journal of Epidemiology*, 150: 476–81.

Ruppen, W., Derry, S., McQuay, H. and Moore, R.A. (2006) Incidence of epidural hematoma, infection, and neurologic injury in obstetric patients with epidural analgesia/anesthesia. *Anesthesiology*, 105(2): 394–9.

Russell, A.R. and Murch, S.H. (2006) Could peripartum antibiotics have delayed health consequences for the infants? *BJOG*, 113: 758–65.

Russell, J.A., Douglas, A.J. and Ingram, C.D. (2001) Brain preparations for maternity: adaptive changes in behavioral and neuroendocrine systems during pregnancy and lactation – an overview. *Prog Brain Res*, 133: 1–38.

Russell, R., Groves, P., Taub, N. et al. (1993) Assessing long term backache after childbirth. *BMJ*, 306: 1299–303.

Russell, S. and Doyle, E. (1997) Paediatric anaesthesia. *BMJ*, 314: 201–3.

Rutishauser, S. (1994) *Physiology and Anatomy*. Churchill Livingstone, Edinburgh.

Sackett, D., Haynes, R.B., Guyatt, G. and Tugwell, P. (1991) *Clinical Epidemiology: A Basic Science for Clinical Medicine*, 2nd edn. Little, Brown, Boston.

Sadler, L., Davison, T. and McCowan, L. (2000a) A randomised controlled trial and meta-analysis of active management of labour. *British Journal of Obstetrics and Gynaecology*, 107: 909–15.

Sadler, L., McCowan, L., White, H. et al. (2000b) Pregnancy outcomes and cardiac complications in women with mechanical, bioprosthetic and homograft valves. *British Journal of Obstetrics and Gynaecology*, 107: 245–53.

Safari, H., Fassett, M., Souter, I. et al. (1998) The efficacy of methylprednisolone in the treatment of hyperemesis gravidarum. *American Journal of Obstetrics and Gynecology*, 179: 921–4.

Saha, P., Stott, D. and Atalla, R. (2009) Haemostatic changes in the puerperium '6 weeks postpartum' (HIP Study): implication for maternal thromboembolism. *BJOG*, 116(12): 1602–12.

Sampson, H.A., Munoz-Furlong, A., Campbell, R. et al. (2006) Symposium on the definition and management of anaphylaxis: summary report. *Journal of Allergy and Clinical Immunology*, 117: 391–7.

Samrén, E.B., van Duijn, C.M., Koch, S. et al. (1997) Maternal use of antiepileptic drugs and the risk of major congenital malformations: a joint european prospective study of human teratogenesis associated with maternal epilepsy. *Epilepsia*, 38: 981–90.

Sanaullah, F., Gillian, M. and Lavin, T. (2006) Screening of substance misuse during early pregnancy in Blyth: an anonymous unlinked study. *J. Obstetrics Gynaecol*, 26: 187–90.

Sari, A., Sheldon, T., Cracknell, A. et al. (2007) Extent, nature and consequences of adverse events: Results of a retrospective case note review in a large NHS hospital. *Quality and Safety in Health Care*, 16: 434–9.

Sarici, S.U., Yurdakök, M., Serdar, M.A. et al. (2002) An early (sixth-hour) serum bilirubin measurement is useful in predicting the development of significant hyperbilirubinemia and severe ABO hemolytic disease in a selective high-risk population of newborns with ABO incompatibility. *Pediatrics*, 109(4): e53.

Sawle, G. (1995) Epilepsy and anti-convulsant drugs, in Rubin, P. (ed.) *Prescribing in Pregnancy*, 2nd edn. BMJ Group, London.

Schaefer, C. (2007a) Anticoagulants and fibrinolytics, in Schaefer, C., Peters, P.W. and Miller, R.K. (eds) *Drugs during Pregnancy and Lactation: Treatment Options and Risk Assessment*, 2nd edn. Elsevier, Oxford.

Schaefer, C. (2007b) Cardiovascular drugs and diuretics, in Schaefer, C., Peters, P.W. and Miller, R.K. (eds) *Drugs during Pregnancy and Lactation: Treatment Options and Risk Assessment*, 2nd edn. Elsevier, Oxford.

Schaefer, C. (2007c) Antiinfectives, in Schaefer, C., Peters, P.W. and Miller, R.K. (eds) *Drugs during Pregnancy and Lactation: Treatment Options and Risk Assessment*, 2nd edn. Elsevier, Oxford.

Schaefer, C. (2007d) Antiepileptics, in Schaefer, C., Peters P.W. and Miller, R.K. (eds) *Drugs during Pregnancy and Lactation: Treatment Options and Risk Assessment*, 2nd edn. Elsevier, Oxford.

Schaefer, C. (2007e) Psychotropic drugs, in Schaefer, C., Peters P.W. and Miller, R.K. (eds) *Drugs during Pregnancy and Lactation: Treatment Options and Risk Assessment*, 2nd edn. Elsevier, Oxford.

Schaefer, C., Peters P.W. and Miller R.K. (eds) (2007) *Drugs during Pregnancy and Lactation: Treatment Options and Risk Assessment*, 2nd edn. Elsevier, Oxford.

Schaefer-Graf, U., Buchanan, T., Xiang, A. et al. (2000) Patterns of congenital anomalies and relationship to initial maternal fasting glucose levels in pregnancies complicated by type 2 and gestational diabetes. *American Journal of Obstetrics and Gynecology*, 182: 313–20.

Schatz, M. (1999) Asthma and pregnancy. *Lancet*, 353: 1202–4.

Schatz, M., Dombrowski, M.P. and Wise, R. (2003) Asthma morbidity during pregnancy can be predicted by severity classification. *J Allergy Clin Immunol*, 112(2): 283–8.

Schatz, M., Dombrowski, M.P., Wise, R. et al. (2004) The relationship of asthma medication use to perinatal outcomes. *J Allergy Clin Immunol*, 113(6): 1040–5.

Schatz, M., Zeiger, R., Harden, K. et al. (1997) The safety of asthma and allergy medications during pregnancy. *Journal of Allergy and Clinical Immunology*, 100(3): 301–6.

Schier, J., Howland, M., Hoffman, R. and Nelson, L. (2003) Fatality from administration of labetalol and crushed extended-release nifedipine. *Annals of Pharmacotherapy*, 37: 1420–3.

Schimmer, B. and Parker, K. (2006) Adrenocorticotropic hormone: adrenocortical steroids and their synthetic analogues, in Brunton, L., Lazo, J. and Parker, K. (eds) *Goodman & Gilman's: The Pharmacological Basis of Therapeutics*, 11th edn. McGraw-Hill, New York.

Schmittner, J., Schroeder, J.R., Epstein, D.H. and Preston, K.L. (2005) Menstrual cycle length during methadone maintenance. *Addiction*, 100(6): 829–36.

Scholz, J., Steinfath, M. and Schulz, M. (1996) Clinical pharmacokinetics of alfentanil, fentanyl and sufentanil. *Clinical Pharmacokinetics*, 31: 275–92.

Schondorfer, C.W. (2007) Heart and circulatory system drugs and diuretics, in Schaefer, C., Peters, P.W. and Miller, R.K. (eds) *Drugs during Pregnancy and Lactation: Treatment Options and Risk Assessment*, 2nd edn. Elsevier, Oxford.

Schreiber, S., Lurtzing, F., Gotze, R. et al. (2003) Extrajugular pathways of human cerebral venous blood drainage assessed by duplex ultrasound. *Journal of Applied Physiology*, 94: 1802–5.

Schwartz, L. (1998) Infertility and pregnancy in epileptic women. *Lancet*, 352: 1952–3.

Schwartz, U., Ritchie, M., Bradford, Y. et al. (2008) Genetic determinants of response to warfarin during initial anticoagulation. *New England Medical Journal of Medicine*, 358(10): 999–1008.

Schwenkhagen, A.M. and Stodieck, S.R. (2008) Which contraception for women with epilepsy? *Seizure*, 17(2): 145–50.

Serretti, A. and Artioli, P. (2004) The pharmacogenomics of selective serotonin reuptake inhibitors. *Pharmacogenomics*, 4(4): 233–44.

Shafik, A. (1993) Constipation: pathogenesis and management. *Drugs*, 45(4): 528–40.

Shah, D. and Reed, G. (1996) Parameters associated with adverse perinatal outcome in hypertensive pregnancies. *J. Human Hypertension*, 10(8): 511–15.

Shaheen, S., Newson, R., Sherriff, A. et al. (2002) Paracetamol use in pregnancy and wheezing in early childhood. *Thorax*, 57: 958–63.

Sharma, P., Day, J. and Webster, S. (1995) Dangerous side-effect of neuroleptic therapy. *Hospital Update*, 21(8): 374–6.

Sharma, S.K., Gajraj, N.M., Sidawi, J.E. and Lowe, K. (1996) EMLA cream effectively reduces the pain of spinal needle insertion. *Reg Anest*, 21(6): 561–4.

Sharma, S.K., Sidawi, J.E., Ramin, S.M. et al. (1997) Cesarean delivery: a randomized trial of epidural versus patient-controlled meperidine analgesia during labor. *Anesthesiology*, 87(3): 487–94.

Sharma, V., Smith, A. and Khan, M. (2004) The relationships between duration of labour, time of delivery and puerperal psychosis. *Journal of Affective Disorders*, 83: 215–220.

Shatrugna, V., Raman, L., Kailash, U. et al. (1999) Effect of dose and formulation on iron tolerance in pregnancy. *National Medical Journal of India*, 12(1): 18–20.

Sheehan, P. (2007) Hyperemesis gravidarum: assessment and management. *Australian Family Physician*, 36(9): 698–701.

Sheenan, A., Cooke, V., Lloyd-Jones, F. et al. (1995) Blood pressure changes during labour and whilst ambulating with combined spinal epidural analgesia. *British Journal of Obstetrics and Gynaecology*, 102: 192–7.

Sheikh, A. and Tunstall, M. (1986) Comparative study of meptazinol and pethidine for the relief of pain in labour. *British Journal of Obstetrics and Gynaecology*, 93: 264–9.

Sheiner, E., Shoham, I., Sheiner, E. et al. (2000) A comparison between the effectiveness of epidural analgesia and parenteral pethidine during labor. *Archives of Gynecology and Obstetrics*, 263(3): 95–8.

Shin, H. and Kim, M. (2006) Subcutaneous tissue thickness in children with type I diabetes. *Journal of Advanced Nursing*, 54(1): 29–34.

Shor, S., Koren, G. and Nulman, I. (2007) Teratogenicity of lamotrigine. *Can Fam Physician*, 53(6): 1007–9.

Shuster, J. (1995) Double diuresis? Drug fever and Jarisch-Herxheimer reaction. *Hospital Pharmacy*, 30(12): 1123A.

Shyken, J. and Petrie, R. (1995) Oytocin to induce labor. *Clinical Obstetrics and Gynecology*, 38(2): 232–45.

Sibai, B. (1996) Treatment of hypertension in pregnant women. *New England Journal of Medicine*, 335: 257–65.

Sibai, B. (1998) Prevention of preeclampsia: a big disappointment. *American Journal of Obstetrics and Gynecology*, 179: 1275–8.

Siega-Riz, A.M., Herring, A.H., Olshan, A.F. et al.; National Birth Defects Prevention Study (2009) The joint effects of maternal prepregnancy body mass index and age on the risk of gastroschisis. *Paediatr Perinat Epidemiol*, 23(1): 51–7.

SIGN (Scottish Intercollegiate Guidelines Network) (2002) *Guidelines for Postnatal Depression and Puerperal Psychosis*. Royal College of Physicians, Edinburgh.

SIGN (Scottish Intercollegiate Guidelines Network) (2003) Contraception, pregnancy and HRT, in *Diagnosis and Management of Epilepsy in Adults*, Guideline 70, www.sign.ac.uk/guidelines/fulltext/70/index.html.

Silverstone, T. and Romans, S. (1996) Long term treatment of bipolar disorder. *Drugs*, 51: 367–82.

Silverton, L. (1993) *The Art and Science of Midwifery*. Prentice Hall, London.

Simhan, H. and Caritis, S. (2007) Prevention of preterm delivery. *New England Journal of Medicine*, 357: 477–87.

Simmons, D. (1997) Persistently poor pregnancy outcomes in women with insulin dependent diabetes. *BMJ*, 315: 263–4.

Simmons, S.W., Cyna, A.M., Dennis, A.T. and Hughes, D. (2007) Combined spinal-epidural versus epidural analgesia in labour. *Cochrane Database of Systematic Reviews*, Issue 3. Art. No.: CD003401. DOI: 10.1002/14651858. CD003401.pub2.

Simpkin, P. (1989) Non-pharmacological methods of pain relief during labour, in Chalmers, I., Enkin, M. and Kierse, M.J. (eds) *Effective Care in Pregnancy and Childbirth*. Oxford Medical, Oxford.

Singh, G., Driever, P.H. and Sander, J.W. (2005) Cancer risk in people with epilepsy: the role of antiepileptic drugs. *Brain*, 128(1): 7–17.

Skidgel, R. and Erdos, E. (2006) Histamine, bradykinin and their antagonists, in Brunton, L., Lazo, J. and Parker, K. (eds) *Goodman & Gilman's: The Pharmacological Basis of Therapeutics*, 11th edn. McGraw-Hill, New York.

Slattery, D.A. and Neumann, I.D. (2008) No stress please! Mechanisms of stress hyporesponsiveness of the maternal brain. *Journal of Physiology*, 586: 377–85.

Slordal, L. and Spigset, O. (2006) Heart failure induced by non-cardiac drugs. *Drug Safety*, 29(7): 567–86.

Smith, A. (1997) Prescribing iron. *Prescribers' Journal*, 37(2): 82–7.

Smith, G. and McEwan, H. (1997) Use of magnesium sulphate in Scottish obstetric units. *British Journal of Obstetrics and Gynaecology*, 104: 115–16.

Smith, G., Pell, J., Pasupathy, D. and Dobbie, R. (2004) Factors predisposing to perinatal death related to uterine rupture during attempted vaginal birth after caesarean section: retrospective cohort study. *BMJ*, 329: 375–7.

Smith, G.N. and Piercy, W.N. (1995) Methyldopa toxicity in pregnancy: a case report. *Am J. Obstet Gynecology*, 172(1 Pt 1): 222–4 .

Smith, P., Anthony, J. and Johanson, R. (2000) Nifedipine in pregnancy. *British Journal of Obstetrics and Gynaecology*, 107: 299–307.

Smith, S., Duell D. and Martin, B. (2008) *Clinical Nursing Skills: Basic to Advanced Skills*, 7th edn. Pearson/Prentice Hall, Englewood Cliffs, NJ.

Smithells, R.W., Shepherd, S., Schorah, C. et al (1980) Possible prevention of neural-tube defects by periconceptual vitamin supplementation. *Lancet*, 8164: 339–40.

Soares, J. Dornhorstt, A. and Beard, R. (1997) The case for screening for gestational diabetes. *BMJ*, 315: 737–9.

Soares-Weiser, K., Bravo Vergel, Y., Beynon, S. et al. (2007) A systematic review and economic model of the clinical effectiveness and cost-effectiveness of interventions for preventing relapse in people with bipolar disorder. *Health Technol Assess*, 11(39): 1–226.

Soens, M.A., Birnbach, D.J., Ranasinghe, J.S. and van Zundert A. (2008) Obstetric anesthesia for the obese and morbidly obese patient: an ounce of prevention is worth more than a pound of treatment. *Acta Anaesthesiologia Scandinavia*, 52(1): 6–19.

Solves, P., Altes, A., Ginovart, G. et al. (1997) Late haemorrhagic disease of the newborn as a cause of intracerebral bleeding. *Annals of Haematology*, 75: 65–6.

Soriano, D., Dulitzki, M., Schiff, E. et al. (1996) A prospective cohort study of oxytocin plus ergometrine compared with oxytocin alone for prevention of postpartum haemorrhage. *British Journal of Obstetrics and Gynaecology*, 103: 1068–73.

Sosa, C.G., Balaguer, E., Alonso, J.G. et al. (2004) Meperidine for dystocia during the first stage of labor: a randomized controlled trial. *American J Obstetrics Gynecol*, 191(4): 1212–18.

Sosa, C.G., Buekens, P., Hughes, J.M. et al. (2006) Effect of pethidine administered during the first stage of labor on the acid-base status at birth. *European J Obstetrics Gynecol Reprod Biol*, 129(2): 135–9.

Souza, A., Amorim, M. and Feitosa, F. (2008) Comparison of sublingual versus vaginal misoprostol for the induction of labour: a systematic review. *BJOG*, 115(11): 1340–9.

Spencer, J. (1995) The management of term labour. *Archives of Disease in Childhood*, 72: F55–61.

Spencer, R. (1993a) Agents affecting the upper gastrointestinal tract, in Spencer, R, Nichols, L., Lipkin, G. et al. (eds) *Clinical Pharmacology and Nursing Management*, 4th edn. Lippincott, Philadelphia.

Spencer, R.T. (1993b) Interactions between food and medications, in Spencer, R.T., Nicolls, L., Lipkin, G. et al. (eds) *Clinical Pharmacology and Nursing Management*. Lippincott, Philadelphia.

Stables, D. (1999) *Physiology in Childbearing*. Baillière Tindall, London.

Steel, J. and Johnstone, F. (1996) Guidelines for the management of insulin-dependent diabetes mellitus. *Drugs*, 52: 60–70.

Steer, P. (1995) Recent advances: obstetrics. *BMJ*, 311: 1209–12.

Steer, P. (1999) Management of preterm labour. Author's reply. *BMJ*, 319: 257.

Steer, P., Biddle, C., Marley, W. et al. (1992) Concentration of fentanyl in colostrum after an analgesic dose. *Canadian Journal of Anaesthesia*, 39: 231–5.

Stevens, L. and Levey, A. (2005) Chronic kidney disease in the elderly: how to assess risk. *New England Journal of Medicine*, 352(20): 2122–4.

Stevenson, M. and Billington, M. (2007) Hypertensive disorders and the critically ill woman, in Billington, M. and Stevenson, M. (eds) *Critical Care in Childbearing for Midwives*. Blackwell, Oxford.

Stienstra, R., Jonker, T., Bourdrez, P. et al. (1995) Ropivacaine 0.25% versus bupivacaine 0.25% for continuous epidural analgesia in labor: a double-blind comparison. *Obstetric Anesthesia*, 80: 285–9.

Stock, M. (1992) Pituitary agents, in Baer, C. and Williams, B. (eds) *Clinical Pharmacology and Nursing*, 2nd edn. Springhouse, Springhouse, PA.

Storey, M. and Jordan, S. (2008) An overview of the immune system. *Nursing Standard*, 23(15/17): 47–56.

Strandberg-Larsen, K., Tinggaard, M., NyboAndersen, A. et al. (2008) Use of nicotine replacement therapy during pregnancy and stillbirth: a cohort study. *BJOG*, 115: 1405–10.

Strang, J., Griffiths, P., Abbey, J. and Gossop, M. (1994) Survey of use of injected benzodiazepines among drug users in Britain. *BMJ*, 308: 1082.

Suri, R.A., Altshuler, L., Burt, V.K. and Hendrick, V.C. (1998) Managing psychiatric medications in the breast-feeding woman. *Medscape Women's Health*, 3: 1–10, http://womenshealth.medscape.com/M.

Surkan, P.J., Peterson, K.E., Hughes, M.D. et al. (2006) The role of social networks and support in postpartum women's depression: a multi ethnic urban sample. *Maternal and Child Health Journal*, 10: 375–83.

Swartjes, J.M. and Van Geijn, H.P. (1998) Pregnancy and epilepsy. *European Journal of Obstetrics, Gynecology and Reproductive Biology*, 79(1): 3–11.

Sweetman, S.C., Blake, P., McGlashan, G. and Parsons, A. (eds) (2007) *Martindale: The Complete Drug Reference*, 35th edn. Pharmaceutical Press, London.

Szal, S., Croughan-Minihane, M. and Kilpatrick, S. (1999) Effect of magnesium prophylaxis and pre-eclampsia on the duration of labor. *American Journal of Obstetrics and Gynecology*, 180: 1475–9.

Tan, B. and Hannah, M. (2000) Prostaglandins versus oxytocin for prelabour rupture of membranes at or near term. *Cochrane Database Systematic Review* (issue 2). Update Software, Oxford.

Tan, L. and Tay, S. (1999) Two dosing regimens for preinduction cervical priming with intravaginal dinoprostone pessary: a randomised clinical trial. *British Journal of Obstetrics and Gynaecology*, 106: 907–12.

Tapson, V. (2008) Acute pulmonary embolism. *New England Journal of Medicine*, 358: 1037–52.

Taylor, D., Paton, C. and Kerwin, R. (2007) *The Maudsley Prescribing Guidelines*, 9th edn. Informa Healthcare, London.

Taylor, G. and Cohen, B. (1985) Ergonovine-induced coronary artery spasm and myocardial infarction after normal delivery. *Obstetrics and Gynecology*, 66(6): 821–2.

Taylor, P. (2006) Agents acting at the neuromuscular junction and autonomic ganglia, in Brunton, L., Lazo, J. and Parker, K. (eds) *Goodman & Gilman's: The Pharmacological Basis of Therapeutics*, 11th edn. McGraw-Hill, New York.

Thapa, P., Whitlock, J., Worrell, K. et al. (1998) Prenatal exposure to metronidazole and risk of childhood cancer. *Cancer*, 83: 1461–8.

Thellin, O. and Heinen, E. (2003) Pregnancy and the immune system: between tolerance and rejection. *Toxicology*, 185(3): 179–84.

Thompson, A. and Hillier, V. (1994) A re-evaluation of the effect of pethidine on the length of labour. *Journal of Advanced Nursing*, 19: 448–56.

Thomson, A., Walker, I. and Greer, I. (1998) Low-molecular weight heparin for immediate management of thromboembolic disease in pregnancy (letter). *Lancet*, 352: 1904.

Thomson, F., Naysmith, M. and Lindsay, A. (2000) Managing drug therapy in patients receiving enteral and parenteral nutrition. *Hospital Pharmacist*, 7(6): 155–64.

Thornton, J.G. (1996) Active management of labour. *BMJ*, 313: 378.

Thorp, J., Hu, D., Albin, R. et al. (1993) The effect of intrapartum epidural analgesia on nulliparous labor: a randomised, controlled, prospective trial. *American Journal of Obstetrics and Gynecology*, 169: 851–8.

Thurlow, J.A., Laxton, C.H., Dick, A. et al. (2002) Remifentanil by patient-controlled analgesia compared with intramuscular meperidine for pain relief in labour. *British Journal of Anaesthesiology*, 88(3): 374–8.

Toft, B. (2009) The dangers of heparin flushes. *Quality and Safety in Health Care*, 18(2): 84–5.

Toglia, M. and Weg, J. (1996) Venous thromboembolism during pregnancy. *New England Journal of Medicine*, 335(2): 108–14.

Tomson, T. and Battino, D. (2007) Pharmacokinetics and therapeutic drug monitoring of newer antiepileptic drugs during pregnancy and the puerperium. *Clinical Pharmacokinetics*, 46(3): 209–19.

Tomson, T. and Hiilesmaa, V. (2007) Epilepsy in pregnancy. *BMJ*, 335(7623): 769–73.

Torbjörn, T. and Vilho, H. (2007). Epilepsy in pregnancy. *BMJ*, 335: 769–73.

Torrance, C. and Jordan, S. (1996) Bionursing: the management of migraine and vomiting. *Nursing Standard*, 19(10): 40–2.

Traynor, J., Dooley, S., Seyb, S. et al. (2000) Is the management of epidural analgesia associated with an increased risk of cesarean delivery? *American Journal of Obstetrics and Gynecology*, 182: 1058–62.

Tryba, M. and Kulka, P. (1993) Critical care pharmacotherapy. *Drugs*, 45: 338–52.

Tsang, R., Chen, I., Friedman, M. et al. (1975) Parathyroid function in infants of diabetic mothers. *Journal de Pediatria*, 86: 399–404.

Tsui, M., Kee, W., Ng, F. and Lau, T. (2004) A double blinded randomised placebo-controlled study of intramuscular pethidine for pain relief in the first stage of labour. *BJOG*, 111: 648–55.

Tucker, J. (2007) Rectal and vaginal drug delivery, in Aulton, M. (ed.) *Aulton's Pharmaceutics*, 3rd edn. Elsevier, Edinburgh.

Tulandi, T., Gelfand, M.M. and Majolo, L. (1985) Effect of prostaglandin E2 on puerperal breast discomfort and prolactin secretion. *Journal of Reproductive Medicine*, 30: 176–8.

Turner, J., Deyo, R, Loeser, J. et al. (1994) The importance of placebo effects in pain treatment and research. *JAMA*, 271: 1609–14.

Twycross, R. (1994) *Pain Relief in Advanced Cancer*. Churchill Livingstone, Edinburgh.

Tytgat, G.N., Heading, R.C., Ller-Lissner, S. et al. (2003). Contemporary understanding and management of reflux and constipation in the general population and pregnancy: a consensus meeting. *Aliment Pharmacol Ther*, 18: 291–301.

Ulrich, M., Kristofferson, K., Rolschau, J. et al. (1999) The influence of folic acid supplement on the outcome of pregnancies in the county of Funen in Denmark, Part III. Congenital anomalies: an observational study. *European Journal of Obstetrics, Gynecology and Reproductive Biology*, 87(2): 115–18.

Upjohn (1990) Hemabate TM sterile solution, carboprost tromethamine, in *Drug Reference*. Upjohn, Crawley.

Urbani, C. and Albonico, A. (2003) Anthelminthic drug safety and drug administration in the control of soil-transmitted helminthiasis in community campaigns. *Acta Tropica*, 86: 215–21.

Uvnäs-Moberg, K., Alster, P., Petersson, M. et al. (1998) Postnatal oxytocin injections cause sustained weight gain and increased nociceptive thresholds in male and female rats. *Pediatric Research*, 43(3): 344–8.

Valenzuela, G., Ramos, S.L., Romero, R. et al. (2000) Maintenance treatment of preterm labor with the oxytocin antagonist atosiban. *American Journal of Obstetrics and Gynecology*, 182: 1184–90.

Van Dijk, K.G., Dekker, G. and van Geijn, H.P. (1995) Ritodrine and nifedipine as tocolytic agents: a preliminary comparison. *Journal of Perinatal Medicine*, 23(5): 409–15.

Van Dongen, P. and de Groot, A. (1995) History of ergot alkaloids. *European Journal of Gynecology and Reproductive Biology*, 60: 109–16.

Van Tonningen, M.R. (2007a) Antiallergic drugs and desensitisation, in Schaefer, C., Peters, P.W. and Miller, R.K. (eds) *Drugs during Pregnancy and Lactation: Treatment Options and Risk Assessment*, 2nd edn. Elsevier, Oxford.

Van Tonningen, M.R. (2007b) Gastrointestinal and antilipidemic agents and spasmolytics, in Schaefer, C., Peters, P.W. and Miller, R.K. (eds) *Drugs during Pregnancy and Lactation: Treatment Options and Risk Assessment*, 2nd edn. Elsevier, Oxford.

Van Way, C. (1999) *Nutrition Secrets*. Hanley and Belfus, Philadelphia.

Van Wijk, F.H., Wolf, H., Piek, J.M. and Büller, H.R. (2002) Administration of low molecular weight heparin within two hours before caesarean section increases the risk of wound haematoma. *BJOG*, 109(8): 955–7.

Vaughan, N. (1995) Treatment of diabetes, in Rubin, P. (ed.) *Prescribing in Pregnancy*, 2nd edn. BMJ Group, London.

Ververs, T.F., van Wensen, K., Freund, M.W. (2009) Association between antidepressant drug use during pregnancy and child healthcare utilisation. *BJOG*, 116(12): 1568–77.

Vesalainen, R., Ekholm, E., Jartii, T. et al. (1999) Effects of tocolytic treatment with ritodrine on cardiovascular autonomic regulation. *British Journal of Obstetrics and Gynaecology*, 106: 238–43.

Viguera, A.C., Emmerich, A.D. and Cohen, L.S. (2008) Case records of the Massachusetts General Hospital. Case 24-2008. A 35-year-old woman with postpartum confusion, agitation, and delusions. *New England Journal of Medicine*, 359(5): 509–15.

Vinod, J., Bonheur, J., Korelitz, B.I. and Panagopoulos, G. (2007) Choice of laxatives and colonoscopic preparation in pregnant patients from the viewpoint of obstetricians and gastroenterologists. *World J Gastroenterol*, 13(48): 6549–52.

Volmanen, P., Sarvela, J., Akural, E. et al. (2008) Intravenous remifentanil vs. Epidural levobupivacaine with fentanyl for pain relief in early labour: a randomised, controlled, double-blinded study. *Acta Anaesthesiol Scand*, 52(2): 249–55.

Von Dadelszen, P., Ornstein, M., Bull, S. et al. (2000) Fall in mean arterial pressure and fetal growth restriction in pregnancy hypertension: a meta-analysis. *Lancet*, 355: 87–92.

Von Kries, R., Gobel, U., Hachmeister, A. et al. (1996) Vitamin K and childhood cancer: a population based case-control study in Lower Saxony. *BMJ*, 313: 199–203.

Wagner, M. (1993) Research shows medication of pain is not safe. *MIDIRS Midwifery Digest*, 3(3): 307–9.

Wahl, R.U. (2004) Could oxytocin administration during labor contribute to autism and related behavioral disorders? A look at the literature. *Medical Hypotheses*, 63(3): 456–60.

Wald, N.J. and Bower, C. (1995) Folic acid and the prevention of neural tube defects. *BMJ*, 310: 1019–20.

Waldenstrom, U. (1999) Experience of labor and birth in 1111 women. *Journal of Psychosomatic Research*, 47: 471–82.

Walker, J. (2000) Severe pre-eclampsia and eclampsia. *Baillière's Best Practice and Research: Clinical Obstetrics and Gynecology*, 14(1): 57–71.

Walker, S.P., Permezel, M. and Berkovic, S.F. (2009) The management of epilepsy in pregnancy. *BJOG*, 116(6): 758–67.

Walkinshaw, S. (2000) Very tight versus tight control for diabetes in pregnancy. *Cochrane Database Systematic Review* (issue 2). Update Software, Oxford.

Wall, R. (2002) Perioperative management of the patient with thyroid disease, in 53rd Annual Refresher Course Lectures, Clinical Updates and Basic Science Reviews Program. Item 135, www.anesthesia.org.cn/asa2002/rcl_source/135_Wall.pdf.

Wallace, A.W. and Amsden, G.W. (2002) Is it really OK to take this with food? *Journal of Clinical Pharmacology*, 42(4): 437–43.

Wallace, E., Chapman, J., Stenson, B. and Wright, S. (1997) Antenatal corticosteroid prescribing: setting standards of care. *British Journal of Obstetrics and Gynaecology*, 104: 1262–6.

Walley, R., Wilson, J., Crane, J. et al. (2000) A double blind placebo controlled randomised trial of misoprostol and oxytocin in the management of the third stage of labour. *British Journal of Obstetrics and Gynaecology*, 107: 1111–15.

Ward, S. and Wisner, K.L. (2007) Collaborative management of women with bipolar disorder during pregnancy and the postpartum: pharmacologic considerations. *Journal of Midwifery & Women's Health*, 52(1): 3–13.

Watkins, L. and Weeks, A.D. (2009) Providing information to pregnant women: how, what and where? *BJOG*, 116(7): 877–9.

Weatherhead, S., Robson, S. and Reynolds, N. (2007) Eczema in pregnancy, *BMJ*, 335: 152–4.

Weiss, G., Klein, S., Shenkman, L. et al. (1975) Effect of methylergonovine on puerperal prolactin secretion. *Obstetrics and Gynecology*, 46(2): 209–10.

Wells, P.G. (2007) Chemical teratogenesis, in Kalant, H., Grant, D. and Mitchell, J. (eds) *Principles of Medical Pharmacology*, 7th edn. Saunders, Toronto.

Welters, I.D. and Leuwer, M. (2008) General anesthetics and therapeutic gases, in Aronson, J.K. (ed.) *Side Effects of Drug Annual* 30. Elsevier, Amsterdam.

Wen, S.W., Demissie, K. and Liu, S. (2001) Adverse outcomes in pregnancies of asthmatic women: results from a Canadian population. *Annals of Epidemiology*, 11(1): 7–12.

Wendel, P., Ramin, S., Barnett-Hamm, C. et al. (1996) Asthma treatment in pregnancy: a randomised controlled study. *American Journal of Obstetrics and Gynecology*, 175: 150–4.

Werler, M., Hayes, C., Louik, C. et al. (1999) Multivitamin supplementation and risk of birth defects. *American Journal of Epidemiology*, 150(7): 675–82.

Werler, M.M., Mitchell, A.A., Moore, C.A. and Honein, M.A.; National Birth Defects Prevention Study (2009) Is there epidemiologic evidence to support vascular disruption as a pathogenesis of gastroschisis? *Am J Med Genet A*, 149A(7): 1399–406.

Westfall, R.E., Janssen, P.A., Lucas, P. and Capler, R. (2006) Survey of medicinal cannabis use among childbearing women: patterns of its use in pregnancy and retroactive self-assessment of its efficacy against 'morning sickness'. *Complement Ther Clin Pract*, 12(1): 27–33.

Wickham, S. (2001) *Anti-D in Midwifery: Panacea or Paradox?* Books for Midwives, Oxford.

Wiklund, I., Norman, M., Uvnäs-Moberg, K. et al. (2009) Epidural analgesia: breast-feeding success and related factors. *Midwifery*, 25(2): e31–8.

Wikner, B.N., Stiller, C.O., Bergman, U. et al. (2007) Use of benzodiazepines and benzodiazepine receptor agonists during pregnancy: neonatal outcome and congenital malformations. *Pharmacoepidemiol Drug Saf*, 16(11): 1203–10.

Wildsmith, J. (1996) Routes of drug administration: intrathecal and epidural injection, *Prescribers' Journal*, 36(2): 110–15.

Wilkinson, G. (2001) Pharmacokinetics, in Hardman, J., Limbard, L., Molinoff, P. et al. (eds) *Goodman & Gilman's: The Pharmacological Basis of Therapeutics*, 10th edn. New York, McGraw-Hill.

Wilkinson, G.R. (2005) Drug metabolism and variability among patients in drug response. *N Engl J Med*, 352(21): 2211–21.

Williams, B., Poulter, N., Brown, M.J. et al. (2004) British Hypertension society guidelines: Guidelines for management of hypertension: report of the fourth working party of the British Hypertension Society. *Journal of Human Hypertension*, 18: 139–85.

Williams, G. (1991) Hypertensive vascular disease, in Wilson, J., Braunwald, E., Isselbacher, K. et al. (eds) *Harrison's Principles of Internal Medicine*, 12th edn. McGraw-Hill, New York.

Wilson, J. (1994) Preventing infection during iv therapy. *Professional Nurse*, 9(3): 388–92.

Winberg, J. (2005) Mother and newborn baby: mutual regulation of physiology and behavior – a selective review. *Developmental Psychobiology*, 47: 217–29.

Winter, C., Macfarlane, A., Deneux-Tharaux, C. et al. (2007) Variations in policies for management of the third stage of labour and the immediate management of postpartum haemorrhage in Europe. *BJOG*, 114(7): 845–54.

Winterbottom, J.B., Smyth, R., Jacoby, A. and Baker, G.A. (2007) Preconception counselling for women with epilepsy to reduce adverse pregnancy outcome (Protocol). *Cochrane Database of Systematic Reviews*, Issue 3. Art No.:CD006645.DOI:10.1002/14651858.CD006645

Wisborg, K., Barklin, A., Hedegaard, M. and Henriksen, T.B. (2008) Psychological stress during pregnancy and still-birth: prospective study. *BJOG*, 115: 882–5.

Wisner, K., Gelenberg, A., Leonard, H. et al. (1999) Pharmacologic treatment of depression during pregnancy. *JAMA*, 282: 1264–9.

Wisner, K.L., Hanusa, B.H., Peindl, K.S. et al. (2004) Prevention of postpartum episodes in women with bipolar disorder. *Biological Psychiatry*, 56: 592–6.

Wissart, J., Parshad, O. and Kulkarni, S. (2005) Prevalence of pre- and postpartum depression in Jamaican women. *BMC Pregnancy Childbirth*, 5: 15, doi: 10.1186/1471-2393-5-15.

Witlin, A., Friedman, S. and Sibai, B. (1997) The effect of magnesium sulfate therapy on the duration of labor in women with mild preeclampsia at term: a randomised, double-blind placebo-controlled trial. *American Journal of Obstetrics and Gynecology*, 176: 623–7.

Wolff, K., Boys, A., Rostami-Hodjegan, A. et al. (2005) Changes to methadone clearance during pregnancy. *Eur J Clin Pharmacol*, 61(10): 763–8.

Wong, C., Walsh, L., Smith, C. et al. (2000) Inhaled corticosteroid use and bone mineral density in patients with asthma. *Lancet*, 355: 1399–403.

Wong, E., Patel, J. and Guzofski, S. (2008) Drugs of abuse, in Aronson, J.K. (ed.) *Side Effects of Drug Annual* 30. Elsevier, Amsterdam.

Workman, B. (1999) Safe injection technique. *Nursing Standard*, 13(39): 47–53.

Worldwide Atosiban versus Beta-agonists Study Groups (2001) Effectiveness and safety of the oxytocin antagonist atosiban versus beta-adrenergic agonists in the treatment of preterm labour. *British Journal of Obstetrics and Gynaecology*, 108: 133–42.

Wright, D. (2002) Medication administration in nursing homes. *Nursing Standard*, 16: 33–8.

Writer, W., Stienstra, R., Eddleston, J. et al. (1998) Neonatal outcome and mode of delivery after epidural analgesia for labour with ropivacaine and bupivacaine: a prospective meta-analysis. *British Journal of Anaesthesia*, 81(5): 713–17.

Wu, Y.W. and Colford, J.M. Jr (2000) Chorioamnionitis as a risk factor for cerebral palsy: a meta-analysis. *JAMA*, 284(11): 1417–24.

Xiong, X., Buekens, P., Fraser, W. et al. (2006) Periodontal disease and adverse pregnancy outcomes: a systematic review. *BJOG*, 113: 135–43.

Yelland, J., Krastev, A. and Brown, S. (2009) Enhancing early postnatal care: findings from a major reform of maternity care in three Australian hospitals. *Midwifery*, 25(4): 392–402.

Yerby, M. (2000) Pharmacological methods of pain relief, in Yerby, M. and Page, L. (eds) *Pain in Childbearing*. Baillière Tindall, Edinburgh.

Yoshida, K., Smith, B. and Kumar, R. (1999) Psychotropic drugs in mothers' milk: a comprehensive review of assay methods, pharmacokinetics and of safety of breast feeding. *Journal of Psychopharmacology*, 13(1): 64–80.

Yuen, P., Chan, N., Yim, S. and Chang, A. (1995) A randomised double blind comparison of syntometrine and syntocinon in the management of the third stage of labour. *British Journal of Obstetrics and Gynaecology*, 102: 377–80.

Zelcer, J., Owers, H. and Paull, D. (1989) A controlled oximetric evaluation of inhalational, opioid and epidural analgesia in labour. *Anaesthesia and Intensive Care*, 17(4): 418–21.

Zeng, L., Cheng, Y., Dang, S. et al. (2008) Impact of micronutrient supplementation during pregnancy on birth weight, duration of gestation, and perinatal mortality in rural western China: double blind cluster randomised controlled trial. *BMJ*, 337: 1211–15.

Zimmerman, S.A., Malinoski, F.J. and Ware, R.E. (1998) Immunologic effects of anti-D (Win Rho-SD) in children with immune thrombocytopenic purpura. *American Journal of Haematology*, 57(2): 131–8.

Zipursky, A. (1996) Vitamin K at birth. *BMJ*, 313: 179–80.

Zuraw, B. (2008) Hereditary angioedema. *New England Journal of Medicine*, 359(10): 1027–36.

Zwart, J.J., Richters, J.M., Ory, F. et al. (2009) Uterine rupture in the Netherlands: a nationwide population-based cohort study. *BJOG*, 116(8): 1069–78.

Index

Page numbers in *italics* refer to the 'quick reference' lists in Appendix 1. Asterisks (*) against page numbers indicate entries in the glossary.